Neurosurgery Research Progress

nova
Medicine & Health
New York

Neurosurgery Research Progress

Reticular Concept of Nervous System Physiology
Oleg Sotnikov, PhD (Editors)
2022. ISBN: 978-1-68507-996-3 (Hardcover)
2022. ISBN: 979-8-88697-350-1 (eBook)

Neuroscience and Technology Transform the Educational Ecosystem
Franco F. Orsucci (Editor)
Nicoletta Sala (Editor)
2022. ISBN: 979-8-88697-157-6 (Hardcover)
2022. ISBN: 979-8-88697-248-1 (eBook)

Advances in Neurosurgery Research
Amit Agrawal, MD, Pradeep Chouksey, MD, Adesh Shrivastava, MD, Sumit Raj, MD and Rakesh Mishra, MD (Editors)
2022. ISBN: 978-1-68507-859-1 (Hardcover)
2022. ISBN: 979-8-88697-061-6 (eBook)

Neurosurgery Research: An Update
Amit Agrawal, MD (Editor)
Pradeep Chouksey, MD (Editor)
Adesh Shrivastava, MD (Editor)
Sumit Raj, MD (Editor)
Rakesh Mishra, MD (Editor)
2022. ISBN: 978-1-68507-837-9 (Hardcover)
2022. ISBN: 979-8-88697-076-0 (eBook)

More information about this series can be found at https://novapublishers.com/product-category/series/neurosurgery-research-progress/

Xianli Lv
Editor

Understanding and Managing Cerebral Aneurysms

nova
Medicine & Health
New York

DOI: https://doi.org/10.52305/MFLO0750

NOTICE TO THE READER

Library of Congress Cataloging-in-Publication Data

Names: Lv, Xianli, editor.
Title: Understanding and managing cerebral aneurysms / editor Xianli Lv, MD, Associate Professor, Department of Neurosurgery, Beijing Tsinghua Changgung Hospital, School of Clinical Medicine, Tsinghua University, Beijing, China.
Description: New York : Nova Science Publishers, [2024] | Series: Neurosurgery research progress | Includes bibliographical references and index. |
Identifiers: LCCN 2024010844 (print) | LCCN 2024010845 (ebook) | ISBN 9798891136083 (hardcover) | ISBN 9798891136830 (adobe pdf)
Subjects: LCSH: Intracranial aneurysms. | Intracranial aneurysms--Treatment.
Classification: LCC RC693 .U53 2024 (print) | LCC RC693 (ebook) | DDC 616.1/33--dc23/eng/20240408
LC record available at https://lccn.loc.gov/2024010844
LC ebook record available at https://lccn.loc.gov/2024010845

Published by Nova Science Publishers, Inc. † New York

Contents

Preface

This book provides a detailed introduction to the characteristics of cerebral aneurysms and the current treatment methods. Cerebral aneurysms are not rare, and they have a high disability and mortality rate. Most patients are unaware that they have a cerebral aneurysm, with the most common being cerebral hemorrhage. The diagnosis and treatment of cerebral aneurysms have been ongoing for more than 100 years. We have achieved excellent results, but there are still many things that we do not know. An increasing number of unruptured cerebral aneurysms are accidentally discovered during neuroimaging examinations. The greatest risk of cerebral aneurysm is the risk of rupture. Due to the extremely high mortality rate, once these aneurysms are detected, systematic treatment is necessary. The earlier a patient is referred to a neurosurgeon or interventional neuroradiologist, the better the outcome will be compared to the patient experiencing rupture. The decision to treat is multifactorial.

Chapter 1 - Intracranial aneurysms (IA) occur in 3-6% of the population. The incidence of aneurysmal subarachnoid hemorrhage (SAH) is 10-15 per 100,000 people per year. Aneurysmal SAH can cause one third of patients to die. Among the survivors, half will return to normal life, and the rest will need support to continue their normal daily activities. Because of the damage caused by SAH, researches have been committed to clarify the pathogenesis of IA, with the aim of increasing the understanding of the disease process. Endovascular coil embolization and flow diversions have become the standard of treatment for these lesions in the majority of cases in comparison to surgical clipping.

Chapter 2 - Anterior communicating (Acom) aneurysms are difficult to understand because of anatomical variations in this region, although they are the most common intracranial aneurysms. This chapter was to classify Acom aneurysms into 5 subgroups (straight, superior, inferior, anterior, and posterior) of orientations according to the axis connecting A1 origin and the base of the aneurysm. This classification of Acom aneurysms distinguishes their characteristics, including the shape, location, orientation, size, probability of occurrence and endovascular treatments. It adds an interesting classification system to the evaluation and treatment of Acom aneurysms.

Chapter 3 - Posterior communicating artery (PcomA) aneurysms are the second most common intracranial aneurysm. They are classified according to the site of origin into "Junctional aneurysms," which could be either at the junction of the internal carotid artery (ICA) and PcomA or at the junction of PcomA and posterior cerebral artery (PCA), and "true PcomA aneurysms" that originate from PcomA itself.

The exact etiology of PcomA aneurysms is yet to be determined. However, some factors are closely related to their development and must be appraised in the evaluation steps. The patient may present with subarachnoid hemorrhage (SAH), partial or complete oculomotor nerve palsy (OMNP), and non-traumatic subdural hematoma (SDH). Individual-based planning must be obtained for each patient to achieve the optimal outcome.

Several morphological parameters have been studied to upgrade the assessment of treatment plans like origin, size, neck, dome, and fetal PcomA. These parameters are carefully analyzed using CTA, MRA, and DSA to determine the management scheme. PcomA aneurysms can be treated by surgical or endovascular approach. Surgical clipping can be approached through a pterional or lateral supraciliary approach, while endovascular treatment includes direct coiling, stent-assisted coiling, and flow diverter methods. The recovery status after surgical or endovascular management depends on multiple factors, including the timeline between the diagnosis and treatment, the existence of SAH with the consequent brain injury, and the degree of OMNP. In general, the morbidity rate of surgically treated PcomA aneurysms is low compared to the other aneurysms in the circle of Willis.

All the stated facts will be discussed in this chapter for the purpose of establishing an accurate assessment of the aneurysm, its management, and the suitable measures for dealing with its possible complications.

Chapter 4 - Middle cerebral artery (MCA) aneurysms are among the most frequent intracranial aneurysms, with bifurcation being the most common site. Their rupture is frequent resulting not only in subarachnoid hemorrhage but also in intracerebral hemorrhage. For the diagnosis of the ruptured aneurysms commonly used radiological examinations are CT, CTA, MRA or DSA. Also, lumbar puncture can be helpful revealing xanthochromia in cases of negative CT. There have been described three main classic surgical methods and one more contemporary, while the clipping technique of the aneurysm is more individualized, though some general principles can be followed. Even though in most centers surgical options are chosen, there are efforts to develop new endovascular methods to treat even complex aneurysms avoiding a surgery.

Chapter 5 - This text presents a case report on the surgical management of a ruptured giant middle cerebral artery (MCA) aneurysm, highlighting the challenges associated with its complex anatomy and the potential complications of conventional treatment approaches. The authors describe an alternative technique utilizing a modified superficial temporal artery-middle cerebral artery (STA-MCA) bypass procedure to overcome these limitations. The modified approach offers advantages such as enhanced maneuverability, utilization of the upper M1 stump for suction decompression, and modification of aneurysm morphology. The technical nuances of the bypass procedure, including meticulous preparations, donor vessel handling, anastomosis techniques, temporary clip removal, and confirmation of success, are discussed in detail. By adopting this innovative technique, the authors aim to optimize surgical outcomes and minimize the risk of ischemic neuronal damage while managing giant MCA aneurysms.

Chapter 6 - This study aimed to analyze the characteristics, embolization techniques, and treatment outcomes in saccular aneurysm of the middle cerebral artery (MCA). Retrospective analysis of data from consecutive MCA saccular aneurysm patients who underwent embolization treatment at three neurosurgical centers from January 2016 to January 2021. The outcomes include thromboembolic and hemorrhagic complications, angiographic outcomes and neurological complications. The hemorrhagic and thromboembolic complications were 5/208 (2.40%) and 9/208 (4.33%) during the procedure, respectively, and 2/208 (0.96%) and 3/208 (1.44%) within 30 days. The major events (mRS>2) occurred in 3/208 (1.44%) during the procedure, and 2/208 (0.96%) within 30 days. The rate of complete embolization and neck remnant of aneurysms was 88.5% initially, 90.4% at 6-12 months, and 92.1% at >12 months. The rates of neurological complication were 6.73%, 1.92%, 2.88%, 1.92%, and 1.44% at initial,

1 month, 6 months, 12 months, and 24 months, respectively. Traditional embolization techniques provide a feasible option for endovascular treatment of MCA saccular aneurysms. Even in the era of flow diverting stents and Woven EndoBridge (WEB), traditional embolization techniques are still not outdated.

Chapter 7 - Distal aneurysms of the intracranial arteries (DAIAs) occur distal to the major branches of the circle of Willis and the vertebrobasilar system. DAIAs are rare, and treatment, including open surgery and endovascular treatment (EVT), is sometimes necessary. Open surgery is challenging for DAIAs due to the deep location and difficulty in preserving the parent artery. EVT, especially reconstructive EVT, can be an alternative surgery for treating DAIAs. However, some DAIAs cannot be reconstructed due to the small size and complicated anatomy of the parent artery. Endovascular parent artery occlusion (PAO), a deconstructive method, plays an important role in treating DAIAs. Because our current understanding of DAIA sacrifice or reconstruction by EVT is insufficient, the authors discuss this issue, including the definition, incidence, pathogenesis, and classification of DAIAs; therapeutic options for DAIAs; reconstructive EVT for DAIAs; status of endovascular PAO; risk of endovascular PAO and balloon occlusion test; option for embolic materials for endovascular PAO; and PAO characteristics of each DAIA in this review. The authors found that, in EVT for DAIAs, although preservation and reconstruction of the parent artery should naturally be the prime objective, in selected cases, PAO was still a valuable option that yielded favorable outcomes.

Chapter 8 - Intracranial dissecting aneurysms are a special type of pathological aneurysm. Unlike a saccular aneurysm, the dissecting aneurysm is usually caused by the damage to the vessel wall structure of cerebral arteries, especially a disruption of the internal elastic lamina, the media with or without the adventitia which leads to a partial protrusion of the adventitia. Stent-assisted coiling embolization is a recommended technique for cases in which vessels are damaged as a result of aneurysms. Surgical clipping is not effective due to the high morbidity and mortality rates. Flow-diversion devices (FDs) have provided good results in the management of dissecting aneurysms. Still, they should be evaluated according to the location of the aneurysm, the type of aneurysm, the patient's age, and the patient's preoperative health condition, weighing the advantages and risks of each treatment strategy, and choosing the best treatment according to the patient's actual situation.

Chapter 9 - Infectious aneurysms might involve aortic arch, proximal supra-aortic vessels downstream to very distal cerebral vasculature. Intracranial infectious aneurysms (IIAs) are relatively rare yet might harbor devastating consequences with a rupture-associated mortality risk ranging between 30-80%. Septic vegetation seeding from an infective endocarditis (IEC) represents the most common source, resulting into intracranial vessel wall damage, necrosis, and aneurysmal formation.

IIAs are typically multiple, fusiform shaped distally indwelling; however, the presentation is widely variable. Moreover, patients usually present late in the course of the disease. Cutting-edge imaging modalities such as multi-detector computed tomography and time of flight magnetic resonance imaging (TOF-MRI) might have improved the diagnostic accuracy of IIAs guided by diversified established features; however digital subtraction angiography (DSA) still represents the gold standard examination. Integrating clinical finding along with the imaging features might aid prompt diagnosis and timely treatment of IIAs. Yet to be considered, IIAs are inherently dynamic where an aneurysm might get instituted and rupture in less than one week; therefore, an earlier stage of aneurysmal development could be easily missed even with serial investigations.

Management of IIAs is still controversial. Taking in consideration their grave natural prognosis, the decision to intervene is influenced furthermore by many variables including patient's general condition, aneurysm size, location and geometry, rupture status, presence of hematoma with significant mass effect and territorial eloquence of the feeding artery. Therefore, a multidisciplinary approach remains the most successful strategy in dealt with these aneurysms.

Therapeutic choices include serial monitoring under antimicrobial coverage, endovascular embolization, parent artery sacrifice and direct surgical excision and debridement. However, observational strategy still carries a high risk of fulminant hemorrhage. Surgical resolution is not without complications.

Chapter 10 - This chapter is an overview of the history of the development and current state of endovascular treatment of cerebral aneurysms. It compares embolization and microsurgical clipping of both ruptured and non-ruptured aneurysms of various localizations. It considers in detail indications for invasive intervention and the issues of angiographic diagnostics. It reviews the capabilities of modern endovascular devices such as coils, balloons and stents. The chapter presents an analysis of coiling techniques including balloon-and stent-assisted options. Stent-assistance is discussed in detail starting from the standard technique to complex stenting options, such as Y-stenting, X-stenting, semijailing, transverse stenting, and the waffle-cone technique. The chapter also reviews indications for the use of flow diverters and their implantation techniques. It considers the methods of prevention and treatment of typical complications in endovascular treatment of cerebral aneurysms and describes the techniques of balloon and chemical angioplasty in the complex treatment of aneurysms while acute period hemorrhage accompanied by severe angiospasm.

Chapter 11 - The treatment of A1 aneurysms through endovascular methods can be difficult. Coiling and assisted coiling are the most commonly used techniques. While flow diverters (FDs) are widely accepted for treating ruptured blister-like and dissecting aneurysms, their efficacy in treating ruptured distal A1 aneurysms requires further investigation. More case studies are needed to determine the safety and effectiveness of using FDs for this purpose. To aim this purpose, the authors report 3 ruptured A1 aneurysms treated with FDs. The authors's case series demonstrate FDs' safety and efficacy profile on ruptured distal A1 aneurysms. Ultimately, deciding the most appropriate treatment method for an A1 aneurysm will depend on carefully considering the individual case and the patient's specific needs.

Chapter 12 - Reconstructive treatment for vertebrobasilar junction (VBJ) aneurysms involves repairing or rebuilding the damaged portion of the blood vessel to prevent future rupture or bleeding. These aneurysms are a rare and complex subgroup of saccular aneurysms and require careful consideration when determining the most appropriate treatment method. Endovascular techniques, such as stent placement or flow diverter deployment, are often utilized in reconstructive treatment. The specific technique will depend on various factors, including the size, location, and type of aneurysm as the patient's overall health and medical history. The current study reported three successful cases of VBJ aneurysms treated through combined reconstructive endovascular methods. These case reports demonstrate that endovascular treatment can effectively achieve a curative result and is associated with good clinical outcomes and low mortality rates. It is important to note that these are individual cases, and the results may not represent all patients. Further research and case studies are needed to establish the safety and efficacy of reconstructive treatment for VBJ aneurysms.

Chapter 13 - V4 aneurysms located in the posterior circulation of the brain can cause uncommon symptoms due to their distinctive position. Although many V4 aneurysms are diagnosed incidentally, there have been case reports of posterior circulation aneurysms causing symptoms due to their anatomic proximity to the brainstem. These symptoms can also be indicative of other medical conditions, so it's important to seek a professional medical evaluation. In some cases, patients with V4 aneurysms may not experience any symptoms at all. The current study reports two cases of V4 aneurysms with uncommon presenting symptoms. The first case was an unruptured V4 aneurysm causing neck pain, and the second one was a V4 aneurysm leading to chronic coughing, which caused a delayed diagnosis of a V4 aneurysm. Both aneurysms were treated with endovascular techniques and the patient's symptoms improved after the treatment.

Chapter 14 - The coil is designed to be tightly packed in the aneurysm cavity, thus blocking the blood flow into the aneurysm and preventing the rupture and growth of the aneurysm. For narrow-neck aneurysms (aneurysm neck<4 mm or body/neck ratio >2), coil embolization is relatively easy to perform. However, when wide-necked aneurysm (aneurysm neck≥4 mm or body/neck ratio ≤2) is encountered, the coil will be easy to protrude from the neck of the aneurysm back to the parent artery, block the blood flow to the distal artery, and increase the risk of thromboembolism complications. Some pioneers began to explore stent-assisted coil embolization, which has become an important technique for the treatment of cerebral aneurysms, and has significantly increased the range of aneurysms that can be treated endovascularly. In this chapter, the stent technique as well as recent new techniques and materials were summarized.

Chapter 15 - Objective: To evaluate the technical feasibility, peri- and post-procedural morbidity and mortality as well as angiographic follow-up of stent-assisted coiling of broad-based cerebral aneurysms using the Enterprise and the Solitaire AB stents.

Methods: Consecutive 77 patients with cerebral aneurysms stented with the Enterprise or Solitaire AB stents were retrospectively studied. Angiographic follow-up (mean 8.25 months) was available in 90.9% of patients.

Results: All stents were successfully deployed. There is a higher acute intra-stent thrombosis complication in Solitaire AB stent placement ($p = 0.012$). However, no significant differences in peri-procedural morbidity and mortality rates ($p = 0.253$), angiographic results ($p = 0.411$), recurrence rate ($p > 0.999$) or long-term neurological deficit ($p = 0.435$), were observed.

Conclusion: Both stents exhibited similar immediate and mid-term results, major neurological morbidities and mortality are low. Thrombogenic complications seems higher in Solitaire AB group.

Chapter 16 - Endovascular treatment has lower morbidity and mortality rates than surgical clipping. Woven Endo Bridge (WEB) device (also called an intrasaccular flow diverter) is a new and effective endovascular embolization method primarily used to treat wide-necked or bifurcated cerebral aneurysms. In WEB-assisted embolization, a specially structured scaffold-like metal cage (WEB) is placed within the aneurysm, and the blood flow is redirected to branch arteries. Thus, blood entry into the aneurysm sac is prevented, and the risk of rupture of the aneurysm is reduced. The advantages of WEB embolization are the shorter embolization time and the reduced need for antiaggregant usage and intra-/peri-aneurysmal manipulations compared to coiling with or without stent placement. With the advancing technical developments (e.g., more visible single-layer wires), WEB devices are a safe alternative to other types of aneurysms or unusual locations (e.g., side-wall, PCOM origin, pericallosal, distal, or para-ophthalmic aneurysms. Adequate occlusion rates of the WEB devices were 84% at five years of follow-up. Complex morphology (e.g., the presence of irregular, multilocular, and/or partially thrombosed sac) and a large (>10 mm) neck or width of the aneurysm were found to be associated with recurrences after the WEB placements.

Chapter 17 - The optimal treatment of unruptured aneurysms in elderly patients remains controversial. The variability of life expectancy, comorbidities, and rupture risk, coupled with the heterogeneity of intravascular and surgical treatment, has led to a lack of clear guidelines and current management is highly personalized. Elderly patients exhibit unique considerations, including weakness, cognitive impairment, vascular disease, shortened life expectancy, and overall worsening prognosis at the time of rupture, which determine the risk and success of endovascular and microsurgical treatments. In this chapter, the natural risk of unruptured aneurysms in the elderly and the factors that affect their treatment strategies will be discussed.

Chapter 18 - This chapter evaluated whether an arterial aneurysm within an arteriovenous malformation (AVM) angioarchitecture is an indication for endovascular embolization in cases of ruptured and unruptured AVM. 94 patients with AVMs managed between August 2015 and August 2017 were retrospectively reviewed. Nineteen AVM-associated arterial aneurysms were detected in the 17 patients (only one patient had multiple aneurysms). Hemorrhage was the most frequent presenting symptom (11 patients, 64.7%). Ten aneurysms were coiled prior to AVM treatment. The remaining nine were obliterated at the time of AVM treatment, with Onyx embolization used for both procedures. None of the patients developed complications. After a mean 10.4 months (range, 3-25 months) of follow-up, excellent outcomes (modified Rankin Scale score [mRS] = 0 to 1) were recorded for 13 patients (76.5%) and good outcomes (mRS = 2) were noted for four patients (23.5%). Endovascular treatment options of arterial aneurysms in AVMs were comprised coil embolization or parent vessel sacrifice using coils or liquid embolics. Embolization of arterial aneurysms on feeding pedicles should be considered prior to or adjunct AVM embolization.

Chapter 19 - Reconstructive interventions on the carotid arteries in patients with intracranial aneurysms requires an individual patient-selected approach, in contrast to certain standards based only on the principles of evidence-based medicine. It should be noted that such situations are not uncommon in neurosurgical practice - the incidence of cerebral aneurysms in the population, according to epidemiological studies, varies from 3 to 5%, and in the group of patients with hemodynamically significant stenosis of the carotid arteries, it is 3.2%. In N. N. Burdenko National Medical Research Center for Neurosurgery experience, cerebral aneurysms were diagnosed in 4.1% of all patients who had indications for carotid endarterectomy. At the same time, due to the wider use of CT angiography as a method of primary diagnosis of steno-occlusive pathology, the number of such clinical cases is increasing every year.

Present clinical guidelines classify such patients in a group of increased risk of carotid endarterectomy, pointing out the disagreement in approaches to the treatment of cerebral aneurysms in combination with internal carotid artery (ICA) stenosis and assigning the first role in making a decision the individual characteristics of each individual patient and the capabilities of the surgical hospital. The complexity of determining the tactics of treating such patients is due to the competition of mutually opposite pathogenetic mechanisms that determine the likelihood of ischemic stroke on the one hand and the risk of aneurysm rupture on the other. This, in turn, leads to antagonism of the methods of potential medical and surgical treatment.

Taking into account the increased risks of perioperative complications of reconstructive surgery, such patients are often redirected from the departments of vascular surgery to neurosurgical hospitals for the primary treatment of cerebral aneurysms, followed by a decision on the issue of carotid endarterectomy. At the same time, this treatment tactic is not always justified, since it does not take into account the individual risks of aneurysm rupture and possible ischemic cerebrovascular accident.

The aim of this chapter is to determine the algorithm for the treatment of patients with a combination of cerebral aneurysms with carotid stenosis.

Chapter 20 - "anatomical basis," or "aptitude and attitude" played a role in the usual surgeon's parlance, technology was diversely understood.

Now, the times are changing, and technology has arrived to play a leading role. Oversight of this situation could lead to a compromise in surgical results and may result in not giving the patient the best of what is available.

Neurosurgery and many other surgical fields have been brought to a new level since the microscope was introduced more than five decades ago.

Books were written, instruments were built, and the neurosurgical universe is now measured in small parts of a millimetre because of the microscope. Microsurgical anatomy has become the norm.

Training hand skills and system-related handling is mandatory for microscopic surgeons nowadays. The starting point for this goal should be related to visual aid systems, new tools, their benefits and limitations, and scientific methods to gain proper confidence and dexterity using them.

Chapter 21 - High resolution Intracranial vessel wall imaging (HR-IVWI) has emerged in recent years as an adjunct to conventional imaging. Although, not studied as extensively as in intracranial atherosclerotic diseases, experiences with HR-IVWI in cerebral aneurysms are growing. HR-IVWI has been found to be helpful in differentiation of a stable from an unstable aneurysm in cases of unruptured cerebral aneurysms. Circumferential aneurysmal wall enhancement (CAWE) has been found to be the only independent predictor of instability of an aneurysm. HR-IVWI might also be used to identify the culprit lesion in subarachnoid hemorrhage (SAH) with multiple aneurysms. Furthermore, HR-IVWI might also be used to determine the source of hemorrhage in patients with angiogram negative non-perimesencephalic SAH. Thus, to conclude, HR-IVWI may serve as an important additional tool in the diagnostic armamentarium of cerebral aneurysms that can guide neurointerventionist regarding the selection and timing of appropriate treatment strategies.

Chapter 22 - Although endovascular devices and treatment techniques are continuously developing, these minimally invasive procedures still carry treatment-specific risks. Before entering the era of flow diverter stents, the standard stent-assisted coiling technique has become a well-established treatment option for most cerebral aneurysms. The placement of permanent stents during coiling is associated with greater durability and higher risk of thromboembolic complications. In addition, permanent stents require platelet inhibition, increasing the risk of haemorrhagic complications. Awareness of complications, their predisposing factors, and their prevention and management can further reduce morbidity and mortality.

Chapter 23 - Postprocedural rupture of intracranial unruptured aneurysms after flow diverter (FD) deployment is catastrophic. At present, the cause of this complication is poorly understood. Therefore, the authors conducted a review. The findings are as follows. The incidence of postprocedural rupture of intracranial unruptured aneurysms after FD deployment is <5%. Although postprocedural aneurysm rupture can occur within days or weeks following FD deployment, it is most likely to occur 1 month after surgery. The causes of postprocedural aneurysm rupture include an increase in intra-aneurysmal pressure caused by a detrimental flow pattern induced by FD deployment, an increase in aneurysmal volume caused by the rapid formation of red thrombi, and progressive destruction of the aneurysm wall by inflammation and autolysis. In patients with postprocedural aneurysm rupture after FD deployment, aneurysm size was an independent risk factor, as large aneurysms had a greater postprocedural rupture rate. To date, there have been no effective means to prevent postprocedural aneurysm rupture after FD deployment, but several management strategies, including steroid administration, adjunctive coiling, overlapping FDs and coiling followed by staged FD deployment, have been attempted. Postprocedural aneurysm rupture after FD deployment may result in fatal hemorrhage and carotid cavernous fistula. If the patient is stable, prompt surgery to reduce intracranial pressure is necessary. Then, the ruptured aneurysm requires isolation from the cerebral circulation by open surgery, covered stent deployment and additional FD deployment. For a carotid cavernous fistula, transvenous embolization can be used. The prognosis of postprocedural aneurysm rupture after FD deployment is poor.

Chapter 24 - Aggressive intensive care of patients with aSAH using invasive neuromonitoring is associated with improved outcomes. In addition to disturbances in ICP and patients with SAH are frequently have derangement of CPP, cerebral blood flow (CBF), cerebral oxygenation, and cerebral energy metabolism. The incidence of intracranial hypertension in aSAH is around 80%. aSAH patients with longer episodes of ICP above 20–25 mmHg have shown to be associated with an increased risk of clinical deterioration, delayed cerebral ischaemia, unfavorable outcome, and mortality. After ventriculostomy ICP should be maintained above 15 mm Hg to reduce the risk of re-bleeding. CPP closer to 70–90 mmHg is associated with better brain tissue oxygenation, cerebral energy metabolism, and favourable outcome in aSAH but the threshold has not been validated through prospective studies. It is possible to individualize autoregulatory CPP-target using derived parameters from ICP waveform such as pressure reactivity index (PRx), mean flow index (Mx), and oxygen reactivity index (ORx). SAH is associated with varied changes in cerebral blod flow (CBF) from hyperemia to vasospasm to ischaemia. Transcranial Doppler (TCD) ultrasonography is a bedside dynamic monitoring tool to screen for the presence and progression of cerebral vasospasm in patients with SAH. It can be differentiated from cerebral hyperemia through Lindegrad index. In patients with SAH, additional applications of the TCD technique include studies of CBF autoregulation integrity by the carotid artery compression test (transient hyperemic response test) or induced hypertension and indirect evaluation of ICP through the use of the pulsatility index. Adequacy of global cerebral blood flow can be assessed using jugular venous oximetry. Very few studies have evaluated the diagnostic or clinical relevance of jugular venous oximetry in the management of patients with SAH. Concomitant use of brain tissue oxygenation monitoring (PbtO2) may further improve the clinical relevance. PbtO2, measured using commercial devices, can be used as a surrogate measure of CBF. PbtO2 monitoring is a reliable technique for early detection of DCI and brain hypoxia in patients with SAH. Treatment of PbtO2 below 1.33 kPa was effective in reducing secondary ischemic damage. Limitations of PbtO2 monitoring are, it provides information only on local tissue changes and its an invasive technique. Near Infrared Spectroscopy (NIRS)is a simple, portable, continuous, real time, non-invasive monitoring of cerebral oximetry. Vasospasm detection, DCI prediction, and prognostication have explicitly been evaluated in the aSAH population using NIRS. Cerebral metabolic dysfunction has been shown to extensively mediate the pathophysiology of brain injury after SAH. Cerebral microdialysis (CMD) is a tool that can measure concentrations of multiple bioenergetics metabolites in brain interstitial fluid. Emerging investigations have suggested that CMD is an effective way to monitor the changes of cerebral metabolic dysfunction after SAH in real-time and can also monitor for the development of vasospasm and delayed neurological deficits. It has been suggested that the use of continuous EEG to assess for non-convulsive seizures in patients who fail to improve. EEG monitoring also helps in detecting cortical spreading depression (CSD) and DCI. Every neuromonitoring technique, in isolation, has limitations. For that reason. The combined use of multiple monitors is termed "multimodality monitoring" (MMM). MMM tools have been developed to enable monitoring of the different steps to achieve cerebral energy metabolism and enables earlier detection of impending brain injury, diagnosis of the specific pathomechanisms and initiation of cause-specific therapies. Precision and personalization in managing Aneurysmal subarachnoid haemorrhage is possible with monitoring targeted therapy.

Chapter 1

Intracranial Aneurysms

Huachen Zhang[1]
Shikai Liang[1]
Kevin Abel Sene[2]
and Xianli Lv[1,*]

[1]Department of Neurosurgery, Beijing Tsinghua Changgung Hospital, School of Clinical Medicine, Tsinghua University, Beijing, China.
[2]International Department, Chifeng University Affiliated Hospital, Chifeng University, Chifeng, China

Abstract

Intracranial aneurysms (IA) occur in 3-6% of the population. The incidence of aneurysmal subarachnoid hemorrhage (SAH) is 10-15 per 100,000 people per year. Aneurysmal SAH can cause one third of patients to die. Among the survivors, half will return to normal life, and the rest will need support to continue their normal daily activities. Because of the damage caused by SAH, researches have been committed to clarify the pathogenesis of IA, with the aim of increasing the understanding of the disease process. Endovascular coil embolization and flow diversions have become the standard of treatment for these lesions in the majority of cases in comparison to surgical clipping.

Keywords: endovascular, Intracranial aneurysm, surgical clipping, flow diversion, coil embolization

Introduction

Intracranial aneurysms (IA) are pathological dilatations of cerebral arteries, which are common vascular diseases affecting about 3%–6% of the general population [1]. Rupture of the weak wall of such aneurysms mainly results in subarachnoid hemorrhage (SAH), which is still disastrous despite progress in diagnosis, management, care, and follow-up. Different types of

* Corresponding Author's Email: lvxianli000@163.com.

In: Understanding and Managing Cerebral Aneurysms
Editor: Xianli Lv
ISBN: 979-8-89113-608-3

intracranial aneurysms can be observed clinically. They are classified on their shape (Figure 1), size, location, and cause. Most intracranial aneurysms are saccular or berry aneurysms, whereas dissecting, fusiform, infectious, and traumatic aneurysms are much rarer [1].

IAs usually occur at the branches or bifurcations of cerebral arteries [2]. The formation of aneurysm is the result of the interaction between hemodynamic factors (such as axial flow impingement and water hammer effect) and structural defects at the top of arterial bifurcation (such as congenital and acquired medial defects, funnel shaped expansion and thinning areas) (Figure 2) [3]. Hypertension, female sex and familial factors also contribute to the formation of aneurysms. The enlargement of aneurysm is caused by the interaction between mechanical factors (such as constant pressure and resonance), which will lead to the pathological process of structural fatigue and aneurysm wall repair [3, 4]. Aneurysm rupture is caused by the same hemodynamic factors that affect the growth [5]. Pathologically, fibrin, leukocyte infiltration, blister-like and slight bleeding may occur before severe rupture. This slight leakage can lead to healing, growth and re-rupture regardless of their size [3].

Anatomy of Intracranial Aneurysm

The human brain has a complex vascular network, and has a rich supply of blood vessels, which provide oxygen and other essential nutrients [6]. The brain is supplied by two internal carotid arteries and two vertebral arteries (Figure 3), connected by the circle of Willis (Figure 4), the central anastomosis lies in the interpeduncular fossa at the bottom of the brain. The internal carotid artery is divided into the anterior cerebral artery and the middle cerebral artery (Figure 2 B and C). The two anterior cerebral arteries are connected by the anterior communicating artery (Figure 5). The basilar artery, formed by the union of two vertebral arteries (Figure 6), branches into two posterior cerebral arteries.

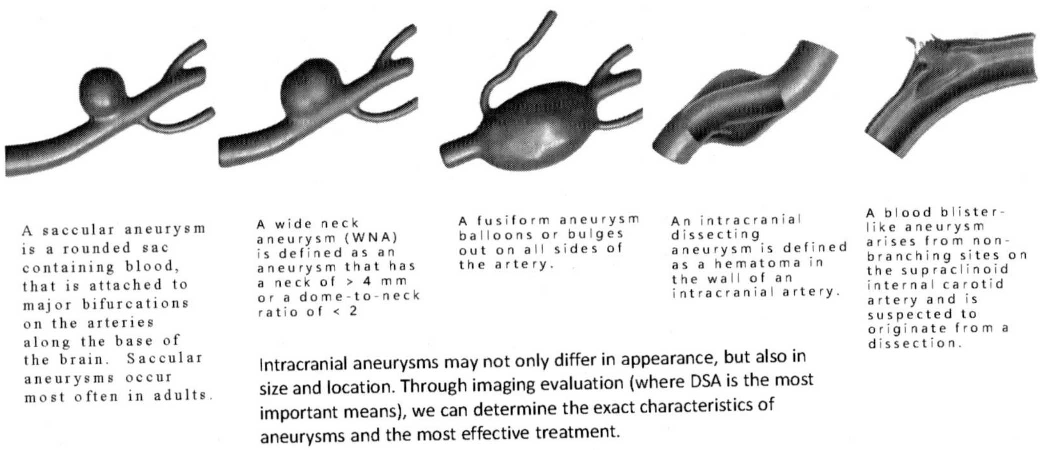

Figure 1. Intracranial aneurysms vary greatly in shape, with five common types.

The posterior communicating artery is a branch of the internal carotid artery connecting with the posterior cerebral artery. The classic arterial circle is bilaterally symmetrical and is a complete vascular ring. This typical configuration and their calibers may vary correlating with genes, which develop in early embryo and persist after birth [2]. They are often hypoplastic, duplicated or even absent. Several studies have shown that these variations play an important role in the development of berry IAs [6]. The incidence of variation of the circle of Willis in the group with aneurysm was significantly higher than that of the control group without aneurysm. There is a clear correlation between the asymmetric proximal segment of the anterior cerebral artery and aneurysm of the anterior communicating artery. There is also a trend of correlation in aneurysm case at the junction of the asymmetric posterior communicating artery and the internal carotid artery [2]. For example, aneurysms of the anterior communicating artery account for 30%–37% of all IAs and are frequently associated with SAH [7]. In IA operation and internal carotid artery ligation, the status of circle is very important to determine the adequacy of cerebral circulation (Figures 7 and 8).

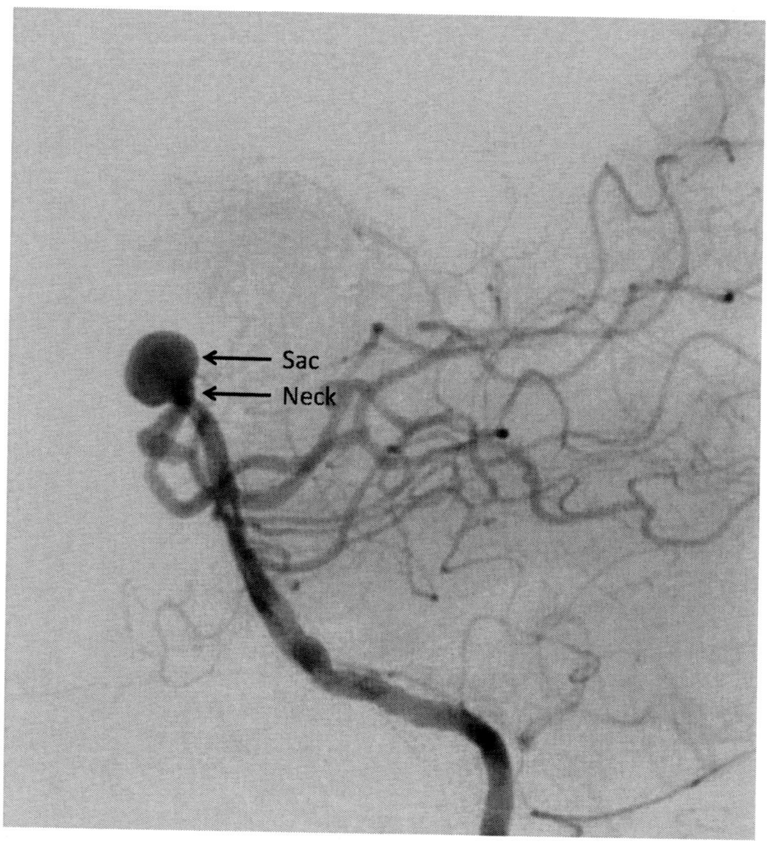

Figure 2. The lateral view of the vertebral artery angiography showed an aneurysm at the bifurcation of the basilar artery. Neck, aneurysmal neck; Sac, aneurysmal sac.

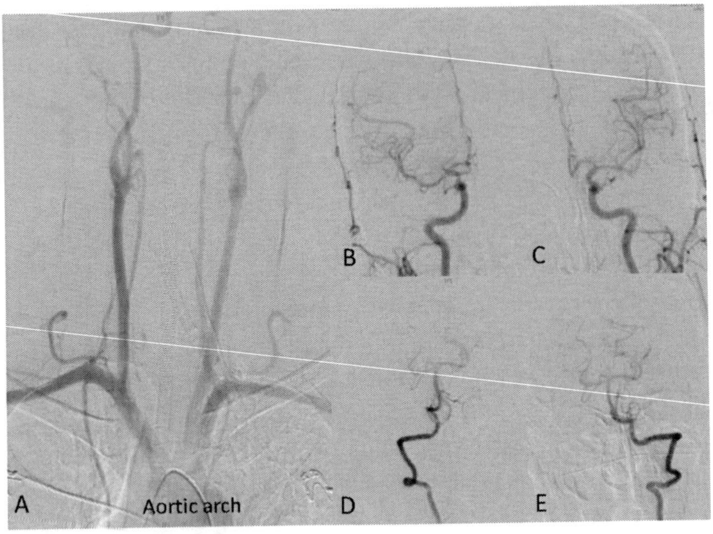

Figure 3. A, aortic arch angiography, anterior posterior view, showed the convexity of the aortic arch gives off three branches; the brachiocephalic trunk, the left common carotid artery and the left subclavian artery. After the sternoclavicular joint, the brachiocephalic trunk divides into the right common carotid artery and the right subclavian artery. B, the frontal view of the right carotid artery angiography. C, the frontal view of the left carotid artery angiography. D, the frontal view of the right vertebral artery angiography. E, the frontal view of the left vertebral artery angiography.

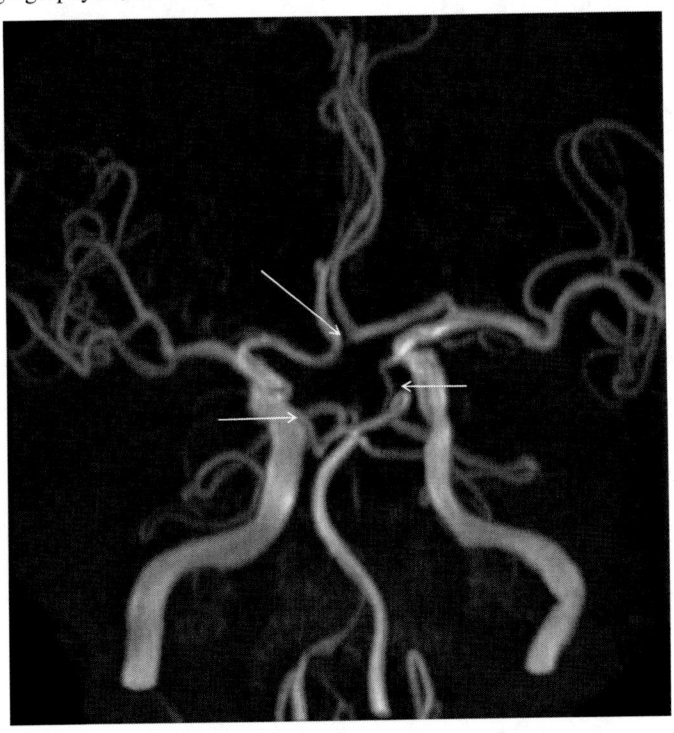

Figure 4. Magnetic resonance angiography showed the arterial ring (circle of Willis) at the bottom of the brain. Acoma, anterior communicating artery; Pcoma, posterior communicating artery.

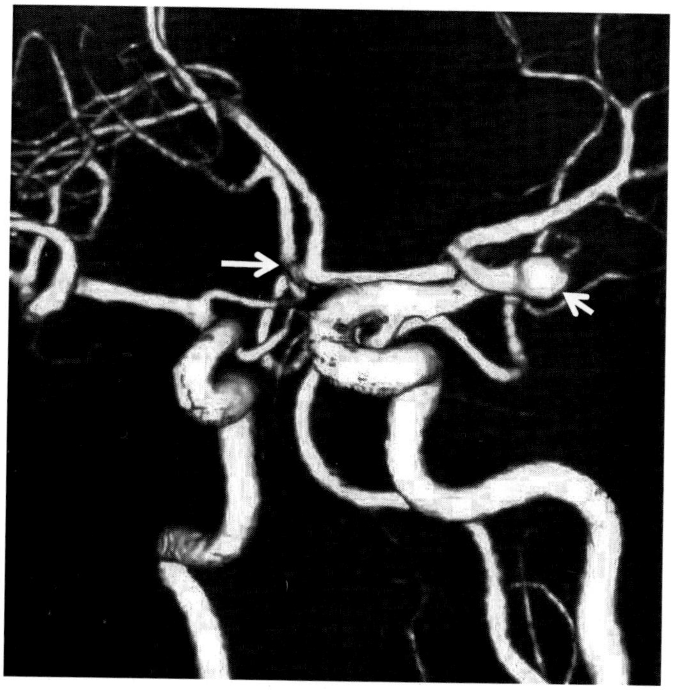

Figure 5. Head CTA examination showed that the left middle cerebral artery bifurcation aneurysm (short arrow) and the two anterior cerebral arteries were connected by the anterior communicating artery (long arrow).

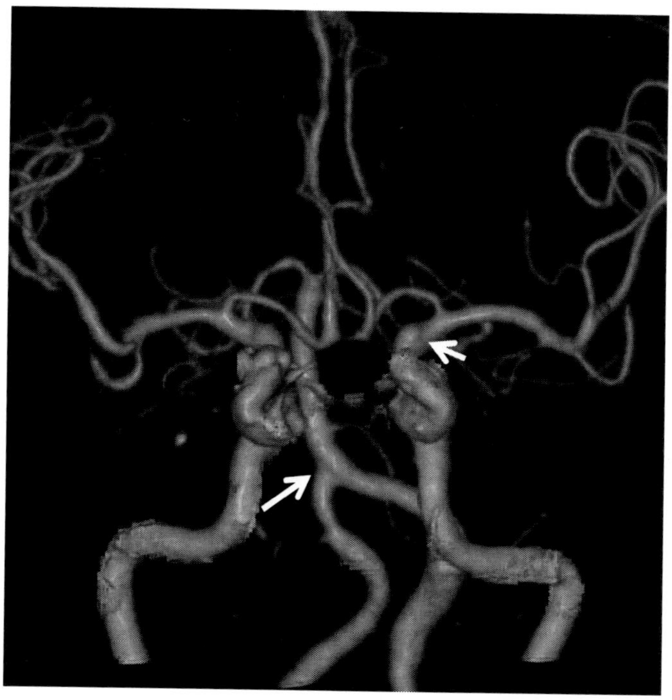

Figure 6. Head CTA examination for SAH suggested a blood blister-like aneurysm of the supraclinoid segment of the left internal carotid artery(short arrow) and the basilar artery, formed by the union of two vertebral arteries, branched into two posterior cerebral arteries (long arrow).

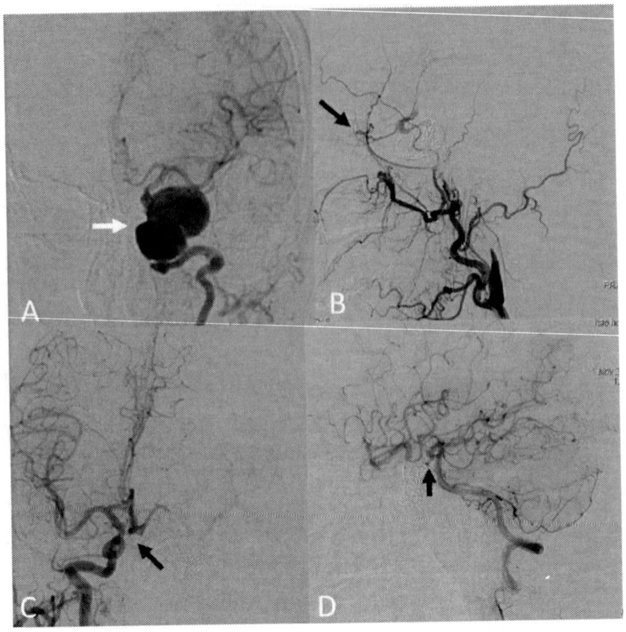

Figure 7. A 68-year-old female with a large cavernous aneurysm of the left internal carotid artery was treated with sacrifice of the left internal carotid artery (A, arrow). The distal branches of the left internal carotid artery were filled sufficient blood through the ophthalmic artery (B, arrow), anterior (C, arrow) and posterior communicating arteries (D, arrow). There was no neurological deficit after operation.

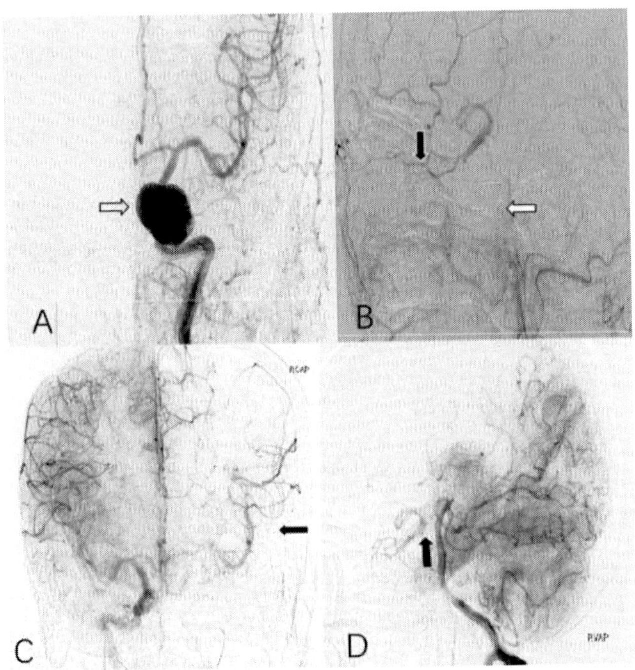

Figure 8. A 61-year-old female with a large cavernous aneurysm of the left internal carotid artery was treated with sacrifice of the left internal carotid artery(A, arrow) using detachable balloons (B, white arrow). The distal branches of the left internal carotid artery were filled insufficient blood through the ophthalmic artery (B, black arrow), anterior(C, black arrow) and posterior communicating arteries (D, black arrow). The patient developed cerebral infarction and hemiplegia after operation.

The hemodynamic changes of the circle of Willis may play a role in the development of IAs. Several authors found that upstream vessel narrowing, similarly to the tapering seen in fire hose nozzles, was shown to lead to flow acceleration and higher velocity toward the bifurcation apex, and to result in increased wall shear stress and related spatial gradients, thus creating favorable hemodynamic conditions for aneurysm initiation and progression. The vessel tapering phenomenon was demonstrated in aneurysms of the anterior communicating artery termed the "fire hose nozzle effect "is also present in case of middle cerebral artery aneurysms [8, 9].

IAs caused by brain trauma are rare, mainly located in supratentorial compartment, and can be classified as "true" or "false" [10, 11]. A true aneurysm is an expansion caused by a partial rupture of the arterial wall. A false aneurysm, or pseudoaneurysm, is formed by a full layer laceration and scar or organized hematoma of brain tissue acts as the aneurysm wall. The interval between the onset of trauma and the diagnosis of traumatic IA is usually several hours to several weeks, because most of them are found by angiography in the acute or subacute stage of head injury [10].

Pathophysiology

Before the rise of genetic sequencing and other genetic tools, epidemiological studies show several correlations between patterns of inheritance with IA formation and rupture [12]. The first- and second-degree relatives of patients of IA or SAH have a 2-4-fold increased risk of developing an IA. In the population of Japan and Finland, the risk of SAH is about three times higher comparing with other ethnic groups. Well known genetic diseases, including autosomal dominant inheritance polycystic nephropathy, Ehlers-Danlos syndrome, Loeys-Dietz syndrome, Marfan syndrome, tuberous sclerosis and fibromuscular dysplasia, are associated with increased risk of IA development. Each of these diseases is characterized by genetic mutations at unique loci, supporting that the pathogenesis of IA may be mediated by a variety of gene products and regulatory proteins. Since then, the research on genetics of IAs has been based on or to elucidate the culprit genes behind these recognized associations or to find new loci related to IA risk. Genome-wide association studies (GWAS) is the key to these efforts. The strongest GWAS to date has utilized single nucleotide polymorphism (SNP) data in thousands of cases and controls to find several susceptible loci including SOX17 and CDKN2A genes. The proteins encoded by these genes regulate endothelial functions and angiogenesis, it supports the hypothesis that genetic variation affecting extracellular matrix or related factors has the greatest impact on IA risk. Histologically, IAs are characterized by a disruption of the inner elastic lamina, thinning of the tunica media with a reduction in the number of vascular smooth muscle cells, and a disorganization of the extracellular matrix. These observed morphological changes lead researchers to focus on expression genes responsible for maintaining the integrity of vascular wall and preventing vascular remodeling after vascular wall injury. Research on genetic basis of IA may produce identification of specific biomarkers and provide new genetic therapies to change IA management.

Risk Factors for Aneurysm Rupture

Many studies have focused on identifying risk factors for rupture of IAs [13]. The size and shape irregularity of aneurysm determined by the presence of blebs have been identified as risk factors for future aneurysm rupture. In addition, the risk score scale (such as population, hypertension, age, size, early SAH and location) has been assigned to evaluate the risk of aneurysms rupture. The identification of specific hemodynamic changes increasing the risk of rupture helps to develop accurate, aneurysm-specific management strategies for growing aneurysms [3]. Some authors have demonstrated the potential of using predictive machine learning models based on specific hemodynamic, geometric and anatomical characteristics of aneurysms to identify small aneurysms with regular shapes that are prone to rupture [5]. The adverse hemodynamic environment characterized by intense concentrated inflow jets, high-speed, complex unstable flow patterns and concentrated, oscillatory, uneven wall shear stress patterns is associated with small and regular aneurysm rupture [5].

Dissecting Aneurysm

Although the incidence rate of intracranial dissecting aneurysms is not high (1-1.5/100,000), the mortality and disability rates are higher than those of intracranial saccular aneurysms, which is the difficulty of endovascular embolization and neurosurgical treatment [14]. Intracranial dissecting aneurysms can occur in any intracranial artery, especially in the vertebrobasilar system as well as internal carotid artery system [14]. The cause of intracranial dissecting aneurysm is due to the sudden rupture and interruption of the elastic layer in the blood vessel (Figure 9). In the chronic dissecting aneurysms, the pathological process is "thrombosis-thrombolysis-thrombosis". The chronic dissecting aneurysm continues to expand and develop, and even forms a huge, thrombotic "serpentine" aneurysm (Figure 10). According to different levels of vascular injury, intracranial dissecting aneurysm can be divided into three stages: the first stage is vascular intima injury, where blood enters between the intima and the media. At this time, the aneurysm may have no symptoms, and may be manifested as headache or cerebral infarction. Headache is caused by vascular wall injury, while cerebral infarction is caused by small perforating vessel injury from the dissected artery. If the vascular injury develops to the vascular media, the blood enters between the vascular media and adventitia. At this time, in addition to the above clinical manifestations, aneurysms are at any time at risk of rupture and bleeding through the adventitia. The occurrence of a blood blister-like aneurysm is one of these cases [15]. If the injury and healing occur repeatedly, the diseased vessels will become tortuous, dilated and irregular in shape (Figure 10). It often leads to cerebral infarction, which can be caused by the blockage of the distal branch of the dissected artery by an embolus, or by the injury of the perforator from the dissected artery (Figure 10D). Therefore, the pathological process and clinical manifestations of intracranial dissecting aneurysms are variable. Because of the damage of arterial wall, it is difficult to treat and the concept of treatment is constantly updated. For example, asymptomatic dissecting aneurysms and manifested as cerebral infarction should be given conservative or aspirin treatment. However, according to the current clinical experience and literature reports, the prognosis of patients is very poor. The clinical outcome is better for the early treatment of some dissecting aneurysms [14, 15].

Endovascular treatment is the main treatment for intracranial dissecting aneurysms [16]. Surgical clipping can't repair the injury of arterial intima and can result of the possible recurrence, continued expansion of aneurysm, or even re-bleeding after surgery. The choice of endovascular methods for intracranial dissecting aneurysms with different locations, shapes and clinical manifestations will be different. The main methods of endovascular treatment are parent artery occlusion and reconstruction of stent or flow diversion [17]. For example, the bleeding dissecting aneurysm will be more aggressive in treatment. The parent artery can be occluded or the stent can be reconstructed with coil embolization. Dissecting aneurysms without bleed may be treated with flow diversion.

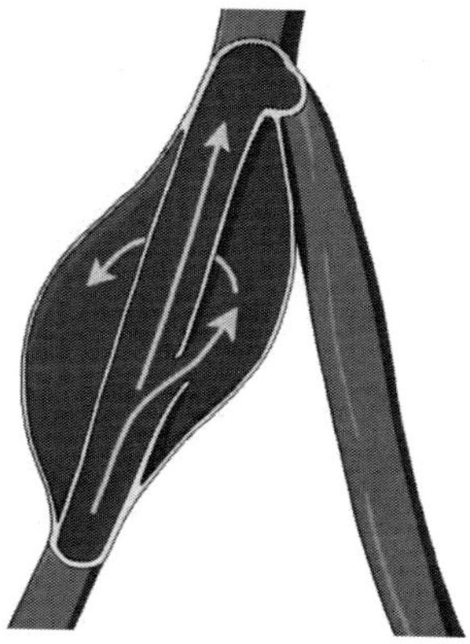

Figure 9. Schematic diagram of the formation of dissecting aneurysm.

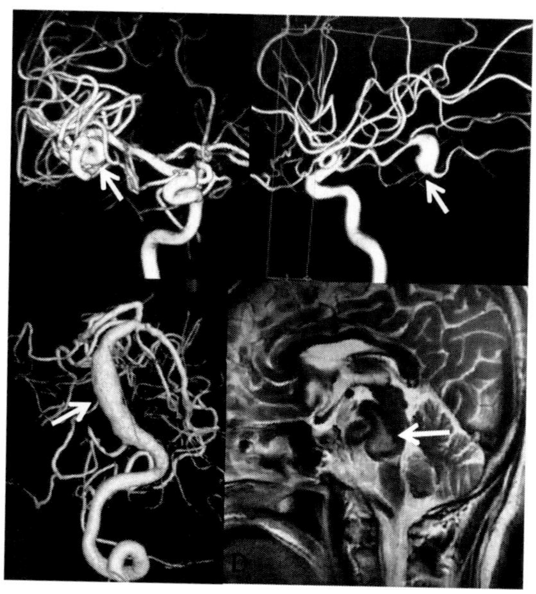

Figure 10. The angiographic images showed chronic arterial dissection in the middle cerebral artery (A, arrow), posterior cerebral artery(B, arrow) and basilar artery(C, arrow). Head MRI examination, T2-weighted, sagittal position, showed basilar artery dissection leading to pons infarction (D, arrow).

Microneurosurgery for Aneurysms

The main treatment principle includes achieving complete IA occlusion while preserving blood flow in the parent, branching, and perforating vessels. The first surgical treatment of an IA was performed in 1933 by Norman Dott [18], who wrapped a ruptured IA, while the first surgical clipping of an IA was performed in 1938 by Walter Dandy [19] (Figure 11). In 1975, Yaşargil and Fox described the microsurgical approaches for IA clipping, such as the pterional craniotomy, which afforded safe and effective exposure of the circle of Willis through the Sylvian fissure with minimal retraction on the frontal and temporal lobes [20]. Indeed, with technological developments in vascular imaging, intraoperative navigation, and fluorescence angiography, this technique remains popular for treating IAs of the anterior circulation [21, 22]. From 1978 to 1983, in a prospective continuous study [23], 1076 patients with ruptured IAs, including 674 women and 402 men, had a median age of 49 years. The location of ruptured aneurysm is: internal carotid artery 285(26.5%), Acom and anterior cerebral artery 383(35.6%), middle cerebral artery 291(27%), basilar and vertebral arteries 83(7.7%) and peripheral or other location 34(3.2%). Compared with other locations, the prognosis of patients with internal carotid aneurysms is significantly better. Under comparable clinical conditions, the prognosis of patients with surgery was significantly improved than that of patients without surgery. The advantages of microneurosurgery have been fully demonstrated. The prognosis of patients with vasospasm was significantly worse. In the first two weeks, daily re-bleeding rate was observed from 0.2% to 2.1%, and the prognosis of patients with re-bleeding was significantly worse than that of patients without re-bleeding. The overall results of 2-year follow-up were: normal 27.5%, mild dementia 15.8%, severe dementia 9.9%, vegetative 1.3%, and mortality 45.5%. A 2018 Systematic Review and Meta-Analysis compared endovascular coiling versus neurosurgical clipping for intracranial aneurysms considering no significant difference in 1 year medical costs, however, the length of stay of endovascular coiling was much shorter than neurosurgical clipping and decreased over time [13].

However, the more recent advance in IA treatment has been the advent of safe and effective endovascular techniques for the treatment of IAs, particularly of the posterior circulation. Acceptance and popularity of endovascular techniques increased in 2002 with the results of the International Subarachnoid Aneurysm Trial (ISAT) [24]. Although both surgical and endovascular IA occlusion technologies are effective for appropriately selected patients, improved technology for endovascular devices and techniques has shifted the balance towards these less invasive techniques with the benefit of reducing operative time, suiting patient preference and tolerability in less healthy patients, and decreased length of in-hospital stay [24]. Nonetheless, open surgical techniques including complex IA treatment with bypass techniques remain vital in the cerebrovascular neurosurgeon's armamentarium for IAs that cannot be treated by endovascular means. The treatment techniques and management guidelines for IAs have thus continued to evolve in recent years, and these rapid developments have forced clinicians to adapt their surgical decision-making.

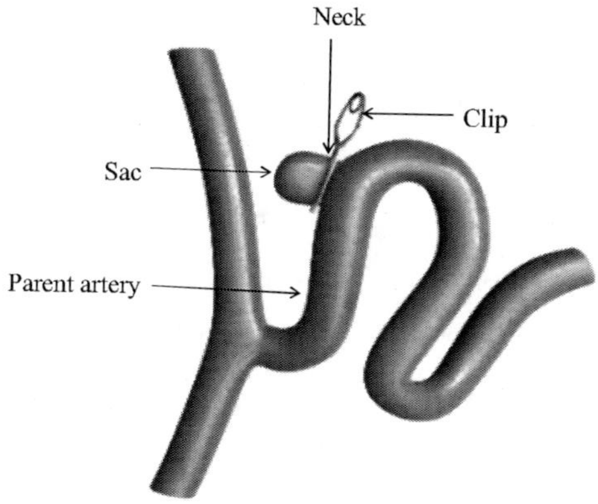

Figure 11. Surgical clipping.

Endovascular Surgery of Cerebral Aneurysms

From 1960s, the detachable balloon technique was first used by Serbinenko [25] and subsequently by Debrun [26]. However, the introduction of Guglielmi endovascular devices overcomes worldwide these old techniques in 1991. The two most significant technological innovations developed for the endovascular treatment of IAs are controlled coil detachment [6, 23] and flow diversion [27]. Coil technology has undergone spectacular development since its inception [5]. Once electrothrombosis was disproven as its underlying mechanism of action [28], alternative detachment modes were developed to facilitate more rapid coil release than could be achieved with electrolysis alone [13, 29]. The clinical availability of three-dimensional and extremely soft finishing coils contributed to the consolidation of coil embolization (Figures 12, 13 and 14) [30, 31]. Stent-assisted coiling enables endovascular management of complex and wide-necked aneurysms with low procedure-related morbidity and mortality (Figure 15 and 16). Stents provide several benefits, e.g., they prevent the protrusion or dislocation of coils into the parent artery, promote vessel wall healing, and some, reduce intra-aneurysmal flow due to a partial flow-divert effect (Figure 17). Other new adjunctive devices include the pCONus, a new neck bridging device, as an adjunct to coil embolization for aneurysms [30].

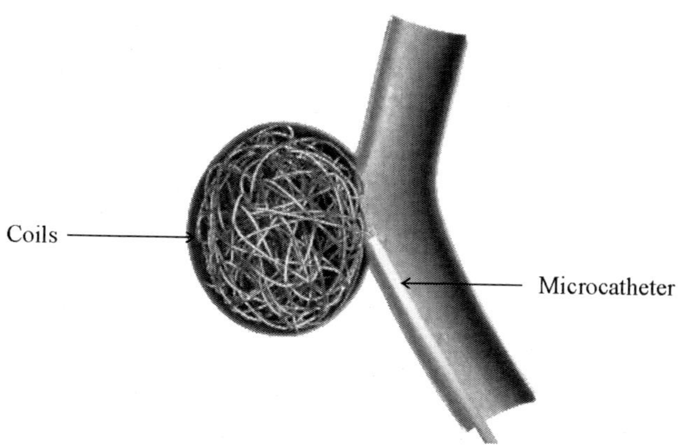

Figure 12. Endovascular coil embolization.

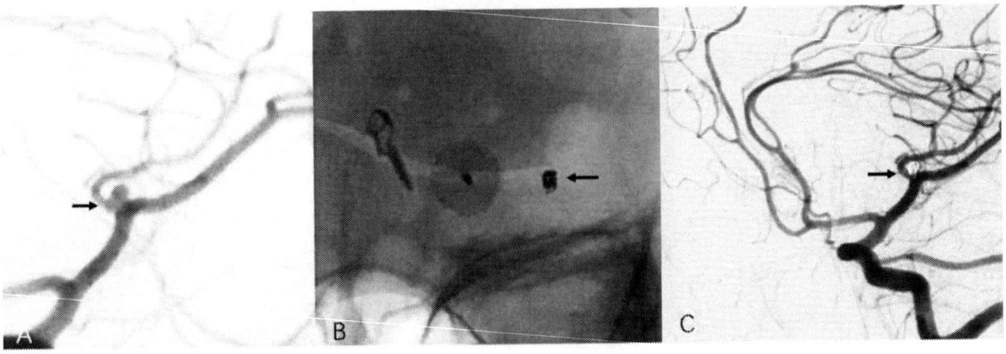

Figure 13. Panels A to C showed the angiographic images of a 52-year-old woman. The left middle cerebral artery bifurcation aneurysm was coiled (arrows) after surgical clipping of the anterior communicating artery aneurysm.

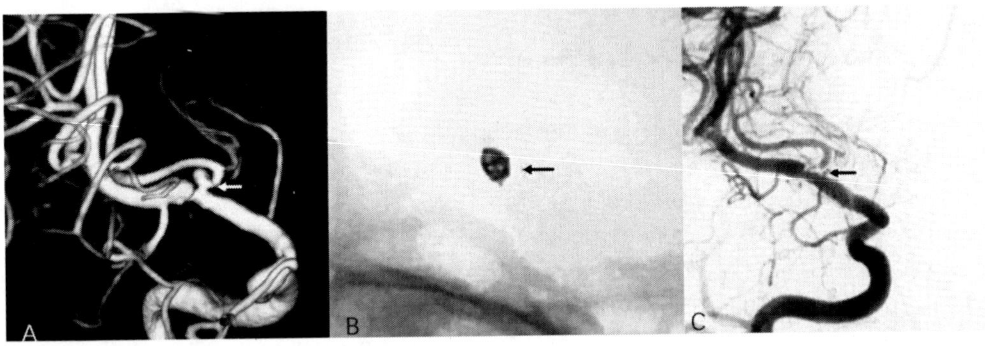

Figure 14. The angiographic images of a 46-year-old male. A, the 3-D reconstruction of the right internal carotid artery injection showed an aneurysm at the bifurcation of the right middle cerebral artery (arrow). B and C, the aneurysm was treated with endovascular coil embolization (arrows).

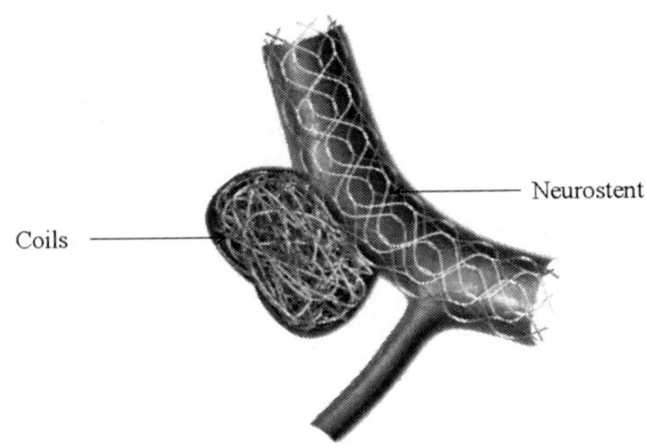

Figure 15. Endovascular stent-assisted coil embolization.

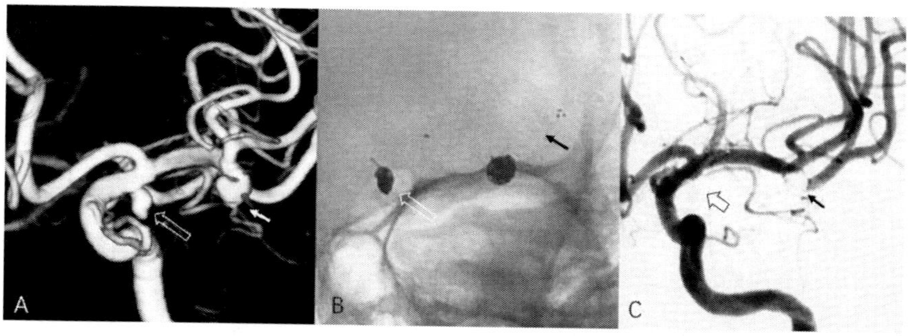

Figure 16. A to C. A 52-year-old female had two cerebral aneurysms. The left anterior choroidal artery aneurysm was treated with endovascular coil embolization (large arrows), and the left middle cerebral artery bifurcation aneurysm was treated with stent-assisted coil embolization (small arrows).

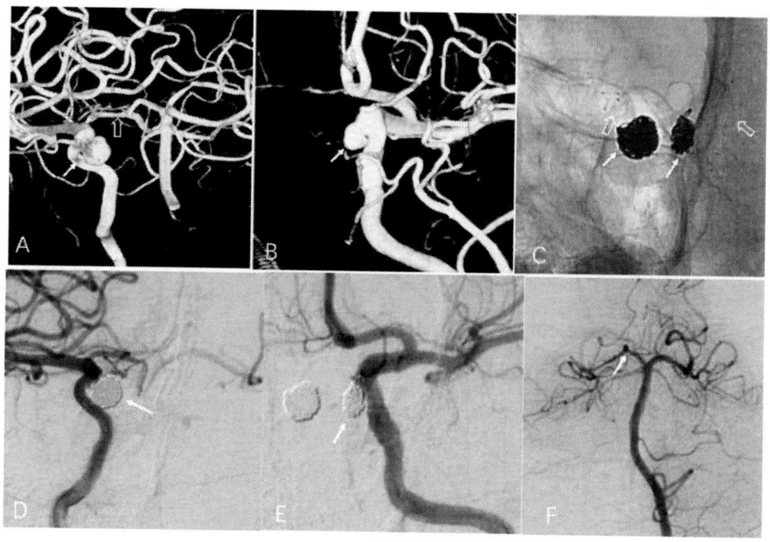

Figure 17. A 53-year-old female with bilateral internal carotid aneurysms underwent stent-assisted coil embolization. A, 3-D reconstruction of right internal carotid artery angiography showed an aneurysm (small arrow) and the opening of the posterior communicating artery (large arrow). B, 3-D reconstruction of left internal carotid artery angiography showed the other aneurysm (small arrow). C, fluoroscopic image showed the 2 neurostents (large arrows) and 2 coil masses (small arrows). The right (D) and left (E) internal carotid artery angiograms showed complete obliteration of the aneurysms (arrows). F, the left vertebral artery angiography showed the right posterior communicating artery (arrow).

Flow diverting stent (FDS) devices are an effective treatment for large, giant and wide-neck intracranial aneurysms. Several different FDS devices are available: The Pipeline (PED & Flex; Medtronic) (Figure 18, 19 and 20), Surpass (Stryker), FRED (flow redirection endoluminal device, MicroVention), SILK (Balt Extrusion), and p64 (Phenox) [17, 27, 28, 31, 32]. The p48 MW and the p64 MW (Phenox) are available with Hydrophilic Polymer Coating (HPC) that reduces the risk of thrombus formation [27]. Recent meta-analyses that evaluated the effectiveness of these FDS devices showed that the overall complete aneurysm occlusion rates were between 76–77.9% at 6 months follow-up, depending on the stents included. The Woven EndoBridge device (WEB) was designed specifically for the treatment of wide neck bifurcation aneurysm, which comprises 26–36% of all intracranial aneurysms [29].

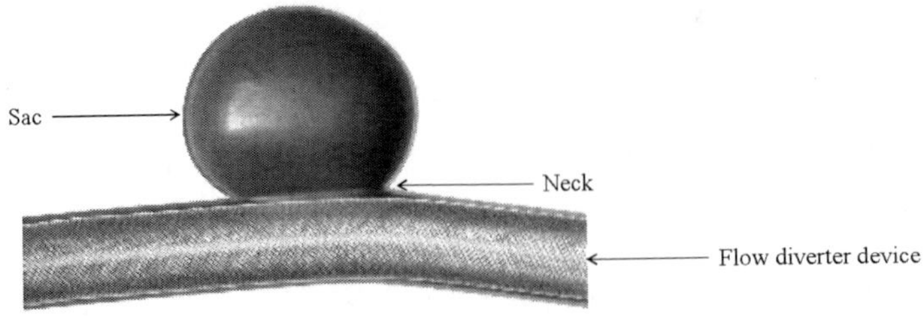

Figure 18. Endovascular intra-luminal flow diversion therapy.

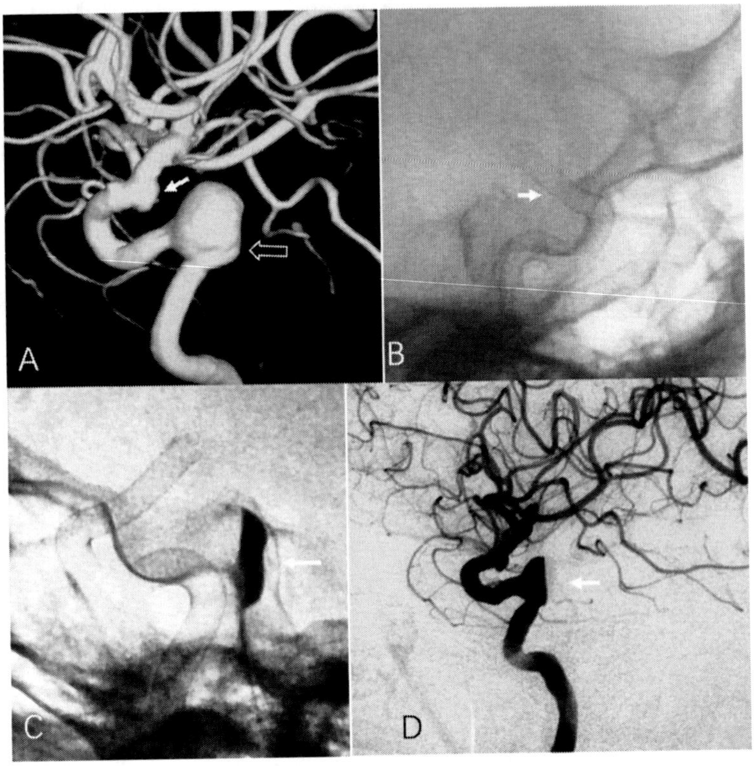

Figure 19. A to D. A 45-year-old female had two internal carotid artery aneurysms. One aneurysm at the clinoid segment and the other at petrous segment of the internal carotid artery was covered with one Pipeline flow diverter in one session (arrows).

Even access approaches within endovascular neurosurgery have seen a major change [33]. Although femoral access was the mainstay for early endovascular access and remains a large part of armamentarium today, alternative routes, such as transradial and transulnar access, have become an important part of our everyday practice.

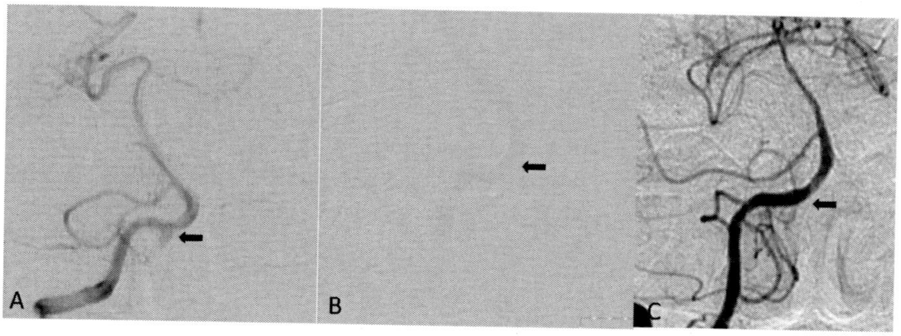

Figure 20. A, the angiographic image of the right vertebral artery injection showed a vertebral artery aneurysm (arrow). B, the aneurysm was treated with one Pipeline flow diverter (arrow). C, the 6-month control angiogram showed that the aneurysm was completely occluded (arrow).

Aneurysm Rupture and Management during Pregnancy

SAH during pregnancy is a rare condition and occurs more often in primiparae and in the third trimester of pregnancy [34]. The hemodynamic and endocrine changes play an important role in the growth and rupture of aneurysms. There are no differences in the clinical course of SAH among pregnant and non-pregnant patients. Intracranial hemorrhage caused by IA is a serious complication of pregnancy, accounting for 5% to 12% of all maternal deaths [35]. Prenatal hemorrhage accounts for 92% of the patients and postpartum hemorrhage accounts for 8% of the patients. 34% of patients had hypertension and/or proteinuria at some time during pregnancy, which sometimes made it difficult to distinguish aneurysmal SAH from eclampsia. The confirmation of the diagnosis is made by CT or lumbar puncture and cerebral angiography. Rupture of IAs is a serious condition, prompt diagnosis and treatment may prevent potentially lethal complications in pregnancy and otherwise. Clipping and endovascular coiling are treatment modalities available [36, 37]. Awake endovascular coiling may be beneficial in such case because it avoided general anesthesia and the use of osmotic diuretics which are potentially hazardous during pregnancy [38]. For those patients with pathological changes who did not undergo treatment, cesarean section did not provide better maternal or fetal outcomes than vaginal delivery. Ruptured IAs should be treated as they would be in patients who are not pregnant, and the delivery method should be based on obstetric considerations [35]. When the aneurysm is successfully handled, the pregnancy can be allowed to progress to term. In these cases, the vaginal delivery is preferred by most clinicians. Caesarean section would be indicated in several circumstances: when the clinical state of mother is severe (coma, brain stem damage), if the aneurysm is diagnosed at term of labour, if the interval between the neurosurgical treatment of aneurysm and labour is less than 8 days [39, 40]. Although SAH during pregnancy can result in disastrous outcomes, the necessity of intracranial screening for high-risk pregnant women is still controversial [39].

Conclusion

IAs often occur in the circle of Willis at the bottom of the brain. From the perspective of some autosomal dominant genetic diseases, the occurrence of aneurysms may be related to gene mutations. The factors of aneurysm rupture include population, hypertension, age, size, early SAH and location. Dissecting aneurysm is a special kind of aneurysms, which is difficult to diagnose and treat. The appearance of flow diversion has significantly improved endovascular treatment of dissecting aneurysms. The treatment of aneurysms has a long history. The exploration of surgical and endovascular treatments started almost at the same time, and both developed rapidly. Endovascular treatment has its unique advantages, including minimally invasive, short procedure time, fast postoperative recovery, and low incidence of epilepsy and postoperative infection. SAH during pregnancy must be distinguished with eclampsia. The treatment of gestational aneurysms should be based on the indications of neurosurgery, and the selection of delivery methods should be based on the indications of obstetrics.

References

[1] Wardlaw JM, White PM. The detection and management of unruptured intracranial aneurysms. *Brain.* 2000 Feb;123 (Pt 2):205-21.

[2] Kayembe KN, Sasahara M, Hazama F. Cerebral aneurysms and variations in the circle of Willis. *Stroke.* 1984 Sep-Oct;15(5):846-50.

[3] Cornelissen BMW, Leemans EL, Slump CH, van den Berg R, Marquering HA, Majoie CBLM. Hemodynamic changes after intracranial aneurysm growth. *J Neurosurg*. 2021 Oct 29:1-7.

[4] Zhang H, Liang S, Lv X. Intra-aneurysmal thrombosis and turbulent flow on MRI of large and giant internal carotid artery aneurysms. *Neuroscience Informatics*. 2021: 1(4): 100027.

[5] Salimi Ashkezari SF, Mut F, Slawski M, Jimenez CM, Robertson AM, Cebral JR. Identification of Small, Regularly Shaped Cerebral Aneurysms Prone to Rupture. *AJNR Am J Neuroradiol*. 2022 Apr;43(4):547-553.

[6] Iqbal S. A comprehensive study of the anatomical variations of the circle of Willis in adult human brains. *J Clin Diagn Res*. 2013 Nov;7(11):2423-7.

[7] Stoeter P, Reulen HJ, Groeger U. CT-findings in hemorrhages from aneurysms of the anterior communicating artery: correlation with angiography and clinical course. *Acta Neurochir (Wien)*. 1987;87(1-2):22-30.

[8] Lauric A, Silveira L, Lesha E, Breton JM, Malek AM. Aneurysm presence at the anterior communicating artery bifurcation is associated with caliber tapering of the A1 segment. *J Neurosurg*. 2021 Oct 15:1-11.

[9] Lauric A, Greim-Kuczewski K, Antonov A, Dardik G, Magida JK, Hippelheuser JE, Kono K, Malek AM. Proximal Parent Vessel Tapering is Associated With Aneurysm at the Middle Cerebral Artery Bifurcation. *Neurosurgery*. 2019 May 1;84(5):1082-1089.

[10] Soria ED, Paroski MW, Schamann ME. Traumatic aneurysms of cerebral vessels: a case study and review of the literature. *Angiology*. 1988 Jul;39(7 Pt 1):609-15.

[11] Lv X, Guo Y, Mao G. 2022. Frontiers in Traumatic Brain Injury. *IntechOpen*. London, United Kingdom.

[12] Laurent D, Small C, Lucke-Wold B, Dodd WS, Chalouhi N, Hu YC, Hosaka K, Motwani K, Martinez M, Polifka A, Koch M, Busl KM, Maciel CB, Hoh B. Understanding the genetics of intracranial aneurysms: A primer. *Clin Neurol Neurosurg*. 2022 Jan; 212:107060.

[13] Karhunen V, Bakker MK, Ruigrok YM, Gill D, Larsson SC. Modifiable risk factors for intracranial aneurysm and aneurysmal subarachnoid hemorrhage: A Mendelian randomization study. *J Am Heart Assoc* [Internet]. 2021;10(22): e022277.

[14] Lv X, Yu J, Zhang W, Zhao X, Zhang H. Acute hemorrhagic cerebral artery dissection: Characteristics and endovascular treatment. *Neuroradiol J*. 2020 Apr;33(2):112-117.
[15] Ye Z, Lv X. The formation mechanism of acute dissection of blood blister-like aneurysm and its implication of endovascular treatment. *Chin Neurosurg J*. 2021 Jun 3;7(1):32.
[16] Lv X, Ge H, Jin H, He H, Jiang C, Li Y. Endovascular treatment of unruptured posterior circulation intracranial aneurysms. *Ann Indian Acad Neurol*. 2016 Jul-Sep;19(3):302-6.
[17] Zhang H, Ren J, Wang J, Lv X. The off-label uses of pipeline embolization device for complex cerebral aneurysms: Mid-term follow-up in a single center. *Interv Neuroradiol*. 2022 Dec 30:15910199221148800. doi: 10.1177/15910199221148800. Epub ahead of print. PMID: 36583531.
[18] Dott NM. Intracranial aneurysms: cerebral arterio-radiography: surgical treatment. *Edinb Med J* 1993;40:T219–T240.
[19] Dandy WE. Intracranial aneurysm of the internal carotid artery: cured by operation. *Ann Surg* 1938;107:654–659.
[20] Yasargil MG, Fox JL. The microsurgical approach to intracranial aneurysms. *Surg Neurol* 1975;3:7–14.
[21] Yasargil MG, Antic J, Laciga R, Jain KK, Hodosh RM, Smith RD. Microsurgical pterional approach to aneurysms of the basilar bifurcation. *Surg Neurol* 1976;6:83–91.
[22] Ormond DR, Hadjipanayis CG. The supraorbital keyhole craniotomy through an eyebrow incision: its origins and evolution. *Minim Invasive Surg* 2013:296-469.
[23] Rosenørn J, Eskesen V, Schmidt K, Espersen JO, Haase J, Harmsen A, Hein O, Knudsen V, Midholm S, Marcussen E, et al. Clinical features and outcome in 1076 patients with ruptured intracranial saccular aneurysms: a prospective consecutive study. *Br J Neurosurg*. 1987;1(1):33-45.
[24] Molyneux AJ, Kerr RS, Yu LM, Clarke M, Sneade M, Yarnold JA, Sandercock P, International Subarachnoid Aneurysm Trial (ISAT) Collaborative Group (2005) International subarachnoid aneurysm trial (ISAT) of neurosurgical clipping versus endovascular coiling in 2143 patients with ruptured intracranial aneurysms: a randomized comparison of effects on survival, dependency, seizures, rebleeding, subgroups, and aneurysm occlusion. *Lancet* 366:809–817.
[25] Serbinenko FA. Balloon catheterization and occlusion of major cerebral vessels. *J Neurosurg* 1974;41 :125-1 45.
[26] Debrun G. Detachable balloon and calibrated leak balloon technique in the treatment of cerebral vascular lesions. *J Neurosurg* 1978;49: 635-649.
[27] Guzzardi G, Galbiati A, Stanca C, Del Sette B, Paladini A, Cossandi C, Carriero A. Flow diverter stents with hydrophilic polymer coating for the treatment of acutely ruptured aneurysms using single antiplatelet therapy: Preliminary experience. *Interv Neuroradiol*. 2020 Oct;26(5):525-531.
[28] Cooper JB, Li B, Kaur G, Gandhi CD, Santarelli JG. Pipeline embolization of ruptured, previously coiled cerebral aneurysms: Case series and considerations for management. *Brain Circ*. 2021 May 29;7(2):111-117.
[29] De Leacy RA, Fargen KM, Mascitelli JR, et al. Wide-neck bifurcation aneurysms of the middle cerebral artery and basilar apex treated by endovascular techniques: a multicenter, core lab adjudicated study evaluating safety and durability of occlusion (BRANCH). *J Neurointerv Surg* 2019;11:31–6.
[30] Pérez MA, Bhogal P, Moreno RM, Wendl C, Bäzner H, Ganslandt O, Henkes H. Use of the pCONus as an adjunct to coil embolization of acutely ruptured aneurysms. *J Neurointerv Surg*. 2017 Jan;9(1):39-44.
[31] Cancelliere NM, Nicholson P, Radovanovic I, Mendes KM, Orru E, Krings T, Pereira VM. Comparison of intra-aneurysmal flow modification using optical flow imaging to evaluate the performance of Evolve and Pipeline flow diverting stents. *J Neurointerv Surg*. 2020 Aug;12(8):814-817.
[32] Rouchaud A, Brinjikji W, Lanzino G, Cloft HJ, Kadirvel R, Kallmes DF. Delayed hemorrhagic complications after flow diversion for intracranial aneurysms: a literature overview. *Neuroradiology*. 2016 Feb;58(2):171-7.
[33] Wilkinson DA, Majmundar N, Catapano JS, Cole TS, Baranoski JF, Hendricks BK, Cavalcanti DD, Frederickson VL, Ducruet AF, Albuquerque FC. Avoiding the Radial Paradox: Neuroendovascular Femoral Access Outcomes After Radial Access Adoption. *Neurosurgery*. 2022 Mar 1;90(3):287-292.
[34] Lv X, Li Y. Progress in diagnosis and treatment of subarachnoid hemorrhage during pregnancy and postpartum [J]. *Chinese Journal of Neurosurgery*, 2015,31 (1): 95-98.

[35] Dias MS, Sekhar LN. Intracranial hemorrhage from aneurysms and arteriovenous malformations during pregnancy and the puerperium. *Neurosurgery*. 1990 Dec;27(6):855-866.

[36] Vatsa R, Sharma JB, Zangmo R, Kumar S, Yadav A. Successful Pregnancy Outcome after Coiling of Ruptured Intracranial Aneurysm. *J Assoc Physicians India.* 2019 Mar;67(3):89-90.

[37] Piotin M, de Souza Filho CB, Kothimbakam R, Moret J. Endovascular treatment of acutely ruptured intracranial aneurysms in pregnancy. *Am J Obstet Gynecol.* 2001 Nov;185(5):1261-2.

[38] Xie F, Hao J, Richard SA, Yang Y, Zou W, Liu HB, Deng M, Zhang C. Awake endovascular coiling of a dissected intracranial aneurysm in a third-trimester twin pregnancy: A case report. *Medicine (Baltimore)*. 2021 Jan 8;100(1): e24239.

[39] Kataoka H, Miyoshi T, Neki R, Yoshimatsu J, Ishibashi-Ueda H, Iihara K. Subarachnoid hemorrhage from intracranial aneurysms during pregnancy and the puerperium. *Neurol Med Chir (Tokyo).* 2013;53(8):549-54.

[40] Mosiewicz A, Jakiel G, Janusz W, Markiewicz P. Leczenie Tetniaków wewnatrzczaszkowych w okresie ciazy [Treatment of intracranial aneurysms during pregnancy]. *Ginekol Pol*. 2001 Feb;72(2):86-92.

Chapter 2

Anatomy and Endovascular Approach for Anterior Communicating Artery Aneurysms

Huachen Zhang[1]
Kevin Abel Sene[2]
and Xianli Lv[1,*]
[1]Department of Neurosurgery, Beijing Tsinghua Changgung Hospital, School of Clinical Medicine, Tsinghua University, Beijing, China
[2]International Department, Chifeng University Affiliated Hospital, Chifeng university, Chifeng, China

Abstract

Anterior communicating (Acom) aneurysms are difficult to understand because of anatomical variations in this region, although they are the most common intracranial aneurysms. This chapter was to classify Acom aneurysms into 5 subgroups (straight, superior, inferior, anterior, and posterior) of orientations according to the axis connecting A1 origin and the base of the aneurysm. This classification of Acom aneurysms distinguishes their characteristics, including the shape, location, orientation, size, probability of occurrence and endovascular treatments. It adds an interesting classification system to the evaluation and treatment of Acom aneurysms.

Keywords: aneurysm, anterior communicating artery, classification, endovascular

Background

The anterior communicating artery aneurysm (Acom) is the most common part of intracranial aneurysms and was observed in 35% of cases [1, 2]. Compared with other cerebral aneurysms, the morphology, anatomy and peripheral vascular structure of Acom aneurysms are the most difficult to understand because of the anatomical variation and complex morphology of Acom [1, 2]. There is a bifurcation between the anterior cerebral artery and Acom, which is the most common location of aneurysms [1, 2].

* Corresponding Author's Email: lvxianli000@163.com.

In: Understanding and Managing Cerebral Aneurysms
Editor: Xianli Lv
ISBN: 979-8-89113-608-3

The formation of an Acom aneurysm is closely related to variations in the Acom complex, such as hypoplasia of the A1 segment on one side or the Acom fenestration. However, just knowing these, is not enough, because in addition to judging on which side Acom aneurysms occur, they may also occur in any direction, and their size and shape will also vary greatly. We need to better understand the anatomical structure of Acom aneurysms in order to better treat them. Endovascular therapy has become an alternative and main choice for surgical clipping [3, 4]. Zhang et al. provided an interesting classification system for the evaluation and endovascular treatment of Acom aneurysms [5]. This classification divided the direction of Acom aneurysms based on the line connecting the A1 origin and the base of the aneurysm into the straight, anterior, inferior, superior and posterior projections. The anatomical structural variations of Acom aneurysms can affect their clinical manifestations and endovascular treatment methods. This anatomical classification is related to the size of the aneurysm body, the size of the aneurysm neck, and the need for stent-assisted treatment. In addition, this classification identified the superior projection subgroup of Acom aneurysms that are more prone to rupture.

Determination of Aneurysm Projection

The projection of the aneurysm was determined by 3-dimensional rotational angiography and reconstruction of the internal carotid artery on the aneurysm side. The direction of the aneurysm was determined by taking the line connecting the A1 origin and the base of the aneurysm as the axis (Figure 1). The line from the base to the dome of the aneurysm (the most distal dome in a bilobed or multilobed Acom aneurysm) is the direction. The straight projection is in the same direction as the axis, the anterior projection is in front of the axis, the inferior projection is downward of the axis, the superior projection is upward of the axis, and the posterior projection is backward of the axis.

Clinical Series

There were 92 patients who were diagnosed with 98 Acom aneurysms over a time span of 2 years (2022–2023) and admitted for endovascular embolization. According to this classification, the most common Acom aneurysms were straight (65.4%) aneurysms, followed by inferior aneurysms (16.3%), superior aneurysms (14.3%), anterior aneurysms (2%), and posterior aneurysms (2%). There were 20 microaneurysms (<2mm), 61 small aneurysms (2–5 mm), 15 medium aneurysms (6–9 mm), and 2 large aneurysms (≥ 10mm). The average size of Acom aneurysms was 3.7 mm, and the average neck size was 1.9 mm. Straight Acom aneurysms have a lower risk of spontaneous bleeding than inferior and superior aneurysms.

The sizes of aneurysms from large to small are: straight (4.1 ± 2.2 mm), anterior (3.5 ± 3.5 mm), inferior (3.4 ± 1.8 mm), posterior (2.5 ± 0.7 mm), and superior (2.0 ± 1.0 mm) (Figure 2). Anterior and posterior aneurysms were more likely to have wide-necked aneurysms. The demand for stent-assisted therapy for superior aneurysms is less, while the possibility of using stent-assisted therapy for other aneurysms is greatly increased.

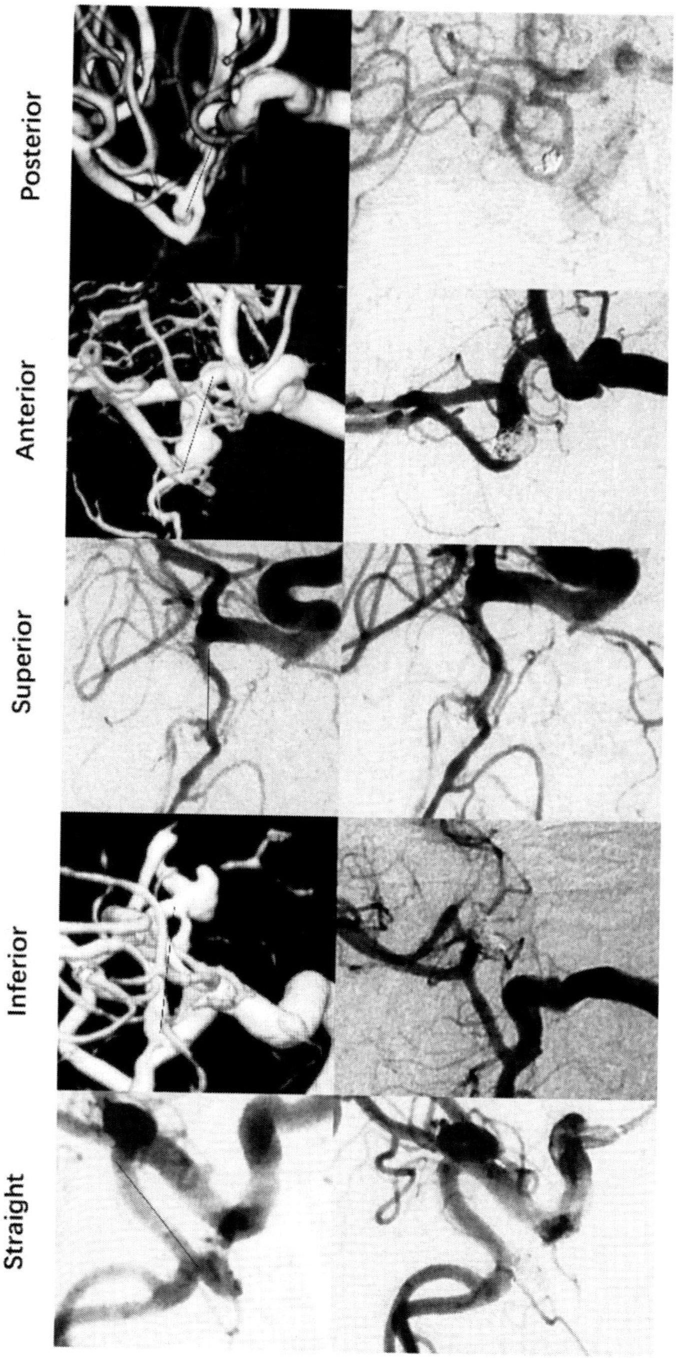

Figure 1. Giving five examples of Acom aneurysms with different directions relative to the axis connecting the A1 origin and the base of the aneurysm. The upper row is the preoperative angiograms, and the lower row is the angiograms after endovascular treatment.

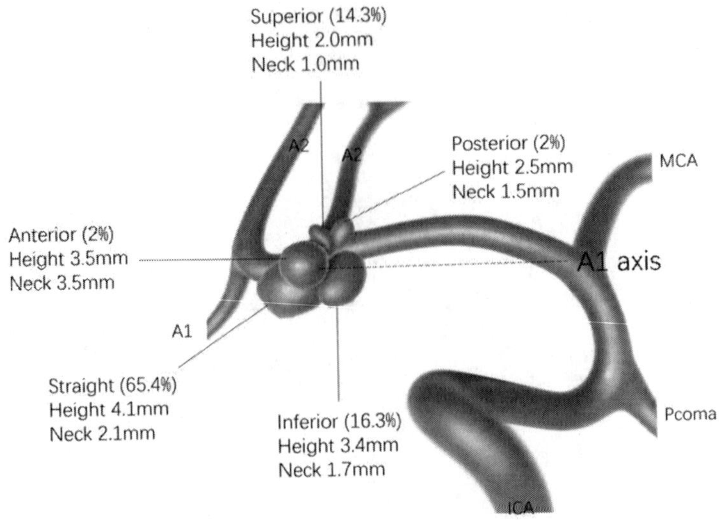

Figure 2. A schematic diagram of the characteristics of Acom aneurysms in different directions. ICA, internal carotid artery; MCA, middle cerebral artery; A1, A1 segment of the anterior cerebral artery; A2, A2 segment of the anterior cerebral artery.

Techniques of Microcatheter and Coil Embolization

According to the different directions of the aneurysm, the head of the microcatheter should have different curvatures. For straight type and superior type, a microcatheter with a straight head is selected. The superior and posterior types are the most difficult, and the tip of the microcatheter should be molded to a very small bending angle. The lower type is the easiest, and the tip of the microcatheter can be bent to 45 °. For microaneurysms, we usually choose the Headway Duo microcatheter (Microvention, USA) and the Nano coil (Stryker, USA).

Techniques for Stents

For wide-necked aneurysms, intracranial stents were routinely selected. According to the market supply, Neuroform Atlas, Leo Baby or LVIS Jr. are preferred. As previously mentioned, antiplatelet therapy is necessary. If thrombosis is found during surgery, tirofiban hydrochloride should be given [3, 4].

Previous Classifications of Acom Aneurysms

The previous classifications of Acom aneurysms are based on surgical findings, such as the relationship between the aneurysm and the axis defined by the artery around the aneurysm [6], the relationship between the aneurysm projection and the A2 segment plane [7], the relationship between the aneurysm projection and A1 segment morphology [8], and the relationship between the aneurysm and the parent vessel [1, 2].

The previous classifications of Acom aneurysms based on intraoperative observations were limited by the choice of surgical approaches and differences in intraoperative anatomical fields. Due to the lack of evaluation of the standard location, the classification derived from surgery is complex and different. The visualization of vascular elements is different from that obtained in autopsy studies. They are not conducive to improving the overall understanding of Acom aneurysms, nor can they be used to guide clinical practice.

Despite adverse reports of endovascular embolization [9], more and more data support endovascular embolization of aneurysms. In a trend matching study of 1332 patients in the United States [10], compared with the clipping cohort, patients with ruptured aneurysms after endovascular embolization had significantly less hydrocephalus within one year. But so far, there is only one Acom aneurysm classification based on flow diversion therapy, and its applicability needs further testing [11]. It is recommended to compare the diameters of two A1 sections: H1 = the same diameter; H2 = <50% diameter difference; H3 = ≥ 50% difference; and Y=no A1 segment. The most suitable anatomical structure for flow diversion treatment seems to be the H1 structure, which is suitable for placement of the shunt from the A1 segment to the A2 segment on the same side. The H3 structure is not suitable for flow diversion treatment. However, further studies are needed to assess the feasibility of this anatomical classification and the reproducibility of the authors' findings.

Although there are successful reports on the use of flow diversion devices to treat Acom aneurysms [3], the application of these devices to Acom aneurysms is still controversial because the diameter of adult A1 is 2.4 mm to 2.6 mm and the length is 12.7 mm [11]. Intra-aneurysm embolization is still the main method to treat Acom aneurysms. Neuro stent-assisted embolization can control Acom aneurysms for a long time, and the growth rate of aneurysms is low after treatment [12]. Double stents, Y-shaped or X-shaped, with assisted coiling can be used as a choice for wide-necked and complex Acom aneurysms [13, 14]. Many new technologies are still aimed at the intra-aneurysm embolization of Acom aneurysms, such as Neuroform Atlas, which was approved by FDA in January 2018 [15], Medina's intra-saccular device [15, 16], the Woven EndoBridge (WEB) device [17], and the PulseRider device [18].

Our classification is based on endovascular techniques for intra-aneurysm embolization. In this study, we classified Acom aneurysms according to their different projections relative to the axis connecting the A1 origin and the base of the aneurysm. This classification is easy to understand, can reflect the anatomical and hemodynamic characteristics of Acom aneurysms in different projections, can provide guidance for neuroendovascular technology, and is convenient for clinical practice. It is necessary to distinguish these types in the diagnosis to adopt different neuroendovascular techniques and treatment plans. Based on this concept, this distinction can also be made in computed tomography angiography (CTA), because the characteristics of aneurysms in different projections have been mastered (Figure 2).

In the surgical treatment study, the authors found that, compared with other Acom aneurysms, the intraoperative rupture rate of upwardly protruding Acom aneurysms was higher (37.5%) and the surgical risk was higher [7]. According to our classification, the superior aneurysms are all ruptured microaneurysms, which can explain the challenges in the treatment of these aneurysms [19]. Acom position is the most common position for ruptured microaneurysms, and it is difficult to achieve a "stable" microcatheter position to safely deliver coils [20]. Proper selection of patients and coils and the use of complex techniques can provide good results for patients with very small aneurysms [21]. In our clinical practice, the use of a

1.5-F microcatheter and Stryker coil greatly improved the safety and effectiveness of treating these microaneurysms.

In the study of Proust et al. [6], the authors proposed that the application of microsurgical clips should be the first choice for the treatment of anterior Acom aneurysms, and for the lesions of posterior Acom aneurysms, endovascular coiling should be selected. The author's direction judgment is based on the axis defined by the pericallosal artery. According to our classification, these two types Acom aneurysms belong to the straight type, which is the most common type of aneurysm and is easy to treat with endovascular embolization. The authors may have missed other rare types of aneurysms in our study.

Unruptured Acom aneurysms should be actively treated, although they are usually small. Although according to ISUIA (International Study of Unruptured Intracranial Aneurysms), the risk of rupture of anterior circulation aneurysms with a diameter <7 mm is the lowest [22], the risk of rupture of Acom aneurysms is twice that of other intracranial aneurysms [23]. Bizlenga et al. also proved this point. They found that anterior circulation aneurysms were not a homogeneous group. Aneurysms of 4 to 7 mm in Acom or the anterior cerebral artery have a similar risk of rupture as posterior circulation aneurysms [24]. They concluded that intervention should be recommended for this high-risk group.

Through different directions, the blood flow may produce different forces, directly impacting the aneurysm wall and ultimately leading to the rupture of aneurysms of different sizes, shapes and acute conditions. The hemodynamics of a cerebral aneurysm were studied using a Doppler guide wire, and it was found that the blood flow velocity in the neck was higher than that in the aneurysm sac [25]. The pulsation near the dome is obviously higher than that of the neck or mother vessel. Pulsation is usually an indicator of peripheral vascular resistance, which is used to describe the increase in flow resistance of an aneurysm sac. Compared with the parent vessel, the typical multi-peak systolic blood flow record of the aneurysm was also found [25]. And, in our clinical practice, endovascular treatment is carefully considered in patients with high SAH grade with ruptured aneurysms because of their poor outcome after endovascular treatment [26].

Conclusion

This classification of Acom aneurysms with the line connecting the A1 origin and the base of the aneurysm as the reference axis makes their characteristics easy to understand, including the shape, location, orientation, size, probability of occurrence and endovascular treatments. This classification can predict the technical requirements of endovascular surgery. It is convenient to establish the overall concept of an aneurysm.

References

[1] Wong H, Banfield J, Hughes N, Shankar JJS. Are Anterior Communicating Aneurysms Truly Anterior Communicating Aneurysms? An Observational Study. *World Neurosurg*. 2019 May;125: e1089-e1092. doi: 10.1016/j.wneu.2019.01.249. Epub 2019 Feb 18. PMID: 30790745.

[2] Hassan T, Elsayed A, Abbas M, Sultan A, Eladawy Y. Proposed Parent Vessel Geometry Based Classification of Anterior Communicating Artery-Located Aneurysms. *World Neurosurg.* 2017 May;101:259-269. doi: 10.1016/j.wneu.2017.01.096. Epub 2017 Feb 4. PMID: 28179173.

[3] Lv X, Jiang C, Wu Z, Jiang W, Wang G. Complex cerebral aneurysms: intra-luminal reconstruction using Pipeline flow-diverting stent and the obliteration mechanism. *Neuroradiol J.* 2020;33(2):91–97.

[4] Lv X, Wang G, Wang J. 2021. Craniospinal Vascular Diseases and Endovascular Neurosurgery. *Nova Science*, NY, USA.

[5] Zhang H, Liang S, Zang B, Lv X. Classification of anterior communicating aneurysms on a basis of endovascular treatments. *Neuroradiol J.* 2023 Nov 1:19714009231212360. doi: 10.1177/1971400 9231212360. Epub ahead of print. PMID: 37914224.

[6] Castaño C, Terceño M, Remollo S, García-Sort MR, Domínguez C. Endovascular treatment of wide-neck intracranial bifurcation aneurysms with 'Y'-configuration, double Neuroform® stents-assisted coiling technique: Experience in a single center. *Interv Neuroradiol.* 2017 Aug;23(4):362-370. doi: 10.1177/1591019917708568. Epub 2017 Jun 6. PMID: 28587530; PMCID: PMC5684913.

[7] Nossek E, Setton A, Karimi R, Dehdashti AR, Langer DJ, Chalif DJ. Analysis of superiorly projecting anterior communicating artery aneurysms: anatomy, techniques, and outcome. A proposed classification system. *Neurosurg Rev.* 2016 Apr;39(2):225-35; discussion 235. doi: 10.1007/s10143-015-0677-4. Epub 2015 Dec 3. PMID: 26631225.

[8] Feng W, Zhang L, Li W, Zhang G, He X, Wang G, Li M, Qi S. Relationship between the morphology of A-1 segment of anterior cerebral artery and anterior communicating artery aneurysms. *Afr Health Sci.* 2014 Mar;14(1):83-8. doi: 10.4314/ahs.v14i1.13. PMID: 26060462; PMCID: PMC4449056.

[9] Liu P, Lv X, Li Y, Lv M. High resolution MRI in treatment decision of anterior communicating artery aneurysm accompanied by visual symptoms: Endovascular treatment or surgical clipping? A report of two cases and literature review. *Interv Neuroradiol.* 2016 Jun;22(3):270-7. doi: 10.1177/1591019915 623559. Epub 2016 Jan 24. PMID: 26809261; PMCID: PMC4984357.

[10] Nia AM, Lall RR, Kan P, Srinivasan VM. Trends and Outcomes of Endovascular Embolization and Surgical Clipping for Ruptured Intracranial Aneurysms: A Propensity-Matched Study of 1332 Patients in the United States. *World Neurosurg.* 2022 May;161:e674-e681. doi: 10.1016/j.wneu.2022.02.077. Epub 2022 Feb 24. PMID: 35218963; PMCID: PMC9081193.

[11] Pagiola I, Mihalea C, Caroff J, Ikka L, Chalumeau V, Yasuda T, Marenco de la Torre J, Iacobucci M, Ozanne A, Gallas S, Marques MC, Carrete H, Frudit ME, Moret J, Spelle L. Flow diversion treatment of aneurysms of the complex region of the anterior communicating artery: which stent placement strategy should 'I' use? A single center experience. *J Neurointerv Surg.* 2019 Nov;11(11):1118-1122. doi: 10.1136/neurintsurg-2019-014858. Epub 2019 Apr 11. PMID: 30975737.

[12] Raslan AM, Oztaskin M, Thompson EM, Dogan A, Petersen B, Nesbit G, Lee DS, Barnwell SL. Neuroform stent-assisted embolization of incidental anterior communicating artery aneurysms: long-term clinical and angiographic follow-up. *Neurosurgery.* 2011 Jul;69(1):27-37; discussion 37. doi: 10.1227/NEU.0b013e31820edbb6. PMID: 21311379.

[13] Castaño C, Terceño M, Remollo S, García-Sort MR, Domínguez C. Endovascular treatment of wide-neck intracranial bifurcation aneurysms with 'Y'-configuration, double Neuroform® stents-assisted coiling technique: Experience in a single center. *Interv Neuroradiol.* 2017 Aug;23(4):362-370. doi: 10.1177/1591019917708568. Epub 2017 Jun 6. PMID: 28587530; PMCID: PMC5684913.

[14] Samaniego EA, Mendez AA, Nguyen TN, Kalousek V, Guerrero WR, Dandapat S, Dabus G, Linfante I, Hassan AE, Drofa A, Kouznetsov E, Leedahl D, Hasan D, Maud A, Ortega-Gutierrez S. LVIS Jr Device for Y-Stent-Assisted Coil Embolization of Wide-Neck Intracranial Aneurysms: A Multicenter Experience. *Interv Neurol.* 2018 Apr;7(5):271-283. doi: 10.1159/000487545. Epub 2018 Apr 3. PMID: 29765397; PMCID: PMC5939862.

[15] Bhogal P, Brouwer PA, Yeo L, Svensson M, Söderman M. The Medina Embolic Device: Karolinska experience. *Interv Neuroradiol.* 2018 Feb;24(1):4-13. doi: 10.1177/1591019917733125. Epub 2017 Sep 28. PMID: 28956513; PMCID: PMC5772534.

[16] Aguilar Perez M, Bhogal P, Martinez Moreno R, Bäzner H, Ganslandt O, Henkes H. The Medina Embolic Device: early clinical experience from a single center. *J Neurointerv Surg.* 2017 Jan;9(1):77-

87. doi: 10.1136/neurintsurg-2016-012539. Epub 2016 Aug 2. PMID: 27484746; PMCID: PMC5264237.

[17] Cortez GM, Akture E, Monteiro A, Arthur AS, Peterson J, Dornbos D, Jabbour P, Gooch MR, Sweid A, Tjoumakaris SI, Delgado Almandoz JE, Kayan Y, Rai AT, Boo S, Fiorella D, Vachhani J, Foreman P, Cress M, Siddiqui AH, Waqas M, Aghaebrahim A, Sauvageau E, Hanel RA. Woven EndoBridge device for ruptured aneurysms: perioperative results of a US multicenter experience. *J Neurointerv Surg*. 2021 Nov;13(11):1012-1016. doi: 10.1136/neurintsurg-2020-017105. Epub 2021 Jan 22. PMID: 33483455.

[18] Srinivasan VM, Srivatsan A, Spiotta AM, Hendricks BK, Ducruet AF, Albuquerque FC, Puri A, Amans MR, Hetts SW, Cooke DL, Ogilvy CS, Thomas AJ, Enriquez-Marulanda A, Rai A, Boo S, Carlson AP, Crowley RW, Rangel-Castilla L, Lanzino G, Chen PR, Diaz O, Bohnstedt BN, O'Connor KP, Burkhardt JK, Johnson JN, Chen SR, Kan P. Early postmarket results with PulseRider for treatment of wide-necked intracranial aneurysms: a multicenter experience. *J Neurosurg*. 2019 Nov 8:1-10. doi: 10.3171/2019.5. JNS19313. Epub ahead of print. PMID: 31703202.

[19] Brzegowy P, Kucybała I, Krupa K, Łasocha B, Wilk A, Latacz P, Urbanik A, Popiela TJ. Angiographic and clinical results of anterior communicating artery aneurysm endovascular treatment. *Wideochir Inne Tech Maloinwazyjne*. 2019 Sep;14(3):451-460. doi: 10.5114/wiitm.2019.81406. Epub 2019 Jan 21. PMID: 31534577; PMCID: PMC6748064.

[20] Liu Y, Wang F, Fu X, Liu Y, Zhang G, Xu K. Clinical and angiographic outcomes following endovascular treatment of very small (3 mm or smaller) intracranial aneurysm: A single-center experience. *Medicine* (Baltimore). 2017 Sep; 96(37):e7475. doi: 10.1097/MD.0000000000007457. PMID: 28906352; PMCID: PMC5604621

[21] Suzuki S, Kurata A, Ohmomo T, Sagiuchi T, Niki J, Yamada M, Oka H, Fujii K, Kan S. Endovascular surgery for very small ruptured intracranial aneurysms. Technical note. *J Neurosurg*. 2006 Nov;105(5):777-80. doi: 10.3171/jns.2006.105.5.777. PMID: 17121145.

[22] International Study of Unruptured Intracranial Aneurysms investigators. Unruptured intracranial aneurysms: risk of rupture and risks of surgical intervention. *N Engl J Med* 1998;339:1725–33.

[23] Mira JM, Costa FA, Horta BL, Fabião OM. Risk of rupture in unruptured anterior communicating artery aneurysms: meta-analysis of natural history studies. *Surg Neurol*. 2006;66 Suppl 3:S12-9; discussion S19. doi: 10.1016/j.surneu.2006.06.025. PMID: 17081844.

[24] Bijlenga P, Ebeling C, Jaegersberg M, Summers P, Rogers A, Waterworth A, Iavindrasana J, Macho J, Pereira VM, Bukovics P, Vivas E, Sturkenboom MC, Wright J, Friedrich CM, Frangi A, Byrne J, Schaller K, Rufenacht D; @neurIST Investigators. Risk of rupture of small anterior communicating artery aneurysms is similar to posterior circulation aneurysms. *Stroke*. 2013 Nov;44(11):3018-26. doi: 10.1161/STROKEAHA.113.001667. Epub 2013 Jul 30. PMID: 23899912.

[25] Benndorf G, Wellnhofer E, Lanksch W, Felix R. Intraaneurysmal flow: evaluation with Doppler guidewires. *AJNR Am J Neuroradiol*. 1996 Aug;17(7):1333-7. PMID: 8871720; PMCID: PMC 8338536.

[26] Zhao B, Yang H, Zheng K, Li Z, Xiong Y, Tan X, Zhong M; AMPAS Study Group. Preoperative and postoperative predictors of long-term outcome after endovascular treatment of poor-grade aneurysmal subarachnoid hemorrhage. *J Neurosurg*. 2017 Jun;126(6):1764-1771. doi: 10.3171/2016.4.JNS152587. Epub 2016 Jul 1. PMID: 27367238.

Chapter 3

Posterior Communicating Artery Aneurysms

Ahmed Muthana[1,*]
Rania H. Al-taie[2,†]
Jaafer Abdul Wahid[3,‡]
Mustafa Ismail[1,§]
Zaid Aljuboori[4,#]
Norberto Andaluz[5,‖]
and Samer S. Hoz[6,|]

[1]University of Baghdad, College of Medicine, Baghdad, Iraq
[2]University of Mustansiriyah, College of Medicine, Baghdad, Iraq
[3]University of Al-Nahrain, College of Medicine, Baghdad, Iraq
[4]Department of Neurosurgery, Geisinger Commonwealth School of Medicine, Geisinger, PA, USA
[5]Department of Neurosurgery, University of Cincinnati College of Medicine, Cincinnati, OH, USA
[6]Department of Neurological Surgery, University of Pittsburgh Medical Center, University of Pittsburgh School of Medicine, Pittsburgh, PA, USA

Abstract

Posterior communicating artery (PcomA) aneurysms are the second most common intracranial aneurysm. They are classified according to the site of origin into "Junctional aneurysms," which could be either at the junction of the internal carotid artery (ICA) and PcomA or at the junction of PcomA and posterior cerebral artery (PCA), and "true PcomA aneurysms" that originate from PcomA itself.

The exact etiology of PcomA aneurysms is yet to be determined. However, some factors are closely related to their development and must be appraised in the evaluation

* Corresponding Author's Email: ahmed.m.najm@gmail.com.
† Corresponding Author's Email: raniahussain03@gmail.com.
‡ Corresponding Author's Email: Jafer.alkhafajy2000@ced.nahrainuniv.edu.iq.
§ Corresponding Author's Email: mustafalorance2233@gmail.com.
# Corresponding Author's Email: Zaljuboori1@geisinger.edu.
‖ Corresponding Author's Email: andalun@ucmail.uc.edu.
| Corresponding Author's Email: hozsamer2055@gmail.com.

In: Understanding and Managing Cerebral Aneurysms
Editor: Xianli Lv
ISBN: 979-8-89113-608-3

steps. The patient may present with subarachnoid hemorrhage (SAH), partial or complete oculomotor nerve palsy (OMNP), and non-traumatic subdural hematoma (SDH). Individual-based planning must be obtained for each patient to achieve the optimal outcome.

Several morphological parameters have been studied to upgrade the assessment of treatment plans like origin, size, neck, dome, and fetal PcomA. These parameters are carefully analyzed using CTA, MRA, and DSA to determine the management scheme. PcomA aneurysms can be treated by surgical or endovascular approach. Surgical clipping can be approached through a pterional or lateral supraciliary approach, while endovascular treatment includes direct coiling, stent-assisted coiling, and flow diverter methods. The recovery status after surgical or endovascular management depends on multiple factors, including the timeline between the diagnosis and treatment, the existence of SAH with the consequent brain injury, and the degree of OMNP. In general, the morbidity rate of surgically treated PcomA aneurysms is low compared to the other aneurysms in the circle of Willis.

All the stated facts will be discussed in this chapter for the purpose of establishing an accurate assessment of the aneurysm, its management, and the suitable measures for dealing with its possible complications.

Keywords: intracranial aneurysms, posterior communicating artery, anatomy, treatment

Key Points

- The neurosurgical anatomy of the posterior communicating artery.
- Posterior communicating artery aneurysm diagnosis and evaluation.
- The value of different diagnostic modalities.
- Decision-making in PcomA aneurysm management.
- Surgical and endovascular management measures.
- Recovery predictors and follow-up plan.

1.1. Posterior Communicating Artery Anatomy

In human anatomy, the posterior communicating artery (PcomA) is vital to brain circulation. It plays a paramount role in connecting the anterior and posterior circulation of the cerebrum, creating the indispensable feeding circle to the brain, the circle of Willis. Figure (1) provides a proposed important concept to establish good understanding of PcomA and its Aneurysms.

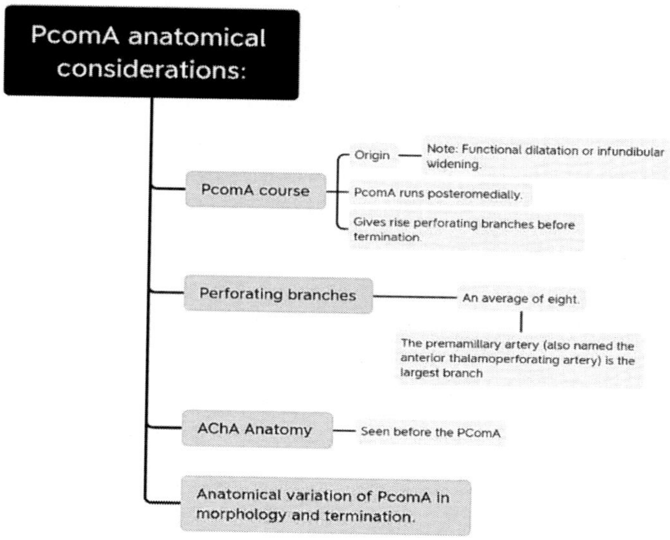

Figure 1. Anatomical considerations of PcomA artery: proposed points to consider while studying anatomy of PcomA. AchA: Anterior choroidal artery.

1.1.1. Course

PcomA is a small branch that originates from the internal carotid artery (ICA) out of its posterolateral wall in the interpeduncular fossa. This origin lies approximately 10 mm distal to the ophthalmic artery and immediately before the origin of the anterior choroidal artery (AChoA). Moreover, it represents a marker of the beginning of the last segment of ICA which is the communicating segment (C7) which eventually bifurcates into a middle cerebral artery (MCA) and anterior cerebral artery (ACA). From the origin, the PcomA runs posteromedially around 12 mm before ending in the posterior cerebral artery (PCA) and thus completing the circle of Willis by creating the main anastomosis between the carotid system and the vertebro-basilar system [1].

1.1.2. Termination

Termination of PcomA is divided into five different types [2]. See Figure 2.

1. *Type I termination*: This is the typical termination of PcomA in which the artery anastomoses with the PCA to divide it into P1 and P2 segments. It is the most found pattern of termination (90%).
2. *Type II termination*: Artery terminates by anastomosing directly with the basilar artery.
3. *Type III termination*: Artery terminates in the fenestration.
4. *Type IV termination:* Artery anastomoses with an extra loop present in the circle of Willis.
5. *Type V termination:* Artery does not anastomose with any artery and directly supply the posterior aspect of cerebrum.

1.1.3. Morphology

It is noteworthy that there are considerable variations in the anatomy of PcomA among the population. These variations have impacts on both surgical and endovascular management plans. The Morphological variations that are encountered in PcomA are aplasia, hypoplasia, fenestration, and fetal PcomA [3]. See Figure 3.

A meta-analysis found that 19% of the population have unilateral hypoplastic or aplastic

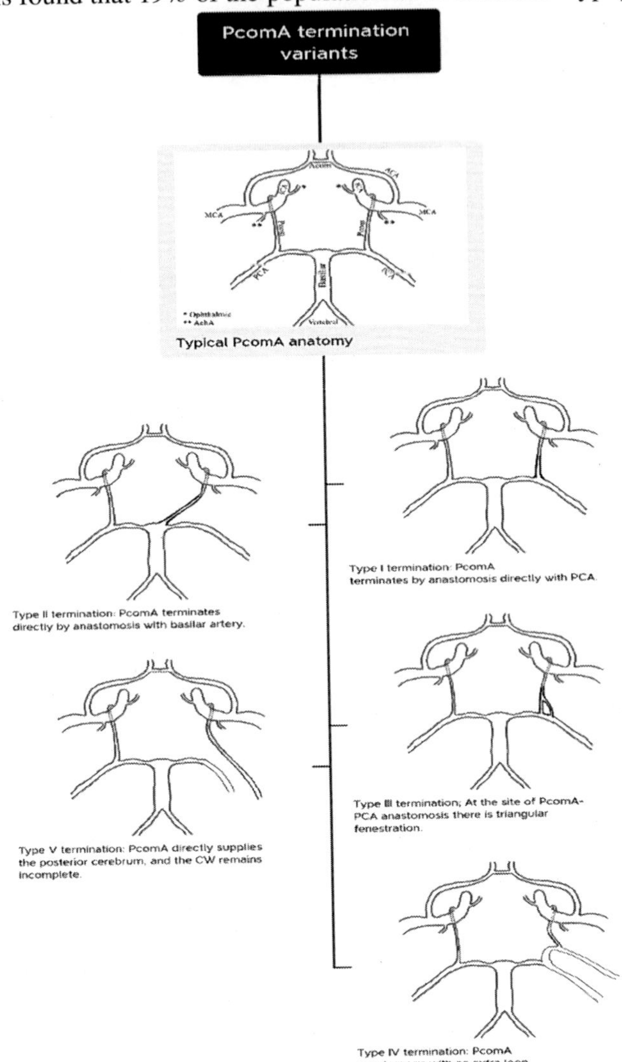

Figure 2. PcomA termination variants: Terminations of PcomA are divided into five different types. Typical PcomA anatomy demonstrated at the top of figure. ICA: Internal carotid artery, ACA: Anterior cerebral artery, MCA: Middle cerebral artery, PCA: Posterior cerebral artery, Acom: Anterior communicating artery.

PcomA and 22% of them have bilateral hypoplastic or aplastic PcomA [4]. Additionally, PcomA can be as large as the posterior cerebral artery (PCA) in a well-known anatomical variant called fetal PcomA. Embryologically, the PcomA continues as the PCA and is a major source of posterior circulation; if this configuration persists in the adult, it is termed a fetal PcomA. To be precise, fetal PcomA has the same caliber as the P2 segment of the PCA and it is associated with an atrophic P1 segment. Consequently, it becomes the primary supply to the PCA. The incidence of the unilateral fetal PcomA variant is 4-29% of patients while bilateral fetal PcomA variants is 1-9% of patients. Fetal PcomA has an important neurosurgical role as it is highly associated with specific types of PcomA aneurysm called "true PcomA aneurysm" (discussed later) [3].

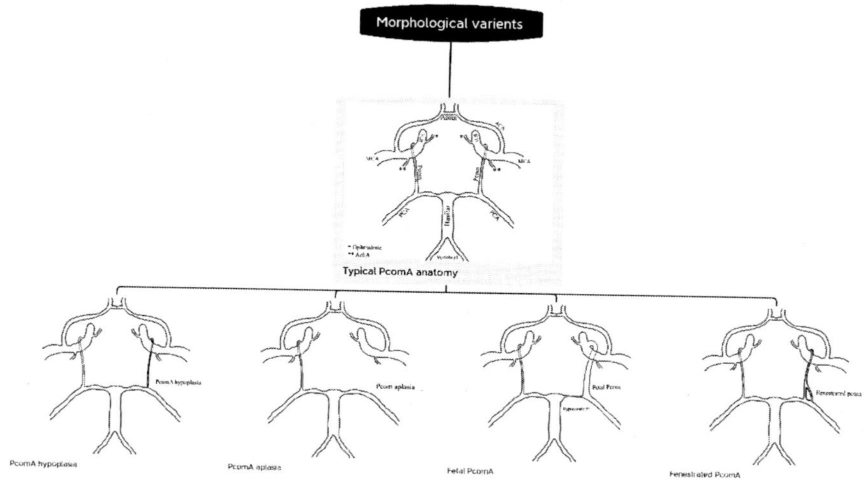

Figure 3. Morphological variant of PcomA: there are four variants highlighted starting from hypoplasia, aplasia, fetal and fenestrated PcomA. Typical PcomA anatomy demonstrated at the top of figure. ICA: Internal carotid artery, ACA: Anterior cerebral artery, MCA: Middle cerebral artery, PCA: Posterior cerebral artery, Acom: Anterior communicating artery.

1.1.4. Perforating Branches

PcomA gives rise to significant perforating branches that range in number from 4-14 branches. These branches include the one that supplies the optic chiasm, oculomotor nerve, ventral thalamus, mammillary body, tuber cinereum, hypothalamus, and internal capsule. The largest one of the perforating branches is the pre-mammillary artery that originates from the middle third of the PcomA [1].

1.1.5. Surrounding Structures

Two important structures related to the PcomA are clinically and surgically important, the oculomotor nerve (OMN) and the anterior choroidal artery (AChoA):

OMN passes inferomedial to the uncus and inferolateral to PcomA to enter the roof of the cavernous sinus through the oculomotor trigone. However, if the PcomA remains as the major origin of the PCA, i.e., fetal PcomA, it courses further laterally above or lateral to the oculomotor nerve. This close relationship greatly contributes to the third nerve palsy which is a common and important clinical manifestation of PcomA aneurysm [5].

AChoA has an important anatomical correlation to PcomA and must be preserved during surgical management of PcomA aneurysm. It originates from the lateral surface of the distal ICA and runs in a posterior course below the optic tract and above the PcomA. It passes through choroidal fissure until it joins the choroid plexus in the temporal horn and atrium of the lateral ventricle. During this course, AChoA provides arterial supply to the optic tract, cerebral peduncle, lateral geniculate body, uncus, and the temporal lobe. These branches supply essential intracranial structures including the optic radiations, globus pallidus, midbrain, thalamus, and retro-lenticular and posterior portions of the posterior limb of the internal capsule. Consequently, preservation of this artery is warranted during surgery of PcomA aneurysm
[1, 6].

1.2. Posterior Communicating Artery Aneurysm

Posterior communicating artery aneurysm represents the second most common intracranial aneurysm. It constitutes about 50% of ICA aneurysms and 25% of all intracranial aneurysms. It is classified according to the site into "Junctional PcomA aneurysm" and "True PcomA aneurysm." The first type is the most common type and mainly originates at the junction of ICA and PcomA (known as ICA-PcomA aneurysm) or less commonly at the junction of PcomA and PCA. The second type is less common and ranges from 4.6 to 13% of all PcomA aneurysms. There is another rare type of PcomA aneurysm that originates at the posterior wall of the ICA without incorporating the origin of the PcomA [7]. This anatomical configuration is important to be determined before planning of the treatment scheme in order to preserve the perforating branches and avoid the risk of complications.

The exact etiology of intracranial aneurysms including PcomA aneurysms is yet to be determined. However, there are some factors that are closely related to their development. These factors include genetic abnormalities, environmental elements, female gender, hemodynamic instability with the value of wall shear stress, atherosclerosis, and social habits like smoking [8]. Regarding the genetic diseases that attribute to the formation of PcomA aneurysms, polycystic kidney disease is associated with inability to encode vascular structural protein in 2 to 10% of patients which in turn leads to the formation of intracranial aneurysms. Additionally, in Marfan syndrome and Ehler-Danlos syndrome, there is arterial fragility due to genetic abnormalities in the formation of collagen fibers [9].

There are several lesions that can mimic the presentation of PcomA aneurysm that must be kept in mind while assessing the diagnosis. For instance, basilar tip aneurysms, cavernous sinus pathology, diabetic neuropathy, multiple sclerosis, myasthenia gravis, head trauma, and brainstem infarction syndromes such as internuclear ophthalmoplegia can all lead to third nerve palsy. Moreover, hypertension, head trauma and herpes simplex virus infection can cause intracranial hemorrhage in the temporal lobe or in the ventricular system. Lastly, on rare occasions, the PcomA aneurysm may present with sudden visual loss with suprasellar intracranial hemorrhage mimicking pituitary apoplexy [9, 10].

1.3. Patho-Anatomy And Morphological Parameters of PcomA Aneurysm

The establishment of well recognized morphological features and anatomical variants associated with PcomA aneurysms leads to upgrade assessment of treatment plan and explore potential markers for rupture risk. This chapter suggests steps and measures to be considered before approaching PcomA aneurysm. See Figure 4.

1.3.1. Origin

Traditionally, the most encountered variation is when the aneurysm originates at the junction of PcomA and ICA, which is termed in literature as "ICA-PcomA aneurysm" or "junctional aneurysm". These aneurysms arise from the ICA sidewall itself and the PcomA originates separately just distal to the neck of aneurysm. This would be the optimal configuration from the treatment point of view. However, in some cases, the PcomA origin is partially incorporated in the aneurysm, in which the PcomA arises at the aneurysm neck, or worse, from the aneurysm dome. In these configurations, the risk of accidental occlusion of the PcomA might be higher irrespective of the treatment method [7].

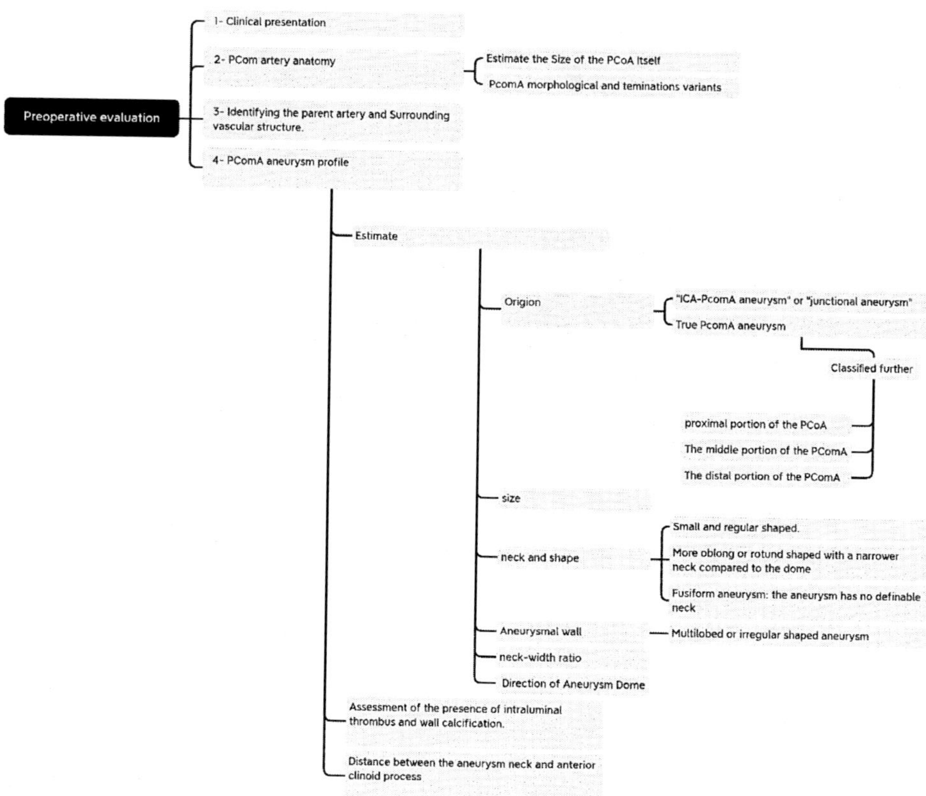

Figure 4. Preoperative evaluation of a patient with PcomA aneurysm: Suggested steps to be evaluated before approaching the aneurysm.

Another variation of PcomA aneurysms that have been recently introduced into the literature is the "true PcomA aneurysm". It was first described by Yoshida et al. in 1979. The neck of this aneurysm arises solely off the PcomA itself. Published literature suggests that these aneurysms constitute 0.1%–2.8% of all intracranial aneurysms and approximately 4.6%-13% of all PcomA aneurysms [11, 12]. These aneurysms can be classified further based on their location as in the proximal PcomA, which is the most common, followed by the middle portion and then the distal portion. These aneurysms are often associated with large or fetal PcomA and treatment of these aneurysms require significant diligence to maintain flow in the PcomA as these aneurysms are more prone to rupture than ICA–PcomA aneurysms [11].

1.3.2. Size

Aneurysm size has been strongly related to the risk of rupture. Ruptured aneurysms tend to be larger than unruptured ones [7]. Large or giant PcomA aneurysms do not occur often. This was also seen in Yasargil's PcomA series [13] which showed only a few large PcomA aneurysms (about 2% of all 173). It was postulated that PcomA aneurysms rarely grow large because of early symptoms of third nerve palsy. Another explanation could be that PcomA aneurysms have a greater rupture risk when compared to other locations of anterior circulation aneurysms, thus they do not reach a large size before rupturing.

1.3.3. Neck

The neck of a PcomA aneurysm is typically narrow in comparison to its dome, and a larger aneurysm neck diameter seems to be related to a higher incidence of rupture. A large portion of unruptured PcomA aneurysms were small and regular shaped, whereas most ruptured ones had a larger aspect ratio and bottleneck factor, meaning they often were more oblong or rotund shaped with a narrower neck compared to the dome. In addition to describing the shape of the aneurysm, the aspect ratio also seems to be related to the aneurysm rupture. However, there are limitations to using this parameter in everyday practice, as we do not know where the clinically significant threshold values lie [14].

1.3.4. Dome Orientation

The aneurysm dome orientation is considered an important factor for microsurgical clipping of these lesions. The most common classification system is the one that has been described by Yasargil [15]. This chapter provides a new classification of the dome orientation of junctional PcomA aneurysm (See Figure 5). In the coronal plane is classified as follows:

- *Inferior dome orientation:* it is the most common projection among PcomA aneurysms. From a sagittal point of view, most of these aneurysms are oriented posteriorly. A study has found that they account for about 50% of PcomA aneurysms. Inferolateral orientation is less common than the pure inferior one, with an incidence of about 20% among PcomA aneurysms. These aneurysms (i.e., inferolateral) often penetrate the Lilliquist membrane pointing into the interpeduncular fossa, especially when directed posteriorly. Additionally, they are also associated with third nerve palsy. Inferomedial orientation is seldom encountered. They are often sidewall aneurysms of the ICA and usually pointed posteriorly.

- *Lateral dome orientation*: pure lateral PcomA aneurysm was found in about 18% of patients with PcomA aneurysm. Sagittally, it is usually pointed anteriorly; here, the origin of the PcomA may be hidden by the aneurysm and the aneurysm may be adherent to the clinoid process, which requires careful dissection so that the fundus may be mobilized and the origin of the PcomA is visualized during application of a clip.
- *Superior dome orientation*: it is a less frequently encountered orientation and is usually directed laterally. Sagittally, posteriorly directed superolateral fundus points into the temporal lobe and is often associated with an intraparenchymal hemorrhage and/or hemorrhage into the temporal horn of the ventricle, anteriorly directed superolateral fundus in which the dome points into the sphenoid ridge. It is highly associated with the risk of rupture and hemorrhage of these aneurysms which may cause SDH. Superomedial orientation is rarely encountered among PcomA aneurysms.
- *Medial dome orientation*: pure medial PcomA aneurysm is rarely encountered as opposed to its lateral counterpart.

For the true PcomA aneurysms, the most encountered dome direction is the inferolateral projection. However, all options are possible, and the dome may project in a variety of directions (see Case 1; Figure 9) The superiorly projecting aneurysms in the middle portion of the PcomA may carry a risk of ischemic surgical complications, as it is the site of origin of the pre-mammillary artery, the largest perforating branch of PcomA. In addition, the oculomotor nerve usually runs below and lateral to the PcomA, meaning that inferolaterally projecting aneurysms may bear a risk of oculomotor nerve injury [7, 16].

1.3.5. PcomA Aneurysmal wall

The multilobed or irregularly shaped aneurysm has a predicted risk of rupture because it indicates a weak and thin wall. To be more specific, there is a 3.5-fold increase in rupture regarding multilobed aneurysms compared to non-multilobed aneurysms (80.3% vs. 22.8%) and a 3-fold increase in the association of irregular PcomA aneurysms compared to smooth surface aneurysms (69.0% vs. 21.8%) [17].

1.3.6. PcomA Fusiform Aneurysm

It is a rare type in which the aneurysm has no definable neck. It has a high morbidity rate owing to the fact that trapping is the only obliteration method and the preservation of perforating arteries is almost impossible. Some authors suggest conducting an extracranial-to-intracranial bypass before the trapping procedure of a fusiform aneurysm [18, 19].

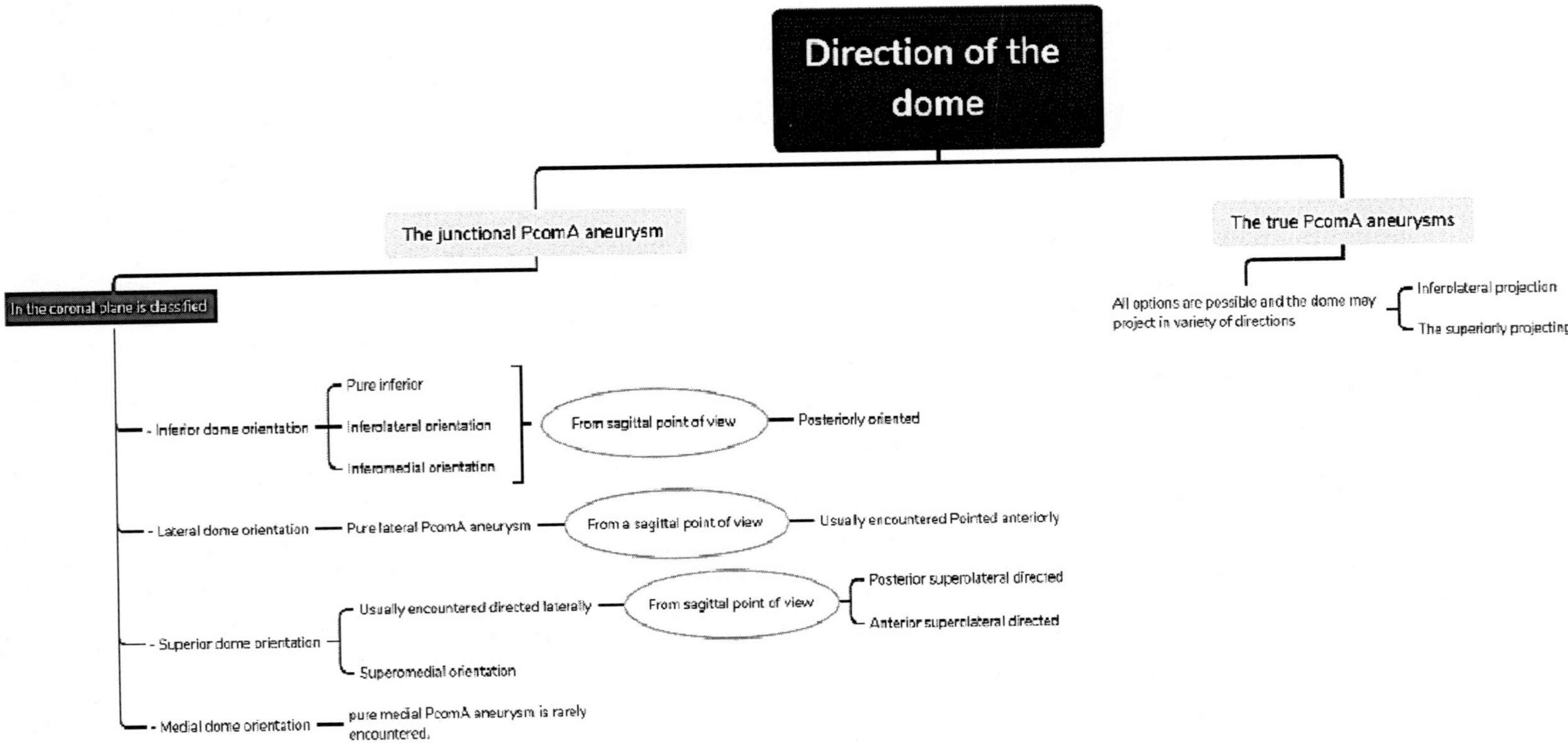

Figure 5. Direction of the dome: A proposed classification of the dome orientation considering the site whether junctional or true PcomA aneurysm. For Junctional aneurysm it is classified in the coronal plane as demonstrated in figure.

1.4. Clinical features of PcomA Aneurysm

Patients who have PcomA aneurysm may present acutely with aneurysmal rupture and its subarachnoid hemorrhage (SAH), or they can present with pathological subdural hematoma (SDH) or with partial or complete oculomotor nerve palsy (see Figure 6). The exact etiology of PcomA aneurysms is not clear, however, there are some factors that are closely related to their presence and must be observed in the evaluation steps. These risk factors include old age, female gender, smoking, alcohol, and hypertension [17, 20]. All of these must be considered in patients who present with signs and symptoms of non-traumatic intracranial hemorrhage.

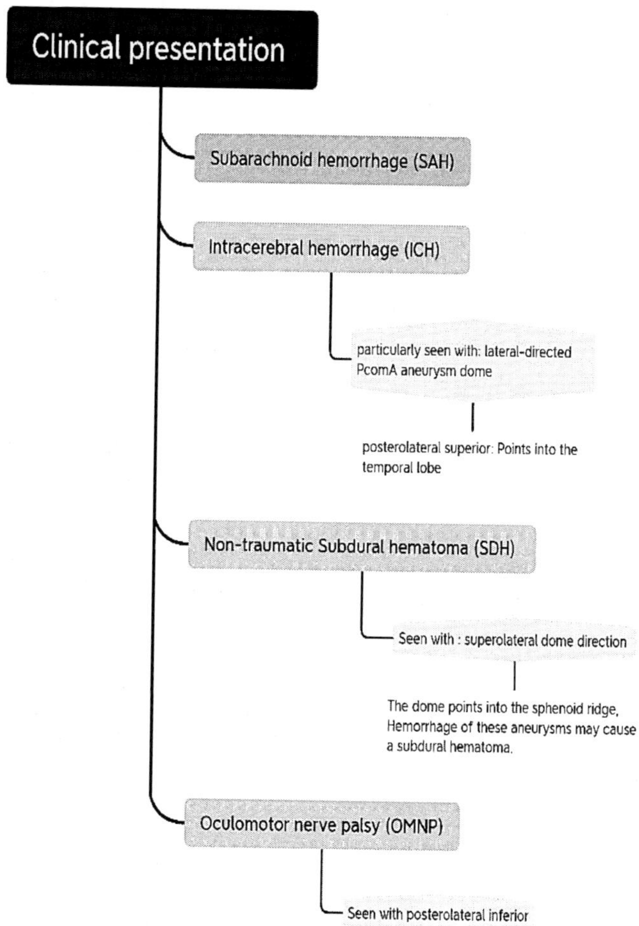

Figure 6. Clinical features of PcomA aneurysm: Patients who have PcomA aneurysm may presented with features of subarachnoid hemorrhage (SAH), subdural hematoma (SDH), intracerebral hemorrhage (ICH) or with partial or complete oculomotor nerve palsy.

1.4.1. Ruptured PcomA aneurysm

The rupture of a PcomA aneurysm is associated with significant morbidity and mortality hence the risk of rupture must be carefully calculated in the management steps. The prevalence of ruptured PcomA aneurysm is high in smaller aneurysms, therefore, small size is not necessarily an indication of a low rupture risk. Other anatomical parameters that indicate aneurysmal rupture are the type of PcomA aneurysms in which true PcomA aneurysms are more prone to rupture than junctional PcomA aneurysms of the same size [11]. Furthermore, an irregular, multilobed PcomA aneurysm with larger height/width ratios and larger flow angles was associated with an increased risk of rupture, whereas perpendicular height was inversely associated with rupture [17]. The rate of PcomA aneurysm rupture resembles that of anterior circulation aneurysms rather than posterior circulation aneurysms [7].

1.4.2. Subarachnoid Hemorrhage (SAH)

As in most intracranial aneurysms, patients with PcomA aneurysm typically present with SAH. The pattern of hemorrhage is mostly involving the basal cistern, or it may be isolated in the temporal lobe, the temporal horn of the lateral ventricle or sylvian fissure, mimicking a middle cerebral artery (MCA) aneurysm [7].

1.4.3. Intracerebral Hemorrhage (ICH)

Intracerebral hemorrhage (ICH) confers additional morbidity to aneurysm rupture, particularly for lateral directed PcomA aneurysms where the hemorrhage is typically in the temporal lobe. The projections of these aneurysms into the temporal lobe make them much more likely to cause ICH upon rupture. Interestingly, smaller volumes, larger maximum height, and smaller aneurysm angles were also significantly associated with ICH. Smaller volume and larger aneurysm maximum height imply a more elongated aneurysm which would be more likely to project into the temporal lobe and result in an ICH. The association of lack of hypertension with ICH may be because hypertension increases rupture risk at a smaller size, that is, prior to the aneurysm is large enough to project into the temporal lobe [14].

1.4.4. Subdural Hematoma (SDH)

Non-traumatic subdural hematoma (SDH) is an infrequent presentation that may be encountered in a PcomA aneurysm. Only 1.3-7.9% of intracranial aneurysms may present with an SDH, and it is important to mention that PcomA aneurysm is responsible for the hemorrhage in 43% of these cases [7].

1.4.5. Rebleeding

The risk of rebleeding in a ruptured PcomA aneurysm must be evaluated in an individual-based manner. There is a 50% risk of re-rupture within the initial six months followed by 3.5% thenceforth. There is an association between hypertension and re-bleeding because blood pressure is more easily transmitted to the dome of aneurysms of primary vessels (i.e., ICA) than secondary vessels (I.e., ACA) [7].

1.4.6. Oculomotor Nerve Palsy (OMNP)

Oculomotor nerve palsy (OMNP) is a relatively common presenting sign of a PcomA aneurysm. In fact, almost 30% of PcomA aneurysms patients have OMNP on presentation and about 80% of aneurysms with OMNP were found to be PcomA aneurysms [7].

The possible mechanisms of OMNP secondary to intracranial aneurysm are [21, 24]:

1. Direct compression of the oculomotor nerve by an aneurysmal mass.
2. The pulsating effect of the aneurysm
3. The irritation of the nerve by the SAH.
4. Combination of all the above-mentioned mechanisms.

There are two manifestations of OMNP, either complete (70%) or partial (30%) OMNP. The usual sequence of the lesion typically involves pupillary dilation followed by ptosis and then an extra-ocular paralysis/paresis. However, up to 17% of patients were present with a pupil sparing OMNP [7]. This condition gives suspicion of surgical rather than medical cause of OMNP. Isolated OMNP (without SAH) is usually secondary to some conformational change in the aneurysmal dome, and it can indicate an impending rupture. The time from pupillary dilation of OMNP to aneurysmal rupture varies from a few days to many months (an average of 29 days) [7, 25].

1.5. Investigation of PcomA Aneurysm and Diagnostic Modalities

The admission non-contrast computed tomography (CT) scan will overlook a significant number of intracranial aneurysms, however, it gives clues about the underlying pathology through the presence of intracranial hemorrhage or cerebral edema. Magnetic resonance angiography (MRA) and Computed tomography angiography (CTA) are considered to be noninvasive imaging tools. Digital subtraction angiography (DSA) is a more invasive technique that gives a three-dimensional reconstruction of the aneurysm. The main aspects that must be focused on in the evaluation of imaging include the aneurysm profile like size, neck-width ratio, surrounding vascular structure, and identifying the parent artery. Moreover, an accurate assessment of the presence of intraluminal thrombus and wall calcification should also be addressed using these imaging techniques. All of which leads to excellent implantation of the management plan.

1.5.1. CTA

It represents the preferable initial study of PcomA aneurysm since it is a noninvasive imaging tool and due to its easy accessibility and rapid acquisition time (see Case 3; Figure 12). This fact made CTA more practical for emergency evaluation of intracranial aneurysms. The interpretation of noninvasive neurovascular imaging is operator dependent, and it requires a well-experienced neuroradiologist.

It has a 67% sensitivity and 100% specificity level. It is noteworthy that positive CTA results control the management strategy which can be either Intra-arterial digital subtraction angiography (IA-DSA) and microsurgical treatment of the PcomA aneurysm or IA-DSA and endovascular treatment [26].

One of the limitations of CTA is the difficulty in identifying aneurysms smaller than 3 mm because it has a low spatial resolution in contrast to DSA, and in case of technical issues, the CTA cannot be repeated immediately [27, 28].

1.5.2. MRA

It is a noninvasive diagnostic modality that has 92% sensitivity and 100% specificity with no radiation risks. The long examination time, low spatial resolution compared to DSA, and high price made this modality only useful as a screening tool for high-risk populations and not routinely used for aneurysm patients [29, 30].

1.5.3. DSA

It is the gold standard technique in diagnosing intracranial aneurysms (see Case 2; Figure 11), however, it is invasive and operator dependent with relatively high complication incidents (4%). Sometimes the images fail to assess crucial morphological parameters of PcomA aneurysms including neck, vessels originating from the sac, intraluminal thrombus, and wall calcifications. Recent studies demonstrated that these obstacles can be conquered using the rotational angiographic technique [31, 32].

1.5.4. Brain Endoscopy

Virtual endoscopic imaging study is valuable in providing information about aneurysms lying in close proximity to bony structures and it has a further advantage in assessing the depth and intraluminal pathology [19, 33].

1.6. Management of PcomA

Management of PcomA aneurysm should be handled with caution. No two cases are the same and the treatment should be tailored to the individual. See Figure 5.

1.6.1. Decision-Making

Most PcomA aneurysms in developed countries occur as accidental discoveries attributed to the widespread availability and usage of noninvasive imaging. As a result, the question of when to observe becomes more critical. The clinical presentation of the patient, the skill of the surgeon, and available resources have the most critical role in the decision. An analysis of the available data on Patients' demographics such as advanced age, smoking, and comorbidities should be considered and the patient's decision to not treat is another factor to appraise. This chapter provides a decision-making algorithm (see Figure 7) for managing PcomA modified from Rangel-Castilla et al. Decision Making in Neurovascular Disease [9].

In patients with single, asymptomatic, small (3-4mm) PcomA aneurysms, CTA or MRA observation follow-up is suggested. However, in patients with symptomatic, multiple, large (>7mm), or growing aneurysms, or family or personal history of aneurysmal SAH, more consideration should be given to treatment than those without [9].

Careful analysis of the patient's history and investigations should be done to differentiate between ruptured and unruptured PcomA aneurysms, as management and interference will differ accordingly (see Case 2; Figure 10). For patients with unruptured PcomA aneurysm, an endovascular approach such as stent-assisted coiling is the management of choice provided the anatomy and morphology of the aneurysm and surrounding vasculatures are manageable by endovascular approach. Otherwise, if the aneurysm is unfavorable for coiling and associated with OMNP or fetal PcomA, then surgical clipping is the treatment of choice [9].

On the other hand, if a PcomA aneurysm rupture has resulted in a large ICH requiring urgent evacuation, craniotomy, and microsurgical clipping should be performed with consideration given to craniectomy, although some may recommend and have reported endovascular management followed by craniotomy and evacuation or a minimally invasive approach to evacuation. In contrast, if no ICH was present after rupture, the patient could be treated by surgical clipping or endovascular means provided the morphology of the aneurysm and anatomy of the approach vessels are amenable to an endovascular approach [9].

1.6.2. Surgical Management of PcomA Aneurysm

PcomA aneurysm surgery is among the most challenging surgeries. Each case should be thoroughly investigated and assessed, beginning with the patient's general condition and on to the detailed anatomy of the aneurysm and surrounding vasculature. As a result, the surgical strategy should be personalized to the individual, and all surgical and post-operative complications should be addressed and discussed with the patient.

Depending on the anatomy of each case, PcomA aneurysm cases can range from simple to exceedingly complicated. Microsurgical clipping has long been the treatment of choice and is a well-described approach. It has both risks and advantages, but in certain cases, particularly in ruptured aneurysms, the benefits outweigh the risks. Over the last few decades, the risk of surgery for ruptured cerebral aneurysms has been gradually reduced. The introduction of the operating microscope, the development of better microsurgical techniques and instruments, advances in anesthetic and intensive care management, improved diagnostic facilities, and the development of vascular neurosurgery as a subspecialty have all contributed to these risk reductions. Furthermore, microsurgical clipping results have improved over the last decade as a result of the centralization of open vascular cases to specialist centers and the introduction of electrophysiologic monitoring and indocyanine green video angiography [34, 36].

Suggested steps and measures of PcomA aneurysm surgery will be discussed below. See Figure 8.

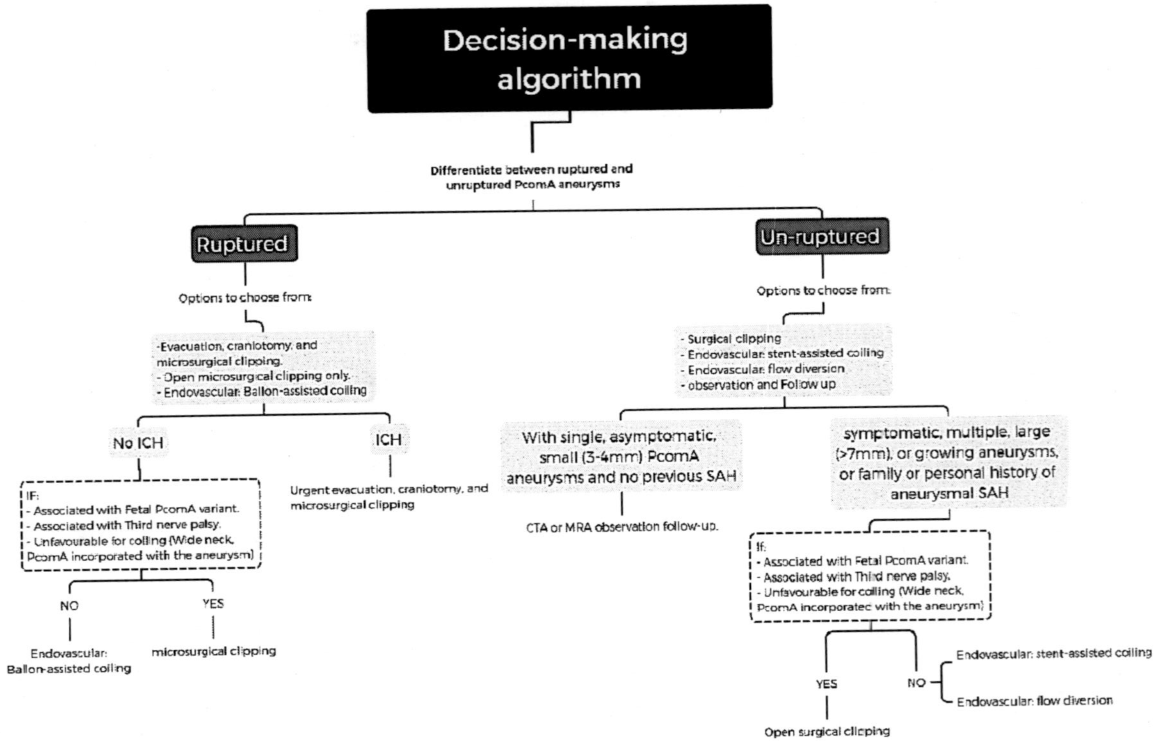

Figure 7. Decision-making algorithm: a proposed algorithm to be considered when managing PcomA. Modified from Rangel-Castilla et al. Decision Making in Neurovascular Disease [9].

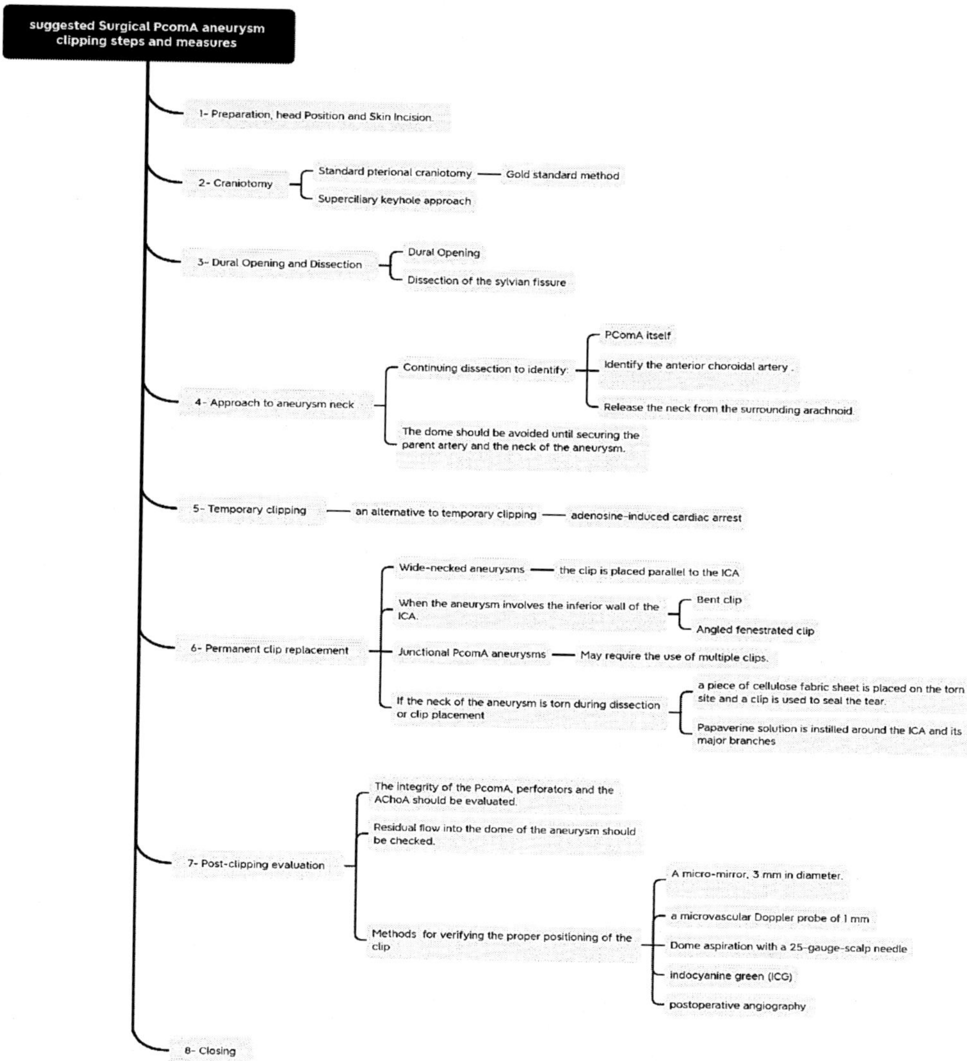

Figure 8. Surgical PcomA aneurysm clipping surgery: suggested steps and measures during surgery.

1.6.2.1. Preparation and Head Positioning

Special care should be taken during the patient's transit to the operating room, and arterial hypertension should be avoided both before and during anesthetic induction. The patient is positioned in a supine position after general anesthesia is administered, with the head fixed in a three-pin clamp. To minimize considerable blood pressure elevation, local anesthetic injection into the scalp pin sites prior to the connection of the device to the skull may attenuate the pain response. After shaving the hair and applying an anti-aseptic technique, the head is covered to disclose only enough of the scalp for the incision to be placed. Scalp electrodes are inserted for the intraoperative recording of somatosensory-evoked potentials during the temporary artery occlusion [34].

1.6.2.2. Craniotomy

1.6.2.2.1. Standard Pterional Craniotomy

The gold standard method has been considered a standard pterional craniotomy because it allows for a wide range of access for the clip-applying forceps [34]. The actions of this this approach are undertaken in this sequence:

1. The neck is extended and rotated to the opposite side by roughly 30 degrees.
2. Following the initial scalp incision, the temporalis muscle is incised, and both skin and muscle are reflected as a single layer, folded over a sponge, and fixed with 3 to 4 scalp hooks.
3. On each side of the sphenoid wing, two burr holes are drilled and joined with a high-speed pneumatic drill.
4. Reflecting the bone flap.
5. To reduce epidural hemorrhage and prevent blood from leaking into the field, the cut edge of the dura is everted and pulled over a sponge with traction sutures.
6. The operating microscope is taken into the field.
7. To achieve a clear view along the cranial base, the sphenoid ridge is drilled down to the superior orbital fissure, and the orbital roof and subtemporal bone are flattened.

1.6.2.3. Superciliary Keyhole Approach

Advantages over standard pterional craniotomy include smaller incision without scalp shaving, smaller craniotomy which reduces the risk of a postoperative epidural hemorrhage, decreased trauma to the body including the temporalis muscle, reduced risk of infection in the operative field, shorter operative time, decreased blood loss, less postoperative pain, and a faster recovery [10].

The sequence of steps in this approach comprises the following:

1. The patient in supine postion, with the head turned 20° contralaterally and slightly extended.
2. A 3.5 cm in length superciliary incision is made from the mid-pupillary line to behind the frontal process of the zygomatic bone.
3. After establishing a single frontobasal lateral bur hole posterior to the temporal line, a small (2 × 2.5 cm) craniotomy is conducted above the orbital ridge with a high-speed drill with a footplate attachment.
4. The frontal floor prominences and a portion of the lesser sphenoid wing are flattened, while the inner border of the craniotomy above the orbital rim is drilled and beveled.

1.6.2.4. Subtemporal Approach

This technique allows for good visualization of the distal portion of the PcomA. Therefore, it is useful for distal true PcomA aneurysm. It has been successfully used for clipping a giant true PcomA aneurysm by reconstructing the PcomA and proximal PCA (18). However, it poses the risk of temporal lobe contusion and venous injury resulting from excessive brain retraction. Additionally, if the aneurysmal neck is located higher than usual, it is difficult to access the aneurysm [16].

1.6.2.5. Anterior Subtemporal Approach

This approach has been described for posteriorly projecting ICA-PcomA aneurysms [37]. Thereafter it was used as an approach to a true PcomA aneurysm in the distal portion [38]. In this approach, the aneurysm can be observed from the more lateral side in comparison with the pterional approach. However, using this method the aneurysms are occasionally hidden under the tentorial edge because of an upward viewing angle from the anterior temporal base [16].

1.6.2.6. Anterior Temporal Approach

This approach enables posterior retraction of the temporal lobe by dissection of the superficial Sylvian vein and the anterior temporal artery from the temporal lobe, and provides the middle surgical corridor of the pterional approach and subtemporal approach [39]. A wider retrocarotid space obtained with this approach provides better visualization of true PcomA aneurysms, particularly in the middle and distal portions. Additional orbitozygomatic osteotomy may allow clipping of high-position true PcomA aneurysms situated higher than 10 mm from the interclinoid line [16, 40].

1.6.2.7. Brain Relaxation

The role of brain relaxation in the fast and atraumatic exposure of PcomA aneurysms in the carotid cistern is significant [34]. It enables easier Transylvanian dissection and the use of retractors to support the loose brain rather than pull the tight brain.

1.6.2.7.1. Method

1. A bolus of mannitol (1 gm/kg body weight) is administered intravenously during the craniotomy. Mannitol may be unneeded in elderly patients, particularly if cortical atrophy is verified on a CT scan.
2. If the preoperative CT indicates excess CSF in the basal cisterns without concomitant hydrocephalus, opening the cisterns can provide appropriate cerebral relaxation.
3. If the preoperative CT scan reveals dilated ventricles, the ipsilateral frontal horn of the lateral ventricle is pierced at Paine's site.
4. If the preoperative CT reveals no ventricular dilatation or CSF gap in the basal cisterns, the CSF is extracted by the pre-inserted spinal catheter.

1.6.2.8. Dissection of the Sylvian Fissure

Because the aneurysm and its associated cerebral arteries are positioned in the carotid cistern, the Sylvian fissure must be dissected. When the brain is totally relaxed and the fissure is filled with CSF or blood, the incision of the arachnoid membrane connecting the fissure is simple and atraumatic. One or more veins bridging the Sylvian fissure may be met and sacrificed if needed. Deep cerebral veins, such as the deep middle cerebral vein, the Rosenthal vein, and the orbital lobe deep vein in the fissure, should be protected to prevent venous infarction. As the fissure is split, the frontal lobe may be gradually mobilized and retracted with the sucker. The dissection is then guided to the chiasmatic cistern that lies beneath the optic nerve. To liberate the frontal and temporal lobes, the bands should be dissected. The Sylvian fissure is opened wide, exposing the M1 and M2 regions of the MCA as well as the carotid bifurcation. Following this surgery, the whole length of the supraclinoid ICA and aneurysm can be revealed with minimum brain retraction. Because the dome of the aneurysm may be attached to the uncus, it may be preferable to retract the temporal lobe only after obtaining proximal arterial control [34].

1.6.2.9. Anterior Clinoidectomy

Anterior clinoidectomy is seldom necessary for PcomA aneurysm clipping [7]. Park et colleagues discovered that only 6 of 96 patients with PcomA aneurysms required clinoidectomy during surgery [41]. He discovered three anatomical characteristics when looking for indicators of possible clinoidectomy:

1. Using CTA measuring the distance between the tip of the anterior clinoid process and the aneurysm's proximal neck. Anterior clinoidectomy is seldom necessary if the gap is larger than 5.8 mm, while it is usually required if the distance is smaller than 4.4 mm.
2. DSA's other anatomical measures are more difficult to measure.
3. The communicating segment of the ICA takes a more lateral path.

1.6.2.10. Approach to the PcomA Aneurysm Neck

Approaching and identifying PcomA aneurysmal necks are considered to be one of the most critical surgical steps, thus, accurate preoperative evaluation of the anatomical characteristics of the aneurysm and whether it is true or junctional aneurysm must be obtained. Each variant has its own approach plan, drawback situations and preventable complications, therefore careful description of them will be discussed as follows.

1.6.2.11. Approach to Junctional PcomA Aneurysm

PcomA aneurysms often arise on the convex side of the ICA and are commonly accompanied with arteriosclerotic changes on the opposite concave side of the ICA. These results aid in identifying aneurysms before they rupture. The proximal component of the PcomA should not be mistaken for an aneurysm. The distal PcomA is commonly identified in the optico-carotid triangle, which is created by the ICA, the optic nerve, and the ACA’s A1 segment. For the fetal type PcomA, because the artery is frequently concealed beneath the ICA or the aneurysm, locating it prior to clip implantation may be difficult. The Anterior choroidal artery can be detected when the dissection progresses toward the carotid bifurcation, and the distal neck of the aneurysm is typically located just proximal to the artery [34].

1.6.2.12. Approach to true PcomA Aneurysm

In order to offer proximal vascular control, the proximal ICA should be identified and dissected free of arachnoid. The ICA is then traced posteriorly to locate the origin of the PcomA, which is generally located on the ICA's posterolateral wall. In contrast to junctional PcomA aneurysms, which may have an apparent aneurysm dome here, the true PcomA aneurysms most commonly occur in what is typically an intra-operative blind spot 2-3 mm posterior to the PcomA's origin at the ICA. To see the neck of the aneurysm, the PcomA should be traced posteriorly into the retro-carotid region. If the aneurysm is located in the proximal region of PcomA and is medially projecting, enlarge the optico-carotid space required [34].

1.6.2.13. Temporary Clipping

When further dissection of the aneurysm's neck seems to be risky, temporary clips may be applied. The anesthesiologist is asked to raise systolic blood pressure to 140-150 mm Hg to protect the brain during a regional circulatory arrest [34].

Temporary clips are placed in the following order: proximal ICA, PcomA, and distal ICA or A1 segment. This is because the fundus may get significant retrograde inflows from a huge PcomA. The somatosensory-evoked potentials are constantly monitored. If the amplitude of evoked potentials decreases, the surgeon is required to open the temporary clips intermittently [34]. As an alternative to temporary clipping, adenosine-induced cardiac arrest can be utilized to temporarily relieve pressure within the aneurysm while a permanent clip is applied [7, 42].

1.6.2.14. Permanent Clip Placement

Once the aneurysm's neck has been identified, it is essential to visualize the surrounding neurovascular systems prior to clip placement. Sharp dissection is used to create planes that separate the aneurysm from the PcomA and AChoA. To improve visualization of the aneurysm, the PcomA should be dissected away from the posterior clinoid if required. It may also be essential to drill a portion of the posterior clinoid to further see the aneurysm's neck [7].

The clip is placed and progressively closed over the neck after space is produced proximal and distal to the aneurysm neck. When the proximal PcomA is hidden behind or under the aneurysm, or when it shares a common neck with the aneurysm, the clip may occlude it. To avoid "dog ear" remnants or ICA stenosis in wide-necked aneurysms, the clip is positioned parallel to the ICA. When using a long clip, care should be taken not to injure the oculomotor nerve. When the aneurysm involves the inferior wall of the ICA, either a bent clip with the blade tips pointing beneath the ICA or an angled fenestrated clip is suitable for full neck obliteration. Because the neck of junctional PcomA aneurysms includes both the ICA and the PcomA, complete aneurysm occlusion may be challenging and may necessitate the application of multiple clips. However, extreme caution should be taken to keep ICA branches away from the clip blades. If the aneurysm's neck is torn during dissection or clip insertion, a piece of cellulose fabric sheet is put over the tear and a clip is used to seal it. After removing the temporary clips, a papaverine solution is infused around the ICA and its main branches to alleviate possible vasospasm produced by manipulation [7, 34].

1.6.2.15. Post-Clipping Evaluation

After successfully clipping the aneurysm, re-evaluation of the PcomA, perforators, and AChoA should be done to ensure that there is no residual flow into the dome of the aneurysm. Several methods for evaluating appropriate clip location have been developed, and if inadequate neck occlusion is discovered, the clip is readjusted after a temporary clip is placed [34]. These techniques are as follows:

1. A micro-mirror: A 3 mm diameter micro-mirror is used to observe the undersurface of the aneurysm neck following clip application to detect any residual aneurysm neck proximal to the clip and to inspect the perforators to ensure they are not trapped in the clip.
2. Microvascular Doppler probe: To confirm the patency of the ICA, PcomA, AChoA, and main perforators, a 1 mm microvascular Doppler probe may use.

3. Aspiration of the clipped aneurysm: To ensure complete clipping, the fundus of the aneurysm distal to the clip is aspirated with a 25-gauge scalp needle linked to a low-power suction line.
4. Postoperative angiography is performed in selected cases of complex or giant aneurysms.

1.6.3. Endovascular Treatment Modalities of PcomA Aneurysm

Endovascular management of PcomA aneurysms is considered to be relatively uncomplicated and technically feasible in most patients. The reasons for the stated fact are the proximal location of PcomA, clear angiographic view of the aneurysm's anatomical parameters compared to MCA and anterior communicating artery aneurysms, and finally the relatively easy access of microcatheter to these aneurysms by using multiple strategies. Therefore, detailed description of the endovascular therapeutic modalities will be discussed as follows:

1.6.3.1. Endovascular Coiling

Endovascular coiling has been increasingly utilized in patients with ruptured and unruptured cerebral aneurysms since 1995. Without the necessity for a craniotomy, this approach allows for the closure of cerebral aneurysms and minimizes the risk of subsequent rupture. This is especially true for PcomA aneurysms due to their close proximity to a first-order intracranial artery. Angiography views of the aneurysm's neck and parent arteries are easier to get in PcomA aneurysms than in other aneurysms. Furthermore, microcatheter access to PcomA aneurysms is often considerably easier than access to paraclinoid ICA aneurysms. The fundus of a PcomA aneurysm is usually parallel to the communicating section of the ICA, but microcatheter access to a paraclinoid aneurysm frequently necessitates a second turn immediately after the carotid siphon. For these reasons, the coiling of PcomA aneurysms tends to be relatively uncomplicated compared to aneurysms located in other parts of the anterior circulation [7, 35].

1.6.3.1.1. Procedure of Aneurysm Coiling

The operation is best performed under general anesthesia. However, if the patients are healthy enough to cooperate, it can be done under local anesthetic in some cases. In nearly all cases, the femoral artery is utilized, while a common carotid artery can be used if the carotid artery cannot be catheterized from the groin due to tortuous proximal arteries. Patients are anticoagulated with intravenous bolus doses of heparin to lower the risk of thrombosis during and after coil insertion [43].

The aneurysms were catheterized using a specially adapted variable stiffness microcatheter (Tracker, Target Therapeutics) inserted through a larger catheter and filled with electrolytically separated platinum coils (Guglielmi detachable coils, Target Therapeutics). The aneurysms are packed so that as much of their lumen occluded while preserving the patency of the parent artery and the PcomA to be remained open [43].

1.6.3.1.2. Limitation of Endovascular Coiling

The main disadvantage of endovascular embolization is the high risk of recurrence [7]. It has been found that PcomA aneurysms are more prone to recanalization after coil embolization, with a 30% greater rate than other aneurysms [44]. Aneurysm size, treatment during the acute phase of rupture, insufficient initial occlusion, and duration of follow-up were all linked with recurrence. Despite the significant recurrence risk, the possibility of rebleeding is rather low. An incomplete initial embolization is the major risk factor for re-hemorrhage. The risk of re-hemorrhage increased from 1.1% in a completely occluded aneurysm to 17.6% in a partially treated aneurysm having untreated residual dome filling [7].

1.6.3.2. Stent-Assisted Coil Embolization

In recent years, the benefit of enhancing coil embolization with stent utilization has been recognized, and it is now established as a valuable and successful way of therapy [45, 48]. The primary function of the stents is to keep the coil from protruding into the parent artery. When effective occlusion fails, it may be used to stabilize protruded coils or to anticipate the flow-diversion effect of the stent in certain aneurysms [46].

Depending on aneurysm configuration and arterial vasculature details, four approaches for stent placement in ICA-PcomA aneurysms have been developed [46, 49].

1. *ICA stenting:* If the aneurysm neck incorporates the distal ICA or the coil protrudes into the distal ICA, the stent should be placed from the distal ICA to the ICA terminus, covering the distal neck of the aneurysm. When the protection of the PcomA by a stent inserted through the ICA is required or when the ICA is of a large caliber, the open cell stents may be of benefit.
2. *ICA-PcomA stenting*: If the aneurysm neck mostly incorporates the PcomA or the coil protrudes into the PcomA, stent placement from the distal ICA to the PcomA preserves PcomA patency. Given that the caliber of the PcomA is sufficient for stent insertion (dominant or fetal type) and the PcomA originates from the distal ICA at an obtuse angle.
3. *PcomA stenting*: If the PcomA requires protection and arises at an acute angle from the ICA or the aneurysm neck, the stent is placed exclusively through the PcomA, with the proximal portion of the stent aligned with the aneurysm neck. Placement from the ICA to the PcomA at an acute-angled origin may cause stent kinking or narrowing ("ovalization"), although malposition or delayed stent migration are risks if only the PcomA is used.
4. *Retrograde stenting*: If the aneurysm neck incorporates both the ICA and the PcomA, and the PcomA originates from the ICA at an acute angle, retrograde stent insertion (through the vertebral artery) may be considered, assuming that the ipsilateral P1 arterial is sufficient to accommodate a microcatheter for stent delivery.

Stent placement may be limited to wide-neck PcomA aneurysms, particularly when the PcomA originates from the ICA or from the aneurysm neck at an acute angle. Because of stent-induced complications such as procedural or delayed thromboembolic infarction and in-stent stenosis, stent protection is not usually suggested as a first-line therapeutic strategy in wide-neck PcomA aneurysms [46].

1.6.3.3. Flow Diversion

Flow diverter devices, such as the SILK stent (Balt Extrusion, Montmorency, France) and the Pipeline Embolization Device (PED) (eV3, Irvine, CA), have emerged as a novel method of interventional treatment and represent a promising new generation of low porosity brain stents with a different mode of action [21]. Flow diversion provides an alternative therapeutic option for complex and large/giant PcomA aneurysms in which endovascular coiling has low rates of occlusion [50, 51]. Furthermore, the presence of an incorporated artery complicates the coiling of the aneurysm, and flow diversion approach provides a solution for certain aneurysms [52].

In contrast to endovascular coiling, which is based on packing the aneurysmal sac, aneurysm occlusion via flow diversion is explained by two mechanisms [50]. First by the effect of flow diversion in inhibiting blood in and outflow through the aneurysm, and second by the reinforcement and repair of the parent artery wall using the stent mesh as a scaffold for intimal generation (scaffolding effect). The interruption of the aneurysm inflow jet significantly reduces shear stresses on the aneurysm fundus, with progressive thrombosis of the aneurysm over time; shrinkage of the aneurysm occurred during healing after the inflammatory response, with the reconstruction of the parent artery lumen while preserving the perforators and side branches. The need for dual antiplatelet therapy during the procedure of flow diversion significantly limits its application, since it is generally contraindicated in acutely ruptured aneurysm [50].

1.6.4. Surgery vs. Endovascular Management of PcomA Aneurysms

There is no significant difference in mortality and morbidity between coiling and clipping patients. Because aneurysms in this location are quite often easier to treat than aneurysms in other locations, the complications of PcomA aneurysms are likely to be substantially lower. According to certain studies, coiling is related to lower mortality and morbidity. However, the complexity of the aneurysms referred to for surgical care has most certainly grown over time. Furthermore, the learning curve and technical advancements in the field of endovascular surgery have grown. Nonetheless, the emergence of stent-assisted embolization has minimized the gap in the complexity of aneurysms referred for surgical vs. endovascular treatment, and many studies have demonstrated that the risk of unfavorable results is increased when an assistive device is utilized [21, 53].

In regard to OMNP, A meta-analysis revealed that there is no significant difference in the complete recovery of OMNP between the clipping and coiling groups, although a tendency in favor of clipping. This is especially true in the case of unruptured PcomA aneurysms. However, in the event of ruptured PcomA aneurysms, clipping was found to be preferable than coiling. The pathophysiological rationale for these findings is yet unknown. It has been proposed that the aneurysmal mass effect and the hematoma around it can be eliminated through surgical clipping. Endovascular coiling, which may add to the mass effect, cannot do this. However, the elimination of aneurysmal pulsation was attributed to the improvement after coiling, which may explain the equivalent of clipping and coiling used in the treatment of OMNP caused by unruptured PcomA aneurysms [21, 53].

1.7. Short-Term and Long-Term Outcome and Recovery Predictors

Due to the wide variety of anatomical characteristics of PcomA aneurysms, the treatment procedure can be one of the easiest or one of the most complicated ones. There is an acceptable chance of recovery after surgical or endovascular management that depends on multiple factors including the timeline between the diagnosis and treatment, the existence of subarachnoid hemorrhage with the consequent brain injury in addition to oculomotor nerve injury. Individual-based planning must be obtained for each patient in order to achieve the optimal outcome. In general, the morbidity rate of surgically treated PcomA aneurysms is low (5%) compared to other aneurysms in the circle of Willis [18]. The surgical and endovascular treatment of PcomA aneurysm have nearly the same outcome on patients. This is true in case of unruptured aneurysm, however, on the other hand, if the ruptured aneurysm results in a large ICH that requires urgent evacuation, the benefits of surgical methods outweigh the endovascular ones. Nevertheless, the endovascular option is about to have an equal outcome in the future as a result of improvement in the technology and training strategies, which is the preferable option for elderly patients who have relevant comorbidities [54, 56].

A recent study demonstrated five morphological parameters associated with stable long-term outcomes in coiled PcomA aneurysms. These parameters include small size PcomA aneurysm, dome-to-neck ration <2, small-sized PcomA artery, ICA-fundus angle of 160-180°, and a posteroinferior dome projection. Regarding the adverse outcome of aneurysmal coiling, incomplete initial embolization is the most significant cause of re-hemorrhage [7, 56].

The recovery of the oculomotor nerve depends on the time to treatment and the degree of pre-operative deficit. Moreover, surgical clipping gives a higher recovery chance than endovascular treatment [54].

1.8. Recurrency of PcomA Aneurysm

The post-clipping recurrence rate is 2.9% while post coiling recurrence rate is 15-33% [57]. The established risk factors of recurrence are the large size of the PcomA aneurysm, wide neck, history of aneurysmal rupture, and the presence of intraluminal thrombus. Moreover, fetal type PCA is considered to be a significant risk factor. To illustrate the previous statement, the presence of fetal type PCA leads to hemodynamic issues that represent the imbalance of blood pressure between the ICA and vertebral basilar system. Patients who present with each of these perils need a more precise follow-up plan and accurate preoperative evaluation [4, 57, 58].

The management of recurrent aneurysms after surgical clipping is complicated due to the technical difficulties that are caused by the existing clip, the formation of scar tissue, and the presence of postoperative adhesions. The endovascular treatment of recurrent aneurysms is more suitable than surgical treatment. Although it could be quite difficult, it carries fewer risks of further comorbidities. Some authors suggest that Stent-assisted coiling could conquer these difficulties [59].

1.9. Follow-up Plan for PcomA Aneurysm Patients

An effective follow-up scheme must equilibrate between efficient risk assessment and avoidance of unnecessary expenses. The important points that must be taken into consideration while addressing the follow-up plan are the aneurysm's features, whether surgical clipping or endovascular treatment was applied, and the patient's own health status. Generally, there is no international guideline upon timetable for follow-up of treated aneurysms. However, patients who have known aneurysmal recurrent risk factors need close attention when formulating a follow-up strategy.

The classical follow-up protocol of surgically and endovascularly treated aneurysms includes an early imaging study at 3-6 months post-treatment followed by a second study after 12 to 24 months of the operation and a third one after 3-5 years of the operation. Some authors advocate for further evaluation of 10 years post-treatment [60].

The imaging studies that are used in the follow-up include digital subtraction angiography (DSA), magnetic resonance angiogram (MRA), and computerized tomographic angiography (CTA). DSA is the gold standard choice, but it is invasive and carries neurological risks after repeated follow-up procedures. MRA is a suitable follow-up tool as it has no radiation risk and is not invasive. However, the presence of intracorporal metallic foreign bodies and patient movement is considered to be limitations factors for its use. Moreover, the appearance of a small residual neck on MRA will lead to performing DSA to confirm the diagnosis and assess the accurate size of the remnant. CTA is frequently performed in the setting of immediate follow-up, but the appearance of artifacts on images that result from the metallic consistency of clips or coils will lead to the covering of the surrounding structures and potential complications. This fact made the DSA a more suitable choice in case MRA is contraindicated [60-62].

1.10. Cases of PcomA Aneurysms

1.10.1. Case 1

1.10.1.1. Pure Posteriorly Directed PcomA Aneurysm [63]

A patient who presented with sudden onset of severe headache, disturbed level of consciousness, left partial oculomotor nerve palsy, and neck stiffness(Figure 9).

1.10.2. Case 2

1.10.2.1. Bilateral PcomA Aneurysms

A 67-years old patient presented with severe headache, vomiting for two days duration and left upper motor weakness grade 4. CT scan revealed SAH in a pattern that raises the suspicion of ruptured right PcomA aneurysm. The ruptured right PcomA aneurysm was urgently treated with surgical clipping while the left aneurysm was treated electively through an endovascular approach in which partial coiling was performed followed by flow diverter deployment. This management plan is based on multiple factors including aneurysmal rupture status, limited availability of endovascular equipment and patient old age. Patient outcome is good (GCS is 15) and no complications are reported (Figure 10).

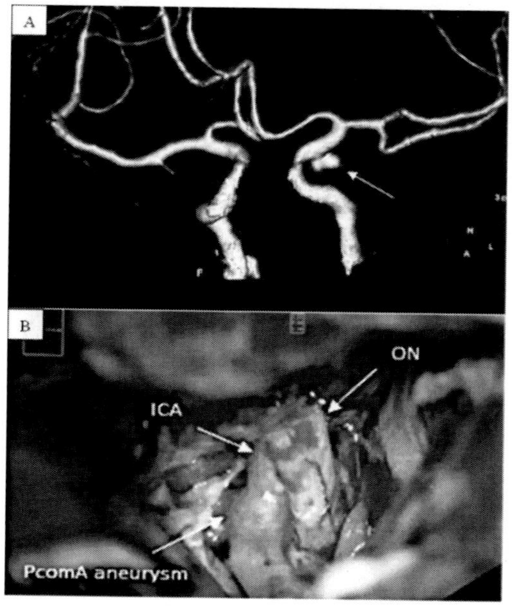

Figure 9. (A) Left anterolateral computed tomography (CT) angiogram showing left pure posteriorly directed PcomA aneurysm. (B) Intraoperative image through the left pterional approach show the aneurysm before clipping with related anatomical structures including optic nerve (ON) and internal carotid artery (ICA).

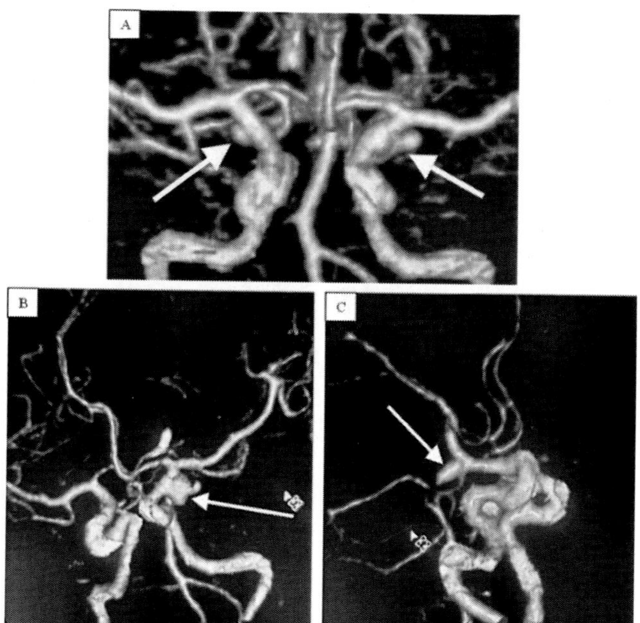

Figure 10. (A) CT angiography revealed bilateral PcomA aneurysms. (B) Shows the left sided PcomA aneurysm which has wide neck and Murphey's teat. (C) Shows the right sided aneurysm which is directed posteriorly.

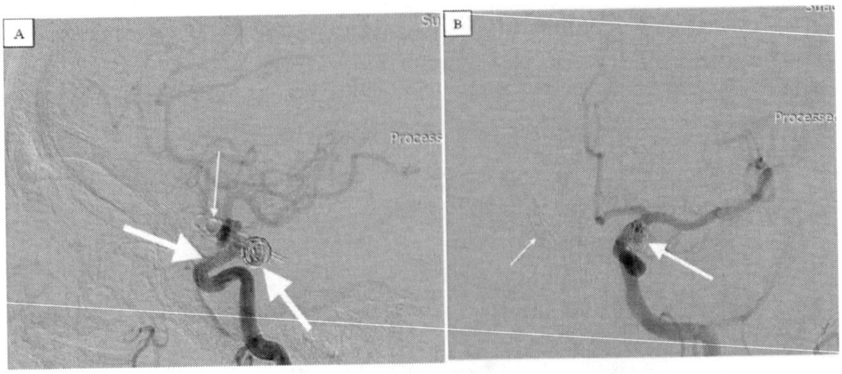

Figure 11. (A) Post operative lateral catheter angiography shows the coil and flow diverter stent in the supra-clinoid carotid artery which is marked by the large arrow. The small arrow represents the superimposed right PcomA aneurysm clip.(B)is PA view catheter angiography of left ICA in which the large arrow shows coiling of left PcomA aneurysm while the small arrow shows the shadow of right PcomA aneurysm clip.

1.10.3. Case 3

1.10.3.1. Left Sided Posteriorly Directed PcomA Aneurysm

A patient presented with left 3rd cranial nerve palsy (Figure 12).

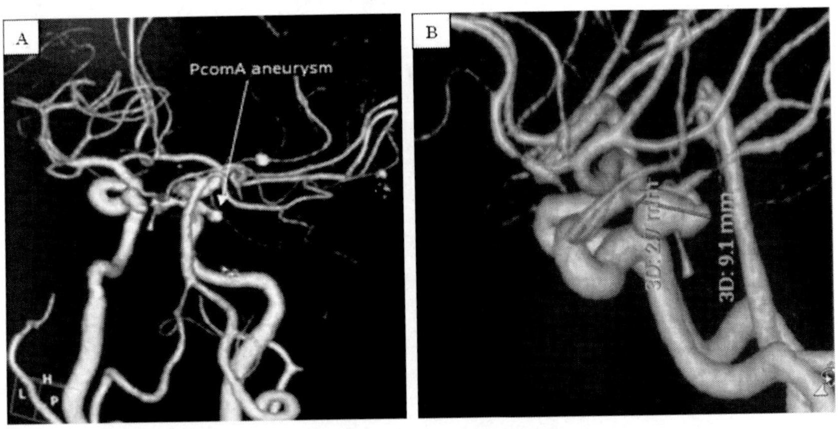

Figure 12. (A-b) CT angiography revealed left sided posteriorly directed PcomA aneurysm.

References

[1] Rhoton AL Jr. The supratentorial arteries. *Neurosurgery*. 2002 Oct;51(4 Suppl):S53-120. PMID: 12234447.

[2] Gunnal S, Farooqui M, Wabale R. Anatomical variability of the posterior communicating artery. *Asian Journal of Neurosurgery*. 2018 Jun;13(02):363-9.

[3] Capone S, Shah N, George-St Bernard RR. A fetal-type variant posterior communicating artery and its clinical significance. *Cureus*. 2019 Jul 2;11(7).

[4] Jones JD, Castanho P, Bazira P, Sanders K. Anatomical variations of the circle of Willis and their prevalence, with a focus on the posterior communicating artery: A literature review and meta- analysis. *Clinical Anatomy*. 2021 Oct;34(7):978-90.

[5] Park HK, Rha HK, Lee KJ, Chough CK, Joo W. Microsurgical anatomy of the oculomotor nerve. *Clinical anatomy*. 2017 Jan;30(1):21-31.

[6] Rhoton Jr AL, Fujii K, Fradd B. Microsurgical anatomy of the anterior choroidal artery. *Surgical neurology*. 1979 Aug 1;12(2):171-87.

[7] Golshani K, Ferrell A, Zomorodi A, Smith TP, Britz GW. A review of the management of posterior communicating artery aneurysms in the modern era. *Surgical neurology international*. 2010;1.

[8] Bourcier R, Chatel S, Bourcereau E, Jouan S, Marec HL, Daumas-Duport B, Sevin-Allouet M, Guillon B, Roualdes V, Riem T, Isidor B. Understanding the pathophysiology of intracranial aneurysm: the ICAN project. *Neurosurgery*. 2017 Apr 1;80(4):621-6.

[9] Rangel-Castilla L, Nakaji P, Siddiqui AH, Spetzler RF, Levy EI. *Decision making in neurovascular disease*. Thieme; 2018.

[10] Park J, Kang DH, Chun BY. Superciliary keyhole surgery for unruptured posterior communicating artery aneurysms with oculomotor nerve palsy: maximizing symptomatic resolution and minimizing surgical invasiveness. *Journal of neurosurgery*. 2011 Oct 1;115(4):700-6.

[11] He W, Gandhi CD, Quinn J, Karimi R, Prestigiacomo CJ. True aneurysms of the posterior communicating artery: a systematic review and meta-analysis of individual patient data. *World neurosurgery*. 2011 Jan 1;75(1):64-72.

[12] Krayenbühl HA, Yaşargil MG, Flamm ES, Tew JM. Microsurgical treatment of intracranial saccular aneurysms. *Journal of neurosurgery*. 1972 Dec 1;37(6):678-86.

[13] Yasargil MG. Management of aneurysms of anterior circulation by intracranial procedures. *Neurological surgery*. 1982;3:1663-96.

[14] Ho A, Lin N, Charoenvimolphan N, Stanley M, Frerichs KU, Day AL, Du R. Morphological parameters associated with ruptured posterior communicating aneurysms. *PLoS One*. 2014 Apr 14;9(4):e94837.

[15] Yasargil MG. Clinical considerations, surgery of intracranial aneurysms and results. *Microneurosurgery*. 1984:224-31.

[16] Masuoka J, Yoshioka F, Furukawa T, Koguchi M, Ito H, Inoue K, Ogata A, Nakahara Y, Abe T. Microsurgical Approach for True Posterior Communicating Artery Aneurysms: Literature Review and Illustrative Case. *Asian Journal of Neurosurgery*. 2022 Aug 25.

[17] Zhang J, Can A, Lai PM, Mukundan S, Castro VM, Dligach D, Finan S, Yu S, Gainer VS, Shadick NA, Savova G. Age and morphology of posterior communicating artery aneurysms. *Scientific reports*. 2020 Jul 14;10(1):1-9.

[18] Matsumoto K, Kuriyama M, Tamiya T, Ohmoto T. Direct clip obliteration of a ruptured giant aneurysm of the posterior communicating artery: case report. *Neurosurgery*. 1997 Oct 1;41(4):939-42.

[19] Unno N, Mitsuoka H, Takei Y, Igarashi T, Uchiyama T, Yamamoto N, Saito T, Nakamura S. Virtual angioscopy using 3-dimensional rotational digital subtraction angiography for endovascular assessment. *Journal of Endovascular Therapy*. 2002 Aug;9(4):529-34.

[20] Huhtakangas J, Lehecka M, Lehto H, Jahromi BR, Niemelä M, Kivisaari R. CTA analysis and assessment of morphological factors related to rupture in 413 posterior communicating artery aneurysms. *Acta neurochirurgica*. 2017 Sep;159(9):1643-52.

[21] Zheng F, Dong Y, Xia P, Mpotsaris A, Stavrinou P, Brinker G, Goldbrunner R, Krischek B. Is clipping better than coiling in the treatment of patients with oculomotor nerve palsies induced by posterior communicating artery aneurysms? A systematic review and meta-analysis. *Clinical Neurology and Neurosurgery*. 2017 Feb 1;153:20-6.

[22] Soni, S. Aneurysms of the posterior communicating artery and oculomotor paresis, J. Neurol. *Neurosurg*. Psychiatry 37 (1974) 475–484.

[23] Giombini, S, Ferraresi, S, Pluchino, F. Reversal of oculomotor disorders after intracranial aneurysm surgery, *Acta Neurochir*. (Wien) 112 (1991) 19–24.

[24] Nam KH, Choi CH, Lee JI, Ko JG, Lee TH, Lee SW. Unruptured intracranial aneurysms with oculomotor nerve palsy: clinical outcome between surgical clipping and coil embolization. *Journal of Korean Neurosurgical Society*. 2010 Aug;48(2):109.

[25] Elmalem VI, Hudgins PA, Bruce BB, Newman NJ, Biousse V. Underdiagnosis of posterior communicating artery aneurysm in non-invasive brain vascular studies. *Journal of neuroophthalmology: the official journal of the North American Neuro-Ophthalmology Society*. 2011 Jun;31(2):103.

[26] Karamessini MT, Kagadis GC, Petsas T, Karnabatidis D, Konstantinou D, Sakellaropoulos GC, Nikiforidis GC, Siablis D. CT angiography with three-dimensional techniques for the early diagnosis of intracranial aneurysms. Comparison with intra-arterial DSA and the surgical findings. *European journal of radiology*. 2004 Mar 1;49(3):212-23.

[27] Chaudhary N, Davagnanam I, Ansari SA, Pandey A, Thompson BG, Gemmete JJ. Imaging of intracranial aneurysms causing isolated third cranial nerve palsy. *Journal of Neuro-ophthalmology*. 2009 Sep 1;29(3):238-44.

[28] Mathew MR, Teasdale E, McFadzean RM. Multidetector computed tomographic angiography in isolated third nerve palsy. *Ophthalmology*. 2008 Aug 1;115(8):1411-5.

[29] Seruga T, Bunc G, Klein GE. Helical High-Resolution Volume-Rendered 3-Dimensional Computer Tomography Angiography in the Detection of Intracranial Aneurysms. *Journal of Neuroimaging*. 2001 Jul;11(3):280-6.

[30] Yasargil MG. Clinical considerations, surgery of intracranial aneurysms and results. *Microneurosurgery*. 1984:224-31.

[31] Hochmuth A, Spetzger U, Schumacher M. Comparison of three-dimensional rotational angiography with digital subtraction angiography in the assessment of ruptured cerebral aneurysms. *American journal of neuroradiology*. 2002 Aug 1;23(7):1199-205.

[32] Waugh JR, Sacharias N. Arteriographic complications in the DSA era. *Radiology*. 1992 Jan;182(1):243-6.

[33] Scherer A, Siebler M, Aulich A. Virtual arterial endoscopy as a diagnostic aid in a patient with basilar artery fenestration and thromboembolic pontine infarct. *American journal of neuroradiology*. 2002 Aug 1;23(7):1237-9.

[34] Lee KC, Lee KS, Shin YS, Lee JW, Chung SK. Surgery for posterior communicating artery aneurysms. *Surgical neurology*. 2003 Feb 1;59(2):107-13.

[35] Molyneux A, Kerr R, International Subarachnoid Aneurysm Trial (ISAT) Collaborative Group. International Subarachnoid Aneurysm Trial (ISAT) of neurosurgical clipping versus endovascular coiling in 2143 patients with ruptured intracranial aneurysms: a randomized trial. *Journal of stroke and cerebrovascular diseases*. 2002 Nov 1;11(6):304-14.

[36] Thiarawat P, Jahromi BR, Kozyrev DA, Intarakhao P, Teo MK, Choque-Velasquez J, Hernesniemi J. Microneurosurgical management of posterior communicating artery aneurysm: A contemporary series from helsinki. *World Neurosurgery*. 2017 May 1;101:379-88

[37] Horiuchi T, Nakagawa F, Tanaka Y, Miyama H, Hongo K. Anterior subtemporal approach for posteriorly projecting posterior communicating artery aneurysms. *Neurosurgical review*. 2007 Jul;30(3):203-7.

[38] Yang Y, Meng X, Song J, Nie X, Zhao C, Su W. Microsurgical treatment of ruptured true posterior communicating artery aneurysm in the distal portion of the posterior communicating artery. *Journal of Craniofacial Surgery*. 2019 Jan 1;30(1):e5-7.

[39] Katsuno M, Tanikawa R, Izumi N, Hashimoto M. A modified anterior temporal approach for low-position aneurysms of the upper basilar complex. *Surgical Neurology International*. 2015;6.

[40] Katsuno M, Tanikawa R. Zygomatic anterior temporal approach for high-position upper basilar aneurysm. *Neurologia medico-chirurgica*. 2019;59(11):430-5.

[41] PARK, Sang Kyu, et al. Preoperative predictive value of the necessity for anterior clinoidectomy in posterior communicating artery aneurysm clipping. *Neurosurgery*, 2009, 65.2: 281-286.

[42] Guinn NR, McDonagh DL, Borel CO, Wright DR, Zomorodi AR, Powers CJ, Warner DS, Lam AM, Britz GW. Adenosine-induced transient asystole for intracranial aneurysm surgery: a retrospective review. *Journal of neurosurgical anesthesiology*. 2011 Jan 1;23(1):35-40.

[43] Byrne JV, Molyneux AJ, Brennan RP, Renowden SA. Embolisation of recently ruptured intracranial aneurysms. *Journal of Neurology, Neurosurgery & Psychiatry*. 1995 Dec 1;59(6):616-20.

[44] Kim MJ, Chung J, Park KY, Kim DJ, Kim BM, Suh SH, Lee JW, Huh SK, Kim YB, Joo JY, Son NH. Recurrence and risk factors of posterior communicating artery aneurysms after endovascular treatment. *Acta neurochirurgica*. 2021 Aug;163(8):2319-26.
[45] Biondi A, Janardhan V, Katz JM, et al. Neuroform stent-assisted coil embolization of wide-neck intracranial aneurysms: strate- gies in stent deployment and midterm follow-up. *Neurosurgery* 2007;61:460 – 68.
[46] Cho YD, Lee WJ, Kim KM, Kang HS, Kim JE, Han MH. Stent-assisted coil embolization of posterior communicating artery aneurysms. *American Journal of Neuroradiology*. 2013 Nov 1;34(11):2171-6.
[47] Peluso JP, van Rooij WJ, Sluzewski M, et al. A new self-expandable nitinol stent for the treatment of wide-neck aneurysms: initial clinical experience. *AJNR Am J Neuroradiol* 2008;29:1405– 08.
[48] Piotin M, Blanc R, Spelle L, et al. Stent-assisted coiling of intracranial aneurysms: clinical and angiographic results in 216 consecutive aneurysms. *Stroke* 2010;41:110 –15.
[49] Lee SJ, Cho YD, Kang HS, Kim JE, Han MH. Coil embolization using the self-expandable closed-cell stent for intracranial saccular aneurysm: a single-center experience of 289 consecutive aneurysms. *Clinical radiology*. 2013 Mar 1;68(3):256-63.
[50] Moubark M, Allah AE, Yosef H, Abdel-Tawab M, Panos P, Othman M. Flow diverter devices in the treatment of posterior communicating artery aneurysms: mid-term clinical and radiological outcomes. *Egyptian Journal of Radiology and Nuclear Medicine*. 2020 Dec;51:1-9.
[51] Slater L-A, Soufan C, Holt M, Chong W (2015) Effect of flow diversion with silk on aneurysm size: a single-center experience. Interv Neuroradiol 21(1): 12–18.
[52] Lubicz B, Lefranc F, Levivier M, Dewitte O, Pirotte B, Brotchi J et al. (2006) Endovascular treatment of intracranial aneurysms with a branch arising from the sac. *Am J Neuroradiol* 27(1):142–147.
[53] Gaberel T, Borha A, di Palma C, Emery E. Clipping versus coiling in the management of posterior communicating artery aneurysms with third nerve palsy: a systematic review and meta-analysis. *World Neurosurgery*. 2016 Mar 1;87:498-506.
[54] Kyriakides T, Aziz TZ, Torrens MJ. Postoperative recovery of third nerve palsy due to posterior communicating aneurysms. *British journal of neurosurgery*. 1989 Jan 1;3(1):109-11.
[55] Leivo S, Hernesniemi J, Luukkonen M, Vapalahti M. Early surgery improves the cure of aneurysm-induced oculomotor palsy. *Surgical neurology*. 1996 May 1;45(5):430-4.
[56] Songsaeng D, Geibprasert S, ter Brugge KG, Willinsky R, Tymianski M, Krings T. Impact of individual intracranial arterial aneurysm morphology on initial obliteration and recurrence rates of endovascular treatments: a multivariate analysis. *Journal of neurosurgery*. 2011 Apr 1;114(4):994-1002.
[57] Lee HJ, Choi JH, Shin YS, Lee KS, Kim BS. Risk factors for the recurrence of posterior communicating artery aneurysm: the significance of fetal-type posterior cerebral artery. *Journal of Stroke and Cerebrovascular Diseases*. 2021 Jul 1;30(7):105821.
[58] Huang DZ, Jiang B, He W, Wang YH, Wang ZG. Risk factors for the recurrence of an intracranial saccular aneurysm following endovascular treatment. *Oncotarget*. 2017 May 5;8(20):33676.
[59] Drake CG, Friedman AH, Peerless SJ. Failed aneurysm surgery: reoperation in 115 cases. *Journal of neurosurgery*. 1984 Nov 1;61(5):848-56.
[60] Reade De Leacy Md, Gal Yaniv Md, Kambiz N. Cerebral Aneurysm Follow-Up: How Standards Have Changed and Why.
[61] Campi A, Ramzi N, Molyneux AJ, Summers PE, Kerr RS, Sneade M, Yarnold JA, Rischmiller J, Byrne JV. Retreatment of ruptured cerebral aneurysms in patients randomized by coiling or clipping in the International Subarachnoid Aneurysm Trial (ISAT). *Stroke*. 2007 May 1;38(5):1538-44.
[62] Lecler A, Raymond J, Rodriguez-Regent C, Al Shareef F, Trystram D, Godon-Hardy S, Ben Hassen W, Meder JF, Oppenheim C, Naggara ON. Intracranial aneurysms: recurrences more than 10 years after endovascular treatment-a prospective cohort study, systematic review, and meta-analysis. *Radiology*. 2015 Oct 1;277(1):173-80.
[63] Ismail M, Alshalchi AK, Badr MM, Abdulameer AO, Algburi HA, Al-Taie RH, Al-Lami S, Al-Khafaji AO, Hoz SS. Impact of dome projection on operative steps during clipping of a ruptured pure posteriorly directed posterior communicating artery aneurysms. *Romanian Neurosurgery*. 2022 Sep 15:355-8.

Chapter 4

Endovascular and Surgical Options for Ruptured Middle Cerebral Artery Aneurysms

Ioannis Koukoulithras[1]
Athanasios Gkampenis[1]
Georgios Fotakopoulos[1]
Spyridon Voulgaris[1,2]
and George A. Alexiou[1,2,*]
[1]Department of Neurosurgery, University of Ioannina, Ioannina, Greece
[2]Neurosurgical Institute, University of Ioannina School of Medicine, Ioannina, Greece

Abstract

Middle cerebral artery (MCA) aneurysms are among the most frequent intracranial aneurysms, with bifurcation being the most common site. Their rupture is frequent resulting not only in subarachnoid hemorrhage but also in intracerebral hemorrhage. For the diagnosis of the ruptured aneurysms commonly used radiological examinations are CT, CTA, MRA or DSA. Also, lumbar puncture can be helpful revealing xanthochromia in cases of negative CT. There have been described three main classic surgical methods and one more contemporary, while the clipping technique of the aneurysm is more individualized, though some general principles can be followed. Even though in most centers surgical options are chosen, there are efforts to develop new endovascular methods to treat even complex aneurysms avoiding a surgery.

Keywords: endovascular, surgery, ruptured, middle cerebral artery, aneurysm

Introduction

The prevalence of middle cerebral artery (MCA) aneurysms among the intracranial aneurysms ranges between 26% and 34%, making MCA the second most common location after ICA, according to a systematic review of Rinkel GJ et al. in 1998 [1]. The aneurysms, located in

* Corresponding Author's Email: galexiou@uoi.gr.

In: Understanding and Managing Cerebral Aneurysms
Editor: Xianli Lv
ISBN: 979-8-89113-608-3

MCA, are among the most common aneurysms to be ruptured, resulting not only in subarachnoidal hemorrhage (SAH) as usual, but also in intracerebral hemorrhage (ICH) or in intrasylvian hemorrhage (ISH) [2, 3]. The majority of the cases of acute SAH (aSAH) with non-traumatic evidence is caused by the rupture of intracranial aneurysm. This trend can be observed in the data of our university hospital in Ioannina, as between 2000 and 2010, 93.7% of non-traumatic SAH was caused by intrancranial aneurysm rupture. MCA aneurysms due to their anatomical properties are more prone than other aneurysms to lead in ICH and their rupture leads in ICH in one third of the cases [2, 4, 5]. The angulation of the aneurysm shows according to Neyazi B et al., a significant correlation with the type and the localization of the hemorrhage [2]. More specifically, frontal angulation was associated with frontal ICH, temporal was associated with temporal ICH, and sylvianally angulated aneurysms were behind the majority of SAH [2].

Among MCA aneurysms, MCA bifurcation is the most common aneurysm site, and are categorized as main bifurcation aneurysms [3, 5]. Fundus projection is an important and helpful factor in the planning of the microsurgical approach for these aneurysms and many neurosurgeons have established and used such classification systems to help them to plan a safe route and avoid the dome of the aneurysm [5, 6]. These classifications, however, do not indicate the appropriate clipping technique and that's why Washington CW et al. in 2014 proposed another classification according to the anatomic visual characteristics of aneurysms [6]. Through this novel shape-based categorization system the researchers were able to propose specific clipping strategies for each aneurysm category [6].

Despite the agreement of the majority of researchers that most of the MCA aneurysms originate from MCA bifurcation, there is not a commonly accepted anatomical classification system [3, 5]. According to Ulm et al. in 2008 MCA aneurysms can be generally classified with respect to their origin into six categories:

1. the ones from M1 bifurcation,
2. these from M1 trifurcation,
3. the ones from the takeoff of lenticulostriate arteries,
4. the ones from branch site of M1 segment temporal arteries,
5. these from M1 frontal branch arteries, and
6. these from distal sites on M2, M3, M4 [3]

According to the guidelines from the European Stroke Organization (ESO) for the management of intracranial aneurysms and subarachnoid hemorrhage, the treatment of aneurysmal SAH should target to the complete occlusion of the ruptured aneurysm to prevent rebleeding [7]. These guidelines also highlight the need for treatment of the ruptured aneurysm as early as technically and logistically possible, if applicable ideally within 72 h after the first symptoms [7]. A relevant meta-analysis demonstrated that patients, who underwent clipping within 72 h and with WFNS 1-3 on admission, had a significantly better outcome than the ones clipped after 72h [7]. The trend was similar in patients with admission worse WFNS scores 4-5, but this was not statistically significant [7].

Symptoms and Clinical Presentation

Ruptured aneurysms are the most common cause of acute subarachnoid hemorrhage [8]. Less commonly these patients presented with intracerebral hematoma or acute subdural hematoma [8]. It is well mentioned that the prognosis of patients with MCA aneurysm rupture is worse when SAH co-existing with intraparenchymal hemorrhage [9]. Approximately 30% of MCA aneurysms rupture combined with intracerebral hemorrhage [10]. The typical presentation of the patients with ruptured aneurysm is a sudden, "thunderclap," and severe headache which peaks in severity within 1-5 minutes [8]. This thunderclap headache should be differentiated with other causes such as migraine attack, exertion, cough etc. Also, the presence of blood in subarachnoid space irritates arachnoid and may cause meningism signs (e.g., neck stiffness). Other symptoms are nausea, vomiting, photophobia, and symptoms of affected brain functions such as seizures, reduced consciousness (ranging from confusion, lethargy to obtundation, and coma), focal neurological deficit (cranial nerves palsy etc.) [8, 11].

Diagnosis of MCA Aneurysm Rupture

The best method for the diagnosis of SAH is the non-contrast head CT scan as soon as possible. According to the NICE guidelines 2022 the CT scan should be done within 6 hours from symptoms onset of the patient to diagnose the SAH [11]. Then a CT Angiography or Digital subtraction angiography (DSA) or Magnetic Resonance Angiography (MRA) could confirm the diagnosis and the site of cerebral aneurysm. If the CT scan doesn't reveal SAH during 6 hours from onset of the symptoms the physician should think other diagnosis. Moreover, if the CT scan performed later than 6 hours and there is high suspicion of aneurysm rupture, the physician should consider lumbar puncture to identify bilirubin (xanthochromia) which confirms SAH and then a CTA or DSA or MRA should be performed [11]. The physician should consider other diagnosis if there is no bilirubin in CSF.

In the MCA aneurysm rupture the CT scan shows diffuse hyperdense SAH. Also, it can be co-existing with intraparenchymal hematoma and/or intraventricular hemorrhage which both have poor prognosis. The volume of intraparenchymal hematoma should be consider because it changes the prognosis and treatment protocol (endovascular or clipping) [12].

Surgical Options for Ruptured MCA Aneurysms

The interventional treatment for ruptured aneurysms should be done as early as possible according to the guidelines from both ESO and NICE to prevent a possible rebleeding [7, 11]. Intracerebral hemorrhage accompanies approximately one third of ruptured MCA aneurysms and given the possible temporal hematoma position and the additional subarachnoid hemorrhage, relatively small hematomas result in significant mass effect [5]. Steiger et al. suggest that the indication for emergency evacuation should be based on the overall patient's medical condition and the hematoma volume, with volumes greater than 20 mL regarded as critical [5]. Especially in case of stuporous or comatose patients H. J. Steiger et al. opt for only a plain CT to acquire the essential information for the surgery, speeding up the presurgical preparations [5]. However, in case of a significant vasospasm as demonstrated on DSA or CTA due to a transfer delay, Cherian J. and Barrow D. L. regarded occasionally logical a postponement of the surgery until postbleed days 11 to 14, namely after the vasospasm window [13].

Preparation

In patients with ruptured aneurysms and aneurysmal SAH, brain edema and/or acute hydrocephalus often limit the working space during early operation [14]. To relax brain and make surgery safer in these patients, cerebrospinal fluid drainage is often indicated, despite anecdotal rupture reports [13]. Intraoperative external ventricular drainage, according to the retrospective study of Pavevesi G. et al. in 2022, constitutes a safe method to increase working space, which allows an immediate brain relaxation facilitating dissection using a simple and safe positioning [14]. However, H. J. Steiger et al. in their book in 2015 do not recommend an external ventricular drain before the evacuation of the hematoma [5]. Moreover, these authors recommend the administration of a bolus of 500-1000 mg of thiopental to drop blood pressure, because in case of a tense dura the opening of the dura will result in a rerupture of the aneurysm [5].

Approaches and Related Positioning

There are three standard approaches for MCA aneurysms and neurosurgeons can also utilize a combination of them or they can change intraoperatively from one technique to another according to encountered difficulties through the dissection [4, 13, 15, 16, 17]. During the proximal sylvian fissure approach the Sylvian fissure is separated in a proximal (medial) to distal (lateral) direction [4, 16]. On the contrary through the distal sylvian fissure approach the opposite direction is used following an M2 branch proximally to the aneurysm, namely a distal to proximal direction [4, 16]. The last classic alternative is the transcortical sylvian fissure approach, which involves a transtemporal dissection by removement of a variable amount of temporal tissue to reach the MCA [4, 15, 16]. However, except these three standard approaches a more focused approach of the sylvian fissure for MCA ruptured and unruptured aneurysms has been evaluated with good results [17].

The Proximal Sylvian Fissure Approach

In the proximal sylvian fissure approach the patient is in supine position, the head is turned contralaterally approximately 30 degrees and extended slightly backwards [4]. After the positioning, neurosurgeons perform a standard pterional craniotomy removing the lateral sphenoid wing and using a pterional flap, whereas careful bone removal reduces the need for retraction [4, 15].

First, optic nerve and carotid artery are identified and the intradural dissection starts in this place opening sharply the arachnoid and letting so cerebrospinal fluid to flow from the optic and carotid cisterns [4]. The need for brain retraction can be minimized through the wide opening of all medial cisterns and separation of both frontal lobes from the optic nerves [4]. If the brain is optimally relaxed, the use of retractors can be avoided, and the surgeon can instead use the suction tip also as a retractor [4]. Otherwise, self-retaining retractors can be placed on the frontal and temporal lobes at 90-degree angles to each other and moved gradually in the separated sylvian fissure along the ICA [4]. Sylvian veins should be protected to avoid possible postoperative hemorrhage and edema and it is preferable to separate the fissure on the frontal side of these veins [4, 13]. After identifying the bifurcation between MCA and ICA the separation is continued along the anteroinferior aspect of the M1 segment, being careful to preserve the lenticulostriate vessels [4]. Using this approach for bifurcation aneurysms means that the sylvian fissure dissection needs to be continued until the MCA bifurcation is identified [4].

The Distal Sylvian Fissure Approach

For this approach the patient positioning can be similar and a pterional craniotomy be used again [10].

The sylvian fissure is either occasionally visible or more commonly indexed by the sphenoid indentation or the sylvian vein, which courses the temporal edge of the fissure [10]. Unless the fissure is perfectly obvious cortical middle cerebral branches can be followed back to their parent arteries in the fissure [4, 10]. According to Heros RC and Fritsch MJ, when the surgeon identifies an M2 branch, he or she can follow it medially on the opposite site of the projection of the aneurysm to expose the MCA bifurcation and the aneurysm [4]. Yaşargil has proposed the inside-out method to enter the sylvian fissure distally, working deeply, and separating the fissure medially following the MCA until the dissection of the fissure [13].

The Superior Temporal Approach

This approach resembles the lateral sylvian approach as the only difference is the entrance, which is now performed at a depth of 1.5 to 2 cm from the surface of the fissure through a cortisectomy in the anterior aspect of the superior temporal gyrus [4]. For this approach the patient is positioned supine with the head rotated 60 degrees and again extended slightly backwards [4, 15]. The incision of the skin begins in front of the tragus at the zygoma level, then curves lightly towards the rear and superior to the ear and after that it continues forward to the edge of the hairline about 2-3 cm laterally from the midline [4, 15]. The craniotomy resembles the standard pterional craniotomy and the lateral aspect of the sphenoid ridge is similarly removed [4]. Nevertheless, the craniotomy is now extended lightly more posteriorly and superiorly than the classic pterional approach [4].

The medial cisterns need not to be opened in this approach, because brain relaxation is not as important as in the transsylvian approaches [4]. The cortisectomy begins approximately 1 cm behind the most anterior point of the sylvian fissure and continues for 2-2.5 cm in the superior temporal gyrus [4, 15]. The cortisectomy is extended medially into the vertical segment of the sylvian fissure over the insula with the use of sunction and bipolar coagulation [4, 13, 15]. After that the opening of the arachnoid, peripheral branches of MCA are identified and followed backwards in MCA bifurcation, which can be fully exposed through a further removal of the mesial superior temporal gyrus [13, 4].

Focused Opening of the Sylvian Fissure

Even though a wide transsylvian approach either distal or proximal has been regarded a classic approach for MCA aneurysms, extensive sylvian dissection can possibly lead in an increased incidence of iatrogenic cerebral and neurovascular injury [17]. Elsharkaway A. et al. in 2013 published their experience using a focused opening technique of the sylvian fissure for 1097 aneurysms, where their technique has proved to be safe and effective for ruptured aneurysms [17].

The position of the patient is supine with the head rotated 15-45 degrees and elevated above the heart level 10-20 cm [17]. Almost in all their surgeries a lateral supraorbital approach was used, whereas for distal MCA aneurysms the approach was altered according to the specific position of the aneurysms and for giant aneurysms pterional approach was elected [17].

The position of the sylvian opening is chosen depending on the location of the aneurysm and the chosen approach angle [17]. The two arachnoid layers are opened with a sharp needle and then going deep into the sylvian fissure the window can be opened can be extended from inside-out with a 10-15 mm opening usually being sufficient [17].

Choosing the Right Approach

Proximal sylvian fissure approach seems the only option for aneurysms of proximal MCA trunk as well as a logical approach for proximally located bifurcation aneurysms if the main MCA trunk is short [4]. That's because in these situations there is the need of the wide opening of the proximal sylvian fissure as the aneurysm is near the limen insula [4].

Distal sylvian fissure approach has the advantage in comparison with the proximal method that less retraction and manipulation of brain and vascular structures is demanded, the risk of injury of the lenticulostriate vessels is lower [4, 10]. Moreover, the commonly more difficult distal anatomy of the aneurysm is first exposed, whereas letting proximal PCA unexposed reduces the risk of exacerbated vasospasm [4]. Also, in the inside-out method of Yaşargil the CSF fills fully the fissure helping in the dissection, but the aneurysm is found before proximal control is accomplished [4, 13]. Nevertheless, this disadvantage rarely can cause a problem, as proximal control can be gained through a further dissection away from the aneurysm following the edge of one division until the distal MCA trunk is exposed [4]. According to the paper of Heros RC and Fritsch MJ, given these facts Heros RC opts for a distal approach in case of a bifurcation aneurysm normal-length MCA or a distal MCA aneurysm, although either a proximal or for a distal fissure approach can be used [4].

The superior temporal gyrus approach provides a direct approach to the MCA bifurcation without exposing widely neither the parasellar region nor the full horizontal segment of the MCA [13]. It is a relatively quick approach with minimal retraction for intracerebral hematomas or very swollen and hyperemic brains during an acute operation, as in both cases problematic identification of the sylvian fissure and congestion of sylvian veins is common [4]. According to Steiger et al. the transtemporal approach is the way to deal with ruptured MCA aneurysms associated with intratemporal hematoma, while for intrasylvian hematomas the approach should be performed cautiously through the sylvian fissure [5]. However, this approach gives no proximal M1 control when exposing the aneurysm initially, while the restricted access to the suprasellar cisterns limits the brain relaxation through CSF evacuation [13]. The greatest drawback of this approach is the predisposition of postoperative seizures, although the risk may be small and poses generally not a problem [4, 13].

Regarding focused sylvian fissure opening according to its developers it seems to be an alternative even for ruptured aneurysms, minimizing the operative time and providing increased safety avoiding iatrogenic injuries of the neighboring neurovascular structures [9]. However, this method demands a relaxed brain, and the use of 3D reconstruction of the CTA data is also of paramount important to accurately classify the aneurysm and find the best route through the sylvian fissure to the aneurysm [17]. Patients with aneurysm rupture may be comatose or stuporous and as we have seen in these cases Steiger et al. performed only a plain CT, as they regarded more imaging time consuming [5]. Moreover, acute operations of very swollen and hyperemic brain may also pose a problem and make the use of a transcortical approach mandatory.

Generally, the choice of the approach seems to depend on the location of the ruptured aneurysm, the position of the hematoma, and the relaxation of the brain. The position of the hematoma on the plain CT can show the projection of the aneurysm dome concerning the bifurcation [5]. More specifically an intratemporal hematoma proves a projection with the dome toward the temporal lobe, a transsylvian hematoma shows that the dome lies within the sylvian fissure, and lastly a frontally located hematoma proves a dome projection toward the frontal lobe [5]. It should be mentioned that the approach may be changed intraoperatively according to the encountered difficulties, whereas combined approaches may be used, e.g., opening first the opticocarotid cistern to provide brain relaxation and proximal control and then continuing with a distal approach [4, 13].

Dissection and Clipping

In case of SAH after the rapture the identification of M2 and M3 branches becomes difficult and abundant irrigation helps to clear the clot faster and increase visibility [4]. Before the dissection of the aneurysm a position, which does not isolate lenticulostriate arteries, in M1 segment should be prepared for temporary clipping [18].

In M1 segment aneurysms frequently appear near one or two lenticulostriate vessels and they are usually small with projection into the frontal lobe [4]. It is significant that the neck of the aneurysm is carefully separated so that the clip blades can be inserted between the vessels and the aneurysm, although the entire aneurysm dome need not to be dissected [4].

For aneurysms of the MCA bifurcation Heros RC and Fritsch MJ perform a complete dissection of the aneurysm complex after the establishing proximal control, whereas they also use a temporary clip as a protection for freshly ruptured aneurysms [4]. Full separation of the aneurysm ensures identification of a possible third division from the bifurcation or from another major division as well as of a perforating vessel arising near the bifurcation [4]. Moreover, full dissection helps in clip placement revealing the trajectory of the aneurysm and increasing freedom in clip application [4]. Before the placement of the permanent clip, it is important the surgeon to inspect the aneurysm ensuring that no lenticulostriate vessels are adherent to the aneurysm [4].

Although clip placement strategy is individualized to the specific aneurysm, some general principles can be applied [13]. Clips should generally be applied parallel to the branch vessels leaving a normal anatomic blood flow but no remnants [13]. Placement of a clip immediately adjacent to a vessel's wall or junction point may lead in kinking or occluding of the arteries [10, 13]. Washington CW et al. have developed a shape-based classification system for aneurysms of MCA bifurcation, which describes four categories also proposing a clipping strategy respectively [6]. Steiger et al. have also proposed their own classification system for

MCA bifurcation aneurysms according to the projection of the aneurysm suggesting clip strategies accordingly [5].

Complex Aneurysms

Multilobed, wide-necked, large, and giant aneurysms constitute a special aneurysm category, where clipping can be really challenging requiring complex reconstruction, multiple clip placement or being not possible at all [4, 13]. Temporary clipping inducing proximal occlusion can increase the success rate of clip placement and reduce the intraoperative rupture risk through the reduction of the aneurysm turgor [13]. Temporary clipping of the dome of a large ruptured MCA aneurysm can control the bleeding spot helping with final dissection, as the mass of the aneurism is reduced through this temporary clipping [13]. In wide-necked, large, and giant aneurysms of MCA if the only problems are their size and the wide neck, they can be usually treated using a series of clips such as fenestrated clips and extra-long clips [13, 4]. In these cases, however, clip may frequently be positioned several millimeters above the neck to ensure adequate wall reconstruction and not to limit flow [13]. If the walls of the aneurysms are calcified or atheromatous as it is common in large, multilobulated aneurysms, tandem-clipping techniques may be used with fenestrated clips distally and nonfenestrated more proximally to the neck [13].

Nevertheless, a calcified and/or atheromatous aneurysm base, as well as in many cases a partially or subtotally thrombosed aneurysm mandates aneurysmorrhaphy before the clipping is made feasible [4]. Full control of the aneurysm complex needs to be gained to procced in temporary trapping and subsequent aneurysmal sac thrombectomy and endarterectomy to make an adequate reconstruction [4, 13].

Endovascular Treatment

Middle cerebral artery (MCA) aneurysm endovascular coiling is still technically difficult due to its complex anatomy, which includes large necks and the integration of significant branches (Figure 1) [19].

One of the most popular methods for treating such complicated lesions is the intracranial stent, which has been shown to be secure and efficient in treating a variety of difficult aneurysms, including unruptured MCA aneurysms (Figures 2 and 3) [20]. However, there was ongoing confusion regarding stenting in ruptured MCA aneurysms, which raises the question of the wisdom of choosing endovascular therapy for this particular type of aneurysm. But it is noteworthy that with the development of treatment methods and expanded experience in recent years, the safety of stenting in ruptured intracranial aneurysms continued to improve.

Smaller vessels can now be stented due to significantly improved stent designs, the introduction of new technologies including intrasaccular and extrasaccular flow diverters (Figure 4), and the development of bioactive and softer coils. These innovations improved the endovascular method for treating a variety of MCA aneurysms. Even with these improvements, subarachnoid hemorrhage death rates in endovascular treatments remained high and posed a significant problem. Also, high rates of procedure complications such as intra-stent thrombosis have been reported in the stent-assisted coiling method [20, 21].

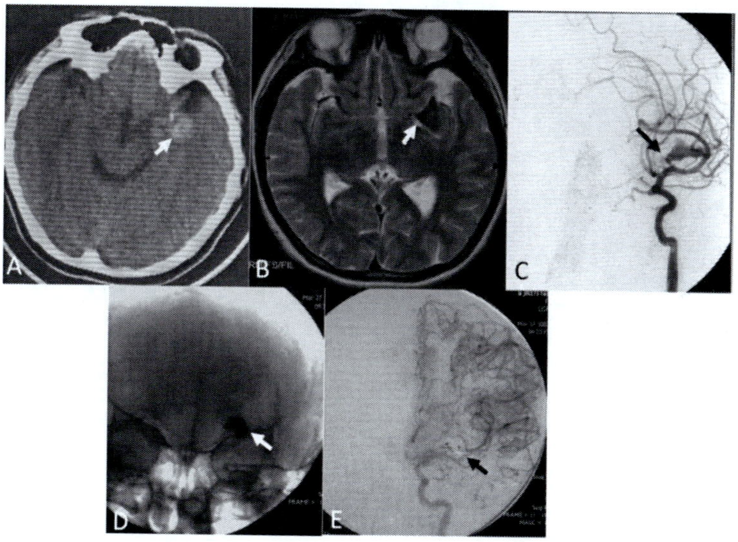

Figure 1. A 15-year-old girl presented with headaches and weakness of the right arm. A, cranial CT scanning showing a large hypertensive mass in the left Sylvian fissure (arrow). B, T2-weighted MR imaging showing a large thrombosed mass in the left Sylvian fissure (arrow). C, oblique view of the left internal carotid artery injection showing a large dissecting aneurysm of a middle cerebral artery branch (arrow). D, unsubtracted image showing the aneurysm and the parent branch of the middle cerebral artery were both occluded with GDCs (arrow). E. frontal view of the left internal carotid artery injection showing the aneurysm and the parent arterial branch were both occluded (arrow). (Courtesy Dr. Xianli Lv M.D. Assoicate Professor Neurosurgery, Department Beijing Tsinghua Changgung Hospital, School of Clinical Medicine, Tsinghua University, Beijing, China).

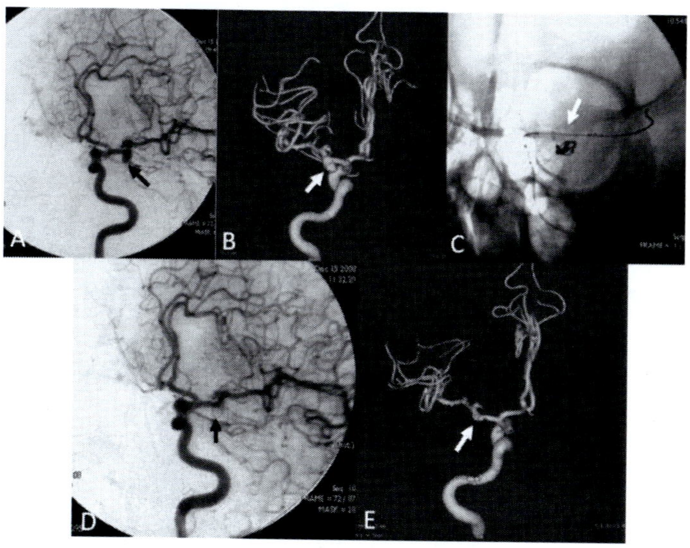

Figure 2. A 48-year-old man presented with an unruptured aneurysm of the middle cerebral artery. A, oblique view of the left internal carotid artery injection showing a M1 segment aneurysm of the middle cerebral artery (arrow). B, 3-D reconstruction of the left internal carotid artery injection showing a 4 mm × 5 mm M1 segment aneurysm of the middle cerebral artery (arrow). C, frontal view of the unsubtracted image showing the aneurysm was treated with 2.5 mm × 15 mm Neuroform stent and coils (arrow). D, oblique view of the left internal carotid artery injection after treatment showing complete occlusion the aneurysm (arrow). E, 3-D reconstruction of the left internal carotid artery after treatment showing complete disappearance of the aneurysm (arrow). (Courtesy Dr. Xianli Lv M.D. Assoicate Professor Neurosurgery, Department Beijing Tsinghua Changgung Hospital, School of Clinical Medicine, Tsinghua University, Beijing, China).

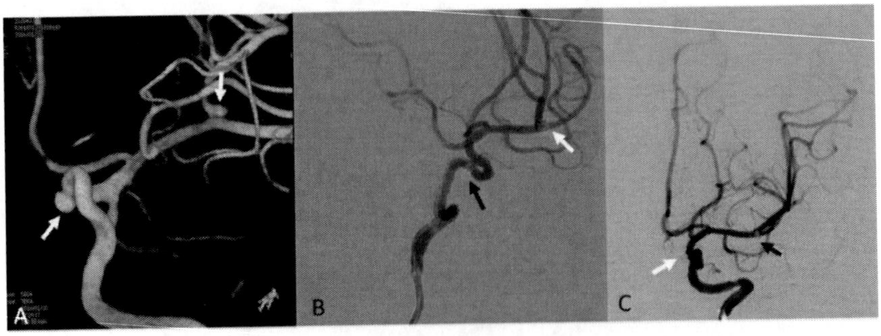

Figure 3. A 45-year-old woman presented with 2 incidental cerebral aneurysms. A, 3-D reconstruction of the left internal carotid artery injection showing 2 aneurysm arising from the middle cerebral artery bifurcation and paraclinoid segment of internal carotid artery (arrows), which were treated with Solitaire AB stents and coils. B, the oblique view of the left internal carotid artery injection showing the Solitaire AB stents and the coil mass (arrows). C, frontal view of the left internal carotid artery injection after coiling showing the 2 aneurysms were occluded completely (arrows). (Courtesy Dr. Xianli Lv M.D. Assoicate Professor Neurosurgery, Department Beijing Tsinghua Changgung Hospital, School of Clinical Medicine, Tsinghua University, Beijing, China).

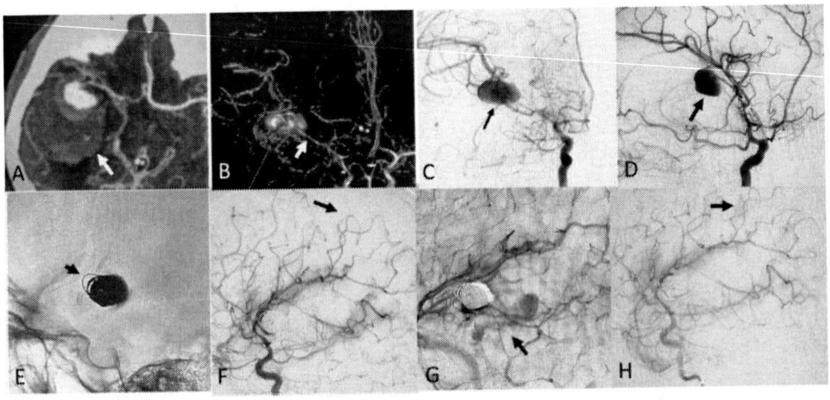

Figure 4. A 28-year-old female had a sudden headache on the the fourth day after delivery. A, enhanced CT scan of the head showed an intracerebral hematoma in the right temporal lobe (arrow). B, CTA showed a giant aneurysm in the M3 segment of the right middle cerebral artery (arrow). The right internal carotid artery angiography, frontal(C) and lateral (D), showed a giant aneurysm in the M3 segment of the right middle cerebral artery. E, non-subtraction image, lateral view, showed flow diverter device and coil mass (arrow). F, postoperative right internal carotid artery angiography showed a slower blood flow of the distal middle cerebral artery (arrow). Slowly inject 7cc 5% tirofiban through a guiding catheter for treatment. F, the right internal carotid artery angiography showed contrast agent exudation at the dome of the aneurysm (arrow). G, after compressing the right internal carotid artery for 5 minutes, another right internal carotid artery angiography showed the disappearance of the aneurysm and the contrast agent leakage, and the blood flow of the distal middle cerebral artery was normal. The patient did not present neurological deficits after treatment. (Courtesy Dr. Xianli Lv M.D. Assoicate Professor Neurosurgery, Department Beijing Tsinghua Changgung Hospital, School of Clinical Medicine, Tsinghua University, Beijing, China).

The Low-profile Visualized Intraluminal Support (LVIS) and Neuroform Atlas devices are novel, closed-cell, self-expanding, single-wire braided, nickel-titanium stents that can be used in complex ruptured aneurysms including aneurysms with wide necks such as MCA [22]. It seems that they provide superior aneurysm neck coverage and side-branch protection, as well as higher metal coverage rates [22]. Better clinical and angiographic outcomes for complex lesions treated with this method have been reported in several recent studies. There are, however, still few reports on its application in the management of ruptured MCA aneurysms. A recent retrospective study including 40 patients with ruptured MCA aneurysms using LVIS stents concluded that it is a safe and effective method as 91,7% of aneurysms occluded and there was a low rate of procedure complications [23].

Clipping versus Coiling of Ruptured MCA Aneurysms

Even today the treatment of ruptured MCA aneurysms remains controversial [24]. There are two methods that can be used: endovascular with coiling and surgical with clipping. In most neurosurgical centers in the world, a "coiling first" tendency has been adopted, although the decision for clipping or coiling depends on several factors [25].

The factors that favor clipping are:

- Young age
- Presence of ICH
- Middle Cerebral Artery (MCA)
- Pericallosal aneurysm
- Wide neck of the aneurysm

On the other hand, the factors that favor coiling are:

- Age above 70 years
- Not presenting ICH
- Posterior circulation aneurysms
- Small aneurysms neck
- Unilobar aneurysm shape

In most centers, MCA aneurysms are treated with surgical clipping in contrast to the treatment of most posterior circulation aneurysms which endovascular treatment has many advantages. Data from our university hospital of Ioannina during the period of 2000 to 2010 showed that 13 ruptured MCA aneurysms were treated surgically and there were no cases with post-operative rebleeding, stenosis or occlusion of the parent arteries. The same data showed also that there was no regrowth in follow-up images acquired more than 1 year after surgery. The endovascular approach to this area is so difficult because of the complex branching pattern of the MCA. Also, the anatomical features of this type of aneurysm include a wide neck and more than one M2 branches into the neck of the MCA aneurysm, so it is considered a contraindication for endovascular treatment [24]. The location of MCA permits easy access during surgery because minimal frontal and temporal lobe retraction can be performed [26].

Till now there are no Randomized Controlled Trials (RCTs) comparing surgical to endovascular approaches for ruptured MCA aneurysms, especially in MCA bifurcation which is the most common area of MCA aneurysms [27]. Most of the comparisons are in retrospective or prospective studies. The first study comparing the two methods was the International Subarachnoid Aneurysm Trial (ISAT) in 2002 [28]. The study showed the superiority of coiling in comparison with clipping, although MCA aneurysms are underrepresented. Only in this subgroup of aneurysms seemed clipping had better outcomes than the endovascular approach. In a single-center series including 38 patients with MCA ruptured aneurysms, surgical treatment had comparable results to coiling. Clipping seemed to be a cheaper and more durable treatment. Although the endovascular approach was more complex, more expensive, and not durable. Also, it has a limitation if there is intracerebral hematoma [29].

In other case series including 90 patients showed that both methods were good alternatives, although complications and retreatment percentages were higher but not statistically significant in the coiling group [30]. Moreover, Taha MM et al. conclude that surgical treatment is as safe as endovascular, although long-term outcomes should be evaluated [31]. It is well mentioned that these case series may suffer from many biases. Last but not least, in the most recent multicenter study including 411 patients clipping was better than coiling in short- and long-term occlusion rates of MCA aneurysms, although surgery was as safe as an endovascular approach [32].

Approximately 44% of ruptured MCA aneurysms present with intracerebral hemorrhage (ICH). A large ICH (>50ml) can cause a significant mass effect so surgical evacuation and clipping is the proffered treatment. Studies have shown that evacuation within 3,5 hours has better outcomes [27]. Also, the study of Zijlstra IA et al. which compare the role of hematoma volume in patients with ruptured MCA aneurysms showed that neurological presentation in the admission and not large hematoma associated with poor outcomes. The neurological presentation was more important than hematoma volume for the decision for decompressive surgery [12].

Conclusion

MCA aneurysms are among the most frequent intracranial aneurysms, with bifurcation being the most common site. Their rupture is frequent resulting not only in SAH but also in intracerebral hemorrhage. For the diagnosis of the ruptured aneurysms commonly used radiological examinations are CT, CTA, MRA or DSA. Even though in most centers surgical options are chosen, there are efforts to develop new endovascular methods to treat even complex aneurysms avoiding a surgery.

Conflict of Interest

None.

Funding

None.

References

[1] Rinkel GJ, Djibuti M, Algra A, van Gijn J. Prevalence and risk of rupture of intracranial aneurysms: a systematic review. *Stroke*. 1998 Jan;29(1):251-6. doi: 10.1161/01.str.29.1.251. PMID: 9445359.

[2] Neyazi B, Siblini A, Frantsev R, Özkan N, Sandalcioglu IE, Sure U, Maslehaty H. The role of the Sylvian fissure configuration and the vascular anatomy on different bleeding patterns in ruptured middle cerebral artery aneurysms. Clin *Neurol Neurosurg*. 2020 Feb;189:105572. doi: 10.1016/j.clineuro.2019.105572. Epub 2019 Oct 31. PMID: 31786430.

[3] Ulm AJ, Fautheree GL, Tanriover N, Russo A, Albanese E, Rhoton AL Jr, Mericle RA, Lewis SB. Microsurgical and angiographic anatomy of middle cerebral artery aneurysms: prevalence and significance of early branch aneurysms. *Neurosurgery*. 2008 May;62(5 Suppl 2):ONS344-52; discussion ONS352-3. doi: 10.1227/01.neu.0000326018.22434.ed. PMID: 18596514.

[4] Heros RC, Fritsch MJ. Surgical management of middle cerebral artery aneurysms. *Neurosurgery*. 2001 Apr;48(4):780-5; discussion 785-6. doi: 10.1097/00006123-200104000-00017. PMID: 11322438.

[5] Steiger HJ, Etminan N, Hänggi D. Aneurysms of the Middle Cerebral Artery. In: *Microsurgical Brain Aneurysms* [Internet]. Berlin, Heidelberg: Springer Berlin Heidelberg; 2015 [cited 2023 Jan 10]. p. 81–9. Available from: http://link.springer.com/10.1007/978-3-662-45679-8_7.

[6] Washington CW, Ju T, Zipfel GJ, Dacey RG Jr. Middle cerebral artery bifurcation aneurysms: an anatomic classification scheme for planning optimal surgical strategies. *Neurosurgery*. 2014 Mar;10 Suppl 1:145-53; discussion 153-5. doi: 10.1227/NEU.0000000000000250. PMID: 24226424.

[7] Steiner T, Juvela S, Unterberg A, Jung C, Forsting M, Rinkel G; European Stroke Organization. European Stroke Organization guidelines for the management of intracranial aneurysms and subarachnoid haemorrhage. *Cerebrovasc Dis*. 2013;35(2):93-112. doi: 10.1159/000346087. Epub 2013 Feb 7. PMID: 23406828.

[8] Cianfoni A, Pravatà E, De Blasi R, Tschuor CS, Bonaldi G. Clinical presentation of cerebral aneurysms. *Eur J Radiol*. 2013 Oct;82(10):1618-22.

[9] Stapleton CJ, Walcott BP, Fusco MR, Butler WE, Thomas AJ, Ogilvy CS. Surgical management of ruptured middle cerebral artery aneurysms with large intraparenchymal or sylvian fissure hematomas. *Neurosurgery*. 2015;76(3):258–264.

[10] Li Z, Hu Q, Zhao L, Huang H, Zhang S, Zheng L, Wang G. Case Report: Ruptured Middle Cerebral Artery Aneurysm With Intrasylvian Hematoma Successfully Treated by Coil Embolization and Minimally Invasive Puncture and Drainage. *Front Neurol*. 2021 Jun 21;12:646990. doi: 10.3389/fneur.2021.646990. PMID: 34234732; PMCID: PMC8256150.

[11] Subarachnoid haemorrhage caused by a ruptured aneurysm: diagnosis and management. London: *National Institute for Health and Care Excellence (NICE)*; 2022 Nov 23. PMID: 36753576.

[12] Zijlstra IA, van der Steen WE, Verbaan D, Majoie CB, Marquering HA, Coert BA, Vandertop WP, van den Berg R. Ruptured middle cerebral artery aneurysms with a concomitant intraparenchymal hematoma: the role of hematoma volume. *Neuroradiology*. 2018 Mar;60(3):335-342. doi: 10.1007/s00234-018-1978-4. Epub 2018 Jan 22. PMID: 29356856; PMCID: PMC5799354.

[13] Cherian, J., & Barrow, D. L. (2022). Surgical Management of Middle Cerebral Artery Aneurysms [Review of Surgical Management of Middle Cerebral Artery Aneurysms]. In *Youmans and Winn Neurological Surgery*. Elsevier.

[14] Pavesi, G., Nasi, D., Moriconi, E. et al. Management and safety of intraoperative ventriculostomy during early surgery for ruptured intracranial aneurysms. *Acta Neurochir* 164, 2909–2916 (2022). https://doi.org/10.1007/s00701-022-05346-z.

[15] Ogilvy CS, Crowell RM, Heros RC. Surgical management of middle cerebral artery aneurysms: experience with transsylvian and superior temporal gyrus approaches. *Surg Neurol*. 1995 Jan;43(1):15-22; discussion 22-4. doi: 10.1016/0090-3019(95)80032-c. PMID: 7701417.

[16] Seibert B, Tummala RP, Chow R, Faridar A, Mousavi SA, Divani AA. Intracranial aneurysms: review of current treatment options and outcomes. *Front Neurol*. 2011 Jul 8;2:45. doi: 10.3389/fneur.2011.00045. PMID: 21779274; PMCID: PMC3134887.

[17] Elsharkawy A, Niemelä M, Lehečka M, Lehto H, Jahromi BR, Goehre F, Kivisaari R, Hernesniemi J. Focused opening of the sylvian fissure for microsurgical management of MCA aneurysms. *Acta*

Neurochir (Wien). 2014 Jan;156(1):17-25. doi: 10.1007/s00701-013-1894-7. Epub 2013 Oct 8. PMID: 24101289.

[18] Chyatte D, Porterfield R. Nuances of middle cerebral artery aneurysm microsurgery. *Neurosurgery*. 2001 Feb;48(2):339-46. doi: 10.1097/00006123-200102000-00020. PMID: 11220377.

[19] Mooney MA, Simon ED, Brigeman S, Nakaji P, Zabramski JM, Lawton MT, et al. Long-term results of middle cerebral artery aneurysm clipping in the barrow ruptured aneurysm trial. *J Neurosurg*. (2018) 130:895– 901. doi: 10.3171/2017.10.JNS172183.

[20] Zhou Y, Yang PF, Li Q, Zhao R, Fang YB, Xu Y, et al. Stent placement for complex middle cerebral artery aneurysms. *J Stroke Cerebrovasc Dis*. (2014) 23:1447–56. doi: 10.1016/j.jstrokecerebrovasdis. 2013.12.054.

[21] Zhao X, Li Z, Fang X, Liu J, Wu D, Lai N. Treatment of ruptured middle cerebral artery aneurysms by endovascular approach: a single-center experience. *Int J Neurosci*. (2017) 127:433–8. doi: 10.1080/ 00207454.2016.1190923.

[22] Fiorella D, Boulos A, Turk AS, Siddiqui AH, Arthur AS, Diaz O, Lopes DK; LVIS investigators. The safety and effectiveness of the LVIS stent system for the treatment of wide-necked cerebral aneurysms: final results of the pivotal US LVIS trial. *J Neurointerv Surg*. 2019 Apr;11(4):357-361. doi: 10.1136/neurintsurg-2018-014309. Epub 2018 Oct 8. PMID: 30297543; PMCID: PMC6582711.

[23] Xue G, Zhou Y, Liu P, Zuo Q, Yang P, Fang Y, Li Q, Zhao R, Xu Y, Hong B, Huang Q, Liu J. Endovascular Treatment of Ruptured Middle Cerebral Artery Aneurysms With a Low-Profile Visualized Intraluminal Support Device. *Front Neurol*. 2021 Jan 28;11:631745. doi: 10.3389/fneur. 2020.631745. PMID: 33584524; PMCID: PMC7876053.

[24] Marcos Dellaretti, Leyzeane Marques do Nascimento, Alan Douglas de Oliveira Lima, Julio Cesar de Almeida, Ricardo Souza Quadros, Efficacy and safety of surgical treatment for middle cerebral artery aneurysms: A retrospective case series, *Interdisciplinary Neurosurgery*, Volume 23,2021,101018, ISSN 2214-7519.

[25] Jeong HW, Seo JH, Kim ST, Jung CK, Suh SI. Clinical practice guideline for the management of intracranial aneurysms. *Neurointervention*. 2014 Sep;9(2):63-71. doi: 10.5469/neuroint.2014.9.2.63. Epub 2014 Sep 3. PMID: 25426300; PMCID: PMC4239410.

[26] Yang, W., Huang, J. Treatment of middle cerebral artery (MCA) aneurysms: a review of the literature. *Chin Neurosurg Jl* 1, 1 (2015). https://doi.org/10.1186/s41016-015-0001-8.

[27] Santiago-Dieppa DR, Pannell JS, Khalessi AA. Endovascular and surgical options for ruptured middle cerebral artery aneurysms: review of the literature. *Stroke Res Treat*. 2014;2014:315906. doi: 10.1155/2014/315906. Epub 2014 Jul 6. PMID: 25097795; PMCID: PMC4109112.

[28] Molyneux A, Kerr R, Stratton I, Sandercock P, Clarke M, Shrimpton J, Holman R; International Subarachnoid Aneurysm Trial (ISAT) Collaborative Group. International Subarachnoid Aneurysm Trial (ISAT) of neurosurgical clipping versus endovascular coiling in 2143 patients with ruptured intracranial aneurysms: a randomised trial. *Lancet*. 2002 Oct 26;360(9342):1267-74. doi: 10.1016/s0140-6736(02)11314-6. PMID: 12414200.

[29] Mohamed Shadad, MD., M. A. M., ABD El-Hameed, MD., E. (2019). 'Ruptured Middle Cerebral Artery Aneurysms: A Single-Center Series Evaluating Microsurgical and Endovascular Treatment', *The Medical Journal of Cairo University*, 87(March), pp. 753-762. doi: 10.21608/mjcu.2019.52533.

[30] Diaz OM, Rangel-Castilla L, Barber S, Mayo RC, Klucznik R, Zhang YJ. Middle cerebral artery aneurysms: a single-center series comparing endovascular and surgical treatment. *World Neurosurg*. 2014 Feb;81(2):322-9. doi: 10.1016/j.wneu.2012.12.011. Epub 2012 Dec 11. PMID: 23238101.

[31] Taha MM, Nakahara I, Higashi T, Iwamuro Y, Iwaasa M, Watanabe Y, Tsunetoshi K, Munemitsu T. Endovascular embolization vs surgical clipping in treatment of cerebral aneurysms: morbidity and mortality with short-term outcome. *Surg Neurol*. 2006 Sep;66(3):277-84; discussion 284. doi: 10.1016/j.surneu.2005.12.031. PMID: 16935636.

[32] Sturiale CL, Scerrati A, Ricciardi L, Rustemi O, Auricchio AM, Norri N, Piazza A, Ranieri F, Tomatis A, Albanese A, Di Egidio V, Farneti M, Mangiola A, Marchese E, Raco A, Volpin L, Trevisi G. Clipping versus coiling for treatment of middle cerebral artery aneurysms: a retrospective Italian multicenter experience. *Neurosurg Rev*. 2022 Oct;45(5):3179-3191. doi: 10.1007/s10143-022-01822-3. Epub 2022 Jun 4. PMID: 35665868; PMCID: PMC9492556.

Chapter 5

Innovative Surgical Strategy for Giant Middle Cerebral Artery Aneurysms: Avoiding Parent Artery Occlusion and Optimizing Outcome

Katsumi Takizawa*, MD
and Kapil Lotanrao Patil, MD
Department of Neurosurgery, Japanese Red Cross Asahikawa Hospital, Asahikawa, Hokkaido, Japan

Abstract

This text presents a case report on the surgical management of a ruptured giant middle cerebral artery (MCA) aneurysm, highlighting the challenges associated with its complex anatomy and the potential complications of conventional treatment approaches. The authors describe an alternative technique utilizing a modified superficial temporal artery-middle cerebral artery (STA-MCA) bypass procedure to overcome these limitations. The modified approach offers advantages such as enhanced maneuverability, utilization of the upper M1 stump for suction decompression, and modification of aneurysm morphology. The technical nuances of the bypass procedure, including meticulous preparations, donor vessel handling, anastomosis techniques, temporary clip removal, and confirmation of success, are discussed in detail. By adopting this innovative technique, the authors aim to optimize surgical outcomes and minimize the risk of ischemic neuronal damage while managing giant MCA aneurysms.

Keywords: surgical strategy, giant, middle cerebral artery, aneurysm

Introduction

Giant middle cerebral artery aneurysms present unique challenges in their surgical management due to their complex anatomy, high risk of rupture, and potential ischemic complications. Surgical intervention is a critical treatment option aimed at preventing rupture, alleviating mass effects, and restoring normal blood flow in the affected vessel. This Chapter provides an

* Corresponding Author's Email: ktaki0820ktaki@gmail.com.

In: Understanding and Managing Cerebral Aneurysms
Editor: Xianli Lv
ISBN: 979-8-89113-608-3

overview of the surgical treatment option we used for giant MCA aneurysms, focusing on techniques to avoid parent artery occlusion.

Surgical management of giant MCA aneurysms involves various approaches, including direct clipping, revascularization procedures, and combination strategies. Direct clipping entails placing a clip across the aneurysm neck to isolate it from normal blood flow. This technique is particularly effective for aneurysms with a wide neck or involving multiple vessels. However, successful clipping and preservation of nearby vessels require meticulous surgical planning and intraoperative decision-making [1].

Revascularization procedures are often employed when direct clipping is not feasible due to the aneurysm's location or complex anatomy. These procedures involve redirecting blood flow through bypass grafts to bypass the aneurysm and restore normal circulation. Superficial temporal artery-middle cerebral artery (STA-MCA) bypass or extracranial-intracranial (EC-IC) bypass is among the techniques used to treat giant MCA aneurysms, facilitating aneurysm exclusion and revascularization of the affected area [2].

Advancements in surgical techniques and technology have expanded the treatment options for giant MCA aneurysms. Intraoperative neurovascular imaging, such as indocyanine green video angiography and intraoperative angiography, enables real-time visualization of blood flow and vessel patency during surgery, enhancing decision-making and improving outcomes. Additionally, using neuro endoscopic-assisted procedures and intraoperative neuronavigation enhances surgical precision and safety.

While surgical treatment of giant MCA aneurysms is technically demanding and carries inherent risks, studies have reported favorable outcomes in terms of aneurysm obliteration rates and patient functional recovery. However, it is important to note that individual patient characteristics, aneurysm morphology, and surgical team expertise significantly influence outcomes [3].

In conclusion, surgical intervention remains a crucial treatment option for giant MCA aneurysms, offering the potential for aneurysm obliteration, restoration of blood flow, and prevention of rupture-related complications. Ongoing advancements in surgical techniques, intraoperative imaging, and adjunctive technologies continue to improve outcomes and expand the possibilities for the successful management of these complex vascular pathologies. Further research and long-term follow-up studies are necessary to refine surgical strategies and optimize patient outcomes.

Case Report

A 67-year-old male patient presented with a complaint of a sudden onset headache and weakness in the left upper and lower limbs. In the emergency department, a CT brain with an angiogram revealed a subarachnoid hemorrhage caused by a ruptured giant right middle cerebral artery aneurysm (Figure 1). The aneurysm was bilobed, with three outflow arteries arising from its wall.

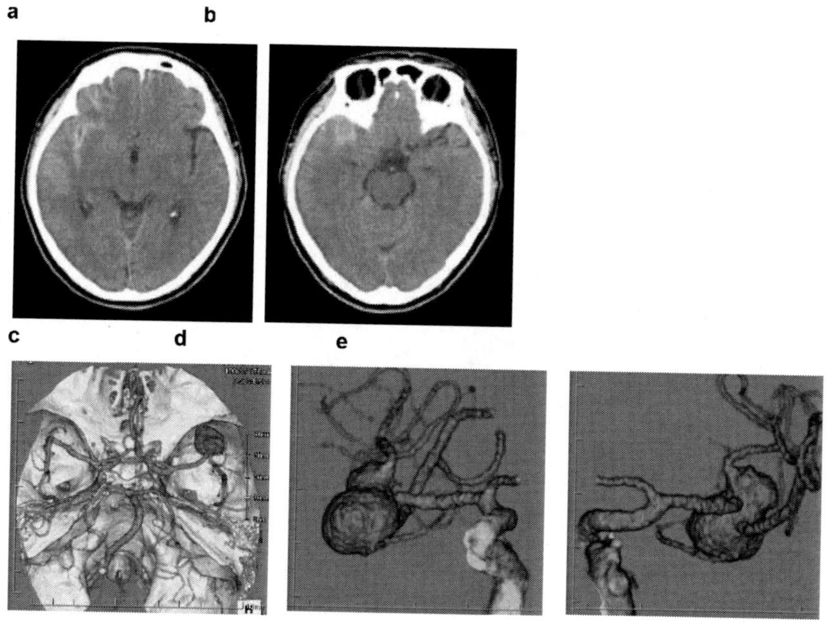

Figure 1. a,b. Non-enhanced CT brain showed subarachnoid hemorrhage along right sylvian fissure .c,d,e. Three-dimensional CT reconstruction shows a bilobed giant right middle cerebral artery aneurysm.

Surgical Treatment

The available treatment options for such an aneurysm include revascularization, clipping of the aneurysm, and/or trapping. For revascularization, the proposed approach is a double barrel STA to MCA bypass (Figure 2).

To avoid parent artery occlusion, a modification was devised. After dissecting the aneurysm and identifying its inflow and outflow, along with the relative anatomy of the perforators intraoperatively, the author decided to perform a STA-MCA bypass (one M2). Additionally, the aneurysm wall was refashioned by applying clips in such a way that blood would be channeled into a remaining branch of the MCA. This approach offers the advantage of freedom of movement for inspection all around, ensuring a proper assessment of the perforators and completeness of occlusion after clip application. In case of any doubt about the progression of the aneurysm, stenting can be considered as an option for further management.

In our technique, we made modifications at the following steps:

1. Instead of performing two STA-MCA bypasses, we performed a single bypass.
2. We utilized suction decompression.
3. We restructured the aneurysm using clip application.

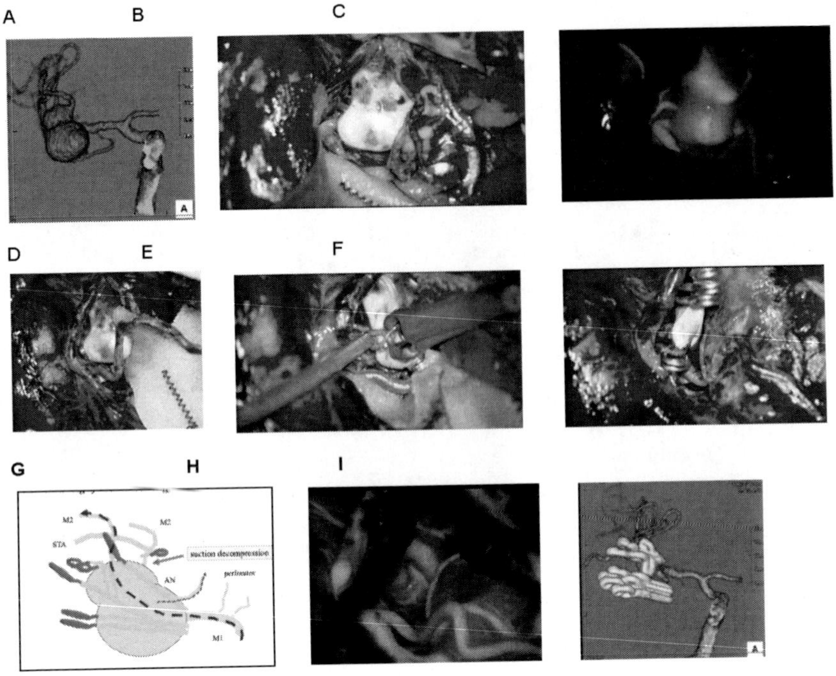

Figure 2. Schematic representation and intraoperative images of clipping and revascularization. A .3D reconstruction of CT angiogram showing internal carotid artery, Anterior cerebral artery, and middle cerebral artery with bilobed aneurysm with inflow and outflow vessels along with perforators. B. intraoperative image of an aneurysm and upper branch M2. C. intraoperative ICG angiography before clipping . D. STA-M2 (upper trunk) bypass. E. suction decompression using upper M2 stump after bypass. F. clip application to reconstruct aneurysm wall for the formation of channel connecting M1 and lower M2. G. schematic representation of surgery strategy. H. ICG angiography post clipping. I. 3D reconstruction demonstrating post-operative CT angiogram.

Technical Nuance of the Bypass Procedure

1. *Preparations:*
   a. Meticulously set up the surgical area using gel foam sheets soaked in a fibrin solution to create an optimal environment.
   b. Avoid the use of cottonoids as they can interfere with the suturing process.
2. *Donor Vessel Preparation:*
   a. Secure the donor vessel precisely with a temporary clip while maintaining its structural integrity.
   b. Flush the vessel with a saline solution containing heparin to minimize residual blood and prevent clot formation.
   c. Implement two 10-0 nylon sutures to secure the heel and toe ends of the vessel meticulously before applying clips on the recipient vessel.
   d. Strategically place the needles in gel foam for easy accessibility and efficiency.
3. *Anastomosis:*
   a. Begin the anastomosis by meticulously suturing the vessels together, starting from the heel end and progressing systematically.

   b. Employ meticulous surgical technique using 10-0 nylon sutures for precise and secure attachment of the vessel walls.
   c. Place intermittent sutures strategically to establish a durable and effective connection between the walls of the donor and recipient vessels.
   d. Ensure meticulous alignment during suturing, directing the sutures from the donor vessel to the recipient vessel.
   e. Evert the suture edge and ensure proper contact between the intima of the donor and recipient vessels.
4. *Temporary Clip Removal:*
   a. Sequentially and controllably remove the temporary clips to restore blood flow progressively.
   b. Begin by removing the clip on the recipient vessel's outflow, followed by the clip on the recipient vessel's inflow, and conclude with the removal of the clip on the donor vessel.
5. *Addressing Bleeding:*
   a. Employ meticulous management techniques to address any minor bleeding that may occur during the procedure.
   b. Utilize gel foam and fibrin glue as effective hemostatic agents to control bleeding and promote clot formation, minimizing the risk of complications.
6. *Confirmation of Success:*
   a. Utilize advanced imaging modalities such as indocyanine green (ICG) video angiography and Doppler studies to objectively assess the success of the bypass procedure.
   b. Visualize and evaluate blood flow within the newly connected vessels to provide objective evidence of a successful bypass.

The Procedure with Advantages to Overcome Limitations and Complication

In our case, we encountered a bilobed aneurysm with three outflow vessels. However, the conventional approach of double barrel anastomosis and trapping presents certain limitations, including the potential for thrombotic occlusion, occlusion of perforators, challenges in confirming the proximal M1 segment, difficulties in clip application, and limited applicability of endovascular techniques.

To overcome these limitations, we employed an alternative strategy. We performed a bypass anastomosis utilizing the superficial temporal artery (STA) with the upper M2 segment.

Advantages of this Approach

1. Enhanced maneuverability: By disconnecting the upper M2 segment, we achieved improved maneuverability, facilitating thorough examination of the aneurysm and its underlying structures. This provided enhanced visualization of the inflow M1 vessel

and the relative positions of the remaining outflow tracts. As a result, we were able to meticulously remodel the aneurysm wall using various clips.

2. Utilization of the upper M1 stump: The upper M2 stump was utilized for suction decompression, affording an additional advantage during the procedure.
3. Modification of aneurysm morphology: By altering the morphology from a bifurcation type to a side wall type, we gained an additional advantage, particularly in terms of facilitating the clip application and the potential utilization of endovascular techniques.

By adopting this alternative approach, our objective was to address the limitations associated with double barrel anastomosis and trapping, while maximizing the procedural benefits and optimizing the feasibility of doing surgical treatment without much-compromising outflow tract leading to ischemic neuronal damage.

Conclusion

Surgical intervention remains a crucial treatment option for giant MCA aneurysms, offering the potential for aneurysm obliteration, restoration of blood flow, and prevention of rupture-related complications. Ongoing advancements in surgical techniques, intraoperative imaging, and adjunctive technologies continue to improve outcomes and expand the possibilities for the successful management of these complex vascular pathologies. Further research and long-term follow-up studies are necessary to refine surgical strategies and optimize patient outcomes.

References

[1] Lawton MT, Spetzler RF. Surgical management of giant intracranial aneurysms: experience with 171 patients. *Clin Neurosurg*. 2005;52:282-294. PMID: 16626069.

[2] Horiuchi T, Tanaka Y, Hongo K. Surgical management of giant middle cerebral artery aneurysms. *Acta Neurochir Suppl*. 2010;107:79-85. doi: 10.1007/978-3-211-99370-5_15.

[3] McDougall CG, Spetzler RF, Zabramski JM, et al. The barrow ruptured aneurysm trial: 6-year results. *J Neurosurg*. 2013;119(1):135-143. doi: 10.3171/2013.3.JNS12683.

Chapter 6

The Characteristics, Embolization Techniques, and Treatment Results in Saccular Aneurysm with the Middle Cerebral Artery

Baorui Zhang[1,*], MD
Wei Wang[1,†], MD
Shangfeng Zhao[1], MD
Dapeng Mo[2], MD
Zhongxue Wu[2], MD
Aihua Liu[2], MD
Jun Kang[1], MD
and Xianli Lv[3], MD
[1]Department of Neurosurgery, Beijing Tongren Hospital, Capital Medical University, Beijing, China
[2]Department of Neurovascular Surgery, Beijing Tiantan Hospital, Capital Medical University, Beijing, China
[3]Department of Neurosurgery, Beijing Tsinghua Changgung Hospital, School of Clinical Medicine Tsinghua University, Beijing, China

Abstract

This study aimed to analyze the characteristics, embolization techniques, and treatment outcomes in saccular aneurysm of the middle cerebral artery (MCA). Retrospective analysis of data from consecutive MCA saccular aneurysm patients who underwent embolization treatment at three neurosurgical centers from January 2016 to January 2021. The outcomes include thromboembolic and hemorrhagic complications, angiographic outcomes and neurological complications. The hemorrhagic and thromboembolic complications were 5/208 (2.40%) and 9/208 (4.33%) during the procedure, respectively, and 2/208 (0.96%) and 3/208 (1.44%) within 30 days. The major events (mRS>2) occurred in 3/208 (1.44%) during the procedure, and 2/208 (0.96%) within 30 days. The rate of complete embolization and neck remnant of aneurysms was 88.5% initially, 90.4% at 6-12

* Corresponding Author's Email: zhangbaorui927@163.com
† Corresponding Author's Email: ww_1498@163.com.

In: Understanding and Managing Cerebral Aneurysms
Editor: Xianli Lv
ISBN: 979-8-89113-608-3

months, and 92.1% at >12 months. The rates of neurological complication were 6.73%, 1.92%, 2.88%, 1.92%, and 1.44% at initial, 1 month, 6 months, 12 months, and 24 months, respectively. Traditional embolization techniques provide a feasible option for endovascular treatment of MCA saccular aneurysms. Even in the era of flow diverting stents and Woven EndoBridge (WEB), traditional embolization techniques are still not outdated.

Keywords: characteristics, embolization, embolization technique, result, saccular aneurysm, middle cerebral artery, aneurysms, recanalization, complication

Abbreviations

CI	confidence interval
MCA	middle cerebral artery
mRS	modified Rankin Scale
OR	odds ratio
RS	Raymond scale
3D	three dimensional

Introduction

Embolization treatment has become an important technique for intracranial aneurysms [1]. However, endovascular treatment of middle cerebral artery (MCA) aneurysm is a controversial topic, because of the particular anatomy such as the location of branches supplying blood to the lateral cortex of the cerebral hemisphere and wide aneurysm neck [2]. Embolization treatment-related complications are serious [3]. In addition, embolization treatment of aneurysm results in a higher frequency (6.1–33.6) of recanalization than surgical clipping [4]. Several studies had indicated that permanent morbidity and mortality were 7.8% and 13.6%, respectively [5, 6]. However, the factors of neurological complications and recanalization of endovascular treatment of MCA aneurysm remained unclear, and the effect of stent-assisted coiling of MCA aneurysms was unknown. Therefore, this study aimed to evaluate the safety and efficacy of embolization treatment of MCA aneurysm, explore the relative factors for neurological complications and recanalization, and evaluate the prognosis after treatment.

Materials and Methods

Patient Population

Retrospective analysis of data on consecutive patients with MCA saccular aneurysms who underwent embolization treatment at three neurosurgical centers: Beijing Tongren Hospital, Beijing Tiantan Hospital, and Beijing Tsinghua Changgung Hospital from January 2016 to January 2021. This study was approved by the ethics committee of three hospitals, and all participants provided informed consent. The exclusion criteria were (1) dissecting aneurysm, fusiform aneurysm, or mycotic aneurysm; (2) intracranial hemorrhage for unknown reasons; (3) follow-up duration <1 month; and (4) aneurysm associated with arteriovenous malformations, arteriovenous fistulas, and moyamoya disease. The patients characteristics included age, sex, hypertension, smoking status, alcohol use, and diabetes mellitus were collected. And aneurysm characteristics included size, wide neck, location (M1, Mbif, Mdist) [7].

Complications and Outcomes

Any thromboembolic and hemorrhagic complications that occurred from treatment and one month or more after treatment were documented. Intraoperative thromboembolic complications include slow filling of blood vessel, thrombus formation, or blood vessel non-filling. Postoperative thromboembolic complications include signs or symptoms of thromboembolism and postoperative imaging for ischemia could comprised computed tomography and/or magnetic resonance imaging.

Intraprocedural contrast extravasation or on postoperative blood on imaging were considered hemorrhagic complications. Those which occurred from the procedure through to follow-up were included and were considered symptomatic if there were symptoms or signs felt to be hemorrhagic.

Follow-Up Outcomes

Angiogram follow-up was routinely performed in patients at 6 months 1 year, 2 years, and so on. Angiographic outcome using digital subtraction angiography (DSA), magnetic resonance angiography (MRA), or computed tomography angiography (CTA) were all considered as available. Aneurysmal occlusion was evaluated with Raymond scale (RS) score (RS1/RS2/RS3; RS1 indicates complete occlusion; RS2, neck remnant; RS3, residual aneurysm) [8]. Aneurysm recanalization was defined as any increase in aneurysmal filling at follow-up [9].

The modified Rankin Scale (mRS) was used to evaluate the functional outcome. The major event was defined as functional outcome with a mRS>2. Neurological complications were defined as changes in neurological status (Compared to preoperative, with an increasing mRS score) through telephone interviews at 1 month, 6 months, 12 months, and 24 months.

Procedure

For patients treated with stent-assisted coiling, dual-antiplatelet therapy (100 mg/d aspirin and 75 mg/d clopidogrel) was administered for unruptured aneurysms at least 3 to 5 days prior to the procedure, and a loading dose of 300 mg aspirin and 300 mg clopidogrel was given for ruptured aneurysms at least 2 hours prior to the procedure.

General anesthesia was used in all patients. After arterial sheath was placed in the femoral artery, systemic heparinization was started with a loading dose of 3000 IU and was maintained with a dose of 1000 IU on an hourly basis. A suitable working projection was determined by 3D rotational angiography. Inside the guiding catheters, microcatheters with proper shapes were introduced over microguidewires and navigated into the aneurysms. After the procedure, the patients were administered clopidogrel (75 mg/d) for 4 to 6 weeks and aspirin (100 mg/d) for at least 6 months.

If wide-neck aneurysm was >4 mm, dome/neck was >2, or coiling alone was difficult, the stent-assisted coiling was performed.

Statistical Analysis

The baseline variables were compared between groups using the $\chi 2$ test or Fisher's exact test for categorical variables. Categorical data are presented as proportions. All data in this study were analyzed using SPSS software (IBM SPSS version 22.0, Armonk, NY, USA). A P-value of <0.05 was considered as statistically significant.

Results

Patient and Aneurysm Characteristics

A total of 208 MCA saccular aneurysms including 56 ruptured aneurysms and 152 unruptured aneurysms were treated with embolization treatment. The basic characteristics of patients with MCA aneurysm are showed in Table 1. There were no differences in sex, age, hypertension, smoking status, alcohol use, hyperlipidemia, diabetes mellitus.

Coiling alone, stent-assisted coiling, and other were performed in 104 (50.0%), 100 (47.6%), and four (1.9%) aneurysms, respectively. Ruptured MCA aneurysms were with higher rate of coiling-alone (Figure 1).

Table 1. The basic Characteristics of patients with MCA aneurysm

Characteristic	Unruptured aneurysms (n = 152)	Ruptured aneurysms (n = 56)	P value
Female	85(55.9)	25(44.6)	0.148
Age (>60 y)	68(44.7)	16(28.6)	0.035
hypertension	86(56.6)	32(57.1)	0.942
smoking status	33(31.7)	13(23.2)	0.817
alcohol use	33(21.7)	16(28.6)	0.301
hyperlipidemia	17(11.2)	3(5.4)	0.206
diabetes mellitus	27(17.8)	6(10.7)	0.217

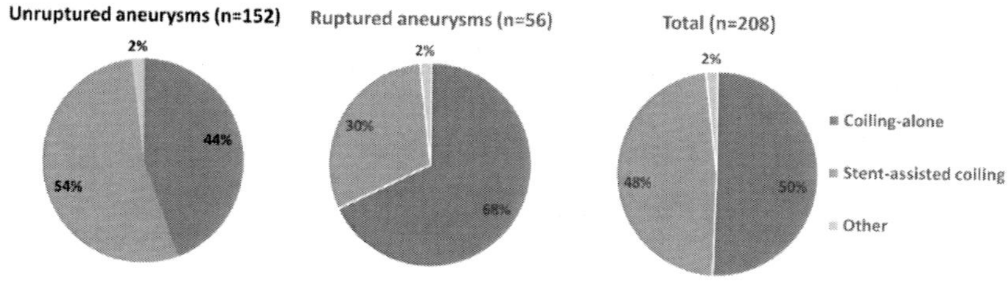

Figure 1. The embolization techniques distribution in MCA saccular aneurysms

The mean maximum aneurysm size was 7.0 mm (median, 5.5 mm; range, 2.3–37.0 mm). There was no significant difference in aneurysm size between ruptured and unruptured aneurysms (Figure 2).

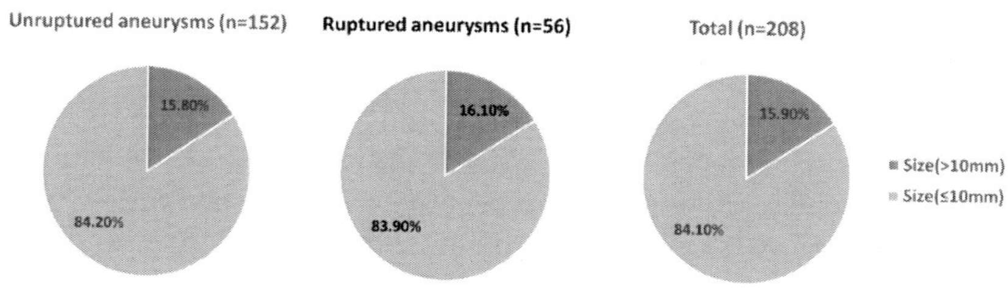

Figure 2. The aneurysm size distribution in MCA saccular aneurysms.

The mean aneurysm neck measured 4.0 mm (median, 2.5 mm; range, 1.2–13.2 mm). There was no significant difference in aneurysm neck size between ruptured and unruptured aneurysms (Figure 3).

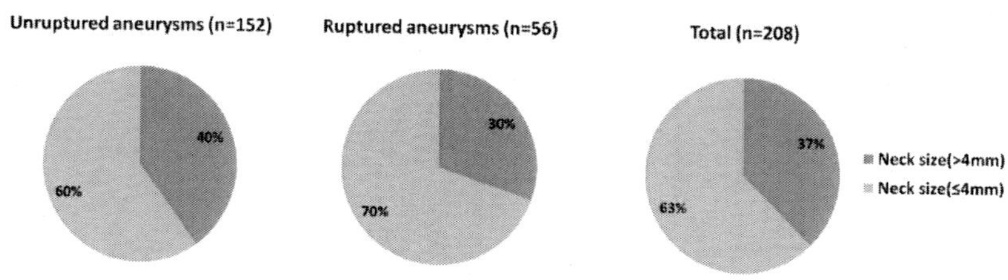

Figure 3. The aneurysm neck size distribution in MCA saccular aneurysms.

A total of 48 (23.1%), 144 (69.2%), and 16 (7.7%) aneurysms were located at the M1 segment, major bifurcation (M1–M2), and distal major bifurcation, respectively (Figure 4).

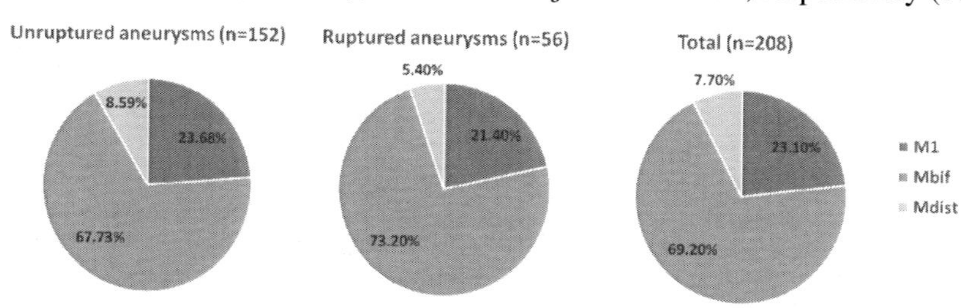

Figure 4. The aneurysm location distribution in MCA saccular aneurysms.

Treatment and Outcomes

Hemorrhagic Complications

Eleven (2.40%) aneurysms with hemorrhagic complications during the procedure, of which two (1.32%) belonged to the unruptured group and three (5.36%) in the ruptured group. Within additional 30 days, one (0.66%) aneurysm with hemorrhagic complications in unruptured group and one (1.79%) aneurysm in ruptured group.

Thromboembolic Complications

Nine (4.33%) aneurysms with thromboembolic complications during the procedure, of which six (3.95%) belonged to the unruptured group and three (5.36%) to the ruptured group. Within additional 30 days, two (1.32%) aneurysms with thromboembolic complications in unruptured group and one (1.79%) aneurysm with thromboembolic complications in ruptured group.

Major Events (mRS>2)

Three (1.44%) aneurysms with major events during the procedure, of which two (1.32%) belonged to the unruptured group and one (1.79%) in the ruptured group. Within additional 30 days, one (0.66%) aneurysm with major events in unruptured group and one (1.79%) aneurysm with major events in ruptured group.

One patient (1.79%) died in Rupture aneurysms group within additional 30 days (Table 2).

Table 2. The outcome after embolization in patients with MCA aneurysms

	Un-rupture aneurysms (n = 152)		Rupture aneurysms (n = 56)		Total (n = 208)
	procedural events	Within additional 30 days	procedural events	Within 30 additional days	
Hemorrhagic	2(1.32)	1(0.66)	3(5.36)	1(1.79)	7(3.37)
Thromboembolic	6 (3.95)	2(1.32)	3(5.36)	1(1.79)	12(5.77)
Total complication	8(5.26)	3(1.97)	6(10.71)	1(1.79)	18(8.65)
major events (mRS > 2)	2(1.32)	1(0.66)	1(1.79)	1(1.79)	5(2.40)
Mortality	0(0.00)	0(0.00)	0(0.00)	1(1.79)	1(0.48)

mRS, modified Rankin Scale.

Initial and Follow-Up Angiographic Outcomes

The complete embolization and neck remnant were achieved in 184/208 (88.5%) aneurysms at initial, 122/135 (90.4%) at 6-12 months, and 58/63 (92.1%) at >12 months after treatment. The mean time to last follow-up was 12.8 months (median, 8 months; range, 1–61 months) (Table 3).

Table 3. Ratio of aneurysm occlusion at follow-up

Raymond-Roy scale	Initial Angiogram (n = 208)	Follow-up at (6-12mo) (n = 135)	Follow-up at (>12mo) (n = 63)
RS 1	126(60.6)	96(71.1)	50 (79.4)
RS 2	58(27.9)	26(19.3)	8(12.7)
RS 3	24(11.5)	13(9 .6)	5(7.9)
RS1and RS2	184(88.5)	122(90.4)	58(92.1)

Raymond scale (RS) score, (RS1/RS2/RS3; RS1 indicates complete occlusion; RS2, neck remnant; RS3, residual aneurysm).

Neurological Complications at Follow-Up

The rates of neurological complication (compared to preoperative, with an increasing mRS score) were 6.73%, 1.92%, 2.88%, 1.92%, and 1.44% at initial, 1 month, 6 months, 12 months, and 24 months, respectively (Figure 5).

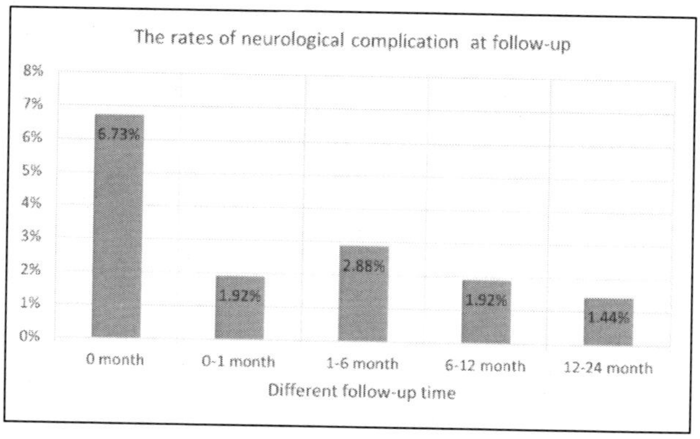

Figure 5. The neurological complications of patients with MCA aneurysm treated with embolization at follow-up.

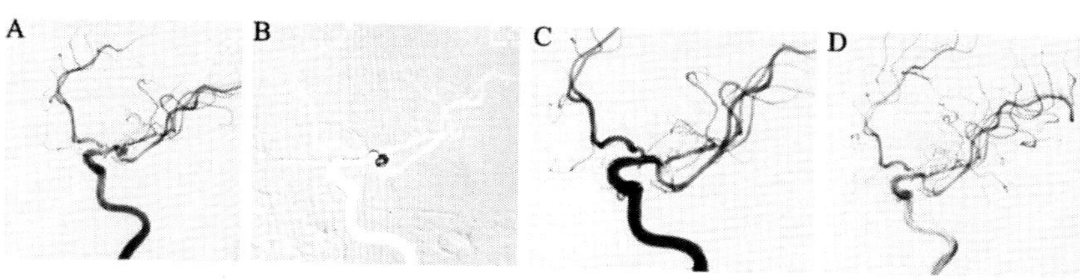

Figure 6. A 45-year-old male with an irregular left MCA bifurcation aneurysm treated with coiling. A: DSA showed irregular aneurysm involving the left MCA bifurcation. B: Single microcatheter technique was used to embolize the middle cerebral artery bifurcation aneurysms. C: The coil was transported through the microcatheter, and the angiogram obtained immediately after embolization treatment demonstrated complete occlusion of the MCA bifurcation aneurysm. D: Left ICA angiogram 6 months after coil embolization showed complete occlusion of the aneurysm without aneurysm recanalization.

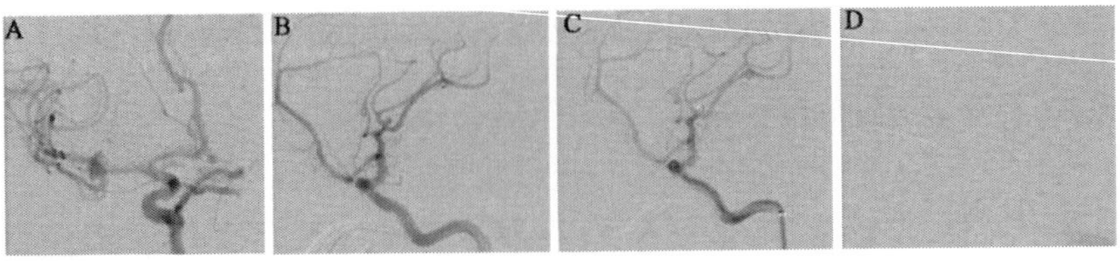

Figure 7. Fifty-seven-year-old woman with bilateral MCA bifurcation aneurysms treated with flow diversion and stent-assisted coiling. A: Right ICA angiogram showed the right MCA bifurcation aneurysm. B: Working position angiogram clearly showed the morphology of the left MCA bifurcation aneurysm. C: Immediate postprocedural right ICA angiogram showed the aneurysm was completely embolized by stent-assisted coil embolization. D: subtraction image showed the right MCA bifurcation aneurysm was treated by flow diversion..

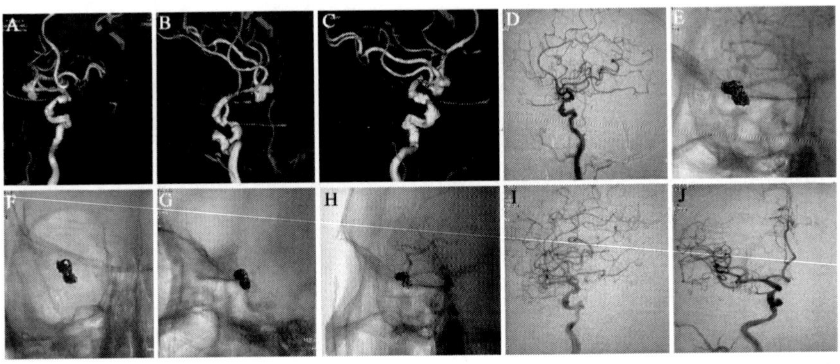

Figure 8. A 67-year-old woman experienced rupture of the right MCA bifurcation aneurysm, with Fisher's grading of 1, and underwent stent-assisted coiling. A-C: Three-dimensional reconstruction clearly showed the irregular shape of the aneurysm and involved branches of the MCA. D-H: LVIS Jr. stent-assisted coil embolization of the aneurysm. Angiography showed dense packing of the aneurysm, LVIS Jr. stent with perfect release, and the parent aneurysm artery patency. I-J: Immediate postprocedural left ICA angiograms showed complete embolization of the MCA bifurcation aneurysm.

Discussion

Middle cerebral aneurysm has been a topic of concern because of its complex anatomic features, complications, and the recanalization after embolization treatment. Anatomic features of MCA aneurysms render embolization treatment difficult, new devices have been and continue to be developed to address these difficulties, including flow diverters, and Woven EndoBridge (WEB). However, this study demonstrated that traditional embolization treatment provides a feasible option for MCA saccular aneurysms, and traditional embolization techniques are still not outdated.

The treatment of MCA aneurysms traditionally chosen microsurgical clipping [10, 11], although many innovative devices have emerged over the past decade with the development of neurointerventional devices. Endovascular coil embolization of MCA bifurcated aneurysms remains an option, even for wide neck, deformed shape, and angiographically unrecognizable branches (Figure 6 to 8). In the Barrow Ruptured Aneurysm Trial (BRAT) and International Subarachnoid Aneurysm Trial (ISAT) studies [12, 13] the results indicated that ruptured aneurysms with better clinical outcomes in the endovascular group. Furthermore, MCA aneurysms were not well represented in these trials, accounting for only 14.2% of all aneurysms in ISAT [13]. Therefore, the prognosis and efficacy of embolization for MCA aneurysms need to be further evaluated. Compared to the study of microsurgical clipping for MCA aneurysms, [14] our study had similar rates of adequate occlusion (92.1% vs 97.2%), but higher thromboembolic complication rates (5.77% vs 0.1%), and comparable proportion of patients with good clinical follow-up outcomes (98.56% vs 99.7%). Compared with other study that MCA aneurysms treated with stenting and coiling, our study has similar radiological outcomes (98.56% vs 100%) and similar clinical outcomes (98.56% vs 100%) [15]. The rates of intraoperative hemorrhagic complications (3.37%), and intraoperative thromboembolism (5.77%) were similar to those in other studies [3, 16].

The Woven EndoBridge is a highly innovative technique for the endovascular treatment of wide-necked bifurcation aneurysms, but it is more suitable for treatment of basilar bifurcation aneurysms, necks size >7 mm, and/or those with a bifurcation angle >180° [17]. The data from landmark WEB (Microvention) cohorts demonstrated an 80% adequate aneurysm occlusion rate [18]. YAN et al. reported the embolization treatment of 57 MCA bifurcation aneurysms with low profile visualized intravascular support (LVIS) stents assisted, [19] the postoperative angiography showed that 45.6% of aneurysms with Raymond 1 occlusions (45.6%), 17.6% of the aneurysms with Raymond 2 occlusions, and two patients (3.5%) experienced perioperative complications, one with a procedure related hemorrhagic event and the other with a procedure-related thromboembolic event. With an average follow-up of 11.7 months after surgery, the angiographic results showed complete occlusion in 78.7%, improvement in 6.4%, stabilization in 10.6%, and recanalization in only 4.3%. Feng et al. reported embolization treatment of 18 MCA aneurysms using LVIS Jr. stents, 8 patients (44.4%) had complete occlusion, 7 patients (38.9%) had residual neck, and 3 patients (16.7%) had partial occlusion at the last angiographic follow-up. One patient had intraoperative stent thrombosis, which disappeared due to intravenous injection of tirofiban [20].

Limitations

Our study has some limitations. First, it was a retrospective study with a small sample size, limiting the generality of the findings. Second, this study analyzed data from three neurosurgery institutions, and although uniform standards were used in data collection, interobserver and reporting biases may still have been introduced. Finally, we do not have data on the long-term follow-up results, so the recurrence rate may be underestimated, requiring a longer follow-up time to draw more reliable conclusions.

Conclusion

Traditional embolization techniques provide a feasible option for endovascular treatment of MCA saccular aneurysms. Even in the era of flow diverting stents and Woven EndoBridge (WEB), traditional embolization techniques are still not outdated.

References

[1] Molyneux A, Kerr R, Stratton I, Sandercock P, Clarke M, Shrimpton J, et al. International subarachnoid aneurysm trial (isat) of neurosurgical clipping versus endovascular coiling in 2143 patients with ruptured intracranial aneurysms: A randomised trial. *Lancet (London, England)*. 2002;360:1267-1274.

[2] Rodríguez-Hernández A, Sughrue ME, Akhavan S, Habdank-Kolaczkowski J, Lawton MT. Current management of middle cerebral artery aneurysms: Surgical results with a "clip first" policy. *Neurosurgery*. 2013;72:415-427.

[3] Brinjikji W, Lanzino G, Cloft HJ, Rabinstein A, Kallmes DF. Endovascular treatment of middle cerebral artery aneurysms: A systematic review and single-center series. *Neurosurgery*. 2011;68:397-402; discussion 402.

[4] Ries T, Siemonsen S, Thomalla G, Grzyska U, Zeumer H, Fiehler J. Long-term follow-up of cerebral aneurysms after endovascular therapy prediction and outcome of retreatment. *AJNR. American journal of neuroradiology*. 2007;28:1755-1761.

[5] Mortimer AM, Bradley MD, Mews P, Molyneux AJ, Renowden SA. Endovascular treatment of 300 consecutive middle cerebral artery aneurysms: Clinical and radiologic outcomes. *AJNR. American journal of neuroradiology*. 2014;35:706-714.

[6] Gory B, Rouchaud A, Saleme S, Dalmay F, Riva R, Caire F, et al. Endovascular treatment of middle cerebral artery aneurysms for 120 nonselected patients: A prospective cohort study. *AJNR. American journal of neuroradiology*. 2014;35:715-720.

[7] Elsharkawy A, Lehečka M, Niemelä M, Kivelev J, Billon-Grand R, Lehto H, et al. Anatomic risk factors for middle cerebral artery aneurysm rupture: Computed tomography angiography study of 1009 consecutive patients. *Neurosurgery*. 2013;73:825-837; discussion 836-827.

[8] Raymond J, Guilbert F, Weill A, Georganos SA, Juravsky L, Lambert A, et al. Long-term angiographic recurrences after selective endovascular treatment of aneurysms with detachable coils. *Stroke*. 2003;34:1398-1403.

[9] Ji W, Liu A, Lv X, Kang H, Sun L, Li Y, et al. Risk score for neurological complications after endovascular treatment of unruptured intracranial aneurysms. *Stroke*. 2016;47:971-978.

[10] Iijima A, Piotin M, Mounayer C, Spelle L, Weill A, Moret J. Endovascular treatment with coils of 149 middle cerebral artery berry aneurysms. *Radiology*. 2005;237:611-619.

[11] Vanzin JR, Mounayer C, Piotin M, Spelle L, Boissonnet H, Moret J. [endovascular treatment of unruptured middle cerebral artery aneurysms]. *Journal of neuroradiology = Journal de neuroradiologie*. 2005;32:97-108.

[12] Lanzino G. The barrow ruptured aneurysm trial. *Journal of neurosurgery*. 2012;116:133-134; discussion 134.

[13] Molyneux AJ, Kerr RS, Yu LM, Clarke M, Sneade M, Yarnold JA, et al. International subarachnoid aneurysm trial (isat) of neurosurgical clipping versus endovascular coiling in 2143 patients with ruptured intracranial aneurysms: A randomised comparison of effects on survival, dependency, seizures, rebleeding, subgroups, and aneurysm occlusion. *Lancet (London, England)*. 2005;366:809-817.

[14] De Leacy RA, Fargen KM, Mascitelli JR, Fifi J, Turkheimer L, Zhang X, et al. Wide-neck bifurcation aneurysms of the middle cerebral artery and basilar apex treated by endovascular techniques: A multicentre, core lab adjudicated study evaluating safety and durability of occlusion (branch). *Journal of neuro-interventional surgery*. 2019;11:31-36.

[15] Zhang X, Wang R, Ding Y, Li W, Ren H, Zhang J. Embolization of unruptured wide-necked aneurysms at the mca bifurcation using the neuroform atlas stent-assisted coiling: A two-center retrospective study. *Frontiers in neurology*. 2023;14:1199390.

[16] Aydin K, Berdikhojayev M, Cay F, Barburoglu M, Nurzhan S, Aygun S, et al. Safety, efficacy, and durability of stent-assisted coiling treatment of m2 (insular) segment mca aneurysms. *AJNR. American journal of neuroradiology*. 2022;43:560-567.

[17] Lv X, Zhang Y, Jiang W. Systematic review of woven endobridge for wide-necked bifurcation aneurysms: Complications, adequate occlusion rate, morbidity, and mortality. *World neurosurgery*. 2018;110:20-25.

[18] Pierot L, Moret J, Barreau X, Szikora I, Herbreteau D, Turjman F, et al. Aneurysm treatment with woven endobridge in the cumulative population of 3 prospective, multicenter series: 2-year follow-up. *Neurosurgery*. 2020;87:357-367.
[19] Yan Y, Zeng Z, Wu Y, Xiong J, Zhao K, Hong B, et al. The use of single low-profile visualized intraluminal support stent-assisted coiling in the treatment of middle cerebral artery bifurcation unruptured wide-necked aneurysm. *Interventional neuroradiology: Journal of peritherapeutic neuroradiology, surgical procedures and related neurosciences*. 2020;26:461-467.
[20] Feng Z, Li Q, Zhao R, Zhang P, Chen L, Xu Y, et al. Endovascular treatment of middle cerebral artery aneurysm with the lvis junior stent. *Journal of stroke and cerebrovascular diseases: The official journal of National Stroke Association*. 2015;24:1357-1362.

Chapter 7

Endovascular Treatment of Distal Aneurysms of the Intracranial Arteries: Sacrifice or Reconstruction

Jinlu Yu*
Department of Neurosurgery, First Hospital of Jilin University, Changchun, China

Abstract

Distal aneurysms of the intracranial arteries (DAIAs) occur distal to the major branches of the circle of Willis and the vertebrobasilar system. DAIAs are rare, and treatment, including open surgery and endovascular treatment (EVT), is sometimes necessary. Open surgery is challenging for DAIAs due to the deep location and difficulty in preserving the parent artery. EVT, especially reconstructive EVT, can be an alternative surgery for treating DAIAs. However, some DAIAs cannot be reconstructed due to the small size and complicated anatomy of the parent artery. Endovascular parent artery occlusion (PAO), a deconstructive method, plays an important role in treating DAIAs. Because our current understanding of DAIA sacrifice or reconstruction by EVT is insufficient, we discuss this issue, including the definition, incidence, pathogenesis, and classification of DAIAs; therapeutic options for DAIAs; reconstructive EVT for DAIAs; status of endovascular PAO; risk of endovascular PAO and balloon occlusion test; option for embolic materials for endovascular PAO; and PAO characteristics of each DAIA in this review. We found that, in EVT for DAIAs, although preservation and reconstruction of the parent artery should naturally be the prime objective, in selected cases, PAO was still a valuable option that yielded favorable outcomes.

Keywords: distal intracranial artery, aneurysm, endovascular treatment, reconstruction, parent artery occlusion

1. Introduction

Distal aneurysms of the intracranial arteries (DAIAs) occur distal to the major branches of the circle of Willis and the vertebrobasilar system and are also called peripheral aneurysms (Figure 1) [1-3]. DAIAs are rare and often spontaneously rupture, so treatment, including open surgery

* Corresponding Author's Email: jlyu@jlu.edu.cn.

In: Understanding and Managing Cerebral Aneurysms
Editor: Xianli Lv
ISBN: 979-8-89113-608-3

and endovascular treatment (EVT), is sometimes needed [3, 4]. Open surgery is challenging for DAIAs due to the irregular morphology, distal location, and involvement of the parent artery [5, 6]. Currently, as an alternative to open surgery, EVT is becoming the most commonly performed treatment for DAIAs [4, 7-9].

Reconstructive EVT is considered the best option for treating DAIAs. However, some DAIAs cannot be reconstructed due to the small size and complicated anatomy of the parent artery. Moreover, parent artery occlusion (PAO), a deconstructive method for treating DAIAs, is vital (Figure 2) [10-13]. Currently, our understanding of EVT for DAIAs is insufficient; therefore, we performed a review.

2. Definition, Incidence, Pathogenesis, and Classification of DAIAs

2.1. Definition

Rhoton and Rodríguez-Hernández established the nomenclature for the distal intracranial artery [14, 15]. In accordance with this proposal, DAIAs in the anterior circulation are located outside the circle of Willis, on or beyond the A2 segment of the anterior cerebral artery (ACA), the M2 segment of the middle cerebral artery (MCA), or the P2 segment of the posterior cerebral artery (PCA); DAIAs in the posterior circulation are located on or beyond the s2 segment of the superior cerebellar artery (SCA), the a2 segment of the anterior inferior cerebellar artery (AICA), or the p2 segment of the posterior inferior cerebellar artery (PICA) [1].

2.2. Incidence

DAIAs are uncommon, and there are various reports on their incidence. In general, the overall incidence of distal aneurysms distributed in the ACA ranges from 1-10%, followed by an incidence of 2-7% in the MCA, 4-5% in the PCA, and 0.6-0.9% in the cerebellar artery [1, 4, 8, 16-20]. Of all these reports, the report by Rodríguez-Hernández et al. was typical. According to our report of 1529 intracranial aneurysms, the overall incidence of DAIAs was 6.5%. Distal ACA aneurysms were more prevalent in distal cerebral arteries, distal PICA aneurysms were more prevalent in distal cerebellar arteries, and the incidence of DAIAs in distal cerebellar arteries was 4.3 times greater than that of DAIAs in cerebral arteries [1].

2.3. Pathogenesis

The pathogenesis of DAIAs, which may include spontaneous dissection, infection, trauma, vasculopathy, a high flow state, irradiation, and congenital collagen deficiency, is unclear [4, 12, 21-27]. In patients with multiple DAIAs, certain congenital etiological factors tend to be involved (Figure 3). DAIAs with these pathogeneses are often unassociated with an arterial branch point and present with fusiform or irregular shapes, large or giant sizes, or even serpentine shapes with intraluminal thrombosis [1, 21, 28-31].

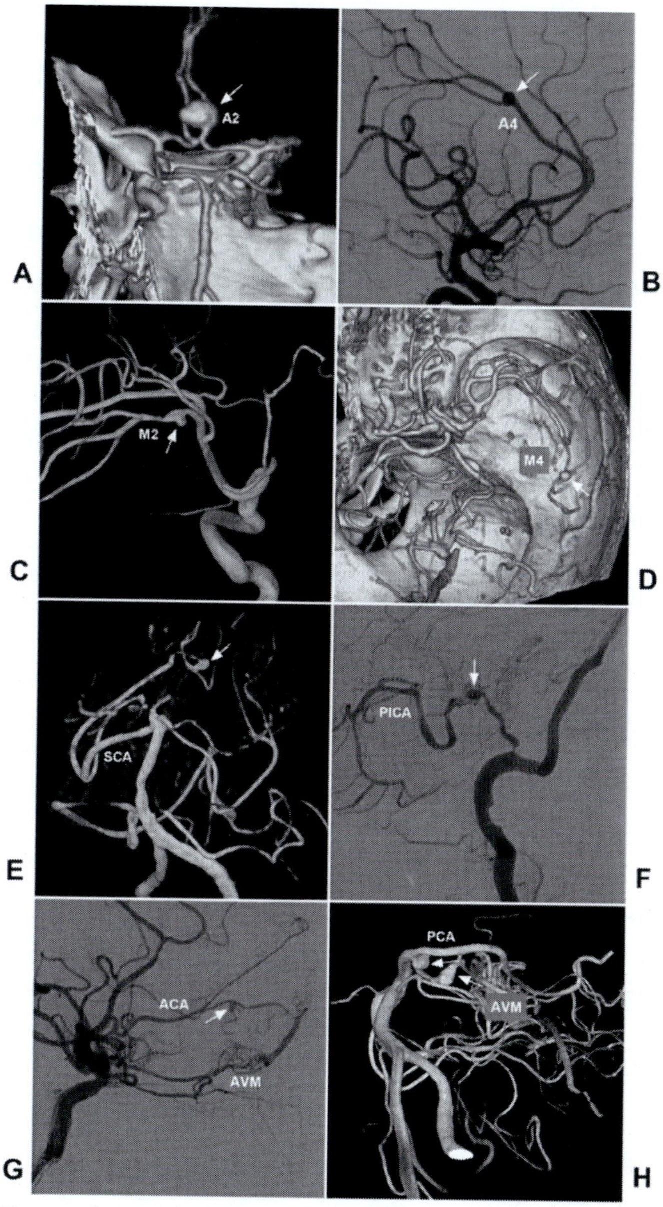

Abbreviations: ACA: anterior cerebral artery, AVM: arteriovenous malformation, CTA: computed tomography angiography, DAIA: distal aneurysm of the intracranial artery, DSA: digital subtracted angiography, MCA: middle cerebral artery, PCA: posterior cerebral artery, PICA: posterior inferior cerebellar artery, SCA: superior cerebellar artery.

Figure 1. Various DAIAs. A: CTA image showing an aneurysm (arrow) at the A2 segment of the ACA. B: DSA image showing an aneurysm (arrow) at the A4 segment of the ACA. C: DSA image showing an aneurysm (arrow) at the M2 segment of the MCA. D: CTA image showing an aneurysm (arrow) at the M4 segment of the MCA. E: DSA image showing an aneurysm (arrow) at the distal SCA. F: DSA image showing an aneurysm (arrow) at the junction of the p2 and p3 segments of the PICA. G: DSA image showing a flow-related aneurysm (arrow) at the branch of the ACA that served as the feeder of the AVM. H: DSA image showing two aneurysms (arrows) at the branch of the PCA serving as the feeder of the AVM.

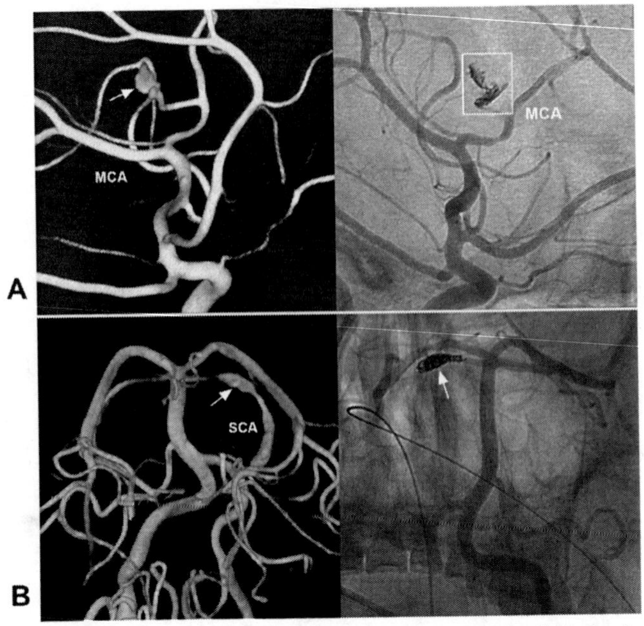

Abbreviations: DAIA: distal aneurysm of the intracranial artery, DSA: digital subtracted angiography, MCA: middle cerebral artery, PAO: parent artery occlusion, SCA: superior cerebellar artery.

Figure 2. Endovascular PAO for DAIA. A: Left panel: DSA image showing a DAIA (arrow) at the M2 segment of the MCA; Right panel: DSA image showing that the DAIA was embolized by Onyx casting (frame). B: Left panel: DSA image showing a DAIA (arrow) at the s2 segment of the SCA; Right panel: Unsubtracted DSA image showing that the DAIA was embolized by coiling (arrow).

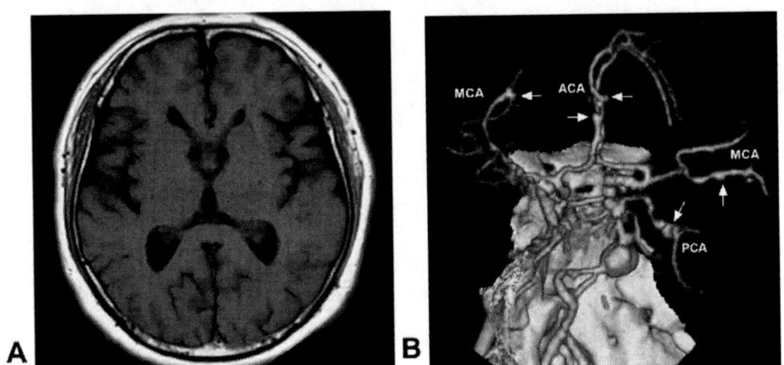

Abbreviations: ACA: anterior cerebral artery, DAIA: distal aneurysm of the intracranial artery, CTA: computed tomography angiography, MCA: middle cerebral artery, PCA: posterior cerebral artery.

Figure 3. Multiple DAIAs. A: Magnetic resonance image showing normal brain tissue. B: CTA image showing that multiple DAIAs (arrows) were distributed at the distal ACA, MCA and PCA.

2.4. Classification

According to the pathogenesis, DAIAs can be divided into spontaneous or infectious and traumatic, true, and false aneurysms. According to their anatomical location, DAIAs can be divided into 4 groups: distal ACA, MCA, PCA and cerebellar aneurysms (Figure 1A-F). DAIAs can also be divided into isolated aneurysms or flow-related aneurysms [32, 33]. Flow-related DAIAs are a response to high hemodynamic stress and may be observed in 5% of brain arteriovenous malformations (BAVMs) (Figure 1G-H) and dural arteriovenous fistulas [1]. In moyamoya disease or intracranial occlusive diseases, aneurysms may be located in collaterals, mainly in the choroidal collateral system. These distal DAIAs are also flow-related aneurysms due to altered hemodynamics and inherent vascular fragility [34-38].

3. Therapeutic Options for DAIAs

3.1. General Overview

To date, no treatment guidelines for DAIAs have been established [2]. However, the elimination of DAIAs and reconstruction of the parent artery must naturally be the prime objective [39-41]. Open surgery, including wrapping, clipping without sacrificing the parent artery, and trapping with or without bypass, can be used to treat DAIAs [42, 43]. However, open surgery potentially increases the risk of complications [4]. For DAIAs, EVT is potentially less hazardous. These techniques can be divided into deconstructive and reconstructive EVTs [44].

3.2. EVT Status

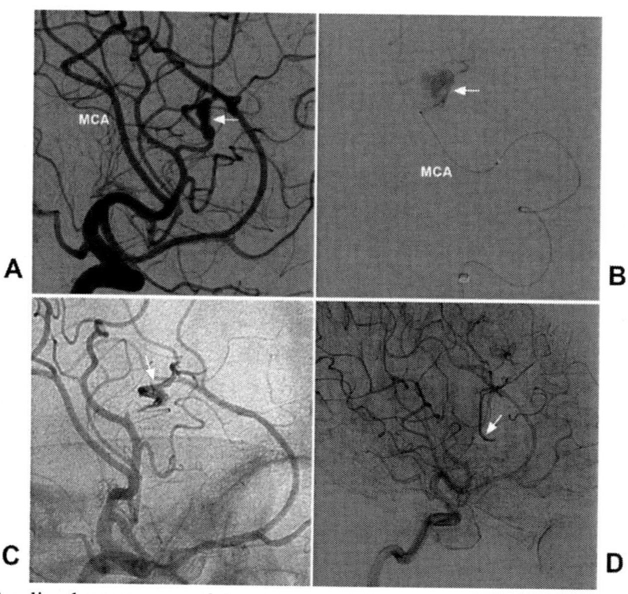

Abbreviations: DAIA: distal aneurysm of the intracranial artery, DSA: digital subtracted angiography, MCA: middle cerebral artery, PAO: parent artery occlusion.

Figure 4. Reliable PAO by casting Onyx for a DAIA. A: DSA image showing an aneurysm (arrow) at the M2 segment of the MCA. B: Superselective angiography of the microcatheter showing the aneurysm (arrow). C: Unsubtracted DSA image showing that both the aneurysm and proximal parent artery were occluded by casting the Onyx (arrow). D: Late arterial phase of DSA image showing retrograde collateral circulation (arrow) of the distal MCA beyond the aneurysm.

Reconstructive EVT for DAIAs, including selective coiling with/without stent assistance to preserve the parent artery or flow diverters (FDs) to reconstruct and preserve the parent artery, is the best option. However, for DAIAs, reconstruction of the parent artery is often difficult due to the small diameter and complicated anatomy of the artery [45]. Deconstructive EVT (PAO) had to be used. Endovascular PAO can be divided into occluding the parent artery and trapping the aneurysm or occluding the proximal parent artery only [7].

Reliable PAO traps the aneurysm as well as a short segment of the adjoining parent artery to avoid recurrence and regrowth of the aneurysm (Figure 4). In theory, PAO of the proximal parent artery may not be sufficient without closure of the aneurysm because the occluded artery can be filled in a retrograde fashion [46]. However, if the DAIAs were not too large or were very distal or had a thin parent artery, PAO of the proximal parent artery could be effective, and thrombosis of the aneurysm was expected.

4. Reconstructive EVT for DAIAs

For DAIAs, coiling assisted by traditional low-metal-coverage stents can be used; however, dissecting aneurysms can recur because intimal tears cannot obtain sufficient protection from traditional stents, especially for traumatic or mycotic pseudoaneurysms with poorly defined necks (Figure 5A) [26, 47, 48].

Recent developments in microneurostents and small FDs have made reconstructive EVT for DAIAs feasible in select cases [39-41]. For unruptured DAIAs, FD deployment is of particular interest because FDs often have a metal coverage rate of more than 30%, which greatly exceeds that of traditional stents.

They can divert the flow away from the aneurysm and allow the perforators to remain patent (Figure 5B) [49, 50]. Several large series and meta-analyses support the safety of FD deployment for the treatment of various DAIAs, even those with parent vessels measuring <2.0 mm in diameter [49-54]. Nevertheless, FD treatment-related complications are not negligible, with an approximate incidence of ischemic events of 15% and a morbidity of 8% [55]. In addition, when the parent artery of the DAIA is too thin or tortuous, FD deployment is not always successful [56]. Even if the FD is successfully deployed in a thin parent artery, the parent artery can become stenotic or occluded (Figure 5C).

For ruptured DAIAs, FD deployment alone is unsafe, and adjunctive coiling is often necessary [57]. However, FD deployment with coiling requires the use of two microcatheters. The parent artery often has difficulty containing two microcatheters, and treating some ruptured DAIAs by FD deployment with adjunctive coiling is difficult.

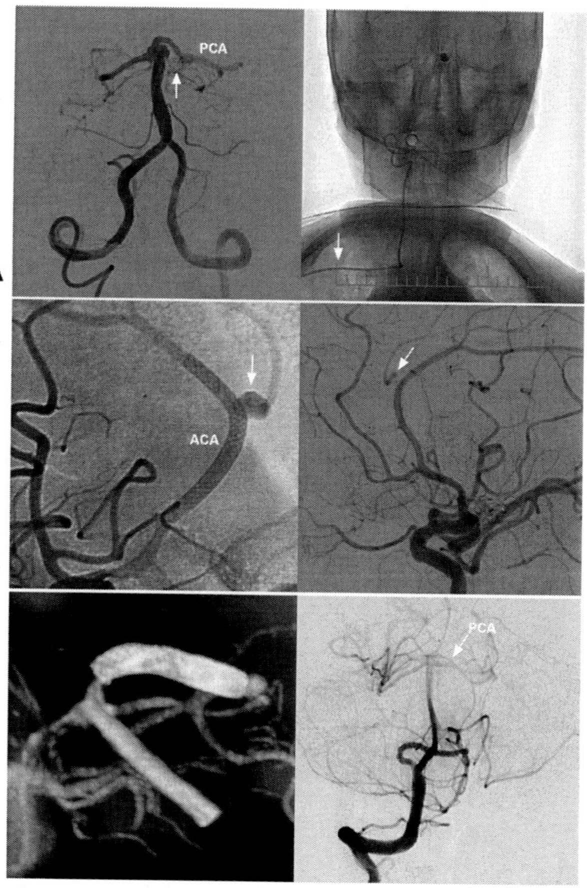

Abbreviations: EVT: endovascular treatment, FD: flow diverter, DAIA: distal aneurysm of the intracranial artery, DSA: digital subtracted angiography, MCA: middle cerebral artery, PCA: posterior cerebral artery.

Figure 5. Reconstructive EVT for DAIAs. A: Left panel: Unsubtracted DSA image showing a dissecting aneurysm (arrow) at the P2 segment of the PCA; Right panel: DSA image showing the aneurysm coiled with the assistance of an Atlas stent (Stryker Neurovascular, Fremont, California, USA). The arrow indicates that EVT was performed via the radial artery. B: Left panel: Unsubtracted DSA image showing an aneurysm (arrow) at the distal ACA; Right panel: Six-month follow-up DSA image showing that the aneurysm (arrow) had shrunk. C: Left panel: Vaso-reconstructive DSA image showing the FD in the PCA; Right panel: DSA image showing that the PCA (arrow) became stenotic and nearly occluded.

5. Risk of Endovascular PAO and the Balloon Occlusion Test

5.1. Risk of Endovascular PAO

Moreover, PAO carries inherent risks due to technique complications, including perforator injury during microwire or microcatheter navigation, and perforator injury is rarely reported [2]. The main risk factor for endovascular PAO is ischemic sequelae of the distal parent artery of the DAIA (Figure 6A). Therefore, the perfusion sufficiency of the eloquent cortex involved in PAO must be considered because acute PAO may not involve a sufficient leptomeningeal network of arteries [58]. In addition, endovascular PAO may require deposition over a length of the parent artery, resulting in occlusion of critical perforating or branching arteries with ischemic injuries of varying severity (Figure 6B) [59].

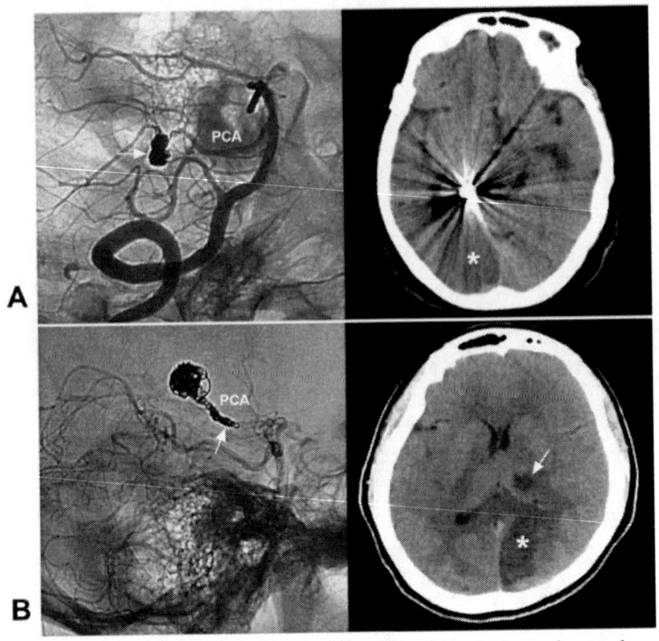

Abbreviations: CT: computed tomography, DSA: digital subtracted angiography, PAO: parent artery occlusion, PCA: posterior cerebral artery.

Figure 6. Risk of endovascular PAO. A: Left panel: Unsubtracted DSA image showing that the aneurysm (arrow) in the distal PCA was coiled; right panel: Postoperative CT image showing infarction in the occipital lobe (asterisk). B: Left panel: Unsubtracted DSA image showing that the aneurysm in the distal PCA was coiled and that the parent artery was occluded too long (arrow); Right panel: Postoperative CT image showing infarctions in the occipital lobe (asterisk) and thalamus (arrow).

5.2. Balloon Occlusion Test

Before performing PAO, the balloon occlusion test (BOT) must be performed to reduce the mean arterial pressure to 70% of the baseline to allow evaluation of neurological deficits [10]. Functional tests similar to those for BOTs, including the superselective Wada test under local anesthesia and the provocative test under general anesthesia, are also recommended [33]. After certain medicines were injected in the region beyond the DAIA through a microcatheter, functional or electrophysiological examinations were performed [2].

Although BOTs and functional tests have been recommended, their results have been unreliable because they may yield false-positive or false-negative results. Therefore, these tests should not be critical for planning endovascular PAO for DAIAs. However, during BOT, the collateral supply and hemodynamic balance between the cortical branches of the distal cerebral and cerebellar arteries can often be evaluated via angiography, revealing retrograde filling of collateral blood flow, which is also important [12].

6. Options for Embolic Materials for Endovascular PAO

The embolization agents used for endovascular PAO include coils, liquid embolic materials (Onyx; Medtronic, Minneapolis, Minnesota, USA), glue (n-butyl cyanoacrylate, NBCA), etc.) (Figure 7) [60, 61]. When the parent artery of the DAIA is thick, PAO by coiling is preferred because the vessels distal to the site of the occlusion are spared, allowing further collateral circulation establishment [32, 62].

When the small size of the parent artery precludes accurate navigation of microcatheters to delivery coils, soft and thin Marathon or Apollo microcatheters (Medtronic, Minneapolis, Minnesota, USA) can be used to access the aneurysm, thus allowing the liquid embolic material to fill the aneurysm and parent vessel [13]. Of the available liquid embolic materials, Onyx is a less adhesive liquid and can be better controlled, which eliminates the risk of the catheter becoming glued to the vessel wall [13, 45].

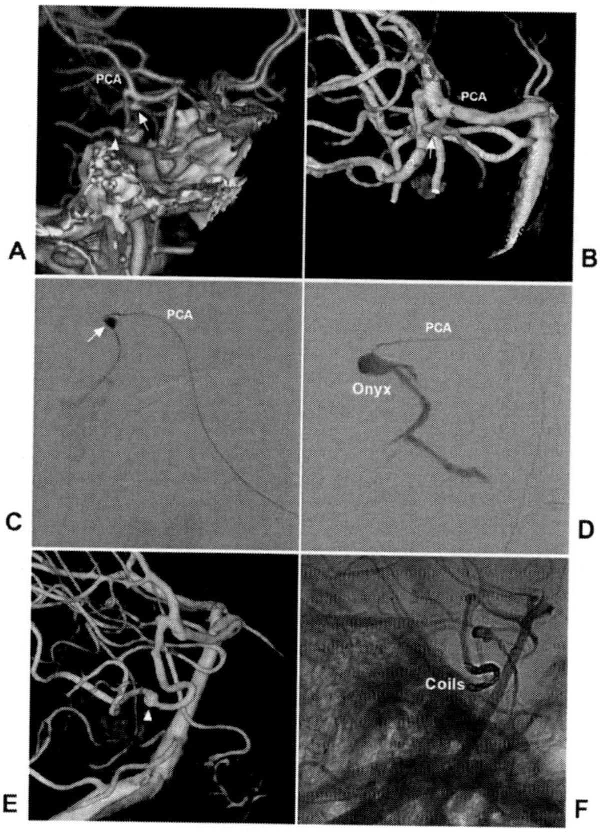

Abbreviations: CTA: computed tomography angiography, DSA: digital subtracted angiography, PAO: parent artery occlusion, PCA: posterior cerebral artery.

Figure 7. Options for embolic materials for endovascular PAO. A: CTA image showing two aneurysms (arrow and arrowhead) distributed at the P2 segment of the PCA and its branch. B: DSA image showing the aneurysm (arrow) at the origin of a branch from the P2 segment trunk. B: Superselective angiography of the microcatheter showing the aneurysm (arrow). D: Roadmap image showing that the aneurysm and distal parent artery were occluded by casting Onyx. E: Three-dimensional DSA image showing the aneurysm (arrowhead) at the branch from the P2 segment trunk. F: Unsubtracted DSA image showing that the proximal segment of the branch from the P2 segment was coiled.

7. PAO Characteristics of Each DAIA

7.1. Distal ACA

PAO for DAIAs on A2-3 segments may carry serious ischemic risks; certainly, PAO is not the first choice because these aneurysms are often saccular at bifurcation, and reconstructive EVT can be performed easily [12, 63-66]. However, if the DAIA on the A2-3 segments is giant and thrombosed, the distal ACA could have slow flow and experience ischemic preconditioning, resulting in an increased likelihood of tolerance to PAO (Figure 8) [12, 30, 67, 68]. For DAIAs in the A4-5 segments, PAO is safe due to the presence of adequate leptomeningeal and pial collaterals from the PCA or MCA (Figure 9) [64, 65, 68, 69]. In PAO, if the branches of the ACA beyond the DAIA are supplied to important functional areas, such as the paracentral artery and precuneal artery, PAO should be performed cautiously [70-72].

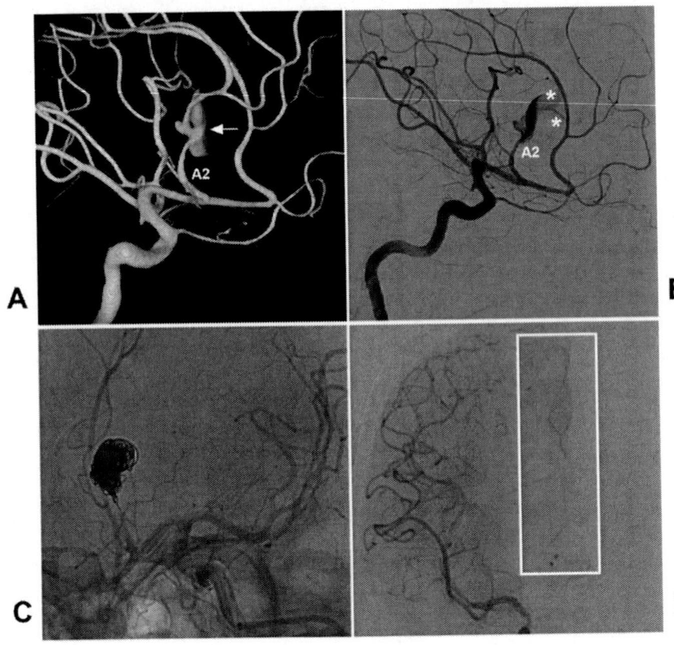

Abbreviations: ACA: anterior cerebral artery, DAIA: distal aneurysm of the intracranial artery, DSA: digital subtracted angiography.

Figure 8. Angiography of ischemic preconditioning of giant ACA DAIA. A: DSA image showing the aneurysm (arrow) at the A2 segment of the ACA. B: DSA image showing the delayed appearance of the branches (asterisks) beyond the aneurysm compared with other branches. C: Unsubtracted DSA image showing that the aneurysm was occluded. D: DSA image showing collateral circulation in the ACA by retrograde filling via the middle cerebral artery.

7.2. Distal MCA

The M2 segment is the most common site affected by a distal MCA aneurysm [19, 73]. Moreover, PAO for DAIAs of the M2 segment should be performed cautiously [12, 74, 75]. If the DAIAs are located on the M2 segment of the inferior trunk and are giant or serpentine with thrombi, the distal MCA may experience ischemic preconditioning, and M2 branch occlusion may be associated with minimal or no deficits (Figure 10) [46].

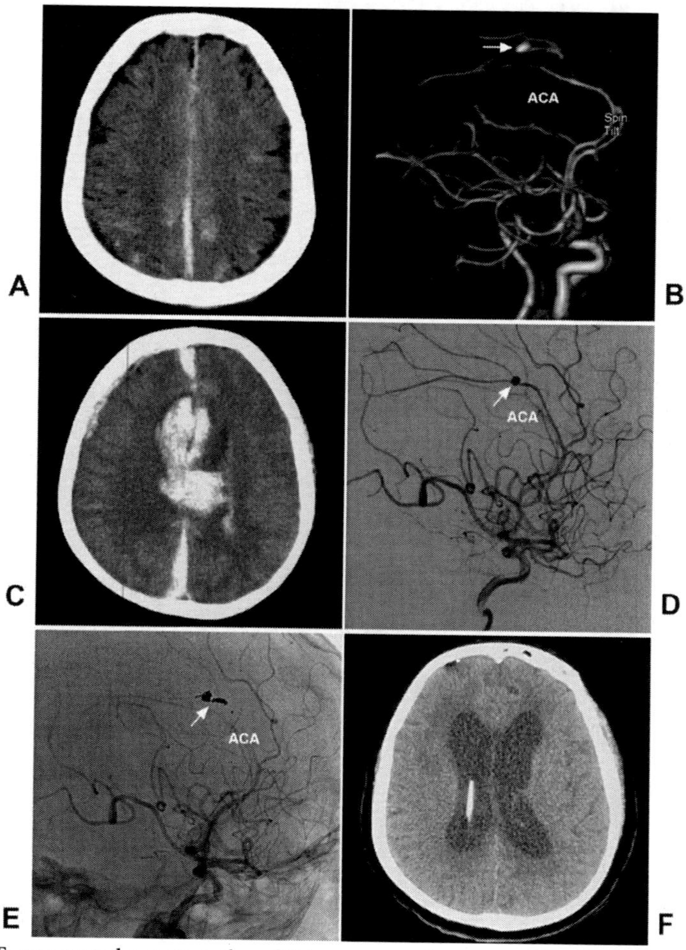

Abbreviations: CT: computed tomography, CTA: computed tomography angiography, ACA: anterior cerebral artery, DAIA: distal aneurysm of the intracranial artery, DSA: digital subtracted angiography, PAO: parent artery occlusion.

Figure 9. Endovascular PAO of ACA-DAIA. A: CT image showing hemorrhage in the longitudinal fissure after traffic injury. B: CTA image showing an aneurysm (arrow) in the distal ACA. C: One day later, CT image showing rehemorrhage in the longitudinal fissure and the formation of a large hematoma. D: DSA image showing a traumatic aneurysm at the A4 segment of the ACA. E: Unsubtracted DSA image showing that the aneurysm and its parent artery (arrow) were occluded by coiling. F: CT image showing that postoperative hydrocephalus was resolved by a ventriculoperitoneal shunt.

PAO for the DAIAs of M3-4 segments can be performed due to adequate leptomeningeal and pial collaterals from the ACA and PCA [46]. However, if the branches of the MCA beyond the DAIAs are supplied to important functional areas, PAO should be performed cautiously [76].

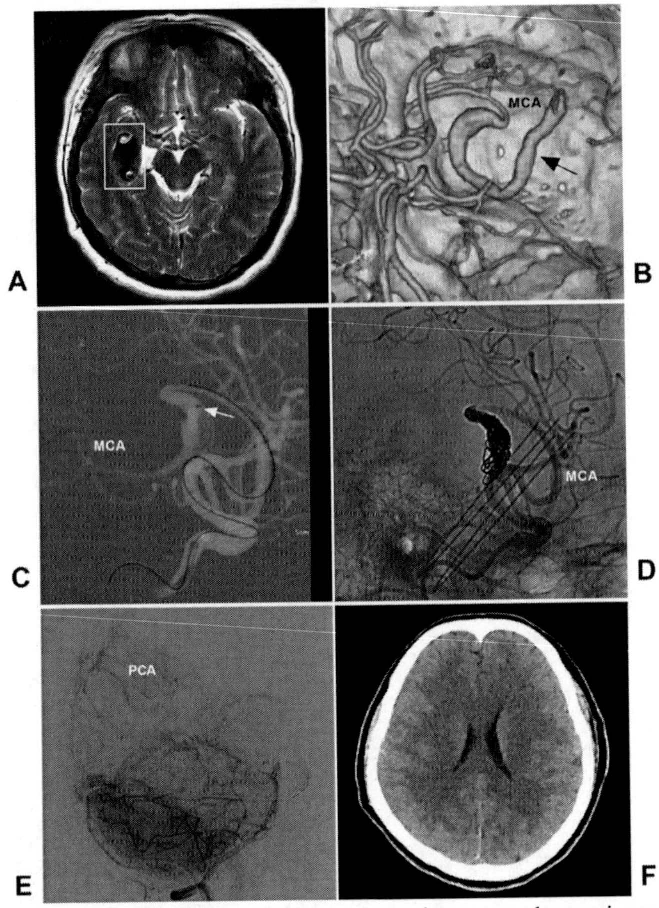

Abbreviations: CT: computed tomography, CTA: computed tomography angiography, MCA: middle cerebral artery, PAO: parent artery occlusion, PCA: posterior cerebral artery.

Figure 10. Endovascular PAO of serpentine MCA DAIA. A: Magnetic resonance imaging showing a circular low-signal lesion with an "eye-side" (frame). B: CTA image showing that the lesion was a serpentine aneurysm (arrow) at the distal MCA. C: Roadmap DSA image showing that the microcatheter used to deliver coils was catheterized into the aneurysm (arrow). D: Unsubtracted DSA image showing that the aneurysm and its parent artery were occluded by coiling and casting the Onyx. E: DSA image of the vertebral artery showing that the occluded distal MCA region was perfused by the PCA. F: Postoperative CT image showing no infarction sign (frame).

7.3. Distal PCA

Potential collateral supply and hemodynamic balance made P2 occlusion safe because the aneurysm occurred after the thalamoperforating vessels arose from the P1 segment [59, 60]. However, when the PCA is fatal, the P2 segment can send out additional perforating arteries, and anastomosis between the MCA and PCA tends to result in less collateral development [77]. At this time, PAO of the P2 segment should be performed cautiously, as PAO of the P2 segment near the P1 segment is dangerous. Due to the rich collateral circulation, PAO for aneurysms in the P3-4 segment is safe [78-80].

7.4. Distal SCA

When the SCA is too thin, reconstructive EVT is difficult [81, 82]. Moreover, PAO has been performed in EVT. The proximal s1 segment of the SCA can send off perforators to the brainstem, and occlusion of the s1 segment can result in brainstem infarction [83]. However, PAO of the s2-s4 segments is safe. In our previous systematic review, 91.2% of DAIAs of the SCA achieved a good outcome after PAO of the distal SCA [84].

7.5. Distal AICA

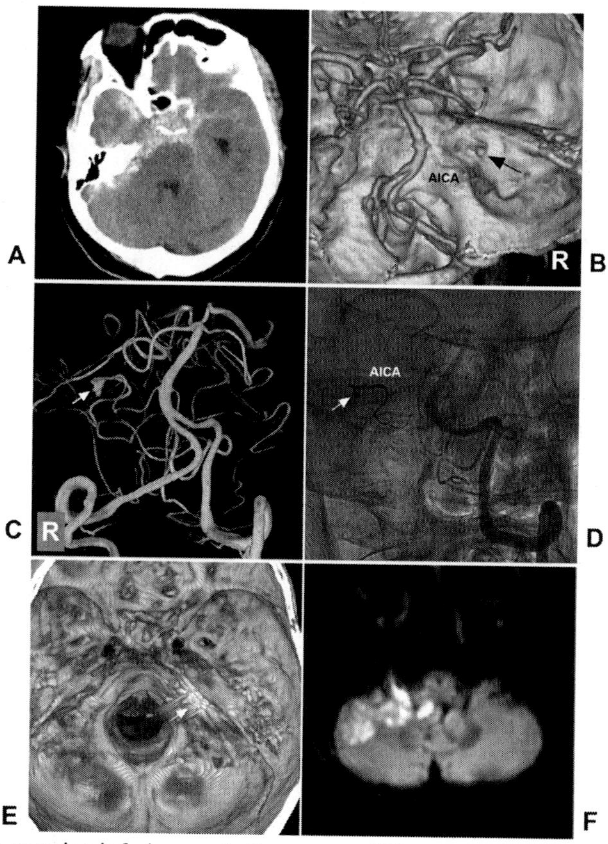

Abbreviations: AICA: anterior inferior cerebellar artery, CT: computed tomography, CTA: computed tomography angiography, DAIA: distal aneurysm of the intracranial artery, DSA: digital subtracted angiography, MR: magnetic resonance, PAO: parent artery occlusion.

Figure 11. Endovascular PAO of AICA-DAIA. A: CT image showing subarachnoid hemorrhage in the cisternal ambiens and suprasellar cistern. B: CTA image showing an aneurysm (arrow) in the distal AICA in the internal auditory canal. C: DSA image showing a dissecting aneurysm at the distal AICA. D: Unsubtracted DSA image showing that the aneurysm and its parent artery (arrow) were occluded by casting the Onyx. E: Xper-CT image showing Onyx casting in the internal auditory canal. F: Magnetic resonance diffuse-weighted imaging showing acute infarction (frame) in the lateral cerebellar hemisphere.

The AICA can be divided into the a1-a4 segments [85, 86]. The a2 segment is divided into the preinternal auditory artery (a2-1) and postinternal auditory artery (a2-2) segments, taking the internal auditory artery as the boundary. The AICA can be divided into proximal (a1 and a2-1) and distal (a2-2, a3 and a4) segments [33]. Moreover, PAO for proximal aneurysms should be performed cautiously, and brainstem infarction and hearing loss must be considered [85]. Moreover, despite the risk of ischemic complications, PAO is acceptable for aneurysms distal to the a2-2 segment (Figure 11). In addition, for aneurysms at the lower or middle branch of duplicate or triplicate AICA trunks, PAO is reasonable and acceptable [33].

7.6. Distal PICA

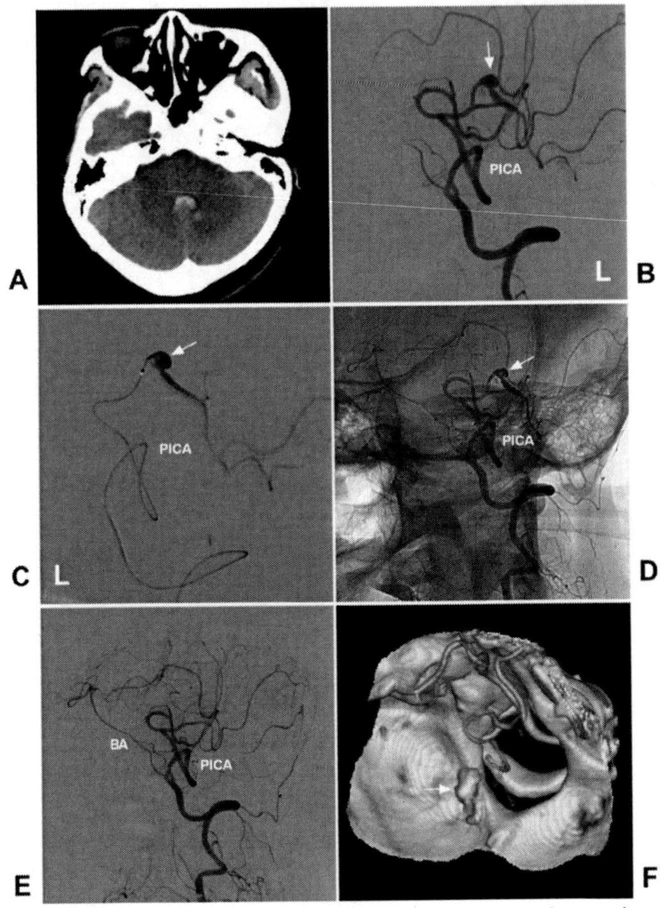

Abbreviations: CT: computed tomography, CTA: computed tomography angiography, DAIA: distal aneurysm of the intracranial artery, DSA: digital subtracted angiography, PAO: parent artery occlusion, PICA: posterior inferior cerebellar artery.

Figure 12. Endovascular PAO of PICA-DAIA. A: CT image showing hemorrhage in the fourth ventricle. B: DSA image showing an aneurysm (arrow) in the distal PICA. C: Superselective angiography showing that the microcatheter accessed the aneurysm (arrow). D: Unsubtracted DSA image showing that the aneurysm and its parent artery (arrow) were occluded by casting the Onyx. E: DSA image showing sufficient other distal branches of the PICA. F: Follow-up CTA showing Onyx casting (arrow).

Ideal EVT comprises complete embolization of the aneurysm while preserving the PICA and perforating arteries [87-89]. However, this is difficult to achieve. For proximal p1 aneurysms, PAO is dangerous due to brainstem infarction [90-92]. While the distal segment of the PICA has a good possibility of collateral flow, PAO can be performed for p2-5 aneurysms (Figure 12) [32, 93]. For some PICA variations, such as those with a double origin or with PICA communicating arteries, aggressive PAO can be performed [32, 94].

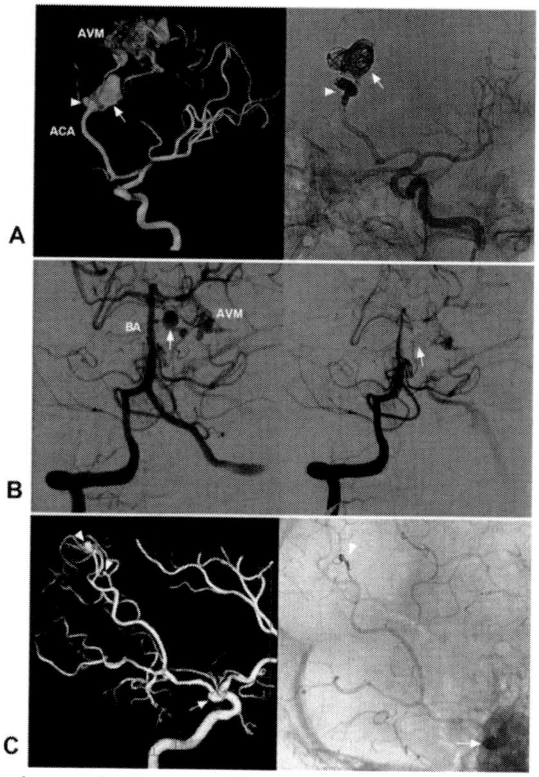

Abbreviations: ACA: anterior cerebral artery, AVM: arteriovenous malformation, BA: basilar artery, DAIA: distal aneurysm of the intracranial artery, DSA: digital subtracted angiography, PAO: parent artery occlusion.

Figure 13. Endovascular PAO of flow-related DAIA. A: Left panel: DSA image showing multiple tandem flow-related aneurysms (arrow and arrowhead) on the ACA as the feeder to an AVM; right panel: Unsubtracted DSA image showing two aneurysms and the parent artery (arrow) were occluded by coiling. B: Left panel: DSA image showing a flow-related aneurysm (arrow) on a BA perforator as the feeder to an AVM; Right panel: Postoperative DSA image showing that the aneurysm was occluded by casting Onyx. C: Left panel: DSA image showing an aneurysm (arrow) in the posterior communicating artery and two aneurysms (arrowheads) in the distal posterior cerebral artery; the ipsilateral middle cerebral artery was occluded; right panel: DSA image showing that the aneurysm (arrow) in the posterior communicating artery was coiled selectively and that two aneurysms (arrowheads) in the distal posterior cerebral artery were occluded by PAO.

7.7. Flow-related aneurysms in BAVM, MMD and MCA occlusion

For flow-related DAIAs, the EVT protocol is similar to that for isolated aneurysms [95, 96]. For a thin or an irregularly shaped parent artery, PAO is sometimes the only choice [97, 98]. Moreover, PEA can be performed more aggressively for isolated aneurysms because the low-pressure shunt permits retrograde flow from the BAVM to the distal segment of the parent artery after the DAIA, which provides time to treat the BAVM (Figure 13A-B) [99, 100].

PAO is often the only choice for treating DAIAs in moyamoya vessels or on collaterals of *MCA occlusion* located on the distal anterior choroidal artery, lenticulostriate artery, distal PCA and middle meningeal artery (Figure 13C) [37, 38]. Due to the small size of moyamoya vessels and their passage, PAO is often the only option and may provide temporary resolution of aneurysms. Our previous study showed that PAO for aneurysms in moyamoya vessels or on collaterals was feasible [101]. However, treatment failure occurred due to inadequate access.

Conclusion

DAIAs are rare. Reconstructive and deconstructive EVTs can treat DAIAs. Reconstructive EVT should naturally be the prime objective. However, when some DAIAs cannot be reconstructed due to the small size and complicated anatomy of the parent artery, endovascular PAO, a deconstructive method, plays an important role in treating DAIAs. By selecting patients appropriately, EVT for DAIAs can result in a good prognosis.

References

[1] Rodríguez-Hernández, A., Z. Zador, R. Rodríguez-Mena, and M. T. Lawton. 2013. "Distal Aneurysms of Intracranial Arteries: Application of Numerical Nomenclature, Predilection for Cerebellar Arteries, and Results of Surgical Management." *World Neurosurg* 80, no. 1-2 (Jul-Aug): 103-12. https://dx.doi.org/10.1016/j.wneu.2012.09.010.

[2] Andreou, A., I. Ioannidis, and A. Mitsos. 2007. "Endovascular Treatment of Peripheral Intracranial Aneurysms." *AJNR Am J Neuroradiol* 28, no. 2 (Feb): 355-61.

[3] Nussbaum, E. S., M. T. Madison, J. K. Goddard, J. P. Lassig, and L. A. Nussbaum. 2009. "Peripheral Intracranial Aneurysms: Management Challenges in 60 Consecutive Cases." *J Neurosurg* 110, no. 1 (Jan): 7-13. https://dx.doi.org/10.3171/2008.6.jns0814.

[4] Rotim, K., B. Splavski, V. Kalousek, M. Jurilj, and T. Sajko. 2020. "Endovascular Management of Intracranial Aneurysms on Distal Arterial Branches: Illustrative Case Series and Literature Retrospection." *Acta Clin Croat* 59, no. 4 (Dec): 712-720. https://dx.doi.org/10.20471/ acc.2020. 59.04.18.

[5] Hendricks, B. K., and R. F. Spetzler. 2020. "Treatment of a Fusiform Anterior Cerebral Artery Aneurysm with an A3-A3 Bypass: 2-Dimensional Operative Video." *Oper Neurosurg (Hagerstown)* 19, no. 4 (Sep 15): E385. https://dx.doi.org/10.1093/ons/opaa143.

[6] Taylor, B. E. S., I. Say, P. Patel, and L. D. Tomycz. 2020. "Microsurgical Clip Ligation of an Unruptured Azygos Bifurcation Aneurysm Indented by the Falx Cerebri: 3-Dimensional Operative Video." *Oper Neurosurg (Hagerstown)* 19, no. 3 (Sep 1): E294. https://dx.doi.org/10.1093/ons/opz393.

[7] Wessels, L., N. Hecht, K. Faust, U. Schneider, M. Czabanka, and P. Vajkoczy. 2021. "Complete or Partial Parent Artery Sacrifice: Effect of Vessel-Occlusion Strategies on Complete Obliteration of Complex Aneurysms." *World Neurosurg* 147 (Mar): e282-e292. https://dx.doi.org/10.1016/j.wneu. 2020.12.050.

[8] Cagnazzo, F., M. Cappucci, C. Dargazanli, P. H. Lefevre, G. Gascou, C. Riquelme, A. Bonafe, and V. Costalat. 2018. "Treatment of Distal Anterior Cerebral Artery Aneurysms with Flow-Diverter Stents: A Single-Center Experience." *AJNR Am J Neuroradiol* 39, no. 6 (Jun): 1100-1106. https://dx.doi.org/10.3174/ajnr.A5615.

[9] Limbucci, N., G. Leone, L. Renieri, S. Nappini, F. Cagnazzo, A. Laiso, M. Muto, and S. Mangiafico. 2020. "Expanding Indications for Flow Diverters: Distal Aneurysms, Bifurcation Aneurysms, Small Aneurysms, Previously Coiled Aneurysms and Clipped Aneurysms, and Carotid Cavernous Fistulas." *Neurosurgery* 86, no. Suppl 1 (Jan 1): S85-s94. https://dx.doi.org/10.1093/neuros/nyz334.

[10] Ganesh Kumar, N., T. R. Ladner, I. S. Kahn, S. L. Zuckerman, C. B. Baker, M. Skaletsky, D. Cushing, M. R. Sanborn, J. Mocco, and R. D. Ecker. 2017. "Parent Vessel Occlusion for Treatment of Cerebral Aneurysms: Is There Still an Indication? A Series of 17 Patients." *J Neurol Sci* 372 (Jan 15): 250-255. https://dx.doi.org/10.1016/j.jns.2016.11.057.

[11] Ishii, A., S. Miyamoto, Y. Ito, T. Fujinaka, C. Sakai, and N. Sakai. 2014. "Parent Artery Occlusion for Unruptured Cerebral Aneurysms: The Japanese Registry of Neuroendovascular Therapy (Jr-Net) 1 and 2." *Neurol Med Chir (Tokyo)* 54 Suppl 2: 91-7.

[12] Biondi, A., B. Jean, E. Vivas, L. Le Jean, A. L. Boch, J. Chiras, and R. Van Effenterre. 2006. "Giant and Large Peripheral Cerebral Aneurysms: Etiopathologic Considerations, Endovascular Treatment, and Long-Term Follow-Up." *AJNR Am J Neuroradiol* 27, no. 8 (Sep): 1685-92.

[13] Chalouhi, N., S. Tjoumakaris, L. F. Gonzalez, D. Hasan, K. Alkhalili, A. S. Dumont, R. Rosenwasser, and P. Jabbour. 2013b. "Endovascular Treatment of Distal Intracranial Aneurysms with Onyx 18/34." *Clin Neurol Neurosurg* 115, no. 12 (Dec): 2528-32. https://dx.doi.org/10.1016/j.clineuro.2013.10.018.

[14] Rodríguez-Hernández, A., A. L. Rhoton, Jr., and M. T. Lawton. 2011. "Segmental Anatomy of Cerebellar Arteries: A Proposed Nomenclature. Laboratory Investigation." *J Neurosurg* 115, no. 2 (Aug): 387-97. https://dx.doi.org/10.3171/2011.3.jns101413.

[15] Rhoton, A. L., Jr. 2002. "The Supratentorial Arteries." *Neurosurgery* 51, no. 4 Suppl (Oct): S53-120.

[16] Sturiale, C. L., W. Brinjikji, M. H. Murad, H. J. Cloft, D. F. Kallmes, and G. Lanzino. 2013. "Endovascular Treatment of Distal Anterior Cerebral Artery Aneurysms: Single-Center Experience and a Systematic Review." *AJNR Am J Neuroradiol* 34, no. 12 (Dec): 2317-20. https://dx.doi.org/10.3174/ajnr.A3629.

[17] Cavalcanti, D. D., A. A. Abla, N. L. Martirosyan, C. G. McDougall, R. F. Spetzler, and F. C. Albuquerque. 2013. "Endovascular Management of Distal Aca Aneurysms: Single-Institution Clinical Experience in 22 Consecutive Patients and Literature Review." *AJNR Am J Neuroradiol* 34, no. 8 (Aug): 1593-9. https://dx.doi.org/10.3174/ajnr.A3408.

[18] Phukan, P., K. Samra, D. Lynser, B. K. Sharma, D. K. Boruah, B. Saikia, and B. K. Singh. 2021. "Endovascular Parent Artery Occlusion for Intracranial Aneurysms Is a Viable, Cost-Effective Alternative: An Institutional Experience from Northeast India." *Acta Med Litu* 28, no. 2: 272-284. https://dx.doi.org/10.15388/Amed.2021.28.2.6.

[19] Tsutsumi, K., T. Horiuchi, A. Nagm, Y. Toba, and K. Hongo. 2017. "Clinical Characteristics of Ruptured Distal Middle Cerebral Artery Aneurysms: Review of the Literature." *J Clin Neurosci* 40 (Jun): 14-17. https://dx.doi.org/10.1016/j.jocn.2016.12.019.

[20] Anil, G., L. Sein, V. Nga, K. Teo, N. Chou, and T. T. Yeo. 2020. "Dissecting Distal Cerebellar Artery Aneurysms: Options Beyond a Parent Vessel Sacrifice." *Neurosurg Rev* 43, no. 2 (Apr): 771-780. https://dx.doi.org/10.1007/s10143-019-01119-y.

[21] Yano, H., M. Sawada, J. Shinoda, and T. Funakoshi. 1995. "Ruptured Dissecting Aneurysm of the Peripheral Anterior Cerebral Artery--Case Report." *Neurol Med Chir (Tokyo)* 35, no. 7 (Jul): 450-3. https://dx.doi.org/10.2176/nmc.35.450.

[22] Watanabe, A., K. Hirano, and R. Ishii. 1998. "Cerebral Mycotic Aneurysm Treated with Endovascular Occlusion--Case Report." *Neurol Med Chir (Tokyo)* 38, no. 10 (Oct): 657-60. https://dx.doi.org/10.2176/nmc.38.657.

[23] Kalousek, V., T. Sajko, B. Splavski, K. Rotim, M. Jurilj, B. Čulo, and A. Rotim. 2020. "Current Endovascular Management of Infected Distal Branch Intracranial Aneurysms: A Case Report and Insight into the Literature." *Acta Clin Croat* 59, no. 4 (Dec): 754-760. https://dx.doi.org/10.20471/acc.2020.59.04.24.

[24] Scotti, G., M. H. Li, C. Righi, F. Simionato, and A. Rocca. 1996. "Endovascular Treatment of Bacterial Intracranial Aneurysms." *Neuroradiology* 38, no. 2 (Feb): 186-9. https://dx.doi.org/10.1007/bf00604818.

[25] Dominguez, L., B. Saway, M. J. Benko, E. Guilliams, E. A. Marvin, and J. J. Entwistle. 2020. "Ruptured Distal Superior Cerebellar Artery Aneurysm after Gamma Knife Radiosurgery for Trigeminal Neuralgia: A Case Report and Review of the Literature." *World Neurosurg* 135 (Mar): 2-6. https://dx.doi.org/10.1016/j.wneu.2019.10.136.

[26] Serrano, F., A. Guédon, J. P. Saint-Maurice, M. A. Labeyrie, V. Civelli, M. Eliezer, and E. Houdart. 2022. "Endovascular Treatment of Infectious Intracranial Aneurysms Complicating Infective Endocarditis: A Series of 31 Patients with 55 Aneurysms." *Neuroradiology* 64, no. 2 (Feb): 353-360. https://dx.doi.org/10.1007/s00234-021-02798-5.

[27] Kaku, Y., J. I. Hamada, J. I. Kuroda, Y. Kai, M. Morioka, and J. I. Kuratsu. 2007. "Multiple Peripheral Middle Cerebral Artery Aneurysms Associated with Behcet's Disease." *Acta Neurochir (Wien)* 149, no. 8 (Aug): 823-7; discussion 827. https://dx.doi.org/10.1007/s00701-007-1226-x.

[28] Wakui, K., Y. Kamijo, K. Seguchi, and T. Sakai. 1992. "Thrombosed Aneurysm of the Middle Cerebral Artery with Occlusion of the Distal Parent Artery--Case Report." *Neurol Med Chir (Tokyo)* 32, no. 11 (Oct): 842-5. https://dx.doi.org/10.2176/nmc.32.842.

[29] Kannoth, S., R. Iyer, S. V. Thomas, S. V. Furtado, B. J. Rajesh, C. Kesavadas, V. V. Radhakrishnan, and P. S. Sarma. 2007. "Intracranial Infectious Aneurysm: Presentation, Management and Outcome." *J Neurol Sci* 256, no. 1-2 (May 15): 3-9. https://dx.doi.org/10.1016/j.jns.2007.01.044.

[30] Senbokuya, N., K. Kanemaru, H. Kinouchi, and T. Horikoshi. 2012. "Giant Serpentine Aneurysm of the Distal Anterior Cerebral Artery." *J Stroke Cerebrovasc Dis* 21, no. 8 (Nov): 910.e7-11. https://dx.doi.org/10.1016/j.jstrokecerebrovasdis.2011.10.019.

[31] Trungu, S., P. Bruzzaniti, S. Forcato, M. Cimatti, and A. Raco. 2017. "Completely Thrombosed Distal Middle Cerebral Artery Aneurysm Mimicking a Cavernous Angioma: Case Report and Review of the Literature." *World Neurosurg* 103 (Jul): 955.e1-955.e4. https://dx.doi.org/10.1016/j.wneu.2017.04.172.

[32] Hou, K., X. Lv, Y. Guo, and J. Yu. 2022a. "Endovascular Treatment of Posterior Inferior Cerebellar Artery Trunk Aneurysm." *Acta Neurol Belg* 122, no. 6 (Dec): 1405-1417. https://dx.doi.org/10.1007/s13760-021-01826-8.

[33] Hou, K., K. Xu, and J. Yu. 2022. "Endovascular Treatment of Anterior Inferior Cerebellar Artery Trunk Aneurysms." *Interv Neuroradiol* 28, no. 5 (Oct): 604-612. https://dx.doi.org/10.1177/15910199211049054.

[34] Harreld, J. H., and A. R. Zomorodi. 2011. "Embolization of an Unruptured Distal Lenticulostriate Aneurysm Associated with Moyamoya Disease." *AJNR Am J Neuroradiol* 32, no. 3 (Mar): E42-3. https://dx.doi.org/10.3174/ajnr.A1993.

[35] Fukuda, N., K. Kanemaru, K. Hashimoto, H. Yoshioka, N. Senbokuya, T. Yagi, and H. Kinouchi. 2019. "Embolization of a Peripheral Cerebral Aneurysm Associated with Intracranial Major Artery Occlusion through a Transdural Anastomotic Artery: Case Report." *Interv Neuroradiol* 25, no. 2 (Apr): 172-176. https://dx.doi.org/10.1177/1591019918801539.

[36] Hou, K., K. Xu, Y. Zhao, and J. Yu. 2022b. "Transdural Anastomotic Aneurysm in Association with Moyamoya Disease: A Rare and Troublesome Neurosurgical Entity." *J Neurol Surg A Cent Eur Neurosurg* 83, no. 1 (Jan): 52-56. https://dx.doi.org/10.1055/s-0041-1723808.

[37] Yang, S., J. L. Yu, H. L. Wang, B. Wang, and Q. Luo. 2010. "Endovascular Embolization of Distal Anterior Choroidal Artery Aneurysms Associated with Moyamoya Disease. A Report of Two Cases and a Literature Review." *Interv Neuroradiol* 16, no. 4 (Dec): 433-41. https://dx.doi.org/10.1177/159101991001600410.

[38] Wiedmann, M. K. H., C. Davidoff, A. Lo Presti, W. Ni, J. K. Rhim, M. Simons, and M. A. Stoodley. 2022. "Treatment of Ruptured Aneurysms of the Choroidal Collateral System in Moyamoya Disease: A Systematic Review and Data Analysis." *J Neurosurg* 136, no. 3 (Mar 1): 637-646. https://dx.doi.org/10.3171/2021.1.jns203936.

[39] Yu, J., and X. Lv. 2021. "Flow Diversion for Intracranial Aneurysms Beyond the Circle of Willis." *Front Neurol* 12: 674966. https://dx.doi.org/10.3389/fneur.2021.674966.

[40] Tsukada, T., T. Izumi, H. Isoda, M. Nishihori, A. E. Kropp, T. Mizuno, and T. Wakabayashi. 2022. "Comparison of Hemodynamic Stress in Healthy Vessels after Parent Artery Occlusion and Flow Diverter Stent Treatment for Internal Carotid Artery Aneurysm." *J Neurosurg* 136, no. 3 (Mar 1): 619-626. https://dx.doi.org/10.3171/2021.2.jns204185.

[41] Brunozzi, D., A. See, M. Rizko, J. Choi, G. Atwal, and A. Alaraj. 2022. "Impact of Cerebral Aneurysm Size on Distal Intracranial Hemodynamics and Changes Following Flow Diversion." *Interv Neuroradiol* 28, no. 3 (Jun): 291-295. https://dx.doi.org/10.1177/15910199211032467.

[42] Gelfenbeyn, M., S. K. Natarajan, and L. N. Sekhar. 2009. "Large Distal Anterior Cerebral Artery Aneurysm Treated with Resection and Interposition Graft: Case Report." *Neurosurgery* 64, no. 5 (May): E1008-9; discussion E1009. https://dx.doi.org/10.1227/01.neu.0000339119.92564.29.

[43] Gruber, A., C. Dorfer, G. Bavinzski, H. Standhardt, H. Ferraz-Leite, and E. Knosp. 2012. "Superselective Indocyanine Green Angiography for Selective Revascularization in the Management of Peripheral Cerebral Aneurysms." *AJNR Am J Neuroradiol* 33, no. 3 (Mar): E36-7. https://dx.doi.org/10.3174/ajnr.A2424.

[44] Eckard, D. A., P. L. O'Boynick, C. M. McPherson, V. R. Eckard, P. Han, P. Arnold, and S. Batnitzky. 2000. "Coil Occlusion of the Parent Artery for Treatment of Symptomatic Peripheral Intracranial Aneurysms." *AJNR Am J Neuroradiol* 21, no. 1 (Jan): 137-42.

[45] Grandhi, R., N. T. Zwagerman, G. Linares, E. A. Monaco, 3rd, T. Jovin, M. Horowitz, and B. T. Jankowitz. 2014. "Onyx Embolization of Infectious Intracranial Aneurysms." *J Neurointerv Surg* 6, no. 5 (Jun): 353-6. https://dx.doi.org/10.1136/neurintsurg-2013-010755.

[46] Baltacioğlu, F., S. Cekirge, I. Saatci, H. Oztürk, A. Arat, N. Pamir, and T. Ozgen. 2002. "Distal Middle Cerebral Artery Aneurysms. Endovascular Treatment Results with Literature Review." *Interv Neuroradiol* 8, no. 4 (Dec 22): 399-407. https://dx.doi.org/10.1177/159101990200800409.

[47] Nonaka, S., H. Oishi, S. Tsutsumi, K. Teranishi, S. Tanoue, Y. Yasumoto, M. Yamamoto, and H. Arai. 2016. "Endovascular Therapy for Infectious Intracranial Aneurysm: A Report of Four Cases." *J Stroke Cerebrovasc Dis* 25, no. 3 (Mar): e33-7. https://dx.doi.org/10.1016/j.jstrokecerebrovasdis. 2015.11.033.

[48] Choi, C. H., W. H. Cho, B. K. Choi, and S. W. Lee. 2006. "Rerupture Following Endovascular Treatment for Dissecting Aneurysm of Distal Anterior Inferior Cerebellar Artery with Parent Artery Preservation: Retreatment by Parent Artery Occlusion with Guglielmi Detachable Coils." *Acta Neurochir (Wien)* 148, no. 3 (Mar): 363-6; discussion 366. https://dx.doi.org/10.1007/s00701-005-0702-4.

[49] Atallah, E., H. Saad, N. Mouchtouris, K. Bekelis, J. Walker, N. Chalouhi, S. Tjoumakaris, M. Smith, R. H. Rosenwasser, H. Zarzour, N. Herial, J. Feghali, M. R. Gooch, S. Missios, A. Sweid, and P. Jabbour. 2019. "Pipeline for Distal Cerebral Circulation Aneurysms." *Neurosurgery* 85, no. 3 (Sep 1): E477-e484. https://dx.doi.org/10.1093/neuros/nyz038.

[50] Ravindran, K., A. Enriquez-Marulanda, P. T. M. Kan, L. Renieri, N. Limbucci, S. Mangiafico, M. M. Salem, A. Y. Alturki, J. M. Moore, C. S. Ogilvy, and A. J. Thomas. 2018. "Use of Flow Diversion for the Treatment of Distal Circulation Aneurysms: A Multicohort Study." *World Neurosurg* 118 (Oct): e825-e833. https://dx.doi.org/10.1016/j.wneu.2018.07.062.

[51] Cagnazzo, F., P. Perrini, C. Dargazanli, P. H. Lefevre, G. Gascou, R. Morganti, D. di Carlo, I. Derraz, C. Riquelme, A. Bonafe, and V. Costalat. 2019. "Treatment of Unruptured Distal Anterior Circulation Aneurysms with Flow-Diverter Stents: A Meta-Analysis." *AJNR Am J Neuroradiol* 40, no. 4 (Apr): 687-693. https://dx.doi.org/10.3174/ajnr.A6002.

[52] Primiani, C. T., Z. Ren, P. Kan, R. Hanel, V. M. Pereira, W. M. Lui, N. Goyal, L. Elijovich, A. S. Arthur, D. M. Hasan, S. Ortega-Gutierrez, E. A. Samaniego, A. S. Puri, A. L. Kuhn, K. Orlov, D. Kislitsin, A. Gorbatykh, M. Waqas, E. I. Levy, A. H. Siddiqui, and M. Mokin. 2019. "A2, M2, P2 Aneurysms and Beyond: Results of Treatment with Pipeline Embolization Device in 65 Patients." *J Neurointerv Surg* 11, no. 9 (Sep): 903-907. https://dx.doi.org/10.1136/neurintsurg-2018-014631.

[53] de Castro-Afonso, L. H., G. S. Nakiri, T. G. Abud, L. M. Monsignore, R. K. Freitas, R. S. de Oliveira, B. O. Colli, A. C. Dos Santos, and D. G. Abud. 2021. "Treatment of Distal Unruptured Intracranial Aneurysms Using a Surface-Modified Flow Diverter under Prasugrel Monotherapy: A Pilot Safety

Trial." *J Neurointerv Surg* 13, no. 7 (Jul): 647-651. https://dx.doi.org/10.1136/neurintsurg-2020-017262.

[54] Bender, M. T., D. A. Zarrin, J. K. Campos, L. M. Lin, J. Huang, J. M. Caplan, R. J. Tamargo, G. P. Colby, and A. L. Coon. 2019. "Tiny Pipes: 67 Cases of Flow Diversion for Aneurysms in Distal Vessels Measuring Less Than 2.0 Mm." *World Neurosurg* 127 (Jul): e193-e201. https://dx.doi.org/10.1016/j.wneu.2019.02.204.

[55] Cagnazzo, F., P. H. Lefevre, I. Derraz, C. Dargazanli, G. Gascou, D. T. di Carlo, P. Perrini, R. Ahmed, J. F. Hak, C. Riquelme, A. Bonafe, and V. Costalat. 2020. "Flow-Diversion Treatment for Unruptured Nonsaccular Intracranial Aneurysms of the Posterior and Distal Anterior Circulation: A Meta-Analysis." *AJNR Am J Neuroradiol* 41, no. 1 (Jan): 134-139. https://dx.doi.org/10.3174/ajnr.A6352.

[56] Lin, N., G. Lanzino, D. K. Lopes, A. S. Arthur, C. S. Ogilvy, R. D. Ecker, T. M. Dumont, R. D. th Turner, M. R. Gooch, A. S. Boulos, P. Kan, K. V. Snyder, E. I. Levy, and A. H. Siddiqui. 2016. "Treatment of Distal Anterior Circulation Aneurysms with the Pipeline Embolization Device: A Us Multicenter Experience." *Neurosurgery* 79, no. 1 (Jul): 14-22. https://dx.doi.org/10.1227/ neu.0000000000001117.

[57] Kang, H., B. Luo, J. Liu, H. Zhang, T. Li, D. Song, Y. Zhao, S. Guan, A. Maimaitili, Y. Wang, W. Feng, Y. Wang, J. Wan, G. Mao, H. Shi, Y. Zhang, and X. Yang. 2022. "Postoperative Occlusion Degree after Flow-Diverter Placement with Adjunctive Coiling: Analysis of Complications." *J Neurointerv Surg* 14, no. 4 (Apr): 371-375. https://dx.doi.org/10.1136/neurintsurg-2021-017445.

[58] Lv, X., W. Li, H. Ge, H. Jin, H. He, C. Jiang, and Y. Li. 2018. "Parent Artery Sacrifice for Ruptured Aneurysms in Acute and Chronic Phases: A Systematic Review." *Neurol India* 66, no. 3 (May-Jun): 695-699. https://dx.doi.org/10.4103/0028-3886.232310.

[59] Essibayi, M. A., S. H. Oushy, Z. Keser, and G. Lanzino. 2022. "Natural History and Management of Posterior Cerebral Artery Aneurysms: A Systematic Review and Meta-Analysis of Individual Patient Data." *Neurosurg Rev* 45, no. 6 (Dec): 3595-3608. https://dx.doi.org/10.1007/s10143-022-01867-4.

[60] Hallacq, P., M. Piotin, and J. Moret. 2002. "Endovascular Occlusion of the Posterior Cerebral Artery for the Treatment of P2 Segment Aneurysms: Retrospective Review of a 10-Year Series." *AJNR Am J Neuroradiol* 23, no. 7 (Aug): 1128-36.

[61] Saravanan, M., A. Clifton, and D. Johnson. 2009. "Onyx Embolization of Distal Aneurysms of the Posterior Circulation." *AJNR Am J Neuroradiol* 30, no. 5 (May): e69; author reply e70. https://dx.doi.org/10.3174/ajnr.A1466.

[62] Gao, X., G. Liang, Z. Li, X. Wang, X. Wei, H. Zhang, S. Feng, and J. Lin. 2012. "Intra-Aneurysmal Onyx Embolization for Distal Aneurysms of the Cerebellar Arteries." *Neurol Res* 34, no. 2 (Mar): 211-6. https://dx.doi.org/10.1179/1743132811y.0000000076.

[63] Cagnazzo, F., A. Fanti, P. H. Lefevre, I. Derraz, C. Dargazanli, G. Gascou, C. Riquelme, R. Ahmed, A. Bonafe, and V. Costalat. 2021. "Distal Anterior Cerebral Artery Aneurysms Treated with Flow Diversion: Experience of a Large-Volume Center and Systematic Review of the Literature." *J Neurointerv Surg* 13, no. 1 (Jan): 42-48. https://dx.doi.org/10.1136/neurintsurg-2020-015980.

[64] Lehecka, M., M. Porras, R. Dashti, M. Niemelä, and J. A. Hernesniemi. 2008b. "Anatomic Features of Distal Anterior Cerebral Artery Aneurysms: A Detailed Angiographic Analysis of 101 Patients." *Neurosurgery* 63, no. 2 (Aug): 219-28; discussion 228-9. https://dx.doi.org/10.1227/01.neu. 0000310695.44670.32.

[65] Lehecka, M., H. Lehto, M. Niemelä, S. Juvela, R. Dashti, T. Koivisto, A. Ronkainen, J. Rinne, J. E. Jääskeläinen, and J. A. Hernesniemi. 2008a. "Distal Anterior Cerebral Artery Aneurysms: Treatment and Outcome Analysis of 501 Patients." *Neurosurgery* 62, no. 3 (Mar): 590-601; discussion 590-601. https://dx.doi.org/10.1227/01.neu.0000317307.16332.03.

[66] Ohno, K., S. Monma, R. Suzuki, H. Masaoka, Y. Matsushima, and K. Hirakawa. 1990. "Saccular Aneurysms of the Distal Anterior Cerebral Artery." *Neurosurgery* 27, no. 6 (Dec): 907-12; discussion 912-3. https://dx.doi.org/10.1097/00006123-199012000-00008.

[67] Türe, U., T. Hiçdönmez, I. Elmaci, and S. Peker. 2001. "Giant Pericallosal Artery Aneurysm: Case Report and Review of the Literature." *Neurosurg Rev* 24, no. 2-3 (Jul): 151-5. https://dx.doi.org/10.1007/pl00012401.

[68] Alurkar, A., L. S. Karanam, S. Oak, and S. Nayak. 2014. "Endovascular Treatment of Fusiform A2 Aneurysm with Parent Artery Occlusion." *Surg Neurol Int* 5, no. Suppl 4: S199-202. https://dx.doi.org/10.4103/2152-7806.137752.

[69] Tanioka, S., F. Ishida, T. Kishimoto, K. Tanaka, S. Shimosaka, and H. Suzuki. 2020. "Prediction of the Extent of Thrombus Formation in the Parent Artery after Endovascular Occlusion of a Distal Anterior Cerebral Artery Aneurysm Using Computational Fluid Dynamics." *J Clin Neurosci* 74 (Apr): 210-212. https://dx.doi.org/10.1016/j.jocn.2019.08.042.

[70] Van Rooij, W. J., and S. B. Van Rooij. 2013. "Endovascular Treatment of Traumatic Pericallosal Artery Aneurysms. A Case Report." *Interv Neuroradiol* 19, no. 1 (Mar): 56-9. https://dx.doi.org/10.1177/159101991301900108.

[71] Tsuji, Y., T. Miki, H. Kakita, K. Sato, T. Yoshida, and F. Shimizu. 2020. "Parent Artery Occlusion for Treatment of a Traumatic Pericallosal Artery Aneurysm: Case Report and Review of the Literature." *World Neurosurg* 140 (Aug): 193-197. https://dx.doi.org/10.1016/j.wneu.2020.04.186.

[72] Nakstad, P., H. Nornes, and H. N. Hauge. 1986. "Traumatic Aneurysms of the Pericallosal Arteries." *Neuroradiology* 28, no. 4: 335-8. https://dx.doi.org/10.1007/bf00333440.

[73] Calvacante, T., S. Derrey, S. Curey, O. Langlois, P. Fréger, E. Gérardin, H. Castel, and F. Proust. 2013. "Distal Middle Cerebral Artery Aneurysm: A Proposition of Microsurgical Management." *Neurochirurgie* 59, no. 3 (Jun): 121-7. https://dx.doi.org/10.1016/j.neuchi.2013.04.007.

[74] Mawad, M. E., and R. P. Klucznik. 1995. "Giant Serpentine Aneurysms: Radiographic Features and Endovascular Treatment." *AJNR Am J Neuroradiol* 16, no. 5 (May): 1053-60.

[75] Cimflova, P., E. Özlük, B. Korkmazer, R. Ahmadov, E. Akpek, O. Kizilkilic, C. Islak, and N. Kocer. 2021. "Long-Term Safety and Efficacy of Distal Aneurysm Treatment with Flow Diversion in the M2 Segment of the Middle Cerebral Artery and Beyond." *J Neurointerv Surg* 13, no. 7 (Jul): 631-636. https://dx.doi.org/10.1136/neurintsurg-2020-016790.

[76] Kivipelto, L., M. Niemelä, T. Meling, M. Lehecka, H. Lehto, and J. Hernesniemi. 2014. "Bypass Surgery for Complex Middle Cerebral Artery Aneurysms: Impact of the Exact Location in the Mca Tree." *J Neurosurg* 120, no. 2 (Feb): 398-408. https://dx.doi.org/10.3171/2013.10.jns13738.

[77] Xu, J., L. Xu, Z. Wu, X. Chen, J. Yu, and J. Zhang. 2015. "Fetal-Type Posterior Cerebral Artery: The Pitfall of Parent Artery Occlusion for Ruptured P_2 Segment and Distal Aneurysms." *J Neurosurg* 123, no. 4 (Oct): 906-14. https://dx.doi.org/10.3171/2014.9.jns1442.

[78] Hou, K., X. Lv, and J. Yu. 2021. "Endovascular Treatment of Posterior Cerebral Artery Trunk Aneurysm: The Status Quo and Dilemma." *Front Neurol* 12: 746525. https://dx.doi.org/10.3389/fneur.2021.746525.

[79] Luo, Q., H. Wang, K. Xu, and J. Yu. 2012. "Endovascular Treatments for Distal Posterior Cerebral Artery Aneurysms." *Turk Neurosurg* 22, no. 2: 141-7. https://dx.doi.org/10.5137/1019-5149.jtn.4079-11.0.

[80] Arat, A., C. Islak, I. Saatci, N. Kocer, and S. Cekirge. 2002. "Endovascular Parent Artery Occlusion in Large-Giant or Fusiform Distal Posterior Cerebral Artery Aneurysms." *Neuroradiology* 44, no. 8 (Aug): 700-5. https://dx.doi.org/10.1007/s00234-002-0747-5.

[81] Acik, V., E. Daglioglu, I. Akmangit, F. Alagoz, B. Sayin, and A. Arat. 2019. "Endovascular Treatment of Superior Cerebellar Artery Aneurysms." *Turk Neurosurg* 29, no. 4: 564-569. https://dx.doi.org/10.5137/1019-5149.jtn.24640-18.3.

[82] Velioglu, M., H. Selcuk, O. Kizilkilic, C. Basekim, N. Kocer, and C. Islak. 2015. "Endovascular Management of Superior Cerebellar Artery Aneurysms: Mid and Long-Term Results." *Turk Neurosurg* 25, no. 4: 526-31. https://dx.doi.org/10.5137/1019-5149.jtn.8611-13.0.

[83] Kim, C. H., Y. D. Cho, S. C. Jung, J. H. Ahn, H. S. Kang, J. E. Kim, W. S. Cho, and M. H. Han. 2014. "Endovascular Treatment for Superior Cerebellar Artery Aneurysms: Morphological Features, Technique, and Outcome." *Neuroradiology* 56, no. 8 (Aug): 647-54. https://dx.doi.org/10.1007/s00234-014-1375-6.

[84] Hou, K., G. Li, X. Wang, K. Xu, and J. Yu. 2019a. "Endovascular Treatment for Peripheral Superior Cerebellar Artery Aneurysms: Current State and Future Considerations." *World Neurosurg* 127 (Jul): 423-433. https://dx.doi.org/10.1016/j.wneu.2019.04.145.

[85] Hou, K., G. Li, B. Xu, K. Xu, and J. Yu. 2019b. "Which Patients with Aneurysms Involving the A1-A2 Segment of the Anterior Inferior Cerebellar Artery Would Benefit from Parent Artery Occlusion?" *World Neurosurg* 126 (Jun): 301-309. https://dx.doi.org/10.1016/j.wneu.2019.03.070.

[86] Hou, K., G. Li, T. Luan, K. Xu, B. Xu, and J. Yu. 2020a. "Anatomical Study of Anterior Inferior Cerebellar Artery and Its Reciprocal Relationship with Posterior Inferior Cerebellar Artery Based on Angiographic Data." *World Neurosurg* 133 (Jan): e459-e472. https://dx.doi.org/10.1016/j.wneu.2019.09.047.

[87] Horiuchi, T., Y. Tanaka, K. Hongo, J. Nitta, Y. Kusano, and S. Kobayashi. 2003. "Characteristics of Distal Posteroinferior Cerebellar Artery Aneurysms." *Neurosurgery* 53, no. 3 (Sep): 589-95; discussion 595-6. https://dx.doi.org/10.1227/01.neu.0000079493.50657.1d.

[88] Chalouhi, N., P. Jabbour, R. M. Starke, S. I. Tjoumakaris, L. F. Gonzalez, S. Witte, R. H. Rosenwasser, and A. S. Dumont. 2013a. "Endovascular Treatment of Proximal and Distal Posterior Inferior Cerebellar Artery Aneurysms." *J Neurosurg* 118, no. 5 (May): 991-9. https://dx.doi.org/10.3171/2012.12.JNS121240.

[89] Lehto, H., A. Harati, M. Niemelä, R. Dashti, A. Laakso, A. Elsharkawy, J. Satopää, R. Billon-Grand, B. Canato, R. Kivisaari, and J. Hernesniemi. 2014. "Distal Posterior Inferior Cerebellar Artery Aneurysms: Clinical Features and Outcome of 80 Patients." *World Neurosurg* 82, no. 5 (Nov): 702-13. https://dx.doi.org/10.1016/j.wneu.2014.06.012.

[90] Shi, L., K. Xu, X. Sun, and J. Yu. 2016. "Therapeutic Progress in Treating Vertebral Dissecting Aneurysms Involving the Posterior Inferior Cerebellar Artery." *Int J Med Sci* 13, no. 7: 540-55. https://dx.doi.org/10.7150/ijms.15233.

[91] Hou, K., and J. Yu. 2022. "Case Report: Can Ruptured Aneurysms in the Hypoplastic and Plexiform Posterior Inferior Cerebellar Arteries Be Safely Occluded?" *Front Neurol* 13: 904863. https://dx.doi.org/10.3389/fneur.2022.904863.

[92] Lewis, S. B., D. J. Chang, D. A. Peace, P. J. Lafrentz, and A. L. Day. 2002. "Distal Posterior Inferior Cerebellar Artery Aneurysms: Clinical Features and Management." *J Neurosurg* 97, no. 4 (Oct): 756-66. https://dx.doi.org/10.3171/jns.2002.97.4.0756.

[93] Hou, K., Y. Guo, B. Xu, K. Xu, and J. Yu. 2018. "Delayed Establishment of Collateral Circulation from Posterior Meningeal Artery after Proximal Occlusion of Posterior Inferior Cerebellar Artery: Case Report and Literature Review." *World Neurosurg* 115 (Jul): 334-337. https://dx.doi.org/10.1016/j.wneu.2018.04.207.

[94] Isokangas, J. M., T. Siniluoto, T. Tikkakoski, and T. Kumpulainen. 2008. "Endovascular Treatment of Peripheral Aneurysms of the Posterior Inferior Cerebellar Artery." *AJNR Am J Neuroradiol* 29, no. 9 (Oct): 1783-8. https://dx.doi.org/10.3174/ajnr.A1218.

[95] Hou, Kun, Yiheng Wang, Wei Li, and Jinlu Yu. 2021. "Endovascular Treatment of Brain Arteriovenous Malformations Involving the Anterior Cerebral Artery." *Med Int* 1, no. 5 (2021/11/01): 22. https://dx.doi.org/10.3892/mi.2021.22.

[96] Hou, K., K. Xu, X. Chen, Y. Wang, K. Li, and J. Yu. 2020c. "Endovascular Treatment for the Flow-Related Aneurysm Originating from an Anterior Inferior Cerebellar Artery Supplying the Cerebellar Arteriovenous Malformation." *Interv Neuroradiol* 26, no. 5 (Oct): 566-574. https://dx.doi.org/10.1177/1591019920954082.

[97] Peluso, J. P., W. J. van Rooij, M. Sluzewski, and G. N. Beute. 2007. "Distal Aneurysms of Cerebellar Arteries: Incidence, Clinical Presentation, and Outcome of Endovascular Parent Vessel Occlusion." *AJNR Am J Neuroradiol* 28, no. 8 (Sep): 1573-8. https://dx.doi.org/10.3174/ajnr.A0607.

[98] Case, D., D. Kumpe, L. Cava, R. Neumann, A. White, C. Roark, and J. Seinfeld. 2017. "Ruptured Distal Posterior Inferior Cerebellar Artery (Pica) Aneurysms Associated with Cerebellar Arterial Venous Malformations (Avms): A Case Series and Review of the Literature Demonstrating the Need for Angiographic Evaluation and Feasibility of Endovascular Treatment." *World Neurosurg* 97 (Jan): 751.e7-751.e13. https://dx.doi.org/10.1016/j.wneu.2016.10.081.

[99] Hou, K., Y. Guo, T. Luan, and J. Yu. 2021. "Parent Artery Occlusion for Flow-Related Aneurysms at the Proximal Segment of the Main Feeding Arteries of Cerebellar Arteriovenous Malformations." *Br J Neurosurg* (Aug 11): 1-8. https://dx.doi.org/10.1080/02688697.2021.1950625.

[100] Hou, K., K. Xu, X. Chen, T. Ji, Y. Guo, and J. Yu. 2020b. "Targeted Endovascular Treatment for Ruptured Brain Arteriovenous Malformations." *Neurosurg Rev* 43, no. 6 (Dec): 1509-1518. https://dx.doi.org/10.1007/s10143-019-01205-1.

[101] Zhou, Zibo, Kan Xu, and Jinlu Yu. 2023. "Parent Artery Occlusion for Ruptured Aneurysms in Moyamoya Vessels or on Collaterals." *Frontiers in Neurology* 14 (2023-January-30). https://dx.doi.org/10.3389/fneur.2023.1085120.

Chapter 8

Intracranial Dissecting Aneurysms

Shikai Liang
Ma Chao
and Xianli Lv*
Department of Neurosurgery, Beijing Tsinghua Changgung Hospital, School of Clinical Medicine, Tsinghua University, Beijing, China

Abstract

Intracranial dissecting aneurysms are a special type of pathological aneurysm. Unlike a saccular aneurysm, the dissecting aneurysm is usually caused by the damage to the vessel wall structure of cerebral arteries, especially a disruption of the internal elastic lamina, the media with or without the adventitia which leads to a partial protrusion of the adventitia. Stent-assisted coiling embolization is a recommended technique for cases in which vessels are damaged as a result of aneurysms. Surgical clipping is not effective due to the high morbidity and mortality rates. Flow-diversion devices (FDs) have provided good results in the management of dissecting aneurysms. Still, they should be evaluated according to the location of the aneurysm, the type of aneurysm, the patient's age, and the patient's preoperative health condition, weighing the advantages and risks of each treatment strategy, and choosing the best treatment according to the patient's actual situation.

Keywords: dissecting aneurysm, flow diverter, pipeline embolization device

Intracranial dissecting aneurysms are uncommon entities associated with high rates of morbidity and mortality [1]. Patients often present with a prodromal headache followed by subarachnoid hemorrhage (SAH) or ischemic stroke [1, 2]. Imaging findings are critical to establishing the diagnosis, as the lesions have a myriad of presentations based on the severity, location, and timing of the dissection [3]. Lesions that present with ischemia are at high risk for future ischemia but have a low risk of future hemorrhage. In contrast, lesions present with hemorrhage have a high rate of rebleeding if left untreated [1, 2]. There are no evidence-based guidelines for medical or surgical management [1]. Several endovascular and surgical techniques have been used to prevent or treat hemorrhage by ligating the parent artery or

* Corresponding Author's Email: lvxianli000@163.com.

In: Understanding and Managing Cerebral Aneurysms
Editor: Xianli Lv
ISBN: 979-8-89113-608-3

reconstructing the vessel wall (Figure 1) [1]. Outcomes are generally poorer in patients with intracranial dissecting aneurysms than in cervical artery dissection (Figure 2), particularly those suffering SAH [1].

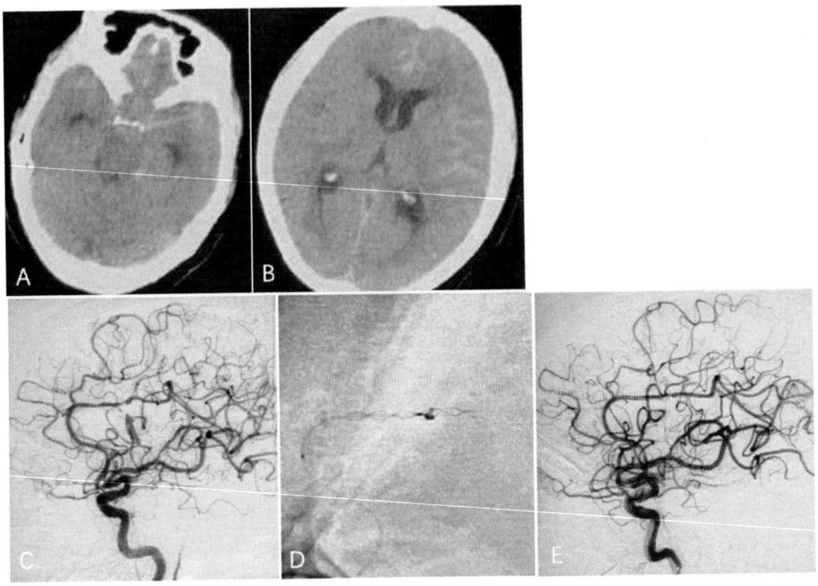

Figure 1. A and B, CT scanning showing subarachnoid hemorrhage in a 61-year-old female patient. C, Internal carotid artery angiogram, lateral view, showing a dissecting aneurysm at the A4 segment of the anterior cerebral artery. D, unsubtracted image, lateral view, showing the aneurysm was treated by Leo baby stent-assisted coiling embolization. E, Postoperative angiogram, lateral view, showing the aneurysm was completely occluded.

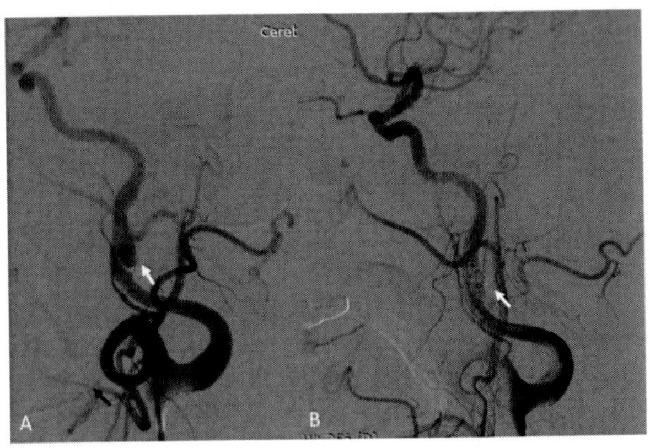

Figure 2. A, Carotid artery angiogram, lateral view, showing a dissecting aneurysm at cervical internal carotid artery (arrow). B, Carotid artery angiogram, lateral view, showing the dissecting aneurysm was treated by Leo stent-assisted coiling (arrow).

Part 1: Etiology and epidemiology

Common causes of dissecting aneurysms may be related to 1) atherosclerotic disease; 2) Inheritance; 3) Vascular structure; 4) Infection; 5) radioactivity; and 6) Others: stenosis of the aortic arch, giant cell arteritis, or trauma [4].

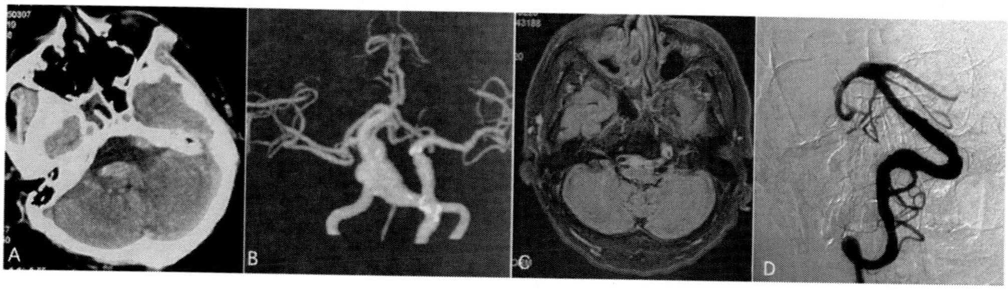

Figure 3. A, CT scanning showing a high-density focal lesion in front of the brainstem. B, CTA examination showing a dissecting aneurysm of vertebrobasilar artery. C, enhanced MRI examination, axial view, T1-weighted, showing an enhanced lesion the front of the brainstem. D, The right vertebral artery angiogram, frontal view, demonstrating an arterial dissection of the vertebrobasilar artery.

The incidence of dissecting aneurysms, previously thought to be rare in the brain, has recently increased as a result of advances in neuroimaging [5]. Dissecting aneurysms may occur in both the anterior circulation artery (anterior cerebral artery (ACA) (Figure 1), middle cerebral artery (MCA)) and posterior circulation artery (posterior cerebral artery, vertebral artery, basilar artery), but are commonly observed in the posterior circulation (Figure 3) [1].

Part 2: Pathological Mechanisms

The available neuropathological specimens usually show disruption of the internal elastic lamina and the media, and it is unclear whether direct bleeding of vasa vasorum (small blood vessels in the wall of larger blood vessels) in the arterial wall is the initial event [6]. Vasa vasorum does not always appear in intracranial arteries, but mainly in the tunica adventitia and proximal intracranial arteries. After 14 days of onset, intramural bleeding is replaced by granulation tissue, followed by compensatory thickening of the intima around the false lumen [6].

In the samples obtained 30 days after the onset of symptoms, it was reported that new blood vessels appeared in the thickened intima, leading to the formation of chronic fusiform shaped aneurysms due to repeated intramural bleeding caused by the rupture of fragile new blood vessels [6]. Different types of intimal injury in intracranial arterial dissection have been reported. A mural hematoma may be caused by an entrance in the false lumen (entry-only lesions) or an entrance and an exit in the false lumen (entry-exit lesions) [1]. The incidence of SAH in entry-only lesions is higher than that in entry-exit lesions [1].

The giant serpentine aneurysms and "blood blister-like" aneurysms (BBAs) are special pathophysiological overlap of intracranial artery dissection. Giant serpentine aneurysm is a rare subtype of intracranial dissecting aneurysm with a distinct appearance. It consists of a partially thrombosed giant intracranial aneurysm ($\geq$ 25 mm) traversed by a patent serpiginous intra-aneurysmal vascular channel (Figures 4 and 5) [7]. This vascular channel is an entry-exit lesion, differentiating it from a giant aneurysm. BBAs located at non-branching sites of intracranial arteries are caused by a direct dilaceration of the internal elastic lamina and media associated arterial dissection (intramural hematoma or double lumen on pathological or MRI examination) (Figure 6) [8].

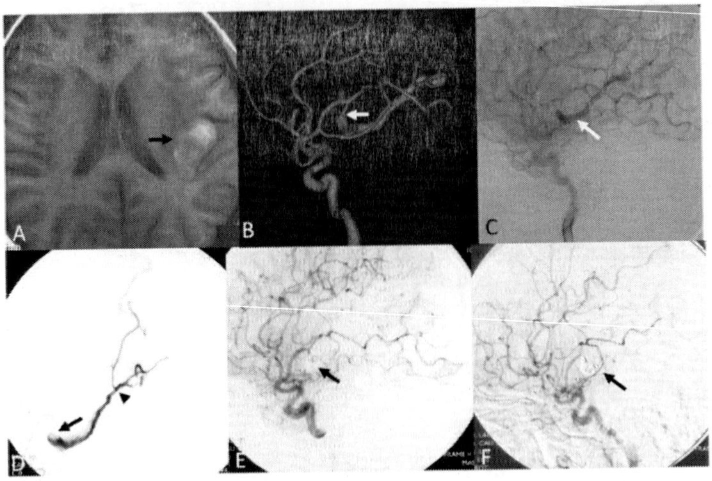

Figure 4. Case presentation of a giant serpentine aneurysm. A 9-year-old boy presented with right limb twitching with numbness for 1 month. A, head MRI examination, axial view, T1-weighted, showing a hyperintense foci in the partially thrombosed aneurysm in the left Sylvian fissure. B, CT angiography showing the serpentine intra-aneurysmal vascular channel. C, the left internal carotid artery angiography, lateral view, late arterial phase, showing the morphology of the patent intra-aneurysm tortuous vascular channel. D, selective angiography of the microcatheter showing the inflow (arrow) and outflow(arrowhead) of the aneurysm. E, after embolization, the left internal carotid artery angiography showed complete occlusion of the aneurysm. F, after 5 months, the left internal carotid artery angiography confirmed complete occlusion of the aneurysm (This case has been published by Lv X, et al. Neuroradiol J. 2007;20(2):237-241).

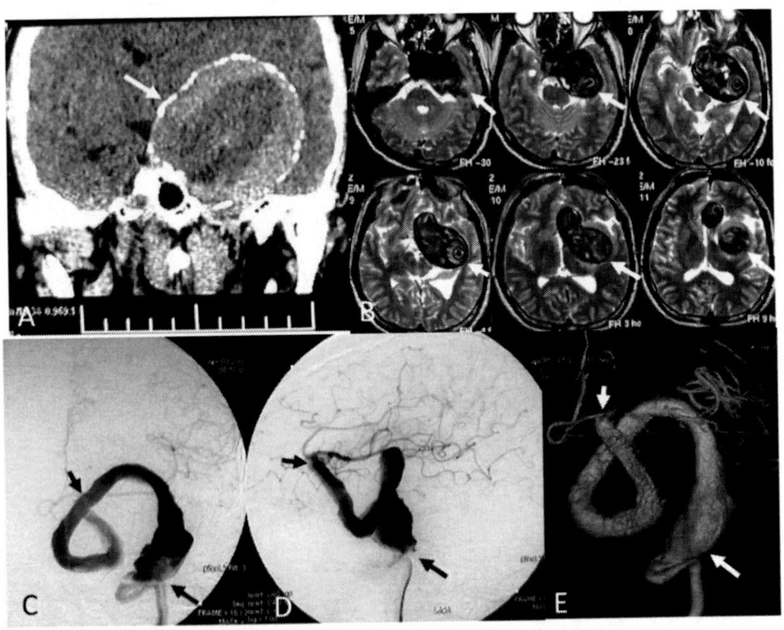

Figure 5. A 38-year-old patient presented with a 2-year history of headaches, left eye blindness and ophthalmoplegia caused by a giant serpentine aneurysm. A, unenhanced coronal CT image showing the large mass in the left frontotemporal region, with central and peripheral calcification (arrow). B, T2-weighted axial images showing a large thrombosed aneurysm in the left frontotemporal region (arrows). C, the left internal carotid artery angiography, frontal view. D, the left internal carotid artery angiography, lateral view. E, 3-D reconstruction of the left internal carotid artery angiography. Showing the morphology of the patent intra-aneurysm tortuous vascular channel and the inflow (long arrow) and outflow(short arrow) of the aneurysm. (This case has been published by Lv X et al. Neuroradiol J. 2020;33(2):105–111).

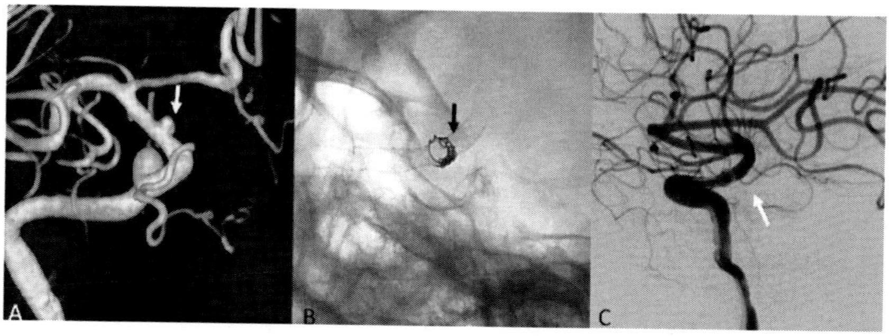

Figure 6. **A** 57-year-old male patient presented with a SAH caused by a BBA.
A, 3-D reconstruction of the right internal carotid artery angiography. Showing the morphology of the BBA (arrow). B, unsubtracted image, lateral view, showing the BBA was treated by the pipeline embolization device (PED; Medtronic Neurovascular, Irvine, California, USA) in combination with coil embolization(arrow). C, the right internal carotid artery angiography, lateral view, showing the BBA was completely occluded.

Part 3: Symptoms

Based on clinical presentation, dissecting aneurysms can be separated into acute or chronic lesions [2, 9]. Understanding the underlying pathological mechanisms associated with these aneurysms is useful for planning appropriate treatment. The two main manifestations are SAH and cerebral ischemia. In most reported series, 50–60% of intracranial arterial dissections cause SAH [10]. SAH occurs if the arterial wall of an intracranial artery dissection in the intradural portion ruptures. Between 30% and 78% of patients with intracranial arterial dissection present with cerebral ischemia (ischemic stroke or transient ischemic attack), without SAH [11].

Other uncommon manifestations of intracranial arterial dissections include isolated headache and symptoms associated with mass effect, which mostly affects the brainstem or cranial nerves [12]. In the case of dissecting aneurysms that were large (≥ 10 mm in diameter) and giant (≥25 mm in diameter), anatomic features are unique [13]. They may be characterized by a predisposition to rupture, resulting in SAH. Mass effect was formed to compress surrounding brain tissue as well as cranial nerves. Ischemic stroke occurs because of its large size, severe damage to vascular tissue (such as thrombosis, calcification, and thinning of blood vessel walls), and susceptibility to the involvement of adjacent perforating arteries.

The ischemic stroke caused by the vertebral basilar artery dissecting aneurysm can present the symptoms of the neurological deficits of low cranial nerves (VIII, IX, X), medulla oblongata as well as the pons [14]. Weakness or hemiplegia of limbs is common in patients with a dissecting aneurysm of the MCA [7].

Part 4: Imaging and Diagnosis

Most dissecting aneurysms expand along the long axis of the artery, and a few can appear elliptical or almost circle on CT and MRI scans, but angiography may show an abnormally dilated and tortuous lumen that can be readily distinguished from saccular aneurysms [3]. A dissecting aneurysm may be located between the endometrium and media or between the media and the adventitia, the parent artery narrowing, and the "string sign" on angiography [3]. The true lumen of the aneurysm and the false lumen may be clear on angiography. In some cases, it is difficult to distinguish between dissecting and fusiform aneurysms based on angiography, and an MRI examination is required. MRI characteristics of dissecting aneurysms were as follows [3]: 1. Endometrial valve located within the vascular lumen; 2. There is a double lumen of the aneurysm; 3. The pseudoaneurysm was found to contain a subacute blood clot, an intramural hematoma. High-resolution MRI can also generally lead to the diagnosis of dissecting aneurysms.

Initially, noninvasive imaging tests such as CTA and MRA allow for the diagnosis of dissecting aneurysms. Digital subtraction angiography (DSA) continues to be the "gold standard" for diagnosing cerebrovascular disease, providing detailed information on the shape and location. The angiographic criteria for detecting dissections are the stagnation of contrast in the aneurysmal pouch, the presence of stenotic segments proximal or distal to the ectasia, and the more likely fusiform appearance. The typical description is the presence of a "pearl-and-string sign," sometimes associated with a pseudoaneurysm.

Part 5: Treatment

Management of dissecting aneurysms includes neurosurgical and endovascular procedures [10-15]. Endovascular therapy consists primarily of simple coiling embolization and balloon-assisted coiling embolization, but these methods often have poor long-term outcomes because of recurrences of the aneurysms [16]. Deconstruction is a good strategy when there are adequate collaterals (Figure 7), though deconstructive techniques carry higher perioperative morbidity than reconstructive techniques (12.0% vs 4.0%, P = 0.04) [17]. Otherwise, surgical trapping and revascularization or endovascular vessel preservation strategies such as overlapping stents, or covered stent is necessary [18]. Currently, FD is a promising device in the management of dissecting aneurysms [19].

Compared with endovascular treatment, neurosurgical treatment has a higher rate of disability and mortality [15]. Neurosurgical treatment has a 24% complication rate [15]. The incidence of disability and mortality was 37.9% and 9.6%, respectively, for large dissecting aneurysms [15]. The disability and mortality rates were 12.9% and 3.0% for non-giant dissecting aneurysms in posterior circulation [15]. Parent artery sacrifice with coil embolization usually has satisfactory results [20, 21]. However, parent artery occlusion is also associated with a risk of cerebral infarction due to insufficient collateral circulation [22]. There is a risk of recurrence of an intra-aneurysm coil embolization, and it is not suitable for independent treatment of dissecting aneurysms [1].

Stent-assisted coiling is also associated with a low rate of complete obliteration and a high rate of complications in treating posterior circulation dissecting aneurysms (Figure 8). A large series study by Shapiro et al. showed a 61% complete obliteration rate and 19% complication rate of stent-assisted coiling for intracranial aneurysms [3]. The study of Rho et al. showed a 67.8% complete obliteration rate and 21.4% complication rate in posterior circulation dissecting aneurysms treated with stents-assisted coiling [23, 24]. However, a recent study showed that stent-assisted coiling for intracranial aneurysms had an aneurysm obliteration rate of 79.8%, an intraoperative complication rate of 7.4%, and a postoperative complication rate of 7.6% [25].

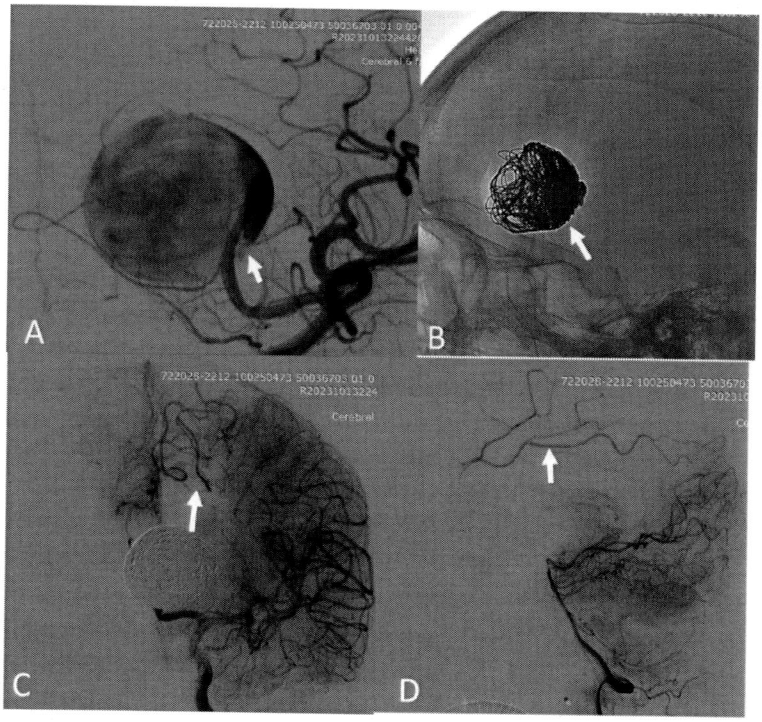

Figure 7. A 57-year-old female patient presented with dizziness. A, the left carotid artery angiogram, oblique view, showing a giant dissecting aneurysm of the left anterior cerebral artery (arrow). B, unsubtracted image, lateral view, showing the aneurysm was treated by deconstructive therapy of the anterior cerebral artery occlusion using coils (arrow). C, the left internal carotid artery angiography, frontal view. D, the left vertebral artery angiography, lateral view. Showing the collateral circulations to the distal anterior cerebral artery (arrows).

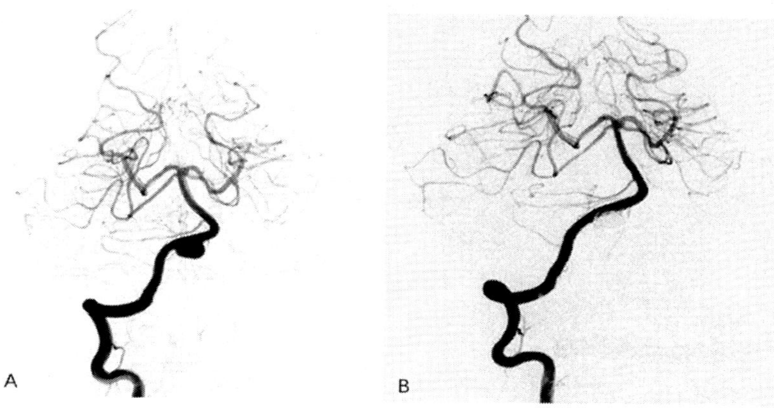

Figure 8. A, the right vertebral artery angiogram, fronal view, showing a dissecting aneurysm of the V4 segment. B, the right vertebral artery angiography, frontal view, showing complete occlusion of the aneurysm after Enterprise stent-assisted coil embolization.

Klisch et al. reported a 70% complete obliteration rate and no related complications in stent-assisted coiling for posterior circulation dissecting aneurysms [26]. These differences may be due to different stent devices used and different aneurysm characteristics.

Flow Diversion Treatment for Dissecting Aneurysms

Due to the high morbidity and mortality associated with microsurgical treatment of those aneurysms, endovascular therapy gained ascendance as the preferred method of treatment. Flow diversion has emerged as a promising treatment option for dissecting aneurysms with a higher occlusion rate compared to other endovascular techniques and a lower complication rate compared to microsurgery [27, 28]. While treatment of saccular and dissecting aneurysms is often associated with comparatively good outcomes, fusiform and dolichoectatic aneurysms should be carefully selected prior to treatment to avoid devastating thromboembolic complications [19]. Occlusion of covered perforating branches showed no correlation with ischemic complications, and appropriate antiplatelet regimen and switching Clopidogrel non-responders to different antiplatelet agents were associated with lower complication rates following flow diversion of dissecting aneurysms [29].

The pipeline embolization device (PED; Medtronic Neurovascular, Irvine, California, USA) with SHIELD technology is a novel PED with phosphocholine surface modifications [30]. It mimics erythrocytes and has shown lower thrombogenicity than the current PED Flex and other FD devices. The PED–SHIELD has similar thrombogenicity to self-expanding stents and aims to reduce thromboembolic events and the number or duration of antiplatelets.

Vertebral Artery Dissecting Aneurysm

Prior studies have demonstrated the efficacy of PED for vertebral artery dissecting aneurysms, with complete embolization rates varying between 66.7%-100% and disability and mortality rates of 0% [27]. The aneurysm involving the posterior inferior cerebellar artery is challenging to treat because of its recurrence and sacrifice of the posterior inferior cerebellar artery. PEDs were effective in treating these aneurysms, and the posterior inferior cerebellar artery was usually preserved after being covered with PED [31]. Thus, FD is considered as a safe and effective treatment for dissecting aneurysms of the vertebral artery.

Vertebrobasilar Artery Dissecting Aneurysm

Vertebrobasilar artery dissecting aneurysms present a significant therapeutic challenge in the vertebral and basilar arteries because of their unfavorable shapes, frequently affecting both the vertebral and basilar arteries. In endovascular coil embolization, there's a frequent recurrence during follow-up, and the outcomes are unpredictable. Recent research indicated that PEDs might be the optimal approach for these aneurysms [32, 33].

Basilar Artery Dissecting Aneurysm

Perforating arteries can usually be observed in basilar artery aneurysms, and their location is usually very close to the brainstem. These characteristics considerably complicate their therapeutic approaches. Whatever neurosurgical or endovascular techniques, there is a high postoperative complication rate. A comprehensive multicenter study highlighted the 13.9% incidence of morbidity and mortality from PED treatments of posterior circulation aneurysms, possibly attributable to the higher proportion of basilar aneurysms in their dataset (Figure 9) [34].

Dissecting Aneurysms of the Main Branch of the Vertebrobasilar Artery

Those dissecting aneurysms arising in the posterior inferior cerebellar artery, the anterior inferior cerebellar artery, the superior cerebellar artery, and the posterior cerebral artery are relatively uncommon, accounting for about 3% of the incidence of aneurysms in the posterior circulation [35-37]. The dissecting aneurysms at the proximal segment of the posterior inferior cerebellar artery or the posterior cerebral artery are often suitable for FD treatment [36,38]. Most of these dissecting aneurysms are treated with simple coiling or stent-assisted coiling embolization techniques [35, 37].

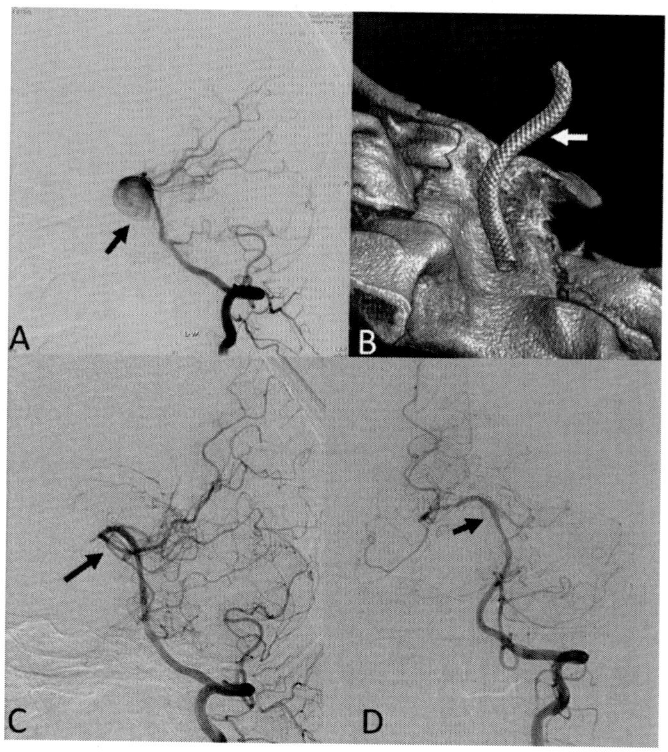

Figure 9. A 20-year-old female patient had headaches. A, the lateral view of vertebral artery angiography showing a giant dissecting aneurysm in the upper segment of the basilar artery (arrow). B. Dyna CT imaging showing that the aneurysm had undergone PED treatment. After 8-month follow-up, the patient did not have any neurological deficits. C, the left vertebral artery angiography, lateral view. D, the left vertebral artery angiography, frontal view. Showing complete occlusion of the aneurysm.

Dissecting Aneurysms of Carotid Circulation

Most studies have focused on dissecting aneurysms occurring in the vertebrobasilar system, with the pathogenesis, clinical features, and neuroradiographic findings. However, treatments for dissecting aneurysms of the carotid artery system are not well documented. Publications concerning dissecting aneurysms of the carotid circulation have been limited to case reports. Several recent case reports have described SAH from a dissecting aneurysm of the intracranial carotid circulation [39]. These reports indicate that the clinical features and pathogenesis of dissecting aneurysms of the intracranial carotid circulation need to be better understood (Figure 10).

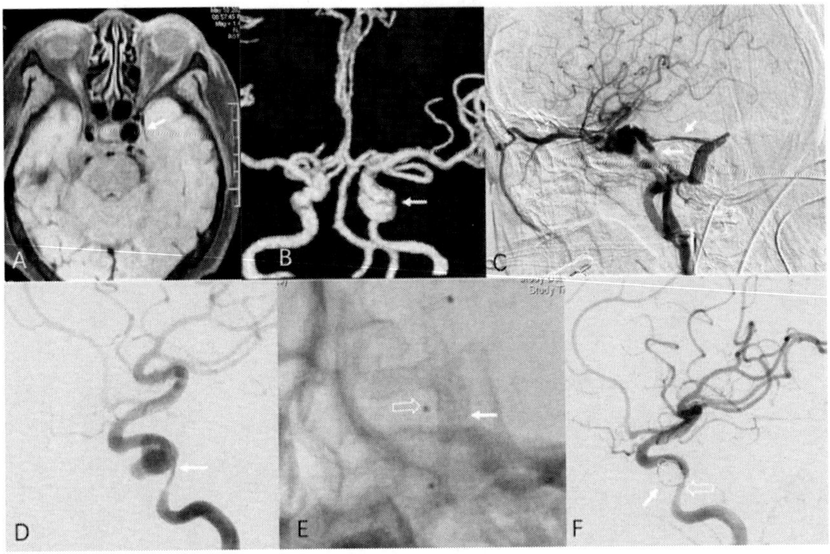

Figure 10. A 41-year-old female patient presented with spontaneous exophthalmos. A, MRI examination, axial view, T1-weighted, showing a flow void signal in the left parasellar region (arrow). B, CTA examination showing an aneurysm of the cavernous segment of the left internal carotid artery (arrow). C, the left internal carotid angiograph, lateral view, showing a carotid cavernous fistula drained through the superior petrosal sinus (short arrow), inferior petrosal sinus(long arrow), and ophthalmic vein(void arrow). D, during treatment, the left internal carotid artery angiography showing a pseudoaneurysm of the cavernous segment of the internal carotid artery with proximal stenosis (arrow). It is considered that the dissecting aneurysm rupture of the internal carotid artery caused the carotid cavernous fistula. E, unsubtracted image showing PED flow diversion (arrow) and coil embolization(void arrow showing the microcatheter for coil embolization) therapy for the lesion. F, at 3-month, follow-up angiography showed complete occlusion of the aneurysm (arrow) and improvement in proximal stenosis(void arrow).

Intracranial dissecting aneurysms of the internal carotid artery are mainly the BBAs of the C2 anterior wall [40]. Because BBA is usually fragile, the rate of intraoperative rebleeding is higher than saccular aneurysm, so the treatment of BBA is still challenging.

Most intracranial dissecting aneurysms of the vertebrobasilar system are associated with SAH. In contrast, those of the carotid system typically present with cerebral infarction caused by arterial stenosis and occlusion [41]. It has also been reported that only 14% of intracranial dissecting aneurysms causing hemorrhage occur in the anterior circulation. Dissecting aneurysms of the intracranial carotid circulation was previously thought to occur primarily in young people presenting with symptoms such as headache, focal neurological deficits, and intracranial hemorrhage [39]. Therefore, the appropriate management of dissecting aneurysms in the anterior circulation remains controversial, especially in patients with cerebral infarction. Some reviews and case reports have compared the outcomes of surgical and medical treatments for these aneurysms. In earlier studies on this topic, such cases were typically reported to have a very poor outcome [39].

It is extremely rare for dissecting aneurysms to develop at the distal intracranial arteries [42]. The M1 segment of the MCA and the A1 segment of the ACA, where many distal dissecting aneurysms arise, have a lot of lenticulostriate perforating arteries. Therefore, dissecting aneurysms of the MCA are often associated with lenticulostriate and branching arteries. Surgical clipping often leads to recurrence or immediate occlusion of branch arteries, which brings great challenges. However, they can be safely covered by FD therapy without leading to strokes and secondary neurological deficits (Figures 11 and 12) [42].

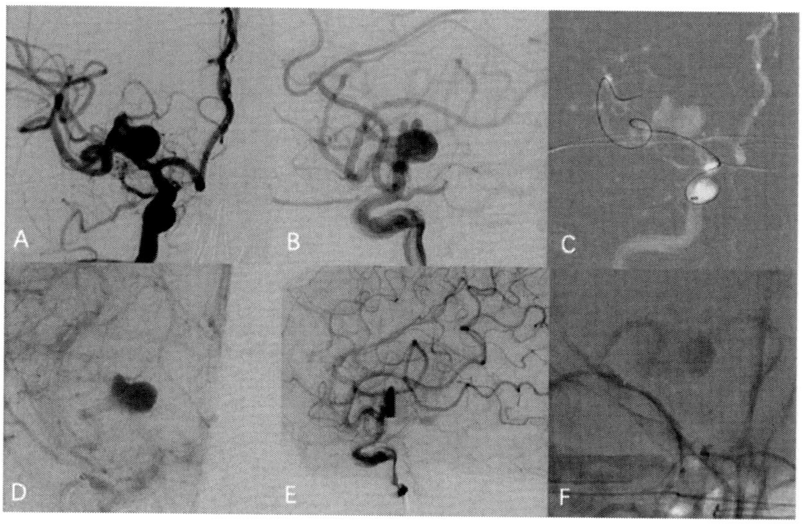

Figure 11. A, the right internal carotid artery angiography, frontal view. B, the right internal carotid artery angiography, lateral view. Showing a giant dissecting aneurysm of the M1 segment of the middle cerebral artery. C, under the road map image, a 0.027-inch microcatheter was navigated by a 0.014-inch microguidewire to reach the distal branch of the middle cerebral artery distal to the aneurysm. D, the right internal carotid artery angiography, frontal view. E, the right internal carotid artery angiography, lateral view. Showing the slowing blood flow in aneurysms after PED therapy. F: unsubtracted image showing the PED.

Dissecting aneurysms for the ACA share common characteristics, including a tendency to affect middle-aged patients, the appearance of serial lesion changes visible on repeated angiograms, and a good prognosis for most patients [43]. Uozumi et al. reviewed 82 cases of dissecting aneurysms for the ACA and demonstrated that 88.6% of cases (A2 and A1 segments) presented with ischemic events [44].

Although the parent arteries of such distal dissecting aneurysms are very small (< 2.5 mm in caliber), tortuous and have multiple branching vessels, the more recent FDs have been designed to be smaller and shorter allowing for easier navigation and deployment of the device [45]. In comprehensive literature reviews concerning the application of PED for the aneurysms of the middle and anterior cerebral arteries, PED demonstrated efficacy in the treatment of distal circulation (MCA and ACA) dissecting aneurysms, with a complication rate of 0-12% and mortality 0-5% [45-48].

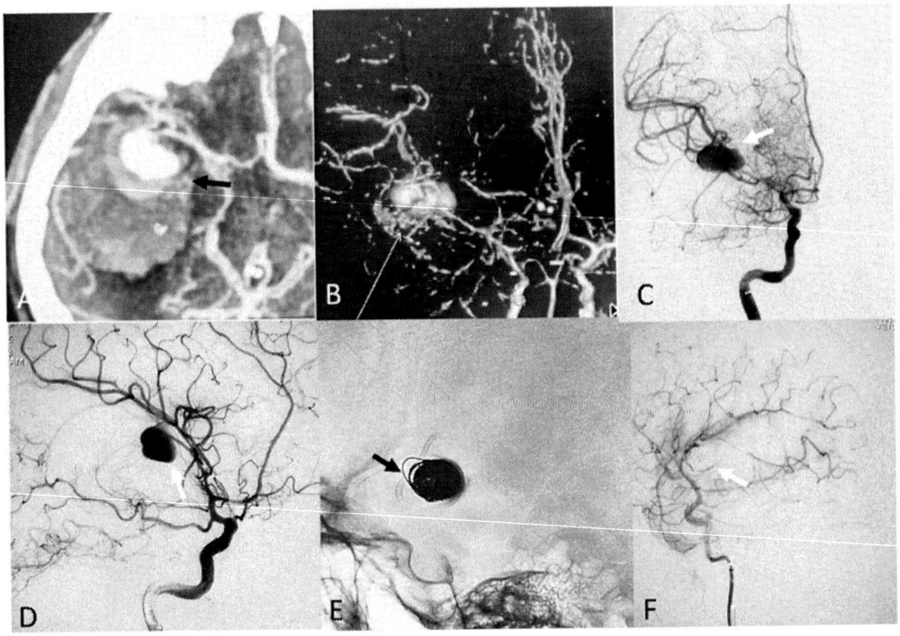

Figure 12. A 28-year-old female patient had headaches 4 days after delivery. A, cranial CT examination showing a hematoma in the right temporal lobe of the brain (arrow). B, the CTA examination showing a giant aneurysm in the M3 segment of the right middle cerebral artery (arrow). The right internal carotid artery angiography, frontal view(C) and lateral view (D), showing a giant dissecting aneurysm in the M3 segment of the right middle cerebral artery(arrows). E, unsubtracted image showing the aneurysm was treated by PED combined with coil embolization (arrow). F, postoperative right carotid angiography, lateral view, showing that the aneurysm was almost completely occluded (arrow). The patient was discharged one week after surgery without any neurological deficits.

Conclusion

Dissecting aneurysms are a special pathologic type of aneurysm wall, in addition to the usual symptoms of aneurysms such as headache, neurological symptoms due to the mass effect of giant aneurysms, SAH following rupture, and stroke due to injury of perforation vessels. The diagnosis was based on noninvasive CTA, MRA, and high-resolution MRI, which showed the structural features of the vessel walls of the aneurysms. Traditional surgical clipping can be considered; however, there is a relatively high recurrence rate, making treatment challenging. Among the many FDs, PED stands out as the most predominant product. It is relatively safe, feasible, and curable for dissecting aneurysms but should be evaluated thoroughly before endovascular treatment, balancing the advantages and risks of each treatment strategy against the patient's actual condition, depending on the location of the aneurysm, the type of aneurysm, the patient's age, and the patient's preoperative health.

References

[1] Debette S, Compter A, Labeyrie MA, Uyttenboogaart M, Metso TM, Majersik JJ, Goeggel-Simonetti B, Engelter ST, Pezzini A, Bijlenga P, Southerland AM, Naggara O, Béjot Y, Cole JW, Ducros A, Giacalone G, Schilling S, Reiner P, Sarikaya H, Welleweerd JC, Kappelle LJ, de Borst GJ, Bonati LH, Jung S, Thijs V, Martin JJ, Brandt T, Grond-Ginsbach C, Kloss M, Mizutani T, Minematsu K, Meschia JF, Pereira VM, Bersano A, Touzé E, Lyrer PA, Leys D, Chabriat H, Markus HS, Worrall BB, Chabrier S, Baumgartner R, Stapf C, Tatlisumak T, Arnold M, Bousser MG. Epidemiology, pathophysiology, diagnosis, and management of intracranial artery dissection. *Lancet Neurol.* 2015 Jun;14(6):640-54. doi: 10.1016/S1474-4422(15)00009-5. PMID: 25987283.

[2] Lv X, Yu J, Zhang W, Zhao X, Zhang H. Acute hemorrhagic cerebral artery dissection: Characteristics and endovascular treatment. *Neuroradiol J.* 2020;33(2):112–117.

[3] Xia S, Wang Y, Lv X, Chen C, Hui J, Wu X, Wang Z, Chen H, Ji J. The use of SNAP and T1-weighted VISTA in cervical artery dissection. *Interv Neuroradiol.* 2023 Jun;29(3):235-242. doi: 10.1177/15910199221082847. Epub 2022 Mar 2. PMID: 35234066; PMCID: PMC10369114.

[4] Urasyanandana K, Songsang D, Aurboonyawat T, Chankaew E, Withayasuk P, Churojana A. Treatment outcomes in cerebral artery dissection and literature review. *Interv Neuroradiol.* 2018 Jun;24(3):254-262. doi: 10.1177/1591019918755692. Epub 2018 Feb 12. PMID: 29433365; PMCID: PMC5967189.

[5] Elsebaie N, Abdelzaher A, Gamaleldin O. Atypical intracranial aneurysms: spectrum of imaging findings in computed tomography and magnetic resonance imaging. *Clin Imaging.* 2022 Mar;83:1-10. doi: 10.1016/j.clinimag.2021.12.003. Epub 2021 Dec 11. PMID: 34915276.

[6] Montalvan V, Ulrich A, Wahlster S, Galindo D. Arterial dissection as a cause of intracranial stenosis: A narrative review. *Clin Neurol Neurosurg.* 2020 Mar;190:105653. doi: 10.1016/j.clineuro.2019.105653. Epub 2019 Dec 30. PMID: 31901612.

[7] Lv X, Li Y, Liu A, Jiang P, Lv M, Wu Z. Endovascular treatment of intracranial giant serpentine aneurysms. *Neuroradiol J.* 2007;20(2):237-241.

[8] Ye Z, Lv X. The formation mechanism of acute dissection of blood blister-like aneurysm and its implication of endovascular treatment. *Chin Neurosurg J.* 2021 Jun 3;7(1):32. doi: 10.1186/s41016-021-00245-1. PMID: 34078466; PMCID: PMC8173849.

[9] Chen L, Yau I, deVeber G, Dirks P, Armstrong D, Krings T. Evolution of a chronic dissecting aneurysm on magnetic resonance imaging in a pediatric patient. *J Neurosurg Pediatr.* 2015 Feb;15(2):192-6. doi: 10.3171/2014.10.PEDS14221. Epub 2014 Dec 5. PMID: 25479578.

[10] Maus V, Mpotsaris A, Dorn F, Möhlenbruch M, Borggrefe J, Stavrinou P, Abdullayev N, Barnikol UB, Liebig T, Kabbasch C. The Use of Flow Diverter in Ruptured, Dissecting Intracranial Aneurysms of the Posterior Circulation. *World Neurosurg.* 2018 Mar;111:e424-e433. doi: 10.1016/j.wneu.2017.12.095. Epub 2017 Dec 23. PMID: 29277587.

[11] Jeon JP, Cho YD, Rhim JK, Park JJ, Cho WS, Kang HS, Kim JE, Hwang G, Kwon OK, Han MH. Stent-Assisted Coil Embolization of Vertebrobasilar Dissecting Aneurysms: Procedural Outcomes and Factors for Recanalization. *Korean J Radiol.* 2016 Sep-Oct;17(5):801-10. doi: 10.3348/kjr.2016.17.5.801. Epub 2016 Aug 23. PMID: 27587971; PMCID: PMC5007409.

[12] Lv X, Jiang C, Li Y, Yang X, Wu Z. Endovascular treatment for pediatric intracranial aneurysms. *Neuroradiology* 2009;51:749-754.

[13] Lv X, Jiang C, Li Y, Yang X, Wu Z. Treatment of giant intracranial aneurysms. *Interv Neuroradiol* 2009;15:135-144.

[14] Lv X, Jiang C, Li Y, Wu Z. Clinical outcomes of lower cranial nerve palsies caused by vertebral artery–posteroinferior cerebellar artery aneurysms after endovascular embolization. *Neurol Res* 2010;32:796-800.

[15] Krag CH, Speiser L, Dalby RB. Long-term outcomes of endovascular simple coiling versus neurosurgical clipping of unruptured intracranial aneurysms: A systematic review and meta-analysis. J Neurol Sci. 2021 Mar 15;422:117338. doi: 10.1016/j.jns.2021.117338. Epub 2021 Feb 9. *Erratum in: J Neurol Sci.* 2021 May 15;424:117411. PMID: 33596532.

[16] Kurata A, Ohmomo T, Miyasaka Y, Fujii K, Kan S, Kitahara T. Coil embolization for the treatment of ruptured dissecting vertebral aneurysms. *AJNR Am J Neuroradiol.* 2001 Jan;22(1):11-8. PMID: 11158881; PMCID: PMC7975530.

[17] Sönmez Ö, Brinjikji W, Murad MH, Lanzino G. Deconstructive and reconstructive techniques in treatment of vertebrobasilar dissecting aneurysms: a systematic review and meta-analysis. *AJNR Am J Neuroradiol.* 2015;36(7):1293-1298.

[18] Lv X, Jiang C, Li Y, Lv M, Zhang J, Wu Z. Intracranial pseudoaneurysms, dissections and carotid-cavernous fistulas: repair with percutaneous implantation of endovascular covered stents. *Interv Neuroradiol* 2008;14:435-440.

[19] Lv X, Yang H, Liu P, Li Y. Flow-diverter devices in treatment of intracranial aneurysms: A Meta-analysis and systematic review. *Neuroradiol J.* 2016;29(1):66-71.

[20] Lv X, Li Y, Jiang C, Wu Z. Endovascular management for P2 aneurysms of the posterior cerebral artery: experience on proximal occlusion of P2 segment. *Interv Neuroradiol* 2009;15:341-348.

[21] Lv M, Lv X, Li Y, Jiang C, Jiang P, Wu Z. Dissecting aneurysm at proximal anterior cerebral artery treated by parent artery occlusion. *Interv Neuroradiol* 2009;15:123-126.

[22] Lv X, Li W, Ge H, Jin H, He H, Jiang C, Li Y. Parent artery sacrifice for ruptured aneurysms in acute and chronic phases: A systematic review. *Neurol India.* 2018 May-Jun;66(3):695-699.

[23] Shapiro M, Becske T, Sahlein D, Babb J, Nelson PK. Stent-supported aneurysm coiling: a literature survey of treatment and follow-up. *AJNR Am J Neuroradiol.* 2012 Jan;33(1):159-63. doi: 10.3174/ajnr.A2719. Epub 2011 Oct 27. PMID: 22033717; PMCID: PMC7966171.

[24] Rho MH, Park HJ, Chung EC, Choi YJ, Lee SY, Won YS, Kim BM. Various techniques of stent-assisted coil embolization of wide-necked or fusiform artherosclerotic and dissecting unruptured vertebrobasilar artery aneurysms for reducing recanalization: mid-term results. *Acta Neurochir (Wien).* 2013 Nov;155(11):2009-17. doi: 10.1007/s00701-013-1866-y. Epub 2013 Oct 1. PMID: 24081786.

[25] Wang J, Vargas J, Spiotta A, Chaudry I, Turner RD, Lena J, Turk A. Stent-assisted coiling of cerebral aneurysms: a single-center clinical and angiographic analysis. *J Neurointerv Surg.* 2018 Jul;10(7):687-692. doi: 10.1136/neurintsurg-2017-013272. Epub 2017 Nov 16. PMID: 29146831.

[26] Klisch J, Eger C, Sychra V, Strasilla C, Basche S, Weber J. Stent-assisted coil embolization of posterior circulation aneurysms using solitaire ab: preliminary experience. *Neurosurgery.* 2009 Aug;65(2):258-66; discussion 266. doi: 10.1227/01.NEU.0000348295.44970.C8. PMID: 19625903.

[27] Kühn AL, Kan P, Massari F, Lozano JD, Hou SY, Howk M, Gounis MJ, Wakhloo AK, Puri AS. Endovascular reconstruction of unruptured intradural vertebral artery dissecting aneurysms with the Pipeline embolization device. *J Neurointerv Surg.* 2016 Oct;8(10):1048-51. doi: 10.1136/neurintsurg-2015-012028. Epub 2015 Nov 6. PMID: 26546600.

[28] Zhang H, Ren J, Wang J, Lv X. The off-label uses of pipeline embolization device for complex cerebral aneurysms: Mid-term follow-up in a single center. *Interv Neuroradiol.* 2022 Dec 30:15910199221148800. doi: 10.1177/15910199221148800. Epub ahead of print. PMID: 36583531.

[29] Suyama K, Nakahara I, Matsumoto S, Morioka J, Tanabe J, Hasebe A, Watanabe S. Efficacy and Safety of Dual Antiplatelet Therapy with the Routine Use of Prasugrel for Flow Diversion of Cerebral Unruptured Aneurysms. *Clin Neuroradiol.* 2023 Oct 17. doi: 10.1007/s00062-023-01355-2. Epub ahead of print. PMID: 37847296.

[30] Bounajem MT, Joyce E, Scoville JP, Seinfeld J, Hoffman J, Grossberg JA, Waiters V, White AC, Nerva J, Burkhardt JK, Tonetti DA, El Naamani K, Gooch MR, Jabbour P, Tjoumakaris S, Ortega Gutierrez S, Levitt MR, Lang M, Ares WJ, Desai S, Mascitelli JR, Kilburg CJ, Budohoski KP, Couldwell WT, Gross BA, Grandhi R. Safety and efficacy of the Pipeline Flex embolization device with Shield Technology for the acute treatment of ruptured internal carotid artery pseudoaneurysms: a multi-institution case series. *Neurosurg Focus.* 2023 May;54(5):E4. doi: 10.3171/2023.2.FOCUS233. PMID: 37127036.

[31] Levitt MR, Park MS, Albuquerque FC, et al. Posterior Inferior Cerebellar Artery Patency after Flow-Diverting Stent Treatment. *AJNR Am J Neuroradiol* 2016;37:487-489.

[32] Natarajan SK, Lin N, Sonig A, et al. The safety of Pipeline flow diversion in fusiform vertebrobasilar aneurysms: a consecutive case series with longer-term follow-up from a single US center. *J Neurosurg*2016;125:111-119.

[33] Munich SA, Tan LA, Keigher KM, et al. The Pipeline Embolization Device for the treatment of posterior circulation fusiform aneurysms: lessons learned at a single institution. *J Neurosurg*2014;121:1077-1084.

[34] Kallmes DF, Hanel R, Lopes D, et al. International retrospective study of the pipeline embolization device: a multicenter aneurysm treatment study. *AJNR Am J Neuroradiol*2015;36:108-115.

[35] Lv X, Ge H, Jin H, He H, Jiang C, Li Y. Endovascular treatment of unruptured posterior circulation intracranial aneurysms. *Ann Indian Acad Neurol* 2016;19:302-6.

[36] Hou K, Lv X, Guo Y, Yu J. Endovascular treatment of posterior inferior cerebellar artery trunk aneurysm. *Acta Neurol Belg*. 2021 Oct 22. doi: 10.1007/s13760-021-01826-8. Epub ahead of print. PMID: 34677822.

[37] Lv X, Ge H, He H, Jiang C, Li Y. Anterior inferior cerebellar artery aneurysms: Segments and results of surgical and endovascular managements. *Interv Neuroradiol.* 2016 Dec;22(6):643-648. Epub 2016 Aug 2.

[38] Huo K, Lv X, Yu J. Endovascular treatment of posterior cerebral artery trunk aneurysm: The status quo and dilemma. *Front Neurol.* 2022 Jan 6;12:746525. doi: 10.3389/fneur.2021.746525.

[39] Sakamoto S, Ikawa F, Kawamoto H, Ohbayashi N, Inagawa T.Acute surgery for ruptured dissecting aneurysm of the M3 portion of the middle cerebral artery. *Neurol Med Chir(Tokyo).* 2003;43:188e191.

[40] Zhang J, Yu M, Lv X. Endovascular treatment of blood blister-like aneurysms of internal carotid artery: Stent-assisted coiling and pipeline flow diversion. *J Clin Neurosci.* 2021 Aug;90:8-13. doi: 10.1016/j.jocn.2021.04.040. Epub 2021 May 21. PMID: 34275585.

[41] Zhang Y, Zhang F, Turhon M, Huang J, Li M, Peng Q, Zheng Z, Liu J, Zhang Y, Liu J, Zhang H, Li T, Song D, Zhao Y, Aisha M, Wang Y, Feng W, Wang Y, Wan J, Mao G, Shi H, Guan S. Treatment of Intracranial Vertebral Artery Dissecting Aneurysms Using Pipeline Embolization Devices: A Multicenter Cohort Study. *Clin Neuroradiol.* 2023 Jun 28. doi: 10.1007/s00062-023-01318-7. Epub ahead of print. PMID: 37380901.

[42] Yu J, Lv X. Flow diversion for intracranial aneurysms beyond the circle of Willis. *Frontiers in Neurology*. 2021;12:1-6.

[43] Mori K, Yamamoto T, Maeda M. Dissecting aneurysm confined to the anterior cerebral artery. *Br J Neurosurg*. 2002 Apr;16(2):158-64. doi: 10.1080/02688690220131787. PMID: 12046736.

[44] Uozumi Y, Katoh H, Tsuzuki N, Toyooka T, Miyazawa T, Nawashiro H, Shima K. Revascularization for anterior cerebral artery dissecting aneurysms--three case reports. *Neurol Med Chir (Tokyo).* 2010 Jan;50(1):49-53. doi: 10.2176/nmc.50.49. PMID: 20098026.

[45] Puri AS, Massari F, Asai T, Marosfoi M, Kan P, Hou SY, Howk M, Perras M, Brooks C, Clarencon F, Gounis MJ, Wakhloo AK. Safety, efficacy, and short-term follow-up of the use of Pipeline Embolization Device in small (<2.5 mm) cerebral vessels for aneurysm treatment: single institution experience. *Neuroradiology*. 2016 Mar;58(3):267-75. doi: 10.1007/s00234-015-1630-5. Epub 2015 Dec 23. PMID: 26700827.

[46] Patel PD, Chalouhi N, Atallah E, Tjoumakaris S, Hasan D, Zarzour H, Rosenwasser R, Jabbour P. Off-label uses of the Pipeline embolization device: a review of the literature. *Neurosurg Focus.* 2017 Jun;42(6):E4. doi: 10.3171/2017.3.FOCUS1742. PMID: 28565978.

[47] Murthy SB, Shah J, Mangat HS, Stieg P. Treatment of Intracranial Aneurysms With Pipeline Embolization Device: Newer Applications and Technical Advances. *Curr Treat Options Neurol.* 2016 Apr;18(4):16. doi: 10.1007/s11940-016-0399-0. PMID: 26923606.

[48] Nossek E, Zumofen DW, Setton A, Potts MB, Raz E, Shapiro M, Riina HA, De Miquel MA, Chalif DJ, Nelson PK. Treatment of distal anterior cerebral artery aneurysms with the Pipeline Embolization Device. *J Clin Neurosci.* 2017 Jan;35:133-138. doi: 10.1016/j.jocn.2016.10.041. Epub 2016 Nov 15. PMID: 27863970.

Chapter 9

Intracranial Infectious Aneurysms: An Exceptional Contender

Mohamed M. Abdelrady[1,2,*], PhD and Mourad C. Elaouni[2], MD

[1]Department of Radiology, Interventional Neuroradiology Unit, Ain Shams University, Cairo, Egypt
[2]Depart of Neuroradiology, Hospital Cavale Blanche, Brest University hospital, Brest, France

Abstract

Infectious aneurysms might involve aortic arch, proximal supra-aortic vessels downstream to very distal cerebral vasculature. Intracranial infectious aneurysms (IIAs) are relatively rare yet might harbor devastating consequences with a rupture-associated mortality risk ranging between 30-80%. Septic vegetation seeding from an infective endocarditis (IEC) represents the most common source, resulting into intracranial vessel wall damage, necrosis, and aneurysmal formation.

IIAs are typically multiple, fusiform shaped distally indwelling; however, the presentation is widely variable. Moreover, patients usually present late in the course of the disease. Cutting-edge imaging modalities such as multi-detector computed tomography and time of flight magnetic resonance imaging (TOF-MRI) might have improved the diagnostic accuracy of IIAs guided by diversified established features; however digital subtraction angiography (DSA) still represents the gold standard examination. Integrating clinical finding along with the imaging features might aid prompt diagnosis and timely treatment of IIAs. Yet to be considered, IIAs are inherently dynamic where an aneurysm might get instituted and rupture in less than one week; therefore, an earlier stage of aneurysmal development could be easily missed even with serial investigations.

Management of IIAs is still controversial. Taking in consideration their grave natural prognosis, the decision to intervene is influenced furthermore by many variables including patient's general condition, aneurysm size, location and geometry, rupture status, presence of hematoma with significant mass effect and territorial eloquence of the feeding artery. Therefore, a multidisciplinary approach remains the most successful strategy in dealt with these aneurysms.

Therapeutic choices include serial monitoring under antimicrobial coverage, endovascular embolization, parent artery sacrifice and direct surgical excision and

* Corresponding Author's Email: mmabdelrady@gmail.com.

In: Understanding and Managing Cerebral Aneurysms
Editor: Xianli Lv
ISBN: 979-8-89113-608-3

debridement. However, observational strategy still carries a high risk of fulminant hemorrhage. Surgical resolution is not without complications.

With technological advances, various embolization tools became readily available encompassing coils, liquid embolic agents as onyx^{TM}, NBCA (n-Butyl Cyanoacrylate), stents and flow diverters. For an efficacious embolotherapy, it might be necessary to occlude the aneurysm in adjunction with the parent artery. Nevertheless, adding to risks of inadvertent embolization, it might be strenuous to navigate safely into distally situated aneurysms within fragile rupture-prone diseased vasculature.

We will take through the natural history, diagnostic features, and management dilemma of IIAs based on our experience in the light of recently published reports.

Keywords: infective endocarditis, intracranial infectious aneurysms, embolization, coiling, flow diverter, parent artery sacrifice

Introduction

The primary descripiton of the infectious aneurysm was presented by Church, 1869 [1]. Subsequently in 1885 and based on the resmeblnace to the 'fresh fungus vegetitaion' at the autopsy specimen, William Osler, an Oxford physician, introduced the earliest nomination of the " mycotic aneurysm" in a 30-year-old male with four aneurysms at the aortic arch that developed because of bacterial endocarditis [2]. Currently, 'intracranial infectious aneurysm' became more scientifically acknowledged than the term 'mycotic' since it refers to any infectious process ending in aneurysmal dilatation with disregard to the causative organism whether of bacterial, viral, parasitic, or fungal origin [3,4].

'Mycotic' or the more properly designated " infectious" aneurysms, represent an infrequent, yet potentially grave local inflammatory cerebrovascular complication of neighboring extracranial, intracranial, remote, or iatrogenic source of infection, like sinusitis complicated by cavernous sinus thrombophlebitis, meningitis, IEC, or a recent craniofacial surgery respectively [5].

The most dreadful complication of IIA is the acute stroke whether ischemic with thromboembolic distal arterial occlusion in an eloquent territory or hemorrhagic in form of subarachnoid, intraventricular, or intracerebral especially in the setting of cardiac surgery where patients get exposed to antithrombotic therapy. On that account, a prompt aneurysmal spotting guided by symptomatic presentation and serial imaging might be inevitable not to miss ghost IIAs [6].

Given invariable natural evolution and initial presentation, management algorithm of IIAs is not yet entirely determined. There is a consensus on timely administration of broad-spectrum antimicrobial therapy as a front-line care till obtaining the results of blood culture. Therapeutic interventions whether endovascular or surgical are still proposed on a case-by-case basis with no clear, evidence-based guidance or selection criteria among the individualized treatment options [7].

Epidemiology

The median age at the time of diagnosis is variable ranging between 35-53 years. Some reports mentioned a relative male predominance while others found no sex predilection. Intracranial infectious aneurysms (IIAs) constitute a distinctive cerebrovascular pathology and account for nearly 0.7–6.5% of all cerebral aneurysms within different series. It might be challenging to demonstrate the global disease burden given the relative rarity of IIAs, the lack of precise population estimates, and the fact that IIAs are commonly clinically silent and antimicrobial responsive, being incidentally depicted in 5-10% of autopsy specimens [8, 9].

According to Morris et al., 2014 [10] IIA are found in nearly 2-4% of patients with infective endocarditis (IEC) that rise to 5-12% in patients with supplemental neurological symptoms. Although the incidence of endocarditis might be declining with the wide-spread use of the antibiotic therapy, left bacterial endocarditis concomitant with intravenous drug abuse, valvular diseases and expansive implantation of prosthetic valves might still represent the most common sources of IIAs. An earlier pooled-cohort analysis found that 65-80% of IIA cases primarily presented with bacterial endocarditis. Other potential causes based on order of frequency were as follow: IV drug abuse, bacterial meningitis, poor oral hygiene, and cavernous sinus thrombosis (CST) [11].

Pathogenesis

Intact vascular endothelium is substantially resistant to bloodborne pathogens; nevertheless, unhealthy tunical layers render the vessel susceptible to penetration by various pathogens. The culprit organism might be of bacterial, viral, fungal, or parasitic origin. Unfortunately, blood and cerebrospinal fluid (C.S.F) cultures depict the causative pathogens in fewer than 50% of the patients. The most frequent pathogens are coagulase-negative staphylococcus aureus and streptococcus haemolyticus species, gram-negative organisms like Salmonella and pseudomonas aeruginosa. While data relevant to s. haemolyticus-mediated IIAs are scarce, coagulase negative staphylococci are culpable for 8% of native valve endocarditis with resultant mortality rate of 25% in the literature. Moreover, methicillin-resistant staphylococci are responsible for 60% of prosthetic valve endocarditis [12]. Other reported viral sources might include varicella zoster virus and HIV-1. The latter has been associated with the childhood arteriopathy [13, 14].

Although fungal pathogens like candida, aspergillus, mycobacterium tuberculosis, and enterococci are relatively less frequent compared to other pathogens, they carry a particularly disatstrous prognosis with very high mortality rate. Fungal IIAs are habitually noted in severly immune-compromised patients with serious conditions like septicemia, AIDS, and Intravenous drug abuse and diabetic cases. Contrasting typical IIAs, fungal ones tend to involve proximal arteries, possibly due to frequent direct extension from skull base [15]. High clinical suspicion and prompt antifungal therapy might improve functional outcomes [16]. Figure 1 demonstartes IIAs caused by IEC and a successful embolization of fungal IIA with endosaccular coils with no technical complications or neurological morbidity.

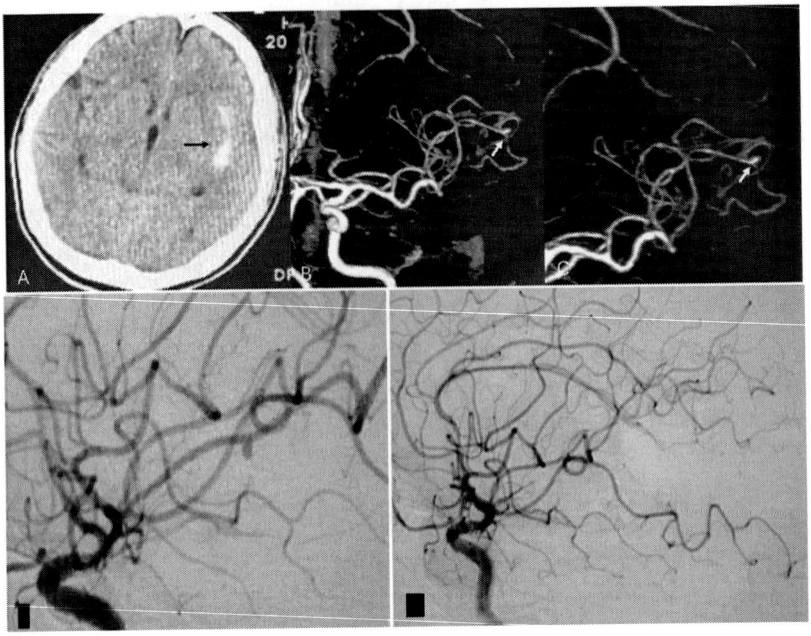

Figure 1. A-C: The 53-years-old female patient had a recurrent fever for 1 month and infective endocarditis for 10 days. She also has type 2 diabetes for 1 year. Blood bacterial culture showed that Staphylococcus aureus was positive, which was a multi drug resistant bacteria (MRSA). She presented sudden onset of headache, nausea and vomiting. A, cranial CT scanning indicated subarachnoid hemorrhage in the left Sylvian fissure (arrow). B and C, CTA of the head indicates an aneurysm at the distal segment of the left middle cerebral artery (arrow). According to the patient's history and CTA images, the diagnosis of infectious aneurysm should be considered. (Courtesy Dr. Xianli Lv M.D. Assoicate Professor Neurosurgery, Department Beijing Tsinghua Changgung Hospital, School of Clinical Medicine, Tsinghua University, Beijing, China). D and E: A 47-year-old immunocompromised patient diagnosed with infective endocarditis (IEC) of fungal origin and maintained on antifungal therapy, recently developed severe headache and drowsiness concomitant with right temporal hematoma and intraventricular haemorrhage on non-contrast brain computed tomography (not shown). Angiography revealed an 2 x 1.5 mm oblong aneurysm at the posterior parietal branch of middle cerebral artery (MCA-M2 segment) (D). Presence of ruptured focal sidewall non-bifurcation aneurysm in a non-eloquent territory with a non-surgical hematoma in the setting of IEC, triggered a prompt endovascular management through coiling-mediated parent artery sacrifice. Primary intrasaccular placement of an Ultrasoft Target® coil (Stryker Neuroendovascular, Kalamazoo, MI, USA) was done followed by another intraluminal coil successfully embolized the aneurysm together with the parent artery (E). Control CT (not shown) revealed focal ischemic infarct related to the territory embolized. Patient returned to normal life with no neurological deficits.

Budohoski et al., 2022 [17] demonstarted a case with Burkitt's lymphoma and graft-versus-host disease who was hospitalized with intracerebral hemorrhage and developed within 8 days a total of 12 anterior circulation IIAs from a disseminated *Scedosporium* infection. Patient died after 6 months because of multiorgan failure despite the aggressive surgical and anti-fungal therapy. The authors underlined the highly angioinvasive nature of the fungal pathogens, that were evident in the form of rapid development of great number of denovo aneurysm, only days after unremarkable angiographic studies adding to swift growth and rupture of consveratively managed IIAs.

IIA might be considered as the second most common neurological sequelae of infective endocarditis (IEC) after embolic strokes. More than 50% of embolic events in the setting of

IEC implicates the cerebral vasculature with 90% of theses within the middle cerebral artery territory. Although there is no current estimate of embolization rate and the individualized risk; however, the incidence might aggravate with an enlarging valvular vegetation and decrease 2-3 weeks following a proprer antimicrobial therapy [18].

The infective organism finds its way to the intracranial vessel wall through a hematogenous spread from a remote extracranial source like bacterial endocarditis, where the septic embolic vegetations preferentially reside with the flow within the branching points of distal middle cerebral vasculature with potential vascular occlusion, infarctions, and parenchymal involvement in the form of cerebritis and abscess formation. Intravascular invasion and lodging are associated with vessel wall degradation manifested by demolition of the internal elastic lamina, marked intimal proliferation and intense polymorphonuclear cells chemotaxis and infiltration of tunica media and adventitia. The above factors together with an outward hydrostatic pressure from the pulsatile blood flow against a weakened thinned arterial wall promote development and further growth of IIAs. Moreover, vascular invasion might be coupled with an interruption of structure wall integrity resulting in obliteration of the smaller penetrating arterioles and ischemic manifestations [19].

Alternatively, organisms might evade the vessel wall through an extravascular direct invasion from an adjacent infective focus such as cavernous thrombophlebitis, invasive sinusitis, orbital cellulitis, brain abscess, meningitis, subdural empyema, and osteomyelitis of the skull per example where the infectious process could be restricted to the neighboring vessel only. Results from animal studies have hypothesized that organisms within the vasa vasorum find its ways into the Virchow–Robin space with subsequent adventitial layer inflammation. Less frequently, IIAs might occur through direct inoculation during trauma or with unidentifiable origin (cryptogenic type) [20].

IIAs are unique in their etiopathogenesis when compared to hemodynamically induced willisian saccular aneurysms that tend to involve areas of low shear stress at base of the brain. They are regarded as 'pseudoaneurysms' ascribed to remote vegetative seedings with infectious microemboli. This theory elucidates the preferential distal location of IIAs at secondary, teritary order branches and the peculiar fusiform or sacculofusiform morphologies harboring an obscure/absent/ wide neck. Moreover, because of disrupted integrity of vascular layers and the subsequent friable thin-walled nature, IIAs are obviously rupture-prone [21].

Despite that IIAs are coupled with an inherent grave prognosis, there are no established angiographic criteria that could predict future developments of IIAs. Goldschmidt et al., 2019 [22] documented within three IIAs cases that septic occlusive embolus with a subsequent ischemic event might be a promoting factor for IIAs development; therefore, contrariwise to the current guidelines, they recommended a short-interval follow-up reinforced by angiography in patients with established infarcts after a septic occlusive embolus. As demonstrated by Hui et al., 2015 [23] hemorrhagic presentation showed a positive correlation with aneurysmal depiction. In their series, IIAs were noticed in 22% of patients presenting with IEC and intracranial hemorrhage compared to 1% in patients presenting only with IEC and absent hemorrhagic manifetstaion. Thus again, angiographic survillence should be pursued in patients with IEC and cerebral hemorhage.

Natural History and Prognosis

Again, with a dearth of population-based analysis, the natural history of IIAs remains undetermined. The development of IIA might occur as rapid as 24 hours till 1 month following septic vegetation embolization. Animal histological sections demonstrated an acute inflammatory response to microbial invasion of the tunica muscularlis with early aneurysm formation at 24 hours following cerebral embolism [24]. In humans, Samaniego et al., 2017 [25] documented a swift formation of IIA aided by digital substraction angiography (DSA) within only 5 days after septic embolization. Accordingly, authors advocated an early DSA in high-risk patients with denovo neurological symptoms or those who are anti-cogulated in anticipation for a cardiac surgery.

IIAs are highly dynamic lesion with a great propensity to either resolve, regress, enlarge, disseminate with formation of denovo aneurysms, or rupture in the worst scenario. Despite technological advancements with improved imaging resolution, some aneurysms stay clinically dormant and remain undetected. With culture-directed therapy other IIAs might show a remarkable symptomatic regression together with reduction in size. However, it is difficult to anticipate the aneurysmal behaviour. Therefore, close serial survillence is warranted within the litertaure if IIAs were managed conservatively with only antimicrobial therapy [26]. On the other hand, although rupture rate of IIAs variates between 2-10% and accounts for only 5% of neurological complications in patients with IEC, aneurysmal rupture might have catastrophic consequences. A recent meta-analysis reported a 13-30% mortality in patients with IIA that is aggravated up to 80% mortality rate if rupture occurs. In a larger review, mortality rates ranged between 30-90% for bacterial and fungal IIAs despite conservative therapy or surgical intervention. The time between the onset of IEC and rupture of IIAs span between 2-5 weeks. Adding to natural history complexity, IIAs size might not truly influence the risk of rupture. Paradoxically, some presume higher risk of rupture in smaller aneurysms. Moreover, no decrease in the rupture incidence with favorably reduced aneurysmal size in patients maintained on antimicrobial therapy [27, 28].

Diagnosis

Considering the dreadful prognosis of IIAs, an instant diagnosis and a prompt treatment would be mandatory. The gold standard diagnostic modality is the pathological demonstration of an infectious organism together with an inflammatory destructive vascular process. Nonetheless, histopathological assessment is feasible only during surgery or as a post-mortem autopsy and is positive in nearly 20% of the specimens. Moreover, prolonged antimicrobial therapy might alter the infectious process so that fibrosis might be the only abnormality delineated histopathologically. Constraints of tissue-based diagnosis promoted the physicians to develop a diagnostic algorithm that could guide diagnosis and treatment of IIAs [29].

Chapot et al., 2002 [30] utilized the following diagnostic criteria: the presence of endocarditis, a positive blood culture and a cerebral aneurysm with the following specifications (1) distal aneurysm, involving segments 2, 3, 4 of the middle or posterior cerebral artery OR (2) proximal affecting segments M1 and P1 in association with at least two of the following criteria (2a) a change in aneurysm size or morphology on consecutive angiograms (2b) presence of another intra- or extracranial IIA, (2c) aneurysmal rupture (2d) arterial occlusion or stenosis adjacent to the aneurysm, and (2e) cerebral infarction due to arterial occlusion at the level of the aneurysm.

The above criteria were criticized for exclusion of aneurysms located at the anterior cerebral artery or the vertebrobasilar circulation, and inclusion of positive blood culture while being cognizant that more than 50% of histological specimen might be devoid of organisms. Among the limitation, restricting the promoting factors for IIAs development to IEC. Whether the endocarditis is an independent predictor of IIAs or not has not been verified in randomized trials; however, even in the light of the notable strong association, it is not advisable to perform neurovascular screening for all patients with endocarditis with disregard to the neurological symptomatology. At the same time, serial imaging might be necessary particularly in patients with neurological deficits and negative primary neurovascular imaging. Ongoing clinical trials like "Neurological Complication of Infective Endocarditis: A Prospective Multi-site Cohort Study with Systematic MRI and Digital Subtraction Angiography" [Clinical Trials. Gov identifier: NCT0515225] might afford a reasonable diagnostic and follow-up cascade.

Kannoth et al., proposed a set of diagnostic criteria including the mandatory criterion (demonstration of intracranial aneurysm by neuroimaging) and 12 supportive criteria categorized into (a) *predisposing infection* that encompass (IEC, meningitis, cavernous sinus thrombophelibitis, and orbital cellulitis), (b) *aneurysm angiographic features* comprising (Multiplicity, distal location, fusiform morphology, and change in aneurysm size or appearance of denovo aneurysms on the follow-up angiogram), and *other features* such as (patient age younger than 45 years, history of recent lumbar puncture, fever at presentation and intraparenchymal hemorrhage on imaging). Meeting the mandatory criterion in addition to one, two, or three supportive criteria were defined as clinically possible, probable, or definite IIA, with reported sensitivity equal to 100%, 100%, 96%, and specificity equal to 39.6%, 87.4%, and 100% respectively [31]. Study limitation included histological confirmation, the gold standard, in only 20% of the cases, sample model validation utilizing the same dataset with low number of recruited cases, and ill-defined diagnostic criteria for IEC which is conventionally diagnosed based on Duke's criteria.

Finally, current definitive diagnosis of IIA necessitaes a histopathological assessment; however, a high clinical index of suspicion together with comprehensive clinical history, laboratory and radiological workup might provide the roadmap for optimized diagnosis, stratification, and proper management of IIAs [32].

Clinical Manifestations

Patients with unruptured IIAs might remain asymptomatic as described in nearly 20% of autopsies of at-risk patients or could present with vague nonspecific symptoms such as sub-acute onset like fever, headache, vomiting, chills, and malaise. However, territorial, or multifocal embolic infarcts with sequential focal neurological deficits (FNDs) as hemiparesis, aphasia could arise following vascular obliteration by septic emboli [33]. According to cloud et al., 2003 [34], transcranial doppler sonography was valuable in detection and monitoring of asymptomatic platelet and thrombus emboli.

In decreasing order of frequency as demonstrated by Singla et al., 2013 [35] presenting symptoms were as follows: headache (83%), fever (67%), vomiting (50%), ocular palsy (25%), seizures (21%), behavioural changes (21%), hemiparesis (21%), drowsiness (17%) and loss of consciousness (17%).

On the other hand, ruptured IIAs could induce intracranial hemorrhage of any kind whether intraparenchymal (IPH), subarachnoid (SAH) or intraventricular (IVH) concomitant with severe relentless focal headache, loss of consciousness, seizures or FNDs. Compared to non-infectious saccular aneurysms presenting classically with a pure SAH, rupture of IIAs habitually presents with IPH in 47.4% of cases. Rarely, IIAs might present with subdural hematoma; a critical observation that should not rule out the necessity for angiography in patients with IEC [36]. Regardless of the symptomatic presentation, the presence of hemorrhage might be the best marker for IIAs existence in patients with IEC. In the study performed by Hui et al., 2015 [23], 22.2% of patients presenting with hemorrhage demonstrated evidence of IIAs in contrast to only 8.5% in patients with non-hemorrhagic presentation.

Laboratory Features

Laboratory findings like leukocytosis, high erythrocyte sedimentation rate (ESR) and raised C reactive protein (CRP) levels could be of diagnostic aid; however, only positive blood culture or histological specimens obtained from the aneurysmal wall could affirm the diagnosis. Still to be considered, blood cultures were positive in approximately one-third of patients with IIA previously screened in an earlier report. However, results could be criticized since samples were obtained after the start of the antimicrobial therapy [37]. A subsequent study [23] found a relatively higher rate of positive blood culture reaching 60% in patients with IIAs. Moreover, it might be strenuous to isolate certain organisms as filamentous fungus, S. apiospermum, with inherent delay in colony formation on mycology culture. Molecular identification aided by gene assays might be of value in this regard.

Imaging Features

IIAs could be visualized on computed tomographic angiography (CTA) or time of flight magnetic resonance angiography (TOF-MRA) as enhancing vascular masses, typically multiple in up to 25-33% of patients, distally situated, and fusiform shaped. Therefore, cautious interpretation of distal vasculature should be performed, not to miss additional IIAs or sequel of septic vegetations. Although typically small in diameter, IIAs tend to change speedily in size or geometry or develop a denovo aneurysm on serial imaging. Because of that dynamic nature, repeat imaging should be performed with any denovo neurological symptomatic alteration.

CTA is a readily available, short duration exam, an exceptional privilege in potentially unstable patients with underlying cardiac failure. CTA might be the most convenient non-invasive frontline diagnostic modality whenever an IA is suspected. It enables an entire visualization of the intracranial vascular tree; so that it could detect relatively smaller IIAs situated within the distal vasculature. Moreover, CT could identify complications of IIAs as possible intracranial hemorrhage and associated vasogenic edema. CT shortcomings might comprise the necessity for the contrast administration and radiation expsure [38]. Compared to the DSA as shown in an earlier study, CTA demonstrated a sensitivity of 83% and specificity of 93%; nonetheless, categorization by aneurysmal size showed a dramatic decline in the CTA sensitivy for aneurysms less than 3 mm in diameter reaching up to 45% as opposed to 95.3% for aneurysms greater than 3 mm [39]. According to Hui et al., 2015 [23]; CTA and MRA detected only 43% and 33% respectively of the angiographically-proven IIAs.

Rupture of IIAs with a subsequent IPH might give rise to the 'connecting vessel' sign which might mimic the 'spot sign,' an imaging biomarker that is commonly utilized to estimate the expansion risk of the sponataneous non-infectious ICH, complicating hypertension, and cerebral amyloid angiopathy. Spot sign is classically described as a round or serpiginous hyperdense spot greater than 1.5 mm within a deep grey matter hematoma (less frequently, within a lobar hematoma) with no connection to an outside vascular structure and more than double the density value of the surrounding hematoma. Other radiological signs have been described in the literature to reinforce the ICH prognostication as'spot and tail' and 'leakage' signs, which refer respectively to spot sign with an enlarged lenticulostriate artery in the case of basal ganglionic hemorrhage, and a relative 10% increase in the HU value of the ICH on delayed images. While imaging features might overlap, patients' clinical profile might discriminate between the two scenarios. Patients with IIAs are younger with a history of drug abuse and, or valvular abnormality compared to elderly hypertensive patients in the spot sign group [40].

Magnetic resonance imaging offers the advantage of greater spatial resolution, better parenchymal demonstration, and the capability of depicting small IIAs yet only down to 4 mm. Moreover, demonstration of T2*-weighted imaging black dots or the more frequently known as microbleeds on the brain surface in patients with IEC, might give a clue to the presence of a thrombosed IIA. More criticially, existence of peri/lesional inflammatory process in the form of encephalitis or meningitis with corresponding contrast enhancement on gadolinium enhanced images might indicate a greater risk for the aneurysmal rupture. These findings might aid the therapeutic decision-making through a proper selection of the timing of cardiac surgery following enhancement disappearance.The limitation of MRI, as compared with CT, might include less accessibility, higher cost, realtively longer acquisition time which augments the susceptibility to motion artifact, and the exemption of patients with implantable cardiac devices and prosthetic valves, which represent known risk factors for IEC and the subsequent development of IIAs [41-44].

Despite being invasive with a 1% potential risk of complications, the DSA still represents the gold standard tool for the diagnosis of IIAs owing to the greater spatial and tempral resolution. Therefore, it would be more appropriately utilized when definitive exclusion is mandatory as in the event of IEC/other source of intarcranial infection in concomitance with intracranial hemorrhage, thrombo-emboilc infaction, any neurological deficit, or negative/ equivocal non-invasive tests. Supplementairly, DSA could be of a great benefit through determinig the natural prognosis and the suitable treatment strategy based on the aneurysmal angiographic feature [45].

Management

Treatment Algorithm

The management of IEC is arduous with a mortality rate of 16-25%. IEC is initially treated conservatively; however, a prompt surgical intervention is mandatory when various complications occur, comprising intractable cardiac failure, persistent/refractory sepsis, large mobile septic vegetations, peripheral embolism, and prosthetic valve endocarditis. The mortality rate of IEC is further augmented when complicated by cerebrovascular disorders as IIAs [46].

Compared to saccular intracranial berry aneurysms, treatment of IIAs is challenging because of the rarity, capricious behavior, inconsistent presentation, and natural evolution. Other than the prompt intitation of the culture-based antimicrobial therapy of the offending organism, there are no standardized treatment algorithms or consensus guidelines on the IIAs management, particularly with the lack of randomized controlled trials, and prospective cohort studies that would influende the clinical decision-making process [47].

Despite being highly individualized and institution-dependent, the current treatment modalities comprise antimicrobial therapy, surgical or endovascular strategy either solely or in combination. Some clinicians propose a conservative treament with serial cerebral angiography monitoring in unruptured IIAs and a shift toward an interventional therapy if the aneurysm rebleed, persist or grow. Others advocate an initial invasive repair in patients with IEC and focal neurological deficits or severely immunocompromised pateints presenting with IIAs [48].

According to Matsubara et al., 2015 [49], the number of endovascular procedures exceeded the surgical repair in the past 15 years with quite satisfactory angiographic and functional outcomes. Endovascular repair is favorable in patients with vulnerable cardiovascular condition who necessiatate an instant cardiac surgery because of the compulsory delay, the demand for anticoagulation, and the reported greater risk of periprocedural cardiac failure. On the other hand, neurosurgery would be more appropriately considered when IIAs are associated with massive IPH or situated with an eloquent territory necessitating an extracranial to intracranial bypass. Unfortuantely, inherent friable nature of the aneurysmal wall and the diseased parent artery could rule out the microsurgical clipping or endosaccular coiling. Parent artery sacrifice might be the optimal therapy; however, it still harbors a considerable neurological risk.

The treatment approach eventually is largely contingent on the aneurysmal rupture status and the sequel of the associated hematoma; however, the decision to treatment might be influenced also by other patient, aneurysmal and cardiac-related variables like patient's age, concomitant comorbidities, number, location, territorial eloquence of IIAs, necessity for revascularization and finally cardiac status in the context of the timing of anticipated cardiothoracic surgery [49]. Based on our experience and the current literature, a detailed management algorithm for IIAs is presented at Figure 2.

Unruptured IIAs (Medical Therapy and Surveillance)

Once diagnosis of unruptured IIAs is validated, a prompt initiation of culture-guided antimicrobial therapy should be performed given the high morbi-mortality associated with the aneurysmal rupture. In the event of negative blood or cerebrospinal fluid (CSF) culture, empirical treatment with antibiotics should be maintained for a minimum of 4-6 weeks.

The decision for the conservative approach is usually adopted in case of unruptured IIAs; especially those deemed to be associated with high interventional morbimortality like fusiform aneurysms that involve the whole vessel circumference and aneurysms situated proximally or within an eloquent vascular territory where parent artery sacrifice would induce a considerable or permanent neurological deficit [50]. Nonetheless, aneurysms should be monitored meticulously with serial angiography to search for denovo aneurysms that might develop even during proper medical therapy and more exigently to evaluate the morphology and the size of the existing aneurysms. The evolution under the conservative therapy is unpredictable, IIAS might rupture in the worst scenario, progressively increase, remain stable, got smaller or disappear. In the former scenarios where the aneurysm is refractory to medical therapy, endovascular or surgical strategy would be justified, and the benefits might outweigh the risks given the grave prognosis associated with the aneurysmal rupture within the latency period. Although rupture risk is less than 2%, the likelihood might be escalated with the anticoagulation, imperative for the concomitant cardiac instability. For that reason, some argue for prophylactic endovascular obliteration or surgical clipping or trapping with disregard to the rupture status or aneurysmal size if the aneurysm is not within an eloquent vascular territory and technically feasible [51].

With that said, the conservative approach showed a variable efficacy throughout the current literature. Brust et al., 1990 [52] reported a complete resolve of medically treated IIAs in the half of cases and a size steadiness in the other half. In a later study conducted by Corr et al., 1995 [53] upon 14 angiographically-monitored patients, 50% showed a favorable outcome divided between 33% cure and 17% size reduction, while 33%, and 17% reported an aneurysmal stability and enlargement respectively. In the study of Bartakke et al., 2002 [54] complete resolution was achieved in 29% of the aneurysms managed conservatively, reduced size in 18.5%, stability in 15%, increased size in 22%, while 15% notably developed supplemental aneurysms. More favorably, Allen et al., 2013 [55] noticed a 64% cure rate with complete regression in patients with IIAs maintained solely on antimicrobial therapy. More recently, Matsubara et al., 2015 [49] with only antimicrobial therapy successfully cured 7 IIAs (6 unruptured, 1 ruptured) with neither rebleeding nor later recurrence. It is speculated that shortened time to the diagnosis of IIAs with advances in imaging resolution and the prompt start of the antimicrobial therapy could be contributory factors in boosting the favorable outcome of IIAs.

Ruptured IIAs

Once IIAs ruptured, a definitive active treatment should follow given associated higher mortality rate; however, the choice between endovascular and surgical approaches is still controversial. Indications and technical success of each modality is highly influenced by the aneurysm site, morphology, territorial eloquence, presence of significant mass effect after the intracranial hematoma (ICH) and the patient's general condition [56].

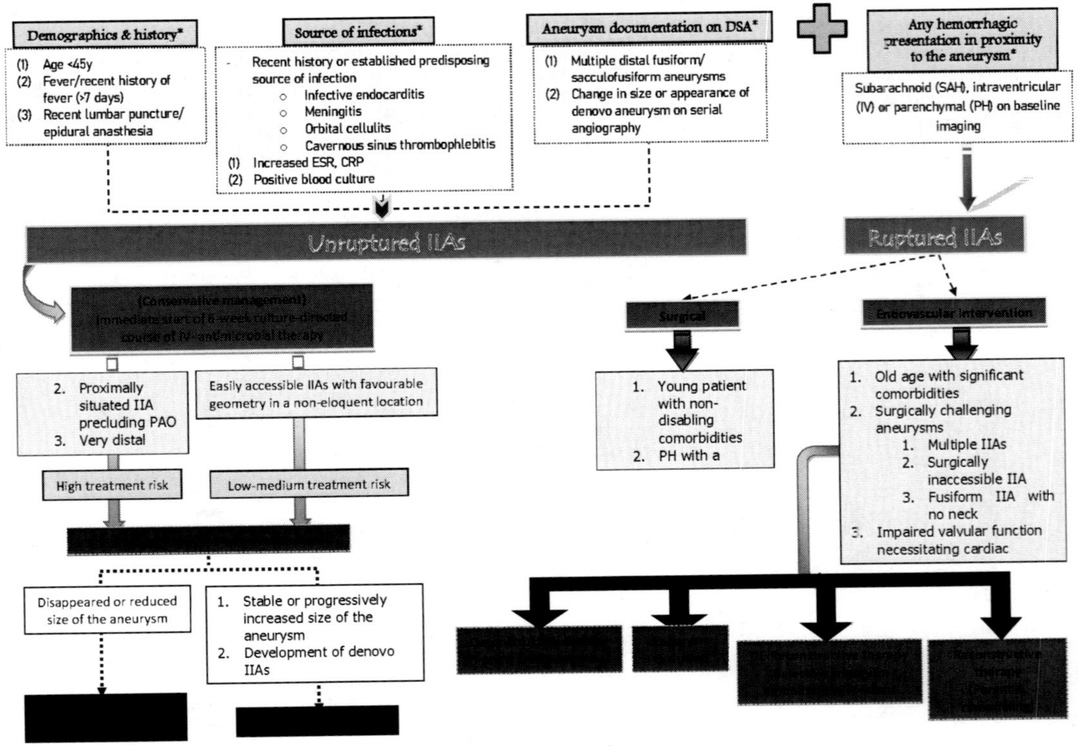

Figure 2. Management algorithm for infectious intracranial aneurysms (IIAs) based on the current literature (Diagnostic criteria from Kannoth et al., 2008*). CRP, c-reactive protein; DSA, digital subtraction angiography; ESR, erythrocyte sedimentation rate; PAO, parent artery occlusion; TTT, treatment.

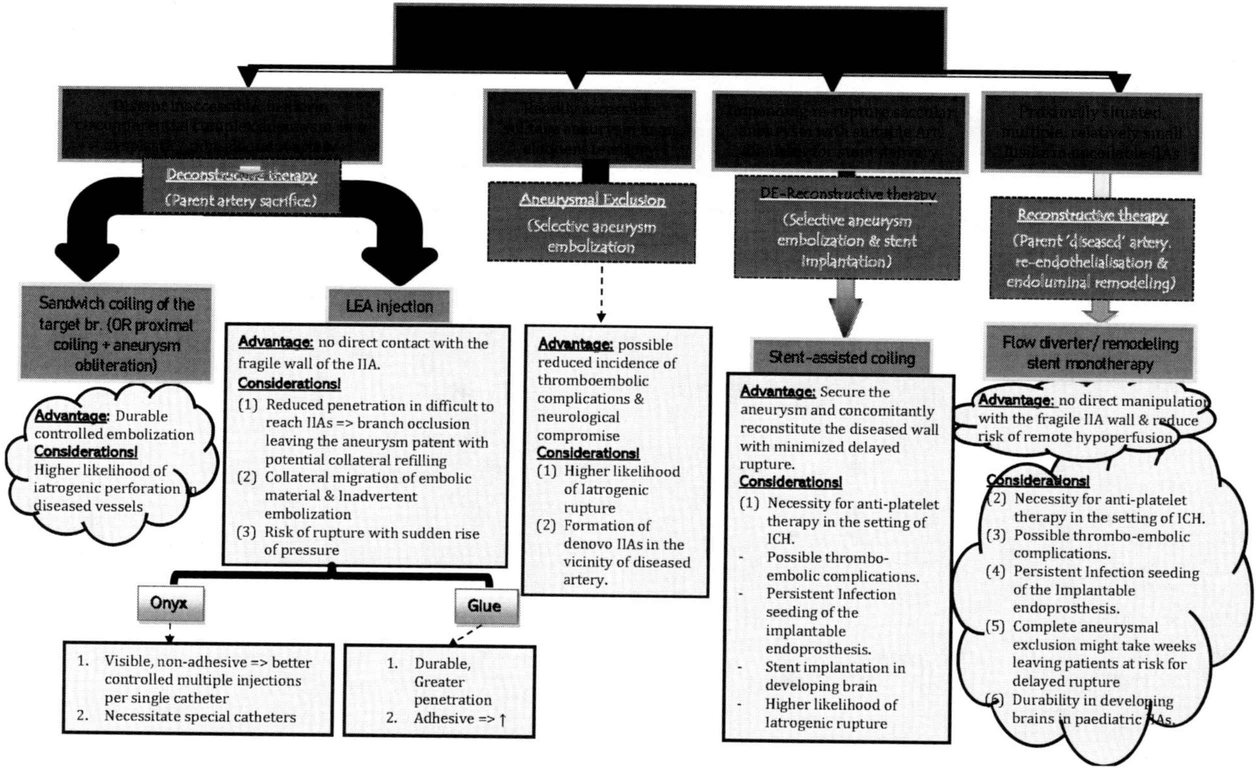

Figure 3. Choice of the pertinent endovascular strategy for treatment of intracranial infectious aneurysms (IIAs). ICH, intracranial haemorrhage; LEA, liquid embolic agent.

Surgical Management

Microsurgical approach might be favored over the endovascular therapy in the case of solitary surgically accessible IIA with an ICH-mediated significant mass effect. However surgical risks might be augmented in patients with large, multiple IIAs or aneurysms situated at an eloquent territory [57].

Neurosurgical options include aneurysmal neck clipping, omentum wrapping, parent artery trapping with/without resection and ICA-ECA bypass, excision with vessel grafting [58]. In 1965, Roach and Drake [59] described the first surgical intervention of ruptured IIAs in which ligation of the aneurysmal sac was not feasible because of the friable nature of the parent vessel with multipoint leakage from infective necrosis. *Simple neck clipping of IIAs* might be regarded the most reasonable approach; nonetheless, it is technically demanding and could easily end in parent artery sacrifice owing to the inherent neck-less fusiform morphology, the friable nature of the aneurysmal wall, disrupted microarchitecture of the parent vessel, and the strenuous identification of the aneurysms in the distal vasculature. In the latter case, frameless stereotactic guidance might be of aid [60]. *Aneurysmal trapping* in concomitance with distal bypass graft might be more appropriate for proximally situated IIAs yet, owing to the small vessel caliber, trapping is not applicable for distal vasculature where IIAs typically reside [61, 62].

The timing of surgical aneurysmal obliteration should be attentively considered in the light of cardiac function since it might substantially complicate the periprocedural management. Cardiac surgery necessitates intraprocedural heparinization and post-operative anti-coagulation, which if performed firstly could boost the probability of the intracranial hemorrhage. Moreover, cardiopulmonary bypass might magnify a pre-existing cerebral ischemic injury through the induced hypotension and augment the cerebral edema in areas of blood–brain barrier disruption. Contrarily, craniotomy might aggravate the risk of periprocedural cardiac failure if performed a head of the cardiac surgery owing to the delay in cardiac repair. Some surgeons proposed the deferral of cerebral surgery provided that no anticipated neurological deficit together with implantation of bioprosthetic valves that do not necessitate a post procedural anticoagulation. Even so, there is no consensus on the optimal interval between the craniotomy and the open cardiac surgery. According to the Japanese Circulation Society in the presence of ruptured IIAs, aneurysmal exclusion should be performed firstly, followed by the cardiac repair with 2-3 weeks apart. An earlier statement from the American Heart Association stated that it is reasonable in patients with IEC with a necessity for a cardiac repair to secure firstly the IIAs, even the non-ruptured ones, by endovascular means [63].

Endovascular

Anciently, endovascular therapy has a limited role in the treatment of IIAs because of the alleged infectious risk associated with the navigation of foreign catheters within infected friable vessels. As per our knowledge, no reported cases of localized abscess formation or severe sepsis after endovascular treatment of IIAs in the literature which might be attributed to the periprocedural antimicrobial therapy.

Nowadays, endovascular therapy has become a valid alternative principally for non-surgically fit patients or in the case of multiple or surgically inaccessible IIAs. With advanced catheter-based innovations and diversity of embolization materials, endovascular therapy is considered potentially safer and more efficacious than open surgical repair, particularly if performed at a teritary high-volume center, and in the absence of significant hematoma with mass effect, increased intracranial pressure, hypotension, incorporation of an eloquent territory.

Endovascular therapy offers several advantages compared to the surgical resolution. It is less invasive with lower potential risks of the general anasthesia (GA) which is of a particular significance when treating patients with IIAs and endocarditis that frequently present with impaired valvular function. In addition, endovascular therapy might permit an expeditious 1–day-apart cardiac valve replacement following IIAs obliteration as compared to the recommended 2-3 weeks following surgical clipping and craniotomy. Moreover, it promotes a speedy reinstitution of the anticoagulant therapy after the cardiac surgery. Therefore, endovascular therapy might be preferable when a prompt cardiac surgery is imperative [64].

Despite the reported safety and ease of access of the endovascular therapy, it is not without risks. Microwire-mediated dissection and perforation might take place with navigation within the friable vasculature. Moreover, the presence of distally situated, fusiform shaped IIAs render the endosaccular access and coiling not attainable in many situations. Gross et al., 2013 [65] reviewed IIAs who were treated by means of endovascular therapy. Coiling was feasible in only 24% of patients in contrast to 71% of parent artery sacrifice aided by detachable balloons or liquid embolic agents. Overall technical success rate was 96% with nearly 9% of intraprocedural complications. Nevertheless, lack of long-term follow up in many studies could contaminate the realistic angiographic success.

The endovascular obliteration of IIAs might be performed with direct aneurysmal exclusion, the deconstructive or the reconstructive strategy in accordance with the location of the aneurysm whether proximal or distal, the eloquence of the vascular territory, and the ease of access (Figure 3).

Deconstructive Therapy

Deconstructive strategy might comprise aneurysmal embolotherapy, parent artery sacrifice or both which could be achieved aided by implantation of detachable coils or injection of liquid embolic agents like n-BCA (N-butyl cyanoacrylate) or non-adhesive agents as Onyx™. Selective endosaccular coiling offers several advantages such as the preservation of the parent artery, the reduction in the time-lag inevitable to fully secure the aneurysm, and the avoidance of the antiplatelet therapy. Nonetheless, certain small-sized, distally situated, irregular aneurysms, as in the case of most IIAs, might not be amenable for coiling because of the strenous distant catheterization or the challenging endosaccular access. Moreover, given the inherent thin, friable, and fragile nature of the infective aneurysmal wall, coiling conveys a greater risk for aneurysmal perforation or rupture [66]. Finally, long-term aneurysmal recurrence and rebleeding could not be ruled out. Ogawa et al., 2016 [67] reported an elderly patient with fungal sinusitis that was complicated by cavernous IIAs. Despite urgent coil embolization, the aneurysm rebled and the patient died. More favorably, Reuschel et al., 2018 [68] illustarted another ruptured IIA at the M3 segment of the MCA which was treated primarily by SACE and 21 months later by parent artery occlusion because of aneurysmal morphological deformation and rebleeding. A review of recent literature for IIAs who were treated by endosaccular coiling is shown in Table 1 [69-90].

Parent artery sacrifice is regarded as the ultimate solution for IIAs, especially when considering the friable aneurysmal sac, the diseased vascular wall, and the small luminal diameter of the parent artery that might prohibit the reconstructive therapy. Nonetheless, it might be the preferrable choice only when managing distant inaccessible, fusiform circumferential complex aneurysms, in a rather dysplastic/ non-eloquent artery [91]. Eddleman et al., 2008 [92] proposed certian criteia when considering arterial sacrifice strategy, which comprise (1) lack of safe microcatherization and aneurysmal access (2) irregular morphology that is inadequate for coiling (3) IIAs is within a non-eloquent territory. Parent artery sacrifice of IIAs in the territory of an eloquent cortex might be associated with a devastating neurological morbiditiy. Therefore, temporary balloon occlusion using a balloon or superselective awake provocative testing induced by sodium amobarbital injection into the target vessel, have been utilized to aid proper selection of patients with a favorable profile that is amenable to embolization with no subsequent neurological impact. According to Matsubara et al., 2015 [49], a considerable number of patients can tolerate parent artery occlusion, especially if they well-tolerated the initial embolic event that preceeded the aneurysmal formarion. Nonetheless, neurological testing itself whether with balloon or pharmacological agents might be associated with thrombo-embolic manifestations, arterial dissection, perforation or seizures, cerebral edema and apnea and unconsciousness that might develop following inadvertent amytal migration to the posterior circulation [93].

Anciently, aneurysmal embolization started with the implantation of detachable balloons. Several reports in the literature illustrated their potential values for the treatment of IIAs. Utilization of detachable coils for intravascular occlusion are favored recently in the event of relatively proximal IIAs as it authorizes a controlled efficacious deployment; yet distal collateral refilling might lead to aneurysmal recurrence; therefore, sandwich coiling might be mandatory for a stable long-lasting and adequate occlusion [94].

Chapot et al., conveniently occluded 18 IIAs with combined aneurysmal coiling and parent artery sacrifice with n-BCA injection. Neither technical complication nor poor functional outcomes were documented in their series. The n-BCA is an adhesive non-absorbable material, which allows for permnant embolization of the aneurysm, together with the parent artery. Despite its efficacy, the inherent rapid polymerization might induce unfortunate gluing of the delivery microcatheter or bleeding upon retrieval (Figures 4-6). Moreover, although the operator might be capable of adjusting the optimum viscosity required for embolization through different concentrations of lipidol: n-BCA mixtures, reduced penetration and inadvertent migration to uninvolved territory are still potential concerns (Figure 7). Moreover, there might be a theoretical rupture risk with a sudden pressure rise in the arterial stump.

On the other hand, and aided with the precipitation process, Onyx, a non-adhesive embolic agent, affords unique charcterisitics when compard with the n-BCA, which includes long precipitation time which might reduce the likelihood of the microcatheter gluing and embolized pedicle avlusion upon microcatheter retrieval, facile angiographic visualization, capability of multi-injections through a single catheter with a rather slow precise control when compared with the n-BCA. These distinctive features might minimize the risk of aneurysmal recurrence through prohibiton of distal collateral refilling that is mediated by complete aneurysmal embolization together with its both afferent and efferent limbs [95]. A review of recent literature for IIAs who were treated by means of parent artery sacrifice is shown in Table 2A-D [96-127].

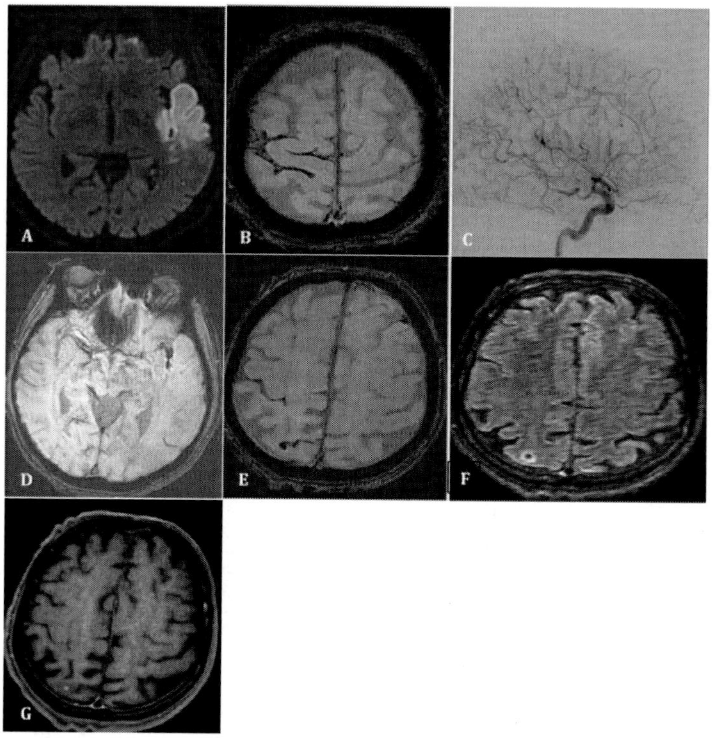

Figure 4. A 65-year-old patient presented with sudden wernicke aphasia with no sensorimotor neurological deficits. Brain computed tomography (CT) showed no recent ischemic or hemorrhagic abnormality (not shown). Two days later, brain diffusion-weighted image (DWI) and susceptibility weighted image (SWI)- magnetic resonance imaging (MRI) revealed respectively a left temporo-insular ischemic infarct (Figure 4A) and right central, precentral cortical hemosiderin deposits (Figure 4B) with no proximal thrombo-embolic clots on vascular imaging. Digital subtraction angiography (DSA) shows no vascular abnormality (Figure 4C; retrospective assessment might reveal start of aneurysmal dilatation). SWI-MRI performed after 2-weeks showed a well-formed clot in the left lower trunk of MCA consistent with the already established infarct (Figure 4D). Right parietal infective vegetation as appeared on SWI (Figure 4E), FLAIR 'fluid-attenuated inversion recovery' (Figure 4F), and the 3D-post gadolinium fat-saturated T1 TSE 'turbo spin echo' (Figure 4G) image.

Reconstructive Therapy

Parent artery preservation could be auspicious over the sacrifice strategy, particularly when the patient harbors bilateral aneurysms or frequently develops denovo aneurysms in an unresolved source of infection. Recent technological advancements in intracranial stents and flow diverters have exceedingly expanded the therapeutic armamentarium of the complex intracranial pseudoaneurysms [128]

Micropore stent implantation could alter intra-aneurysmal flow dynamics with progressive thrombosis of focal IIAs, promote vessel wall remodeling together via providing scaffolds for vessel wall neointimal re-endothelialization [129].

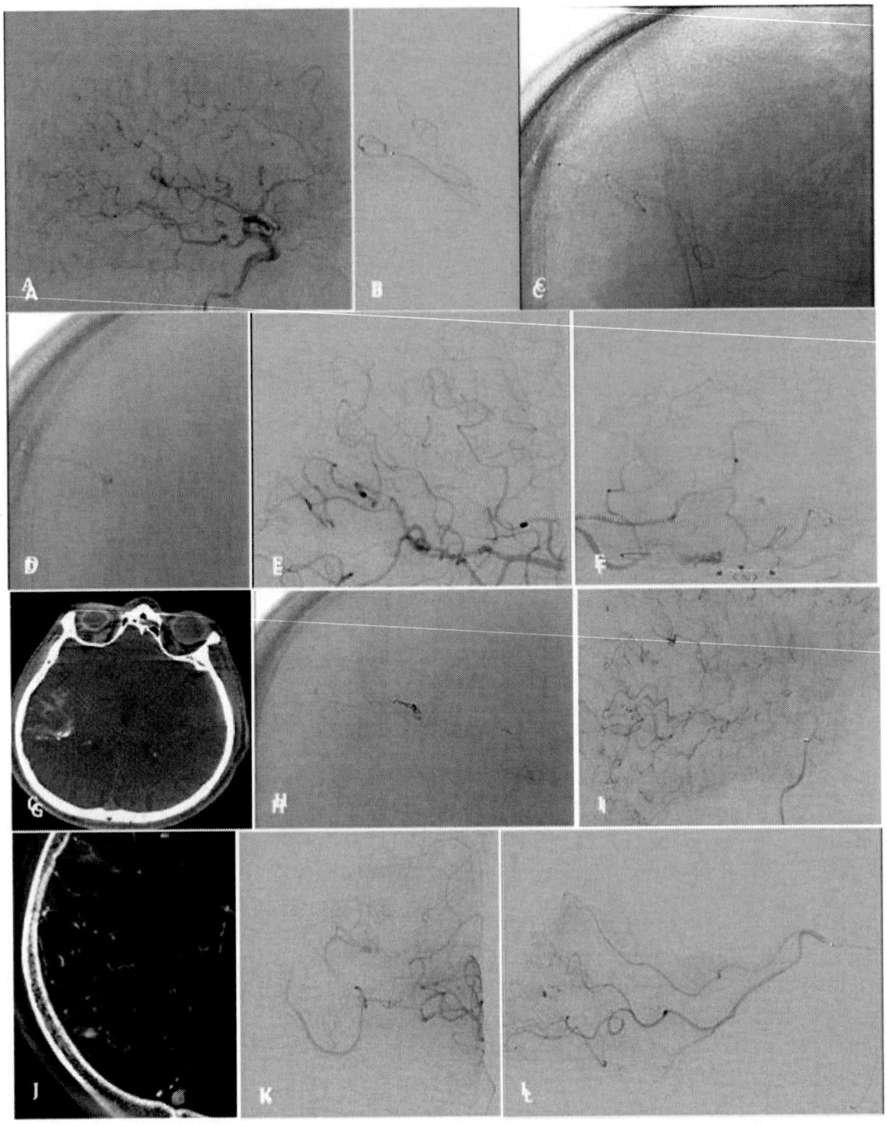

Figure 5. Right internal carotid artery (ICA)-digital subtraction angiography (DSA, lateral projection) revealed a right distal M3 intracranial infectious aneurysm (IIA) at the posterior parietal branch of the middle cerebral artery (Figure 5A). Given the distal location, sacculofusiform morphology, non-eloquence of the territory involved, parent artery sacrifice with n-BCA (n butyl cyanoacrylate) embolization was planned. A Magic 1.2F microcatheter was navigated distally over a .007 Hybrid micro guidewire as near as safely feasible to the aneurysmal sac within the target artery (Figure 5B, 5C) followed by injection of the liquid embolic agent (LEA) (Figure 5D). Control DSA revealed target branch obliteration, yet unfortunately with two points of arterial laceration at the point of LEA injection (Figure 5E) and more proximally at the M1 segment of the middle cerebral artery (MCA) (Figure 5F), possibly related to microcatheter retrieval, although not being so forceful. Immediate Computed tomography revealed a mild sylvian subarachnoid hemorrhage (Figure 5G). An urgent 5-minute balloon tamponade successfully controlled the proximal bleeding yet, failed to control the distal one for which prompt coiling was performed (Figure 5H). Control DSA followed by on table Dyna CT showed collateral refilling of the aneurysm by the anterior cerebral artery (ACA) (Figure 5I, 5J). Multiple trials to catheterize the feeding branch failed (Figure 5K, 5L).

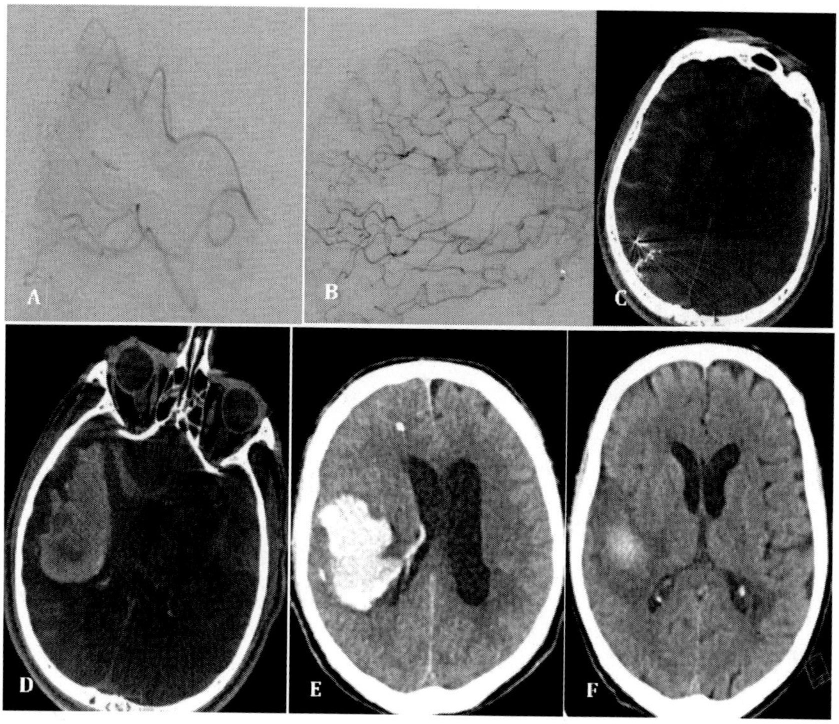

Figure 6. Super selective and right internal carotid artery (ICA) control angiographies after trials of catheterization the anterior cerebral artery (ACA) branch demonstrated a spontaneous occlusion of the aneurysm with no further action taken (Figure 6A, 6B). Control CT revealed no aneurysmal refilling, however with expansion of intracranial hematoma (Figure 6C, 6D). Sequential resolution of the hematoma was noted on the post-ictal 5 day and 1-month follow-up CT scans (Figure 6E, 6F); however, the patient remained hemiplegic with hemianesthesia and persistent leftwards head deviation at 1 month post-procedurally.

Sugg et al., 2006 [130] reported a middle-aged male patient with an IEC that was complicated by basal ganglionic ischemic stroke and SAH. DSA revealed a fusiform dilatation of the supraclinoid segment of the internal carotid artery (ICA) and M1 segment of the middle cerebral artery (MCA) with superimposed focal side-wall aneurysms that progressively enlarged and developed an accessory lobule on the 11-day post-ictus repeat DSA despite broad-spectrum antibacterial and antifungal therapy. Presence of multiple fusiform IIAs at non-branching points with progressive increase in size and deformation in morphology triggered the diagnosis of IIAs that necessitated an immediate neuro-interventional obliteration. Aneurysms were successfully excluded from the cranial circulation by placement of Neuroform® stent (Stryker Neuroendovascular, Kalamazoo, MI, USA). Immediate Angiographic cure was attributed to the "compaction or collapse" of the interrupted diseased wall layers. No follow-up was declared except improved cognition a few days post-procedurally with no denovo appearance of neurological deficits.

Despite presumed efficacy, administration of periprocedural antiplatelets that is necessary to maintain stent patency still poses a notable limitation. Moreover, latency period is necessary before complete aneurysmal obliteration is achieved, which could predispose the patient to aneurysmal re-rupture. Finally, long-term flow diversion effect of the self-expandable nitinol stent is questionable particularly as a monotherapy. Covered stents might serve as a feasible strategy for the prompt management of IIAs; however, flow diverters might be presumptively advantageous in the setting of very lengthy fusiform IIAs where flow must be maintained to eloquent small side branches and tiny perforators, which inherently might be coupled with a relatively considerable lag in the aneurysmal occlusion with a potential spontaneous re-rupture [131].

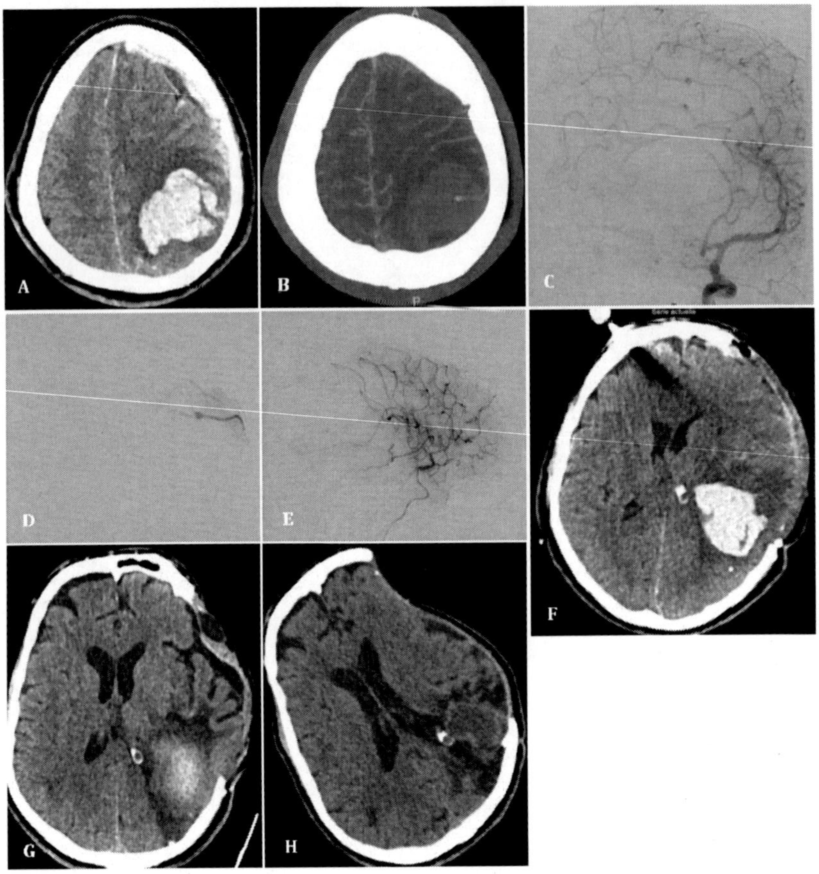

Figure 7. A middle-aged patient with a history of mechanical aortic valve replacement and an infective endocarditis because of E. faecalis, presents with sudden headache, malaise followed by loss of consciousness (GCS 3) and generalized tonic-clonic seizures. Initial brain computed tomography (CT) scan revealed a left subdural collection, left parietal subcortical hematoma with a subsequent mass effect denoted by subfalcine herniation, rightwards midline deviation, and obstructive hydrocephalus (Figure 1A). A connecting vessel sign with a left high parietal distal infectious middle cerebral artery aneurysm on vascular Imaging (Figure1B). The patient underwent an emergent decompressive cranicectomy and sent to the angiosuite. Under general anesthesia, angiography confirmed the presence a left M2-M3 middle cerebral artery (MCA) fusiform aneurysmal at the anterior parietal artery (Figure 1C). A 167 cm-Headway® microcatheter was navigated over a Traxcess® microwire near to the aneurysm followed by injection of 50% diluted Glubran (Figure 1D). Control angiography revealed successful obliteration of the aneurysm together with the parent artery, yet with inadvertent migration of embolic material to the posterior parietal branch of the left MCA (Figure 1E). Post-procedural control CT revealed a stable volume and morphology of the intracranial hematoma with partial regression of the mass effect (Figure 1F). Sequential resolution of the hematoma as denoted on 1 and 3-month follow-up CT scans with a subsequent porencephalic cavitation (Figure 1G., Figure 1H). During hospitalization, patient showed a marked clinical improvement (discharged 3 months post-procedurally on GCS 12) for physiotherapy. Cranioplasty was planned 2 months afterwards.

With that said, Appelboom et al., 2010 [132] first described the utility of the endoluminal flow-diverter in the management of IIAs. A 10-year-old girl presented with meningitis that was complicated by intracavernous large IIA manifested by cranial nerve III palsy. The aneurysm was totally excluded at 3-m DSA after placement of a SILK® flow diverter (Balt extrusion, Montmorency, France) with a concomitant significant amelioration of patient's symptoms. Authors set certain recommendations that are established nowadays to enhance aneurysmal thrombosis, alleviate symptoms related to neurological compression, and to prevent long-term recurrence. They recommended to push on the stent during the delivery to enhance metal coverage area and select a stent length that is at least 3 times the summation of parent vessel diameter and aneurysmal neck size to boost stent stability.

Flow-diverter implantation proved its angiographic and clinical efficacy in subsequent reports in both adults and children (youngest in 2-year-old) with no reported technical complications. Moreover, further advancements in the hydrophilic surface coating of the flow diverter reduced potential thrombogencity and fastened the re-endothelilization process [133]. A review of recent literature for IIAs who were treated by means of reconstructive therapy is shown in Table 3 [134-136].

De-Reconstructive Therapy

A combination of deconstructive and reconstructive strategies might be accomplished through the stent-assisted coiling technique. Ding et al., 2014 [137] illustrated a case of bacterial endocarditis from Streptococcus mitis and episodic diplopia attributable to a 3-mm ruptured IIA of the pericallosal branch of the anterior cerebral artery (ACA). The aneurysm was well-secured with Neuroform®-mediated stent-assisted coil embolization (SACE) as evident on the 3-m follow-up magnetic resonance angiography, and the patient was neurologically intact. Although SACE might offer a superior aneurysmal occlusion over mono-stenting therapy, the placement of endosaccular coils within the fragile IIA might aggravate the risk of the iatrogenic wall perforation and stent thrombotic occlusion via protruded or misplaced coil loops. On the other hand, OuYang et al., 2019 [138] presented an interesting case of infectious ICA pseudoaneurysm that was treated by SACE; however, the aneurysm re-ruptured after 2 months and unfortunately the patient died; which might doubt the long-term safety and efficacy of SACE.

From the same strategic perspective Yen et al., 2007 [134] described a case of meningitis after an upper respiratory infection and positive blood culture for Streptococcus constellates. Brain MRI revealed bilateral intracavernous IIAs of the ICA with luminal stenosis. Despite proper culture-directed antimicrobial therapy, the patient developed bilateral ophthalmoplegia that persisted even with prolonged medical therapy. Aided by balloon-mounted coronary stents, both IIAs were successfully treated with SACE with complete obliteration on the 6m-angiographic control and restoration of the stenotic portion to the nearly normal caliber. Bilateral ophthalmoplegia had ameliorated significantly leaving only mild unilateral sixth cranial nerve palsy. Although balloon expandable stents (BES) are associated with a higher radial outward force and greater metal coverage ratio compared to self-expandable stents, navigating a stiff BES through friable vasculature might exacerbate the condition via provoking a vascular spasm, dissection, perforation, or even rupture. A review of recent literature for IIAs who were treated by means of reconstructive therapy is shown in Table 4.

Table 1. IIA exclusion by Selective endosaccular coiling

Author, year	Age, Sex	Etiology	Presenting N. Symptoms	Aneurysm				He.	Device	occlusion status	Comp.	Outcome
				Sum	Site	Form	Rupture					
Chun, 2001 [66]	39, F	--	--	2	Distal MCA Distal MCA	Saccular	Yes Yes	SAHICH	Coiling Inaccessible	Yes	Hemi-paresis	Fair-GOS 3
	44, F	IEC	Sudden headache	1	L distal MCA		Yes	SAH	Coiling	Yes	None	Good-GOS 5
	42,M	--	--	1	ACA, pericallosal		Yes	SAH	Coiling	N/A	None	Dead
Chapot, 2002 [30]	39, M	IEC		1	R Proximal MCA	--	Yes	ICH	Coils + Balloon	Complete	None	Disability
	62, M	IEC	Infarction	2	L Proximal MCA	--	Yes	ICH	Coils	Complete	None	Disability
	26, M	IEC	Infarction	1	L proximal PCA	--	Yes	NA	Coils	Complete	None	NI
	55, M	IEC		1	R Proximal MCA	--	NO	--	Coils	Complete	None	NI
Erdogan, 2004 [26]	53,M	IEC	Headache, fatigue, nausea, vomiting	1	L distal MCA (3mm)	Saccular	Yes	SAH	Coils	Complete	None	Good-NI
Lasjaunias, 2005 [69]	14,M	IEC	Systemic embolic episodes from the valve including cerebral emboli	1	L ACA	--	No	No	Coils	Complete	None	--
Nakahara, 2006 [70]	56, M	IEC	Low grade fever	2	R distal PCA (9.2 mm) L distal ACA (5.7 mm)		No No	No No	Coils Coils + PAO	Complete	None	Good_NI
Eddleman, 2007 [71]	9, M	IEC	Comatose	1	R PCA-Superior aspect of P3 (10×5×8 mm)	Saccular Multi-lobed	Yes	IVH	Coils	Complete	None	Good-NI
Wajnberg, 2008 [48]	39, M	IEC	CNIII palsy	1	Basilar tip	--	NO	--	Coils	Complete	None	Good-NI
	33, F		Disorientation	1	L distal MCA	saccular	Yes	ICH	Coils	Complete	None	Good-NI
Dhomne, 2008 [72]	20, F	IEC	Hemiparesis, aphasia	2	MCA trifurcation distal MCA	Saccular Saccular	Yes	SAH	Coils Untreated	Complete Reduced		Partial
Trivedi, 2008 [73]	20, F	Pregnant, IEC	confusion, dysphasia, R monoparesis, tonic-clonic seizure => coma	1	L distal MCA (2 mm)	--	Yes	IPH IVH	Coils	Complete	None	Good- mRS2 (R monoparesis; slight expressive dysphasia
Van de Beek, 2008 [74]	22, M	IEC	Blurred vision => haemorrhagic septic emboli	1	R MCA-distal parietal branch (2 mm)	--	Yes	IPH	Coils	Complete	Re-hemorrhage	Good-cognitive slowness
Kim, 2010 [75]	62, F	cavernous sinus thrombo-phlebitis	R proptosis, complete 3rd,4th, 6th CN palsies	1	R cavernous ICA (15 mm)	Saccular	No	--	Coils	Complete	None	Good-NI (improved visual acuity, № extra-ocular movement)

Author, year	Age, Sex	Etiology	Presenting N. Symptoms	Aneurysm				He.	Device	occlusion status	Comp.	Outcome
				Sum	Site	Form	Rupture					
Ray, 2010 [76]	79, F	Bacteraemia	Unresponsive	1	Right PCA (4 x 7mm)	Saccular	Yes	SAHIVH	Coils	Nearly complete	None	Good-GOS 4
Altekin, 2011 [77]	29, M	IEC	headache, diplopia, ataxia	1	R PCA – P2/3	Saccular	Yes	IPH	Coils	Complete	None	Good-NI
Martindale, 2011 [78]	33, F	IEC	Confusion, R arm numbness		L MCA - M3 superior division	Fusiform	No	No	coils	Complete	None	Good-mild R paresthesia
Regelsberger, 2011 [5]	38, M	IEC	Acute headache, weakness	1	Distal bifurcation MCA – Fronto-insular branch	--	Yes	IPH	Coils	Complete	None	Good-NI
Saraf, 2012 [79]	--,--	IEC	--	1	MCA-distal M1	--	--	--	Coils	Complete	None	Good-NI
Allen, 2013 [55]	--, --	Fungal meningitis (1) Crohn's disease on steroids (1) Multiple myeloma on Chemotherapy (1) Unreported (4)	--	2	R MCA-M1 ACA	--	No YES	No --		Complete Untreated	--	Death-Rupture ACA Aneurysm
				1	L MCA - M1		--	--	--	--	None	--
				1	L cavernous		--	--	--	--	None	--
				4	Unreported		--	--	--	--	None	--
Takemoto, 2014 [80]	--	-- --	-- SAH, infarction	2	Posterior circulation	--	No Yes	No SAH	Coils Coils	Complete Complete	None None	Good Poor – GOS 3
Chimparlee, 2014 [81]	16,F	Sub acute IEC	Sudden severe headache	1	Basilar tip (18 mm)	Saccular	Yes	SAH	Coils	Complete	None	Good-NI
Lotan, 2014 [39]	23, F	IEC	L hemiparesis, Facial palsy, upper quadranopsia (AIS)	1	R MCA –M2	Saccular	Yes	SAH	Coils	Complete	None	Good –mRS 0
Yoon, 2014 [82]	44, F	Meningitis following TSS	Post-operative Fever, CSF leak	1	R PCA-P1	Saccular	Yes	SAHIVH	Coils	Complete	None	Death
Matsubara, 2015 [49]	51, F	Meningitis	Mass effect	1	Cavernous ICA (5.5 mm)	Saccular	No	No	Coils	Complete	None	Good –mRS 0
Ogawa, 2016 [67]	85,M	Fungal sinusitis	L ophthalmoplegia, L facial pain (V1)	1	L cavernous ICA (14x14x15 mm)	Multi-lobed	Yes	SAH	Coils	--	Rebleed	Death
Champeaux, 2017 [83]	19,M	IEC	Sudden loss of consciousness	1	L PCA – P2/3 junction (5 mm)	Saccular	Yes	SAH	Coils	Complete	None	Good – NI (Independent)
Wang, 2017 [84]	25,M	Endocarditis	L hemiparesis, Dysarthria (AIS)	1	R MCA-M2 (5x3 mm)	Saccular	Yes	SAH IVH	Coils	Partial (Ray-mond III)	None	Good-mild dysarthria, L facial droop, L hemiparesis (mRS 2)

Table 1. (Continued)

Author, year	Age, Sex	Etiology	Presenting N. Symptoms	Aneurysm				He.	Device	occlusion status	Comp.	Outcome
				Sum	Site	Form	Rupture					
Park, 2017 [85]	62,M	Immune-suppression	Pneumonia, coma	3	L ACA-callosomarginal (5.2 mm) L MCA-distal M2 (5 .5 mm)	Sacculo-fusiform	Yes	SAH ICH IVH	Coils	Complete	None	Fair-GOS 3
	--	--	--	--	--	--	--	--	Coils	--	--	--
Zhong, 2017 [86]	17,M	IEC, meningitis	Headache, fever	1	L cavernous ICA	--	--	--	Coils	Complete	None	--
Kiss, 2018 [87]	19,M	IEC	Anterograde amnesia	1	L PCA	--	Yes	IPH	Coils	Complete	None	Good-NI
Goldschmidt, 2019 [22]	Late 20, -	IEC	Fever, new onset headache, L small parietal stroke	1	L MCA – M4 parietal branch	--	No	No	Coils	Complete	None	Good-NI
	Young adult	IEC	Shortness of breath, chest pain, reduced consciousness level	1	Basilar top	Irregular	Yes	SAH	Coils	Complete	None	Death_cardiac failure
Hall, 2019 [88]	8, M		High fever, altered mental status, headache	2	Left MCA anterior branch (3.4, 9.8 mm)	Fusiform Saccular	No	No	Coils	Complete	None	Good
Lee, 2020 [89]	37,M	Infected LVAD	Altered mental status, fever => non fluent aphasia, encephalopathy	1	R MCA-M3-4 junction	Fusiform bilobed	Yes	SAH	Coils	--	--	--
				3	R MCA	--	--	--	Untreated	--	--	
Matsuzono, 2021 [12]	63, F	IEC	Aphasia, dysarthria	1	L MCA –M2/3	Fusiform	Yes	SAH	Coils	Complete	None	Good _NI
Panagiotopoulos, 2021 [90]	51, F	Maxillofacial infection after CTH	Intermittent refractory epistaxis	1	L para-ophthalmic ICA (9 x 20 mm)	Multi-lobulated	Yes	Cavernous	Coils	Complete	None	Good _NI

Abbreviations: ACA, anterior cerebral artery; AIS, acute ischemic stroke; CN, cranial nerve; CSF, cerebrospinal fluid; CTH, chemotherapy; F, female; GOS, Glasgow outcome score; He., haemorrhage; ICA, internal carotid artery; IEC, infective endocarditis; IIA, infectious intracranial aneurysm; ICH, intracranial haemorrhage; IPH, intraparenchymal hematoma; IVH, intraventricular haemorrhage; L, left; LVAD, left ventricular assisted device; M, male; MCA, middle cerebral artery; mRS, modified Rankin Scale; NI, neurologically intact; №, normal; PAO, parent artery occlusion; PCA, posterior cerebral artery; R, right; SAH, subarachnoid haemorrhage; TSS, Trans-sphenoidal surgery.

Table 2A. Deconstructive embolization of IIAs by PAO aided by detachable balloons & others

Author, year	Age, Sex	Etiology	Presenting symptoms	Aneurysm characteristics				He.	Device	Occlusion status	Complication	Outcome
				No.	Site	Form	Rupture					
Hurst et al, 2001 [15]	73,M	Fungal sinusitis	Headache, decreased vision, epistaxis	1	R cavernous ICA	Fusiform	Yes	Yes	Detachable balloon + coil	Complete occlusion	Aneurysm extension, fatal SAH, R MCA infarct	Death
Chun, 2001 [66]	44,M	Sinusitis	SAH	1	Vertebrobasilar junction	Fusiform	Yes	SAH		Complete	Stroke, coma	Poor-GOS 2
Yuen, 2004 [96]	46, F	Active ethmoidal sinusitis.	Worsening headache, CN III, VI palsies	1	L cavernous ICA	Fusiform	No	No	Detachable Balloon	Complete	Temporo-parietal infarction	Death (herniation)
Crossland, 2005 [97]	49, F	Petrositis	Transient L arm paresis, headache => VI, IX-XII CNP	1	R petrous ICA	Sacculo-fusiform	No	No		Complete	None	Fair-total permanent total R vocal fold palsy
Hot, 2007 [98]	61,M	Sphenoidal sinusitis - HCL	Headache, epistaxis, cough, low grade fever	5	R cavernous ICA	Multi-lobulated	No	No	Balloon (Cervical ICA) + Coils	Complete	None	Good
Wang, 2007 [99]	41, --	Sinusitis in AIDS-pt.	Severe, recurrent epistaxis	1	L cavernous ICA	Irregular	Yes	SSH	Detachable Balloon+ coils	Complete (Trapping)	None	Death (AIDS-related)
Watanabe, 2008 [100]	15, -	Otitis media in IC patient	L temporal Hgc infarct, otorrhagia	1	L petrous ICA	Saccular	No	No	Detachable Balloon	Complete (Trapping)	None	Good
Esenkaya, 2016 [101]	62, F	Pan sinusitis, cortical abscess	Cavernous sinus mass effect (ptosis, diplopia)	1	L cavernous ICA (30 mm)	Saccular	No	No				Good-mRS 0
Chapot, 2002 [30]	44, M	IEC			R distal MCA		No	--	autologous clot	Complete	None	NI
	31, F	IEC			L distal MCA		No	--	PVA	Complete	None	NI

Abbreviations: AIDS, acquired immune deficiency syndrome; CN, cranial nerve; CNP, cranial nerve palsy; F, female; GOS, Glasgow outcome score; HCL, hairy cell leukaemia; He., haemorrhage; IC, immunocompromised; ICA, internal carotid artery; IEC, infective endocarditis; IIA, infectious intracranial aneurysm; L, left; M, male; MCA, middle cerebral artery; mRS, modified Rankin Scale; NI, neurologically intact; PAO, parent artery occlusion; PVA, Polyvinyl alcohol; R, right; SAH, subarachnoid haemorrhage; SSH, sphenoid sinus haemorrhage.

Table 2B. Deconstructive embolization of IIAs by PAO aided by non-selective coils

Author, year	Age, Sex	Etiology	Presenting symptoms	Aneurysm characteristics				He.	Device	Occlusion status	Comp.	Outcome
				No	Site	Form	Rupture					
Chun, 2001 [66]	55,M	--	SAH, ICH	1	Distal PCA	Fusiform	Yes	SAH ICH	Coils	Complete	None	Good
Chapot, 2002 [30]	44, M	IEC	Extensive AIS	1	R proximal MCA	Fusiform	Yes	SAH	Coils		None	Disability
Quisling, 2003 [102]	19, M	Sinusitis => Cavernous thrombosis	L residual VI palsy, L decreased vision	3	L giant ophthalmic (26 x 17.5 x 21 mm) 2 x L cavernous	Saccular	No	No	Coils + detachable balloon	Complete	None	Good- improved vision
Hara, 2006 [103]	62, M	IEC	Coma, hypotension	1	L orbitofrontal bifurcate. A3-ACA (11 mm)	Saccular	Yes	ICH IVH	Coils	Complete	None	Poor- dependent
Van RooiJ, 2006 [104]	27, M	AIDS, endocarditis	--	1	P4-PCA (8 mm)	--	Yes	SAH	Coils	Complete	None	Death
Amano, 2010 [105]	85, M	Otitis media	Vernet's syndrome	1	R extracranial ICA	Irregular	No	No	Coils	Complete	None	Fair-mod.CNP
Saraf, 2012 [79]	--	Meningitis	--		Distal basilar artery	--	--	--	Coils	Complete	None	Good
	--	Fungal sphenoiditis, cavernous sinusitis	--		Intracavernous ICA	--	--	--	Coils	Complete	None	Good
Sorkin, 2013 [106]	14, F	Subacute bacterial endocarditis	L acute hemiparesis, facial asymmetry, altered mental status => R MCA infarct	1	R distal M1 (19x 16 mm)	Saccular	Yes	ICH	Coils	Complete	None	Good_intact speech, cognition, residual L hemiparesis
Matsubara, 2015 [49]	27, F	Sepsis	Mass effect	1	Cavernous ICA (15 mm)	Fusiform	No	No	Coils (trapping)	Complete	None	Good-mRS1
	57, M	Sinusitis	Infarction => SAH	1	P1-P2 PCA (11 mm)	Fusiform	Yes	SAH		Complete	Asympt. bleeding	Poor-mRS5
LV, 2016 [107]	45, M	IEC	Headache	2	L M3-MCA (5 mm) R M4-MCA (7.8 mm)	--	No No	--	Coils Coils	Complete	None	Good
Fusco, 2016 [50]	24, F	IEC	Asymptomatic	1	L distal MCA (5.3x4.7 mm)	Saccular	No	No	Coils	Complete	None	Good
	33, F	IEC	Fever, night sweats, back pain, right hand numbness	1	L MCA-M3 (4 mm)	Fusiform	No	No	Coils	Complete	None	Good
Esenkaya, 2016 [101]	3, F	RFs: Poor dental health, IV drug abuse, Fugal infection, MV operation, Pacemaker,	Fever, headache, confusion, Nausea and vomiting, Hemiparesis, seizures, slurred speech	2	R M3-MCA (4 mm) R M3-MCA (3 mm)	Fusiform	Yes	IPH	Coils	Complete	None	Good-mRS 1
	2,M			1	R M3 MCA (4 mm)	Fusiform	Yes	IPH	Coils	Complete	None	Good-mRS 2
	38,F			1	R M2 MCA (8 mm)	Fusiform	Yes	SAH	Coils	Complete	None	Good-mRS 1
	63,M			1	R P3 PCA (15 mm)	Fusiform	Yes	IPH	Coils	Complete	None	Good-mRS 0
	47,M			1	R P3 PCA (9 mm)	Fusiform	Yes	IPH	Coils	Complete	None	Good -mRS1

Author, year	Age, Sex	Etiology	Presenting symptoms	Aneurysm characteristics				He.	Device	Occlusion status	Comp.	Outcome
				No	Site	Form	Rupture					
	39,M	LVAD, poor general health, unknown		2	L M3 MCA (6 mm) L M4 MCA (3 mm)	Fusiform	Yes	IPH	Coils	Complete	None	Fair -mRS 3
	65, F			1	L M3/4-MCA (2 mm)	Fusiform	Yes	IPH	Coils	Complete	None	Fair -mRS 3
Nonaka, 2016 [108]	63,M		Headache Asymptomatic	1	Distal MCA Distal MCA		Yes No	SAH No	Coils (saccular) Coils	Complete Complete	Recanalization None	mRS 3
	37, F		Hemiparesis Asymptomatic	1 1	Distal MCA Distal PCA		Yes No	ICH No	Coils Coils	Complete Complete	None None	mRS 1
	47,M		Infarction, hemianopia	1	L distal PCA - P3/4		No	No	Coils	Complete	None	mRS 0
	24,M		Headache	1	Distal MCA		Yes	ICH	Coils	Complete	None	mRS 0
Park, 2017 [85]	-- --	-- --	-- --	3	-- --	-- --	-- --	-- --	-- --	-- --	-- --	-- --
Ando, 2019 [64]	36, F	IEC	--	1	Distal PCA (10 mm)	Saccular	Yes	ICH	Coils	Complete	None	mRS 2
	43, M	IEC	Sudden headache, sensory aphasia	3	Proximal MCA (50 mm)	Fusiform	No	No	Coils	Complete	None	mRS 3
	51, M	IEC	Sudden headache, R hemianopia	2	Distal MCA (3.5 mm) Distal PCA (5 mm) Distal PCA (3.5 mm) Distal PCA (2 mm)	Fusiform Saccular Saccular Fusiform	Yes Yes Yes Yes	SAH ICH ICH ICH	Coil_trapping Coil_endosac Coil_trapping Coil + nBCA trapping	Complete Complete Complete Complete	None	mRS 2 (persistent hemianopia)
Sharma, 2019 [109]	10,M	Orbital cellulitis	L Ptosis, Ophthalmoplegia	2	L cavernous ICA (12 x 15x 22 mm) R petrous apex ICA	Lobulated	NO NO	No	Coils	Complete	None	Good-CNIII partial improved
Brown and Fulks, 2020 [110]	--, M	Probable IIA on top of R M2 superior br. occlusion	Severe headache, decreased level of consciousness + recent stroke sequel	1	R superior br.-MCA!!	--	Possibly	SAH !!	Coils	Complete	None	Good
Somboonnithiphol,2020 [111]	8m, F	Meningitis	Seizures, altered consciousness	1	Proximal Basilar artery	Fusiform lobulated	Yes	SAH IVH	Coils	Complete	None	Good-NI
Phukan, 2021 [94]	45,M	--	Headache	1	L M4-MCA (5 mm)	--	Yes	ICH	Coils	Complete	None	Good-NI
	56,M	--	headache, weakness	1	L M4-MCA (4 mm)	--	Yes	ICH		Complete	None	Good-NI
	.25M	--	Seizure, weakness	1	L M4-MCA (40 mm)	--	Yes	ICH		Complete	None	Good-NI
	25, F	--	Headache	1	R parietooccipital–PCA (5 mm)	--	Yes	SAH		Complete	None	Good-NI
Dai, 2022 [112]	18, M	Cavernous thrombosis	Fever, chills, headache => L VI palsy	1	L cavernous ICA	Saccular	No	No	Coils	Complete	None	Good-NI

Table 2B. (Continued)

Author, year	Age, Sex	Etiology	Presenting symptoms	Aneurysm characteristics				He.	Device	Occlusion status	Comp.	Outcome
				No	Site	Form	Rupture					
Prandi, 2022 [113]	40,M	IEC	altered mental status and dyspnoea	2	R MCA – M2/3 L MCA	Fusiform --	Yes Yes	SAH IPH	Coils (+endosaccular) None	Complete	None	Death-recurrent rupture from another L MCA IIA + MI

Abbreviations: ACA, anterior cerebral artery; AIDS, acquired immune-deficiency syndrome; AIS, acute ischemic stroke; Asympt., asymptomatic; CNP, cranial nerve palsy; comp., complications; F, female; He., haemorrhage; ICA, internal carotid artery; IEC, infective endocarditis; IIA, infectious intracranial aneurysm; ICH, intracranial haemorrhage; IPH, intraparenchymal hematoma; IVH, intraventricular haemorrhage; L, left; LVAD, left ventricular assisted device; M, male; MCA, middle cerebral artery; MI, myocardial infarction; mRS, modified Rankin Scale; MV, mitral valve; NI, neurologically intact; PAO, parent artery occlusion; PCA, posterior cerebral artery; R, right; RF, risk factors; SAH, subarachnoid haemorrhage.

Table 2C. Deconstructive embolization of IIAs by PAO aided by injection of LEA (n-BCA)

Author, year	Age, Sex	Etiology	Presenting symptoms	Aneurysm characteristics				He.	Device	Occlusion status	Comp.	Outcome
				No.	Site	Form	Rupture					
Uchiyama, 2001 [114]	5, F	Craniofacial Post-operative Comp.	Unresponsive, fixed dilated pupil, dense hemiplegia	1	L MCA-distal anterior temporal branch (4-5 mm)	Saccular	Yes	IPH	n-BCA (67%)	Complete	None	Good- persistent L CNIII palsy, R hemiparesis
Asai, 2002 [63]	21, M	IEC	Weakness, dysarthria	2	R ACA L MCA	-- --	Yes No	IPH --	nBCA nBCA + coils	Complete Complete	None	Improved hemiplegia
Chapot, 2002 [30]	28, M	IEC		1	L distal PCA		Yes	SAH	nBCA	Complete	None	Good-NI
	57, F	IEC		2	L distal MCA L distal PCA		Yes No	ICH No	nBCA nBCA	Complete	None	Good-NI
	41, M	IEC		1	L distal PCA		No	No	nBCA	Complete	None	Good-NI
	31, F	IEC		1	L distal PCA		Yes	ICH	nBCA + coils	Complete	None	Good-NI
	34, F	IEC		1	R distal PCA		No	No	nBCA	Complete	None	Good-NI
	43, M	IEC		1	R distal PCA		Yes	ICH	nBCA	Complete	None	Good-NI
	45, M	IEC		1	R distal MCA		Yes	ICH	nBCA	Complete	None	Disability
	62, M	IEC		1	R distal MCA		Yes	ICH	nBCA	Complete	None	Disability
	55, M	IEC		2	L distal MCA L distal MCA		Yes Yes	SAH SAHICH	nBCA nBCA	Complete Complete	None	Good-NI
Misser, 2005 [115]	24, M	IEC	Sudden headache	1	R precentral branch -MCA	--	Yes	SAHIPH, IVH	nBCA	Complete	None	Improved
Kannoth, 2007 [29]	9, M	IEC	--	1	Distal MCA	--	No	No	nBCA	Complete	None	Good

Author, year	Age, Sex	Etiology	Presenting symptoms	Aneurysm characteristics				He.	Device	Occlusion status	Comp.	Outcome
				No.	Site	Form	Rupture					
Wajnberg, 2008 [48]	40, M	IEC	Sudden headache	1	L PCA-P3/Parietooccipital branch (~1 mm)	Saccular	Yes	SAH ICH IVH	nBCA 33%	Complete	None	Death (Sepsis, ARDS)
	59, M		Sudden occipital pain	1	L PCA – P2	Bi-lobulated	Yes	SAH IVH		Complete	None	Death (SAH-related)
	54, M		Sudden headache, disorientation	1	L PICA – vermian branch	--	Yes	SAH IVH		Complete	None	Good-GOS 4
Sarica, 2008 [116]	6, --	Primary infectious aneurysm	Sudden headache, nausea, vomiting, high fever	1	L PCA-P4 segment	Saccular	Yes	IPH, IVH	nBCA (25%)	Complete	None	Good-NI
Dhomne, 2008 [72]	28, F	IEC	Hemiparesis	1	Angular MCA br.	--	Yes	IPH	nBCA (50%)	Complete + PAO	None	Partial
	52, F		Headache,vomiting, high-grade fever	1	PCA br.	--	Yes	IPH				Complete
	41, M		Hemiparesis, headache	1	Angular MCA br.	--	Yes	SAH				Complete
	38, M		Altered sensorium	1	Precentral MCA br.	--	Yes	IPH IVH				Rebleed, death
	35, F		Headache,vomiting		PCA br.	--	Yes	IPH				Complete
	35, F		Headache, vomiting, fever		Precentral MCA br.	--	Yes	IPH				Complete
	32, F		Headache		PCA br.	--	Yes	IPH				Complete
	35, M		Altered sensorium		Angular MCA br.	--	Yes	IPH				Rebleed, death
	33, M		Hemiparesis		Posterior parietal branch	--	Yes	IPH				Complete
	36, M		Hemiparesis		Posterior parietal branch	--	Yes	IPH				Complete
	20, M		Headache, vomiting, fever	1	Angular MCA br.	--	Yes	IPH	nBCA (50%) + coils		hemi-paresthesia	Complete
	35, M		Aphasia, hemiparesis		Posterior parietal branch - MCA	--	Yes	IPH			None	Partial
Bhattacharyya, 2009 [19]	17, M	IEC	High grade fever and sudden right sided hemiparesis	1	L parieto-occipital (PCA)	Irregular	Yes	IPH	nBCA (25%)	Complete	None	No new FNDs
	27, F	IEC	Headache, fever, R LL paresis, aphasia	1	L frontal branch (MCA)	Irregular	Yes	IPH	nBCA	Complete	None	Aphasia
Saraf, 2012 [79]	12, M	IEC	Sudden headache, giddiness	2	R MCA-frontal br.	Saccular	Yes	IPH IVH	nBCA	Complete	None	Good-
		Meningitis			Distal anterior choroidal	--	--	--	nBCA	Complete	None	
Saraf & Limaye, 2013 [117]	24, M	Intracranial tuberculoma	Mild generalized headache	1	L distal MCA-frontal branch	Saccular	Yes	IPH	nBCA + intra-saccular coils	Complete	None	Good

Table 2C. (Continued)

Author, year	Age, Sex	Etiology	Presenting symptoms	Aneurysm characteristics				He.	Device	Occlusion status	Comp.	Outcome
				No.	Site	Form	Rupture					
Matsubara, 2015 [49]	21, M	IEC	ICH Infarction	2	Distal ACA (1 mm) Distal MCA (1.5 mm)	Fusiform Fusiform	Yes NO	ICH	nBCA (trapping) nBCA + coil (trapping)	Complete Complete	None	Good-mRS 1
	56, M	IEC	ICH	1	Distal MCA (5 mm)	Saccular	Yes	ICH	nBCA trapping	Complete	Transient ischemia	Death
	68, M	IEC	SAH	1	Distal SCA (7.5 mm)	Fusiform	Yes	SAH	nBCA	Complete	None	Good -mRS0
	35, M	IEC		1	Distal MCA (7 mm)	Saccular	NO	No	nBCA +coil (trapping)	Complete	None	Good -mRS0
	23, M	Sepsis	ICH --	2	Distal MCA (8mm) Distal MCA (1 mm)	Saccular Fusiform	Yes No	ICH	nBCA	Complete Untreated	Asympt. perforation None	Poor-mRS5
	64, M	IEC	SAH	1	Distal MCA (5 mm)	Fusiform	Yes	SAH	nBCA (trapping)	--	--	Fair-mRS3
LV, 2016 [107]	29, F	IEC	--	1	R M3-MCA (3.6 mm)	--	Yes	ICH	nBCA + Coils	Complete	None	Good
	28,M	IEC	Sudden headache, unconsciousness	1	L M4-MCA (4 mm)	Saccular	Yes	ICH	nBCA + IA Coil	Complete	None	Hemiparesis
	48,M	IEC	Severe headache, aphasia	1	R M4-MCA (1 mm)	Saccular	Yes	ICH	nBCA	Complete	None	Good
Park, 2017 [85]	-- 49, M	-- Periodontitis, IEC	-- Sudden headache, fever, myalgia	5	L recurrent A. Heubner (5 mm) L MCA- distal angular br. (5.6 mm) Other 3 aneurysm	-- Saccular --	No Yes --	-- ICH --	r.BCA	Complete	Infarction Non --	Good Good, GOS5 --
Cheng-Ching, 2017 [118]	NR	IEC (n = 8) Infected LVAD (n = 1)	FND (n = 3) Encephalopathy with no FNDs (n = 1) No neurological symptoms (n = 5)	1	R P3-PCA 1.4×1.2 mm	--	NO	--	nBCA (33%-50%)	Complete	None	No FNDs (n=6) NNND (n=3) 1 R upper monoparesis 1 HH 1 hemiparesis, hemineglect
				1	L P4-PCA 3×2.5 mm	--	Yes	IPH		Complete	None	
				1	R M4-MCA 2.9×2.6 mm	--	NO	--		Complete	None	
				2	R M4-MCA 5×5 mm R callosomarginal 1.5×1.4 mm	--	Yes	IPH		Complete	None	
				2	R P4-PCA 1×0.9 mm R P4-PCA 1.6×1.2 mm	--	Yes --	IPH		Complete	None	
				2	R M4-MCA 1.7×1.5 mm L M4-MCA 1.8×1.1mm	--	Yes --	IPH		Complete	None	
				1	R M4-MCA 3.8×3.2 mm	--	NO	--		Complete	None	
				1	R M4-MCA 2.3x2.4 mm	--	NO	--		Complete	None	
				1	R M4-MCA 2.5×2.5 mm	--	NO	--		Complete	None	

Boukobza, 2019 [119]	54, M	IEC	Headache, fever	1	R PCA-distal bifurcation (3 mm)	Saccular	Yes	SDH	nBCA	Complete	None	Good
	42, M	IEC	headache, 2ry generalized status epilepticus	1	L distal PCA	Fusiform			nBCA	Complete	None	Good
Pastor-Cabeza, 2020 [120]	48, F	EVD trajectory-related	Ruptured vermian AVM with 2ry hydrocephalus	1	R ACA–A3 callosomarginal branch (5 mm)	Saccular	NO	--	nBCA (25%)	Complete	None	mRS 3 (not-IIA related)
Okuda, 2022 [121]	37, M	Candidemia with LVAD	Sudden dizziness	2	R middle internal frontal R ant. internal frontal as.	Saccular	Yes	SAH IPH	nBCA (20%)	Complete	None	Good-NI

Abbreviations: ACA, anterior cerebral artery; ARDS, acute respiratory distress syndrome; Asympt., asymptomatic; AVM, arteriovenous malformation; comp., complications; EVD, external ventricular drain; F, female; FND, focal neurological deficit; GOS, Glasgow outcome score; He., haemorrhage; HH, homonymous hemianopia; IA, intra-aneurysmal; IEC, infective endocarditis; IIA, infectious intracranial aneurysm; ICH, intracranial haemorrhage; IPH, intraparenchymal hematoma; IVH, intraventricular haemorrhage; LEA, Liquid embolic agent; L, left; LL, lower limb; LVAD, left ventricular assisted device; M, male; MCA, middle cerebral artery; mRS, modified Rankin Scale; n-BCA, N-butyl cyanoacrylate; NI, neurologically intact; NNNDs, No new neurological deficits; NR, non-reported; PAO, parent artery occlusion; PCA, posterior cerebral artery; PICA, posteroinferior cerebellar artery; R, right; SAH, subarachnoid haemorrhage; SCA, superior cerebellar artery; SDH, subdural haemorrhage.

Table 2D. Deconstructive embolization of IIAs by PAO aided by injection of LEA (Onyx)

Author, year	Age, Sex	Etiology	Presenting symptoms	Aneurysm characteristics				He.	Device	Occlusion status	Comp.	Outcome
				No.	Site	Form	Rupture					
Eddleman, 2008 [92]	16, F	Bacterial endocarditis	R hemiparesis	1	L M3-MCA (4 x 4 mm)	Saccular	Yes	SAHIPH	Onyx 18	Complete	None	NNND
	4wk. F	Bacterial endocarditis	--	1	L anterior br.-MCA (4 x 6 mm)	Saccular	Yes	SAH	Coils + Onyx 18		None	NNND
La Barge, 2009 [122]	53, --	--	--	1	L parietooccipital A.	--	--	--	Onyx 18	Complete	None	Good_mRS 2 NNND
	68, F	Infectious endocarditis	Fever, chills, rapid neurological deterioration	1	R Posterior temporal A.	Fusiform	Yes	SAH IVH IPH				
Zhao, 2010 [123]	18, M	Infectious endocarditis	Sudden seizure with transient loss of consciousness.	1	L P3-PCA (11 x 14 mm)	Irregular	No	No	Onyx 18 (Intra-aneurysmal)	Complete	None	NNND
Chalouhi, 2013 [124]	40, M	Infectious endocarditis	Loss of consciousness	2	L distal ACA 2 mm (ICH-related, 2 mm) L M2 bifurcation –MCA	--	Yes No	SAHIPH	Onyx 18 untreated	Complete	None	Death (complete Heart block)
	--	--	--	2	--	--	--	--	--	--	--	--
Jadhav, 2013 [95]	61, --	Infectious endocarditis		1	R distal anterior temporal MCA (6 mm)	Saccular	No	IPH	Onyx - 34	Complete	Vessel perforation	--
	30,			1	L MCA (4 mm)	--	No	--			None	
Zanaty, 2013 [11]	--	--	--	1	L M2-MCA	--	--	--	Onyx-18	Complete	None	Good-mRS 0
	--	--	--	1	L Distal ACA	--	--	--				
	--	--	--	1		--	--	--				

Table 2D. (Continued)

Author, year	Age, Sex	Etiology	Presenting symptoms	Aneurysm characteristics				He.	Device	Occlusion status	Comp.	Outcome
				No.	Site	Form	Rupture					
Gross and Puri, 2013 [65]	47, M	Tooth abscess	LOC, AMS	1	R distal MCA	Fusiform	Yes	SAH IPH	Onyx	Complete	None	NI
Grandhi, 2014 [91]	24, --	Septic endocarditis	--	1	L M4 - MCA (2 mm)	--	Yes	SAH	Onyx 18 or 34	Complete	None	NNND
	32, --			1	R P4 - PCA (3 mm)		Yes	IVH IPH			None	
	43, --			2	R M3 - MCA (3 mm)		Yes	IVH IPH			None	
					L M4-MCA (3 mm)						Cardiac arrest	
	61, --			2	R M3- MCA (8mm)		Yes	SAH			None	
					R M3-MCA (6 mm)						None	
	45, --			2	R M3-ACA (2.5 mm)		Yes	IPH			None	
	46, --				R M3-ACA (3mm)		No	No			None	
	42, --			1	L A3-ACA (16 mm)		No	No			None	
	55, --			1	R P3 - PCA (2.5 mm)		Yes	IPH			None	
	28, --			6	L A3-ACA (2 mm)		Yes	SAH			IPH	
					L M3-MCA (3 mm)							
					L M3-MCA (4 mm)							
					R M3-MCA (1.5 mm)							
					R M3-MCA (1 mm)							
					L M4-MCA (2 mm)							
Esenkaya, 2016 [101]	11,M	--	--	1	L M4-MCA (7 mm)	Fusiform	Yes	SDH	ONYX	Complete	None	Good-mRS 0
	51,F	--	--	1	L M3 MCA (3 mm)	Fusiform	Yes	IPH	ONYX	Complete	None	Good-mRS 0
	53,F	--	--	1	R P3 PCA (5 mm)	Fusiform	Yes	SAH	ONYX	Complete	None	Good-mRS 0
Remirez, 2017 [125]	55, M	LVAD infection	Worsening pulsatile headache	1	R MCA -temporal branch (7.5 x 4.8 x 5.1-mm)	Saccular	Yes	SAH	Onyx (Intra-aneurysmal)	Complete	None	--
Brimley, 2019 [126]	36, F	Infective endocarditis	Fatigue, fever, altered mental status => headache	2	R distal MCA Basilar tip (5 x 2.5 mm)	Saccular Saccular	No Yes	SAH	Onyx 18 Coil (Balloon-assisted)	Complete Complete	None	Good-NNNDs
Avallone, 2021 [127]	69, M	Infectious endocarditis	Multiple seizures and left-sided weakness	1	R frontal br. M4 – MCA (1mm)	Saccular	Yes	SAHIVH	Onyx 18	Complete	None	Good-NNNDs

Abbreviations: ACA, anterior cerebral artery; AMS, altered mental state; comp., complications; F, female; He., haemorrhage; IIA, infectious intracranial aneurysm; IPH, intraparenchymal hematoma; IVH, intraventricular haemorrhage; LEA, Liquid embolic agent; L, left; LOC, loss of consciousness; LVAD, left ventricular assisted device; M, male; MCA, middle cerebral artery; mRS, modified Rankin Scale; NI, neurologically intact; NNNDs, No new neurological deficits; PAO, parent artery occlusion; PCA, posterior cerebral artery; R, right; SAH, subarachnoid haemorrhage; SDH, subdural haemorrhage.

Table 3. Reconstructive embolization of IIAs by placement of a stent/flow diverter

Author, year	Age, Sex	Etiology	Presenting symptoms	Aneurysm characteristics				He.	Device	Aneurysm status	Comp.	Outcome
				No.	Site	Form	Rupture					
Sugg. et al, 2006 [130]	47, M	Infective endocarditis	Severe headache, R hemiplegia	2	L Supra-clinoid ICA L M1 – MCA	Sacculo-fusiform	Yes	SAH	SES (Neuroform)	Not reported (NR)	None	NI
Yen et al, 2007 [134]	46, M	Cavernous sinus thrombo-phlebitis	Headache, double vision, neck stiffness, malaise, high fever=> ptosis, ophthalmoplegia	2	Bilateral cavernous ICA	--	No	No	BMS (4 x 19 Helistent)	Complete	None	Mild R limited ocular movement
Appelboom et al., 2010 [132]	10, F	Meningitis	R diplopia, ptosis, mydriasis (CN III palsy) => CN IV palsy	1	R cavernous ICA (22 ×15×10 mm)	Saccular	No	No	FD (4 x 25 Silk)	Complete	None	NI
Lee et al, 2015 [135]	46, M	Sinusitis, orbital cellulitis	Worsening temporal Headache, decreased vision, photophobia	1	R ICA	Irregular	No	No	FD (4.5 X 30 PED)	--	None	Persistent Ptosis, No R eye movement
Han et al, 2016 [129]	21, M	Meningitis	Headache, vomiting & VII palsy => TIA	1	R Petrous ICA (15 x 8mm)	Sacculo-fusiform	No	No	BMS (6 x 25 mm)	Complete	None	VII palsy
Kobets et al, 2017 [128]	41, F	Cavernous sinus thrombosis	Visual loss, ophthalmoplegia => aggravated CNIII palsy	1	R cavernous ICA (13×12×5 mm)	Saccular	No	No	FD 3 x 10 PED + 3.5 x 10 PED	Complete	None	NI
Ares et al, 2018 [133]	2, M	Endocarditis	Vomiting, diminished level of consciousness	1	Basilar apex aneurysm (6 mm).	Multi-lobulated	Yes	SAH	PED (2.5×16)	Complete	None	NI
Goldschmidt, 2019 [22]	Infant, --	IEC, IST	multiple punctuate pontine strokes, NIHSS 3	1	Basilar tip aneurysm	Irregular	No	No	FD	Complete	No	NI
Sharma, 2019 [110]	3, F	Orbital cellulitis	L diplopia	2	L cavernous ICA R cavernous ICA	Saccular Fusiform	No No	No	FD	NR	NR	NR
Imamura et al, 2019 [131]	35, M	Bacterial meningitis	L retro-orbital pain, ptosis, diplopia, headache, fever	--	L cavernous ICA Rest left untreated	--	No	No	PED	Complete	None	NI
Aguilar-Perez et al, 2020 [136]	50, M	—	SAH	2	R M2-M3_MCA L MCA	Fusiform	Yes Yes	SAH	FD (3x18 p48 MW HPC) PAO	Persistent filling (Stable)	None	Poor (mRS 5)
Samples et al, 2021 [47]	10, F	Sinusitis => cerebral abscess	Headaches, lethargy, fever => L IPH & trans-tentorial herniation	2	L M1-MCA 1.6 × 0.9 distal 4.05 x4.28 proximal	--	Yes	IPH	CE (proximal aneurysm) + FD (2.5×14 PED)	Complete	None	Good – Near full motor recovery + regain speaking
Neth, 2022 [16]	70, F	Angioinvasive fungal infection	Encephalopathy, L pupil-sparing CN III palsy	1	L cavernous ICA (11 mm)	Multi-lobulated	No	No	Telescoping PED	--	Catast-rophic IPH, IVH	Death

Abbreviations: BMS, balloon mounted stent; CN, cranial nerve; Comp., complications; F, female; FD, flow diverter; He., haemorrhage; ICA, internal carotid artery; IEC, infective endocarditis; IIA, infectious intracranial aneurysm; IPH, intraparenchymal hematoma; IST, immune-suppressive therapy; IVH, intraventricular haemorrhage; L, left; M, male; MCA, middle cerebral artery; NI, neurologically intact; NIHSS, national institute of health stroke scale; NR, non-reported; PED, pipeline embolization device; R, right; SAH, subarachnoid haemorrhage; SES, self-expandable stent; TIA, transient ischemic attack.

Table 4. De-Reconstructive embolization of IIAs by stent assisted coil embolization (SACE)

Author, year	Age, Sex	Etiology	Presenting symptoms	Aneurysm characteristics				He.	Device	Aneurysm status	Comp.	Outcome
				No.	Site	Form	Rupture					
Ding et al, 2014 [137]	35, M	Bacterial endocarditis	Intermittent diplopia	3	Pericallosal A3–A4 Junction L M3 –MCA R M4-MCA	--	Yes No No	IPH No No	SACE (2.5 x 15 Neuroform EZ) Untreated Untreated	Complete Shrinkage Shrinkage	None	NI
OuYang, 2019 [138]	49, M	Recent sinus surgery	Repeated epistaxis, headache, dizziness	1	L cavernous ICA	--	NO	No	SACE	Complete _recurrence after 2 months	Cavernous sinus syndrome	Death-sudden massive epistaxis

Abbreviations: Comp., complications; He., haemorrhage; ICA, internal carotid artery; IIA, infectious intracranial aneurysm; IPH, intraparenchymal hematoma; L, left; M, male; MCA, middle cerebral artery; NI, neurologically intact; R, right; SACE, stent-assisted coil embolization.

Conclusion

Although represent a relatively rare entity; intracranial infectious aneurysms are associated with inherent grave prognosis, with mortality reaching up to 80% following disastrous rupture.

Serial investigation and careful interrogation of vasculo-parenchymal imaging should be considered in clinically suspicious patient with a recent history of endocarditis. An interdisciplinary case-individualized approach is advised for a superior control of IIAs.

Obliteration of the aneurysmal sac together with sacrifice of the parent artery might be the most definitive cure strategy.

Appropriate selection of the access system, choice of embolization agents' type/concentration, wedging of the delivery micro catheter, and the distance from the aneurysmal sac are cardinal pertinent variables when endovascular management is envisaged.

Disclaimer

None.

References

[1] Church WS. Aneurysm of the right cerebral artery in a boy of thirteen. (1869) *Transactions of the Pathological Society of London*. 20: 109.

[2] Osler W. The Gulstonian Lectures, on Malignant Endocarditis. (1885) *British Medical Journal*. 1 (1262): 467-70.

[3] Kim Y. W. (2010). Infected aneurysm: current management. *Annals of vascular diseases*, *3*(1), 7–15. https://doi.org/10.3400/avd.AVDctiia09003.

[4] Elouardi, A., Elyoubi, S., Kibassim, E., Elhafidi, A., Boulmakoul, SE., Majdoub, A., Messouak, M. (2022). Ruptured mycotic aneurysm of the common Femoral artery complicating a mitral valve infective endocarditis. Cirugía Cardiovascular, 29, 103–105. doi: 10.1016/j.circv.2021.12.010.

[5] Regelsberger, J., Elsayed, A., Matschke, J., Lindop, G., Grzyska, U., van den Boom, L., & Venne, D. (2011). Diagnostic and therapeutic considerations for "mycotic" cerebral aneurysms: 2 case reports and review of the literature. *Central European neurosurgery*, *72*(3), 138–143. https://doi.org/10.1055/s-0031-1279756.

[6] Shi, H., Parikh, N. S., Esenwa, C., Zampolin, R., Shah, H., Khasiyev, F., Valenzuela, I., Lavine, S., Gutierrez, J., & Willey, J. (2021). Neurological Outcomes of Patients With Mycotic Aneurysms in Infective Endocarditis. *The Neurohospitalist*, *11*(1), 5–11. https://doi.org/10.1177/1941874420931233.

[7] Ducruet, A. F., Hickman, Z. L., Zacharia, B. E., Narula, R., Grobelny, B. T., Gorski, J., & Connolly, E. S., Jr (2010). Intracranial infectious aneurysms: a comprehensive review. *Neurosurgical review*, *33*(1), 37–46. https://doi.org/10.1007/s10143-009-0233-1.

[8] Hamisch, C. A., Mpotsaris, A., Timmer, M., Reiner, M., Stavrinou, P., Brinker, G., Goldbrunner, R., & Krischek, B. (2016). Interdisciplinary Treatment of Intracranial Infectious Aneurysms. *Cerebrovascular diseases (Basel, Switzerland)*, *42*(5-6), 493–505. https://doi.org/10.1159/000448406.

[9] Desai, B., Soldozy, S., Desai, H., Kumar, J., Shah, S., Raper, D. M., & Park, M. S. (2020). Evaluating the Safety and Efficacy of Various Endovascular Approaches for Treatment of Infectious Intracranial Aneurysms: A Systematic Review. *World neurosurgery*, *144*, 293–298.e15. https://doi.org/10.1016/j.wneu.2020.07.228.

[10] Morris, N. A., Matiello, M., Lyons, J. L., & Samuels, M. A. (2014). Neurologic complications in infective endocarditis: identification, management, and impact on cardiac surgery. *The Neurohospitalist*, *4*(4), 213–222. https://doi.org/10.1177/1941874414537077.

[11] Zanaty, M., Chalouhi, N., Starke, R. M., Tjoumakaris, S., Gonzalez, L. F., Hasan, D., Rosenwasser, R., & Jabbour, P. (2013). Endovascular treatment of cerebral mycotic aneurysm: a review of the literature and single center experience. *BioMed research international*, 2013, 151643. https://doi.org/10.1155/2013/151643.

[12] Matsuzono, K., Ishiyama, Y., Higaki, A., Namba, K., Aoyama, Y., Igarashi, T., Miura, K., Ozawa, T., Mashiko, T., Koide, R., Tanaka, R., Harada, K., Kario, K., Kawai, K., & Fujimoto, S. (2021). Successful endovascular coiling of infectious cerebral aneurysm following *Staphylococcus haemolyticus* endocarditis. *The Journal of international medical research*, *49*(11), 3000605211058857. https://doi.org/10.1177/03000605211058857.

[13] O'Donohue, J. M., & Enzmann, D. R. (1987). Mycotic aneurysm in angiitis associated with herpes zoster ophthalmicus. *AJNR. American journal of neuroradiology*, *8*(4), 615–619.

[14] Mazzoni, P., Chiriboga, C. A., Millar, W. S., & Rogers, A. (2000). Intracerebral aneurysms in human immunodeficiency virus infection: case report and literature review. *Pediatric neurology*, *23*(3), 252–255. https://doi.org/10.1016/s0887-8994(00)00179-x.

[15] Hurst, R. W., Judkins, A., Bolger, W., Chu, A., & Loevner, L. A. (2001). Mycotic aneurysm and cerebral infarction resulting from fungal sinusitis: imaging and pathologic correlation. *AJNR. American journal of neuroradiology*, *22*(5), 858–863.

[16] Neth BJ, Cohen Cohen S, Trejo-Lopez J, et al. Neurological rarities, Mycotic aneurysm. Pract Neurol 2022; 22:407–409. http://dx.doi.org/10.1136/practneurol-2021-003260.

[17] Budohoski, K. P., Raygor, K., Cook, D., Henrich, T., & Abla, A. A. (2022). Rapid sequential development and rupture of mycotic aneurysms within a period of days in a patient with graft-versus-host disease and angiotropic *Scedosporium apiospermum* infection. *Surgical neurology international*, *13*, 242. https://doi.org/10.25259/SNI_970_2021.

[18] Heiro, M., Nikoskelainen, J., Engblom, E., Kotilainen, E., Marttila, R., & Kotilainen, P. (2000). Neurologic manifestations of infective endocarditis: a 17-year experience in a teaching hospital in Finland. *Archives of internal medicine*, *160*(18), 2781–2787. https://doi.org/10.1001/archinte.160.18.2781.

[19] Bhattacharyya, A., Mittal, S., Yadav, R. R., Jain, K., Gupta, B., Parihar, A., Handique, A., Jain, K., & Phadke, R. V. (2009). Endovascular management of infective intracranial aneurysms with acrylic glue. A report of two cases. *Interventional neuroradiology: Journal of peritherapeutic neuroradiology, surgical procedures and related neurosciences*, *15*(4), 443–447. https://doi.org/10.1177/159101990901500412.

[20] Burke, D. J., & Jadhav, A. (2020). Cavernous Thrombophlebitis Secondary to Cavernous Internal Carotid Mycotic Aneurysm. *The Neurohospitalist*, *10*(3), 221–223. https://doi.org/10.1177/1941874419892441.

[21] Kuo I, Long T, Nguyen N, Chaudry B, Karp M, Sanossian N. Ruptured intracranial mycotic aneurysm in infective endocarditis: a natural history. *Case Rep Med.* 2010; 2010:168408. doi:10.1155/2010/168408.

[22] Goldschmidt, E., Faraji, A. H., Salvetti, D., Zussman, B. M., & Jadhav, A. (2019). Intracranial vessel occlusion preceding the development of mycotic aneurysms in patients with endocarditis. *BMJ case reports*, *12*(12), e015480. https://doi.org/10.1136/bcr-2019-015480.

[23] Hui, F. K., Bain, M., Obuchowski, N. A., Gordon, S., Spiotta, A. M., Moskowitz, S., Toth, G., & Hussain, S. (2015). Mycotic aneurysm detection rates with cerebral angiography in patients with infective endocarditis. *Journal of neurointerventional surgery*, *7*(6), 449–452. https://doi.org/10.1136/neurintsurg-2014-011124.

[24] John, S., Walsh, K. M., Hui, F. K., Sundararajan, S., Silverman, S., & Bain, M. (2016). Dynamic Angiographic Nature of Cerebral Mycotic Aneurysms in Patients With Infective Endocarditis. *Stroke*, *47*(1), e8–e10. https://doi.org/10.1161/STROKEAHA.115.011198.

[25] Samaniego, E. A., Ortega, S., Stander, L., & Leira, E. C. (2017). Development of a cerebral mycotic aneurysm within 5 days. *Neurology. Clinical practice*, *7*(5), 449–450. https://doi.org/10.1212/CPJ.0000000000000315.

[26] Erdogan HB, Erentug V, Bozbuga N, Goksedef D, Akinci E, Yakut C (2004) Endovascular treatment of intracerebral mycotic aneurysm before surgical treatment of infective endocarditis. *Tex Heart Inst* J 31(2):165–167.

[27] Alawieh, A., Chaudry, M. I., Turner, R. D., Turk, A. S., & Spiotta, A. M. (2018). Infectious intracranial aneurysms: a systematic review of epidemiology, management, and outcomes. *Journal of neurointerventional surgery*, *10*(7), 708–716. https://doi.org/10.1136/neurintsurg-2017-013603.

[28] Kiwan, R., Son, M., Mayich, M., Boulton, M., Pandey, S., & Sharma, M. (2022). Ruptured intracranial infectious aneurysms: Single Canadian center experience. *Surgical neurology international*, *13*, 185. https://doi.org/10.25259/SNI_69_2022.

[29] Kannoth, S., Iyer, R., Thomas, S. V., Furtado, S. V., Rajesh, B. J., Kesavadas, C., Radhakrishnan, V. V., & Sarma, P. S. (2007). Intracranial infectious aneurysm: presentation, management and outcome. *Journal of the neurological sciences*, 256(1-2), 3–9. https://doi.org/10.1016/j.jns.2007.01.044.

[30] Chapot, R., Houdart, E., Saint-Maurice, J. P., Aymard, A., Mounayer, C., Lot, G., & Merland, J. J. (2002). Endovascular treatment of cerebral mycotic aneurysms. *Radiology*, *222*(2), 389–396. https://doi.org/10.1148/radiol.2222010432.

[31] Kannoth, S., Thomas, S. V., Nair, S., & Sarma, P. S. (2008). Proposed diagnostic criteria for intracranial infectious aneurysms. Journal of neurology, neurosurgery, and psychiatry, 79(8), 943–946. https://doi.org/10.1136/jnnp.2007.131664.

[32] Hage, Z. A., Naidech, A. M., & Bendok, B. R. (2008). Diagnosing intracranial infectious aneurysms with a simple model. Journal of neurology, neurosurgery, and psychiatry, 79(8), 853. https://doi.org/10.1136/jnnp.2008.147603.

[33] Peters, P. J., Harrison, T., & Lennox, J. L. (2006). A dangerous dilemma: management of infectious intracranial aneurysms complicating endocarditis. *The Lancet. Infectious diseases*, *6*(11), 742–748. https://doi.org/10.1016/S1473-3099
(06)70631-4.

[34] Cloud, G. C., Rich, P. M., & Markus, H. S. (2003). Serial MRI of a mycotic aneurysm of the cavernous carotid artery. *Neuroradiology*, *45*(8), 546–549. https://doi.org/10.1007/s00234-003-1021-1.

[35] Singla, A., Fargen, K., Blackburn, S., Neal, D., Martin, T. D., Hess, P. J., Beaver, T. M., Klodell, C. T., & Hoh, B. (2016). National treatment practices in the management of infectious intracranial aneurysms and infective endocarditis. *Journal of neurointerventional surgery*, *8*(7), 741–746. https://doi.org/10.1136/
neurintsurg-2015-011834.

[36] Khan, A., Waqas, M., Nizamani, W. M., & Bari, M. E. (2017). Ruptured mycotic aneurysms: Report and outcomes of two surgically managed patients. *Surgical neurology international*, *8*, 144. https://doi.org/10.4103/sni.sni_78_17.

[37] Lee, S. M., Park, H. S., Choi, J. H., & Huh, J. T. (2013). Ruptured mycotic aneurysm of the distal middle cerebral artery manifesting as subacute subdural hematoma. *Journal of cerebrovascular and endovascular neurosurgery*, *15*(3), 235–240. https://doi.org/10.7461/jcen.2013.15.3.235.

[38] Wang, T. K. M., Griffin, B., Cremer, P., Shrestha, N., Gordon, S., Pettersson, G., & Desai, M. (2020). Diagnostic Utility of CT and MRI for Mycotic Aneurysms: A Meta-Analysis. *AJR. American journal of roentgenology*, *215*(5), 1257–1266. https://doi.org/10.2214/AJR.19.22722.

[39] Lotan, E., Orion, D., Bakon, M., Kuperstein, R., & Greenberg, G. (2014). Ruptured intracranial mycotic aneurysm in infective endocarditis: radiological and clinical findings. *The Israel Medical Association journal: IMAJ*, *16*(5), 317–319.

[40] Caton, M. T., Jr, Wiggins, W. F., & Nunez, D. (2020). The "connecting vessel" sign: an imaging biomarker to differentiate ruptured infected (mycotic) intracranial aneurysm mimicking the CTA spot sign. *Emergency radiology*, *27*(3), 259–268. https://doi.org/10.1007/s10140-020-01749-6.

[41] Goulenok, T., Klein, I., Mazighi, M., Messika-Zeitoun, D., Alexandra, J. F., Mourvillier, B., Laissy, J. P., Leport, C., Iung, B., Duval, X., & IMAGE study group (2013). Infective endocarditis with

symptomatic cerebral complications: contribution of cerebral magnetic resonance imaging. *Cerebrovascular diseases (Basel, Switzerland)*, *35*(4), 327–336. https://doi.org/10.1159/000348317.

[42] Hess, A., Klein, I., Iung, B., Lavallée, P., Ilic-Habensus, E., Dornic, Q., Arnoult, F., Mimoun, L., Wolff, M., Duval, X., & Laissy, J. P. (2013). Brain MRI findings in neurologically asymptomatic patients with infective endocarditis. *AJNR. American journal of neuroradiology*, *34*(8), 1579–1584. https://doi.org/10.3174/ajnr.A3582.

[43] Kin, H., Yoshioka, K., Kawazoe, K., Mukaida, M., Kamada, T., Mitsunaga, Y., Ikai, A., & Okabayashi, H. (2013). Management of infectious endocarditis with mycotic aneurysm evaluated by brain magnetic resonance imaging. *European journal of cardio-thoracic surgery: Official journal of the European Association for Cardio-thoracic Surgery*, *44*(5), 924–930. https://doi.org/10.1093/ejcts/ezt101.

[44] Migdady, I., Rice, C. J., Hassett, C., Zhang, L. Q., Wisco, D., Uchino, K., & Cho, S. M. (2019). MRI Presentation of Infectious Intracranial Aneurysms in Infective Endocarditis. *Neurocritical care*, *30*(3), 658–665. https://doi.org/10.1007/s12028-018-0654-1.

[45] Walkoff L, Brinjikji W, Rouchaud A, Caroff J, Kallmes DF. Comparing magnetic resonance angiography (MRA) and computed tomography angiography (CTA) with conventional angiography in the detection of distal territory cerebral mycotic and oncotic aneurysms. *Interv Neuroradiol.* 2016;22(5):524-528. doi:10.1177/1591019916653247.

[46] Fujita, W., Daitoku, K., Taniguchi, S., & Fukuda, I. (2010). Infective endocarditis with cerebral mycotic aneurysm: treatment dilemma. *General thoracic and cardiovascular surgery*, *58*(12), 622–625. https://doi.org/10.1007/s11748-009-0581-3.

[47] Samples, D. C., Ravindra, V. M., Thoms, D. J., Tarasiewicz, I., & Grandhi, R. (2021). Successful flow diversion treatment of ruptured infectious middle cerebral artery aneurysms with the use of Pipeline Flex with Shield technology. *Interventional neuroradiology: Journal of peritherapeutic neuroradiology, surgical procedures and related neurosciences,* 27(2), 225–229. https://doi.org/10.1177/1591019921990506.

[48] Wajnberg, E., Rueda, F., Marchiori, E., & Gasparetto, E. L. (2008). Endovascular treatment for intracranial infectious aneurysms. *Arquivos de neuro-psiquiatria*, *66*(4), 790–794. https://doi.org/10.1590/s0004-282x2008000600002.

[49] Matsubara, N., Miyachi, S., Izumi, T., Yamanouchi, T., Asai, T., Ota, K., & Wakabayashi, T. (2015). Results and current trends of multimodality treatment for infectious intracranial aneurysms. *Neurologia medico-chirurgica*, *55*(2), 155–162. https://doi.org/10.2176/nmc.oa.2014-0197.

[50] Fusco, M. R., Stapleton, C. J., Griessenauer, C. J., Thomas, A. J., & Ogilvy, C. S. (2016). Endovascular treatment of intracranial infectious aneurysms in eloquent cortex with super-selective provocative testing: Case series and literature review. *Interventional neuroradiology: Journal of peritherapeutic neuroradiology, surgical procedures and related neurosciences*, *22*(2), 148–152. https://doi.org/10.1177/1591019915617326.

[51] Nakahara, I., Taha, M. M., Higashi, T., Iwamuro, Y., Iwaasa, M., Watanabe, Y., Tsunetoshi, K., & Munemitsu, T. (2006). Different modalities of treatment of intracranial mycotic aneurysms: Report of 4 cases. *Surgical neurology*, *66*(4), 405–410. https://doi.org/10.1016/j.surneu.2006.01.021.

[52] Brust JC, Dickinson PC, Hughes JE, Holtzman RN (1990) The diagnosis and treatment of cerebral mycotic aneurysms. *Ann Neurol* 27(3):238–246.

[53] Corr P, Wright M, Handler LC (1995) Endocarditis-related cerebral aneurysms: radiologic changes with treatment. *AJNR Am J Neuroradiol* 16(4):745–748.

[54] Bartakke S, Kabde U, Muranjan MN, Bavdekar SB (2002) Mycotic aneurysm: an uncommon cause for intra-cranial hemorrhagea. *Indian J Pediatr* 69(10):905–907.

[55] Allen, L. M., Fowler, A. M., Walker, C., Derdeyn, C. P., Nguyen, B. V., Hasso, A. N., Ghodke, B. V., Zipfel, G. J., Cross, D. T., 3rd, & Moran, C. J. (2013). Retrospective review of cerebral mycotic aneurysms in 26 patients: focus on treatment in strongly immunocompromised patients with a brief literature review. *AJNR. American journal of neuroradiology*, *34*(4), 823–827. https://doi.org/10.3174/ajnr.A3302.

[56] Akimoto, K., Yanaka, K., Nakamura, K., Takeda, H., Saura, M., Takada, M., Hosoo, H., Matsumaru, Y., & Ishikawa, E. (2022). Simultaneous intracerebral and subarachnoid hemorrhages caused by multiple infectious intracranial aneurysms treated endovascularly and by microsurgical clipping:

illustrative case. *Journal of neurosurgery. Case lessons, 3*(7), CASE21685. https://doi.org/10.3171/CASE21685.

[57] Konovalov, A., Sharipov, O., Shekhtman, O., Gadzhiagaev, V., & Kalinin, P. (2021). Surgical treatment of ruptured right middle cerebral artery mycotic aneurysm and central nervous system aspergillosis: Clinical case and literature review. *Surgical neurology international, 12*, 555. https://doi.org/10.25259/SNI_843_2021.

[58] Furui, M., Sakaguchi, S., Yoshida, T., Kakii, B., Uchino, G., Asanuma, M., & Uchida, N. (2021). Surgical Treatment for Primary Mycotic Aneurysms Using Endovascular Therapy, Focusing on Patient Selection: Single-Center Experience. *Surgical infections, 22*(7), 713–721. https://doi.org/10.1089/sur.2020.363.

[59] Roach, M. R., and Drake, C. G. Ruptured cerebral aneurysms caused by microorganisms. *N. England J. Med.*, 278: 240, 1965.

[60] Lüders, J. C., Steinmetz, M. P., & Mayberg, M. R. (2005). Awake craniotomy for microsurgical obliteration of mycotic aneurysms: technical report of three cases. *Neurosurgery, 56*(1 Suppl), E201. https://doi.org/10.1227/01.neu.0000144491.14623.92.

[61] Rennert, R. C., Budohoski, K. P., Mortimer, V. R., & Couldwell, W. T. (2022). Double bypass for mycotic middle cerebral artery aneurysm. *Surgical neurology international, 13*, 333. https://doi.org/10.25259/SNI_569_2022.

[62] Graffeo, C. S., Srinivasan, V. M., Cole, T. S., & Lawton, M. T. (2022). Double-barrel STA-MCA bypass and partial trapping of a ruptured mycotic MCA aneurysm with flash fluorescence technique. *Neurosurgical focus: Video, 6*(1), V15. https://doi.org/10.3171/2021.10.FOCVID21163.

[63] Asai, T., Usui, A., Miyachi, S., & Ueda, Y. (2002). Endovascular treatment for intracranial mycotic aneurysms prior to cardiac surgery. *European journal of cardio-thoracic surgery: official journal of the European Association for Cardio-thoracic Surgery, 21*(5), 948–950. https://doi.org/10.1016/s1010-7940(02)00092-1.

[64] Ando, K., Hasegawa, H., Kikuchi, B., Saito, S., On, J., Shibuya, K., & Fujii, Y. (2019). Treatment Strategies for Infectious Intracranial Aneurysms: Report of Three Cases and Review of the Literature. *Neurologia medico-chirurgica, 59*(9), 344–350. https://doi.org/10.2176/nmc.oa.2019-0051.

[65] Gross, B. A., & Puri, A. S. (2013). Endovascular treatment of infectious intracranial aneurysms. *Neurosurgical review*, 36(1), 11–19. https://doi.org/10.1007/s10143-012-0414-1

[66] Chun, J. Y., Smith, W., Halbach, V. V., Higashida, R. T., Wilson, C. B., & Lawton, M. T. (2001). Current multimodality management of infectious intracranial aneurysms. *Neurosurgery*, 48(6), 1203–1214. https://doi.org/10.1097/00006123-200106000-00001.

[67] Ogawa, Y., Sato, M., Tashiro, M., Miyazaki, M., Nagata, K., Takahashi, N., Kasahara, K., Izumikawa, K., Yano, H., & Mikasa, K. (2016). Rapid development of a mycotic aneurysm of the intracranial artery secondary to *Scedosporium apiospermum* sinusitis. *Medical mycology case reports, 14*, 30–32. https://doi.org/10.1016/j.mmcr.2016.11.001.

[68] Reuschel V, Groll M, Quäschling U, et al. Middle cerebral artery (M3) aneurysm: atypical primary morphology and early recurrence after stent-assisted coil occlusion during the long-term left ventricular assist device treatment, accompanied by temporary septicemia; parent vessel occlusion as the final treatment with good clinical outcome. In: Henkes H, Lylyk P, Ganslandt O. (eds) *The aneurysm casebook: a guide to treatment selection and technique.* Cham: Springer International Publishing, 2018. doi: 10.1007/978-3-319-70267-4_76-1.

[69] Lasjaunias, P., Wuppalapati, S., Alvarez, H., Rodesch, G., & Ozanne, A. (2005). Intracranial aneurysms in children aged under 15 years: review of 59 consecutive children with 75 aneurysms. *Child's nervous system: ChNS : official journal of the International Society for Pediatric Neurosurgery, 21*(6), 437–450. https://doi.org/10.1007/s00381-004-1125-x

[70] Nakahara, I., Taha, M. M., Higashi, T., Iwamuro, Y., Iwaasa, M., Watanabe, Y., Tsunetoshi, K., & Munemitsu, T. (2006). Different modalities of treatment of intracranial mycotic aneurysms: Report of 4 cases. *Surgical neurology, 66*(4), 405–410. https://doi.org/10.1016/j.surneu.2006.01.021.

[71] Eddleman, C., Nikas, D., Shaibani, A., Khan, P., Dipatri, A. J., Jr, & Tomita, T. (2007). HydroCoil embolization of a ruptured infectious aneurysm in a pediatric patient: case report and review of the

literature. *Child's nervous system : ChNS : official journal of the International Society for Pediatric Neurosurgery*, *23*(6), 707–712. https://doi.org/10.1007/s00381-006-0264-7.

[72] Dhomne, S., Rao, C., Shrivastava, M., Sidhartha, W., & Limaye, U. (2008). Endovascular management of ruptured cerebral mycotic aneurysms. *British journal of neurosurgery*, *22*(1), 46–52. https://doi.org/10.1080/02688690701593561.

[73] Trivedi, M. P., Carroll, C., & Rutherford, S. (2008). Infective endocarditis complicated by rupture of intracranial mycotic aneurysm during pregnancy. *International journal of obstetric anesthesia*, *17*(2), 182–187. https://doi.org/10.1016/j.ijoa.2007.07.007.

[74] Van de Beek, D., Rabinstein, A. A., Peters, S. G., Cloft, H., & Wijdicks, E. F. (2008). Staphylococcus endocarditis associated with infectious vasculitis and recurrent cerebral hemorrhages. *Neurocritical care*, *8*(1), 48–52. https://doi.org/10.1007/s12028-007-9002-6.

[75] Kim, U. S., Kim, J. S., Kwon, O. K., & Hwang, J. M. (2010). Complete visual recovery after mycotic aneurysm embolization complicated by cavernous sinus thrombophlebitis. *Korean journal of ophthalmology: KJO*, *24*(5), 322–324. https://doi.org/10.3341/kjo.2010.24.5.322.

[76] Ray, W. Z., Diringer, M. N., Moran, C. J., & Zipfel, G. J. (2010). Early endovascular coiling of posterior communicating artery saccular aneurysm in the setting of Staphylococcus bacteremia: case report and review of the literature. *Neurosurgery*, *66*(4), E847. https://doi.org/10.1227/01.NEU.0000367617.56186.90.

[77] Altekin, R. E., Karakas, M. S., Yanikoglu, A., Ozbek, S. C., Akdemir, B., Demirtas, H., Deger, N., & Cekirge, I. S. (2011). Aortic valve endocarditis and cerebral mycotic aneurysm due to brucellosis. *Journal of cardiology cases*, *4*(3), e179–e182. https://doi.org/10.1016/j.jccase.2011.07.008.

[78] Martindale, J. L., & Hayden, E. M. (2012). Neurologic complaints in a patient with infective endocarditis. *The Journal of emergency medicine*, *43*(6), e429–e433. https://doi.org/10.1016/j.jemermed.2011.05.026.

[79] Saraf, R., Shrivastava, M., Siddhartha, W., & Limaye, U. (2012). Intracranial pediatric aneurysms: endovascular treatment and its outcome. *Journal of neurosurgery. Pediatrics*, *10*(3), 230–240. https://doi.org/10.3171/2012.5.PEDS1210.

[80] Takemoto, K., Tateshima, S., Golshan, A., Gonzalez, N., Jahan, R., Duckwiler, G., & Vinuela, F. (2014). Endovascular treatment of pediatric intracranial aneurysms: a retrospective study of 35 aneurysms. *Journal of neurointerventional surgery*, *6*(6), 432–438. https://doi.org/10.1136/neurintsurg-2013-010852.

[81] Chimparlee, N., Jittapiromsak, P., Tantivatana, J., & Chattranukulchai, P. (2014). Classical complication of infective endocarditis: ruptured, large mycotic cerebral aneurysm. *BMJ case reports*, *2014*, bcr2013202275. https://doi.org/10.1136/bcr-2013-202275.

[82] Yoon, K. W., Cho, C. S., & Lee, S. K. (2014). Large intracranial aneurysm after transsphenoidal surgery for pituitary macroadenoma. *Journal of Korean Neurosurgical Society*, *55*(3), 160–163. https://doi.org/10.3340/jkns.2014.55.3.160.

[83] Champeaux, C., Walker, N., Derwin, J., & Grivas, A. (2017). Successful delayed coiling of a ruptured growing distal posterior cerebral artery mycotic aneurysm. *Neuro-Chirurgie*, *63*(1), 17–20. https://doi.org/10.1016/j.neuchi.2016.10.005

[84] Wang, J. L., Hinduja, A. P., & Powers, C. J. (2017). Successful coil embolization of a ruptured mycotic aneurysm that developed three days after septic embolic infarction: Case report and review of the literature. *Journal of clinical neuroscience: Official journal of the Neurosurgical Society of Australasia*, *39*, 95–98. https://doi.org/10.1016/j.jocn.2017.01.021.

[85] Park, W., Ahn, J. S., Park, J. C., Kwun, B. D., & Lee, D. H. (2017). Treatment Strategy Based on Experience of Treating Intracranial Infectious Aneurysms. *World neurosurgery*, *97*, 351–359. https://doi.org/10.1016/j.wneu.2016.09.119.

[86] Zhong, X., Li, X., Shao, S., Yang, X., & Fan, X. (2017). A case of infectious intracranial dissecting aneurysm. *Neurology India*, *65*(2), 405–407. https://doi.org/10.4103/neuroindia.NI_1223_15.

[87] Kiss, G., & Braunberger, E. (2018). Emergency Valve Replacement Under Minimal Cardiopulmonary Bypass for a Patient With Infective Endocarditis and Large Brain Hematoma: A Case Report. *A&A practice*, *10*(6), 144–147. https://doi.org/10.1213/XAA.0000000000000665.

[88] Hall, J. M., McElroy, B. J., Arora, P. K., & Mohandas, S. (2019). Intracranial Mycotic Aneurysm Complicating Streptococcus pneumoniae Infection. *The Journal of pediatrics*, *211*, 223–223.e1. https://doi.org/10.1016/j.jpeds.2019.03.031.

[89] Lee, T., Buletko, A. B., Matthew, J., & Cho, S. M. (2020). Bloodstream infection is associated with subarachnoid hemorrhage and infectious intracranial aneurysm in left ventricular assist device. *Perfusion*, *35*(2), 117–120. https://doi.org/10.1177/0267659119858853.

[90] Panagiotopoulos, V., Theofanopoulos, A., Kourakli, A., Symeonidis, A., Krisela, V., Mastronikolis, N. S., & Zampakis, P. (2021). Ruptured infectious ICA pseudoaneurysm into the sphenoid sinus after maxillofacial infection, successfully treated by selective embolization. *Surgical neurology international*, *12*, 191. https://doi.org/10.25259/SNI_52_2021.

[91] Grandhi, R., Zwagerman, N. T., Linares, G., Monaco, E. A., 3rd, Jovin, T., Horowitz, M., & Jankowitz, B. T. (2014). Onyx embolization of infectious intracranial aneurysms. *Journal of neurointerventional surgery*, 6(5), 353–356. https://doi.org/10.1136/neurintsurg-2013-010755.

[92] Eddleman, C. S., Surdell, D., DiPatri, A., Jr, Tomita, T., & Shaibani, A. (2008). Infectious intracranial aneurysms in the pediatric population: endovascular treatment with Onyx. *Child's nervous system: ChNS : official journal of the International Society for Pediatric Neurosurgery*, 24(8), 909–915. https://doi.org/10.1007/s00381-008-0614-8

[93] Davis, M. C., Deveikis, J. P., & Harrigan, M. R. (2015). Clinical Presentation, Imaging, and Management of Complications due to Neurointerventional Procedures. *Seminars in interventional radiology*, *32*(2), 98–107. https://doi.org/10.1055/s-0035-1549374.

[94] Phukan, P., Samra, K., Lynser, D., Sharma, B. K., Boruah, D. K., Saikia, B., & Singh, B. K. (2021). Endovascular Parent Artery Occlusion for Intracranial Aneurysms is a Viable, Cost-Effective Alternative: An Institutional Experience from Northeast India. *Acta medica Lituanica*, 28(2), 272–284. https://doi.org/10.15388/Amed.2021.28.2.6.

[95] Jadhav, A. P., Pryor, J. C., & Nogueira, R. G. (2013). Onyx embolization for the endovascular treatment of infectious and traumatic aneurysms involving the cranial and cerebral vasculature. *Journal of neurointerventional surgery*, 5(6), 562–565. https://doi.org/10.1136/neurintsurg-2012-010460.

[96] Yuen, T., Laidlaw, J. D., & Mitchell, P. (2004). Mycotic intracavernous carotid aneurysm. *Journal of clinical neuroscience: official journal of the Neurosurgical Society of Australasia*, 11(7), 771–775. https://doi.org/10.1016/j.jocn.2004.02.004.

[97] Crossland, G. J., De, R., Higgins, J. N., & Axon, P. R. (2005). Two stage management of petrositis with associated mycotic aneurysm of the intrapetrous carotid artery. The *Journal of laryngology and otology*, 119(6), 479–482. https://doi.org/10.1258/0022215054273214.

[98] Hot, A., Mazighi, M., Lecuit, M., Poirée, S., Viard, J. P., Loulergue, P., Suarez, F., Dupont, B., Merland, J. J., & Lortholary, O. (2007). Fungal internal carotid artery aneurysms: successful embolization of an Aspergillus-associated case and review. *Clinical infectious diseases: an official publication of the Infectious Diseases Society of America*, 45(12), e156–e161. https://doi.org/10.1086/523005.

[99] Wang, H., Rammos, S., Fraser, K., & Elwood, P. (2007). Successful endovascular treatment of a ruptured mycotic intracavernous carotid artery aneurysm in an AIDS patient. *Neurocritical care*, 7(2), 156–159. https://doi.org/10.1007/s12028-007-0072-2.

[100] Watanabe, T., Okada, T., Okada, C., Onishi, T., Watanabe, H., Okamoto, Y., Kitamura, Y., Manabe, S., Matsubara, S., Kageji, T., & Iwai, A. (2009). An aspergillotic aneurysm of the internal carotid artery following allogeneic bone marrow transplantation: successful management with catheter coil embolization and long-term antifungal agents. *Transplant infectious disease : an official journal of the Transplantation Society,* 11(1), 49–53. https://doi.org/10.1111/j.1399-3062.2008.00336.x.

[101] Esenkaya, A., Duzgun, F., Cinar, C., Bozkaya, H., Eraslan, C., Ozgiray, E., & Oran, I. (2016). Endovascular treatment of intracranial infectious aneurysms. *Neuroradiology,* 58(3), 277–284. https://doi.org/10.1007/s00234-015-1633-2.

[102] Quisling, S. V., Mawn, L. A., & Larson, T. C., 3rd (2003). Blindness associated with enlarging mycotic aneurysm after cavernous sinus thrombosis. *Ophthalmology*, *110*(10), 2036–2039. https://doi.org/10.1016/S0161-6420(03)00737-1.

[103] Hara, Y., Hosoda, K., Wada, T., Kimura, H., & Kohmura, E. (2006). Endovascular treatment for a unusually large mycotic aneurysm manifesting as intracerebral hemorrhage - case report. *Neurologia medico-chirurgica*, 46(11), 544–547. https://doi.org/10.2176/nmc.46.544.

[104] Van Rooij, W. J., Sluzewski, M., & Beute, G. N. (2006). Endovascular treatment of posterior cerebral artery aneurysms. *AJNR. American journal of neuroradiology*, 27(2), 300–305.

[105] Amano, M., Ishikawa, E., Kujiraoka, Y., Watanabe, S., Ashizawa, K., Oguni, E., Saito, A., Nakai, Y., Ikeda, H., Abe, T., Uekusa, Y., & Matsumura, A. (2010). Vernet's syndrome caused by large mycotic aneurysm of the extracranial internal carotid artery after acute otitis media--case report. *Neurologia medico-chirurgica*, 50(1), 45–48. https://doi.org/10.2176/nmc.50.45.

[106] Sorkin, G. C., Jaleel, N., Mokin, M., Dumont, T. M., Eller, J. L., & Siddiqui, A. H. (2013). Ruptured mycotic cerebral aneurysm development from pseudoocclusion due to septic embolism. *Surgical neurology international*, *4*, 144. https://doi.org/10.4103/2152-7806.121109.

[107] Lv, N., Zhou, Y., Yang, P., Li, Q., Zhao, R., Fang, Y., Xu, Y., Hong, B., Zhao, W., Liu, J., & Huang, Q. (2016). Endovascular treatment of distal middle cerebral artery aneurysms: Report of eight cases and literature review. *Interventional neuroradiology: Journal of peritherapeutic neuroradiology, surgical procedures and related neurosciences*, *22*(1), 12–17. https://doi.org/10.1177/1591019915617317

[108] Nonaka, S., Oishi, H., Tsutsumi, S., Teranishi, K., Tanoue, S., Yasumoto, Y., Yamamoto, M., & Arai, H. (2016). Endovascular Therapy for Infectious Intracranial Aneurysm: A Report of Four Cases. *Journal of stroke and cerebrovascular diseases: the official journal of National Stroke Association*, *25*(3), e33–e37. https://doi.org/10.1016/j.jstrokecerebrovasdis.2015.11.033.

[109] Sharma, K., Kanaujia, V., Agarwal, R., Singh, V., & Mishra, P. (2019). Mycotic Aneurysm of Intracavernous Internal Carotid Artery Presenting as Cavernous Sinus Syndrome. *Asian journal of neurosurgery*, *14*(2), 547–549. https://doi.org/10.4103/ajns.AJNS_39_18.

[110] Brown, P., & Fulks, D. (2020). An unusual ischaemic presentation of thrombosed intracranial mycotic aneurysm with subsequent subarachnoid haemorrhage. *BMJ case reports*, 13(10), e237044. https://doi.org/10.1136/bcr-2020-237044.

[111] Somboonnithiphol, K., Chanthanaphak, E., Singhara Na Ayudhaya, S. P., Khongkhatithum, C., & Sirilert, B. (2021). Successful endovascular treatment of pediatric basilar infectious (mycotic) aneurysm: a case report and review of the literature. *Child's nervous system : ChNS : official journal of the International Society for Pediatric Neurosurgery*, 37(8), 2687–2693. https://doi.org/10.1007/s00381-020-04917-8.

[112] Dai, Y. L., Chen, V. M., Hedges, T. R., III, & Malek, A. (2022). Lemierre syndrome associated mycotic cavernous sinus thrombosis and carotid aneurysm after COVID-19. *American Journal of Ophthalmology Case Reports*, *27*, 101642. https://doi.org/10.1016/j.ajoc.2022.101642.

[113] Prandi, F. R., Anastasius, M. O., Matsoukas, S., Zhang, L., Scaggiante, J., Fifi, J. T., Romeo, F., & Lerakis, S. (2022). Concurrent cardiac and central nervous system complications of acute infective endocarditis: case report. *European heart journal. Case reports*, *6*(8), ytac337. https://doi.org/10.1093/ehjcr/ytac337.

[114] Uchiyama, C. M., Brockmeyer, D. L., Cherny, W. B., Jacobs, J. J., & Walker, M. L. (2001). Ruptured intracranial mycotic aneurysm: an unusual infectious complication following craniofacial surgery. *Pediatric neurosurgery*, *35*(2), 94–98. https://doi.org/10.1159/000050397.

[115] Misser SK, Lalloo S, Ponnusamy S (2005) Intracranial mycotic aneurysm due to infective endocarditis—successful NBCA glue embolisation. S Afr Med J 95(6):397–399, 403–4.

[116] Sarica, F. B., Erdoğan, B., Tufan, K., Cekinmez, M., Kizilkiliç, O., Sen, O., & Altinörs, M. N. (2008). Endovascular treatment of primary infectious aneurysm in childhood: a case report. *Turkish neurosurgery*, *18*(1), 47–51.

[117] Saraf, R., & Limaye, U. (2013). Ruptured intracranial tubercular infectious aneurysm secondary to a tuberculoma and its endovascular management. *British journal of neurosurgery*, *27*(2), 243–245. https://doi.org/10.3109/02688697.2012.717986.

[118] Cheng-Ching, E., John, S., Bain, M., Toth, G., Masaryk, T., Hui, F., & Hussain, M. S. (2017). Endovascular Embolization of Intracranial Infectious Aneurysms in Patients Undergoing Open Heart

Surgery Using n-Butyl Cyanoacrylate. *Interventional neurology*, *6*(1-2), 82–89. https://doi.org/10.1159/000455806.

[119] Boukobza, M., Duval, X., & Laissy, J. P. (2019). Mycotic intracranial aneurysms rupture presenting as pure acute subdural hematoma in infectious endocarditis. Report of 2 cases and review of the literature. *Journal of clinical neuroscience: official journal of the Neurosurgical Society of Australasia*, *62*, 222–225. https://doi.org/10.1016/j.jocn.2018.12.035.

[120] Pastor-Cabeza, M., González-Crespo, A., Tardáguila, M., Blanco Ibañez de Opacua, A., Remollo, S., Domínguez, C. J., Rimbau, J. M., & Rodríguez-Hernández, A. (2020). Iatrogenic Intracranial Aneurysm After External Ventricular Drain Placement: Traumatic or Mycotic Origin? Case Report and Literature Review. *World neurosurgery*, *143*, 214–218. https://doi.org/10.1016/j.wneu.2020.07.179

[121] Okuda, T., Nishimura, A., Arimura, K., Iwaki, K., Fujino, T., Ushijima, T., Sonoda, H., Tanoue, Y., Shiose, A., & Yoshimoto, K. (2022). Endovascular therapy for intracranial infectious aneurysms associated with a left ventricular assist device: illustrative case. *Journal of neurosurgery. Case lessons*, *3*(11), CASE21559. https://doi.org/10.3171/CASE21559.

[122] La Barge, D. V., 3rd, Ng, P. P., Stevens, E. A., Friedline, N. K., Kestle, J. R., & Schmidt, R. H. (2009). Extended intracranial applications for ethylene vinyl alcohol copolymer (Onyx): mycotic and dissecting aneurysms. Technical note. *Journal of neurosurgery*, 111(1), 114–118. https://doi.org/10.3171/2009.1.JNS08845.

[123] Zhao, P. C., Li, J., He, M., & You, C. (2010). Infectious intracranial aneurysm: endovascular treatment with onyx case report and review of the literature. *Neurology India*, 58(1), 131–134. https://doi.org/10.4103/0028-3886.60429.

[124] Chalouhi, N., Tjoumakaris, S., Gonzalez, L. F., Hasan, D., Alkhalili, K., Dumont, A. S., Rosenwasser, R., & Jabbour, P. (2013). Endovascular treatment of distal intracranial aneurysms with Onyx 18/34. *Clinical neurology and neurosurgery*, 115(12), 2528–2532. https://doi.org/10.1016/j.clineuro.2013.10.018.

[125] Remirez, J. M., Sabet, Y., Baca, M., Maud, A., Cruz-Flores, S., Rodriguez, G. J., Mukherjee, D., & Abbas, A. (2017). Mycotic Intracranial Aneurysm Secondary to Left Ventricular Assist Device Infection. *Journal of vascular and interventional neurology,* 9(3), 23–25.

[126] Brimley, C., Griessenauer, C. J., Dalal, S., Schirmer, C., & Goren, O. (2019). Acute Development and Rupture of a Basilar Tip Mycotic Aneurysm. *World neurosurgery*, S1878-8750(19)30090-7. Advance online publication. https://doi.org/10.1016/j.wneu.2018.12.211.

[127] Avallone, S. V., Levy, A. S., & Starke, R. M. (2021). A rare case of Streptococcus anginosus infectious intracranial aneurysm: Proper management of a poor prognosis. *Surgical neurology international*, 12, 487. https://doi.org/10.25259/SNI_730_2021.

[128] Kobets, A. J., Scoco, A., Nakhla, J., Brook, A. L., Kinon, M. D., Baxi, N., & Altschul, D. (2018). Flow-Diverting Stents for the Obliteration of Symptomatic, Infectious Cavernous Carotid Artery Aneurysms. *Operative neurosurgery (Hagerstown, Md.)*, 14(6), 681–685. https://doi.org/10.1093/ons/opx166.

[129] Han, M. S., Jung, S. H., Kim, T. S., & Joo, S. P. (2016). Reconstructive Endovascular Treatment of an Intracranial Infectious Aneurysm in Bacterial Meningitis: A Case Report and Review of Literature. *World neurosurgery*, 90, 700.e1–700.e5. https://doi.org/10.1016/j.wneu.2016.02.031.

[130] Sugg, R. M., Weir, R., Vollmer, D. G., & Cacayorin, E. D. (2006). Cerebral mycotic aneurysms treated with a neuroform stent: technical case report. *Neurosurgery,* 58(2), E381. https://doi.org/10.1227/01.NEU.0000195116.49114.2B.

[131] Imamura, H., Sakai, N., & Alexander, M. J. (2019). Flow-Diverter Stenting of Intracavernous Internal Carotid Artery Mycotic Aneurysm. *Journal of stroke and cerebrovascular diseases: the official journal of National Stroke Association*, 28(7), e81–e82. https://doi.org/10.1016/j.jstrokecerebrovasdis.2019.04.026.

[132] Appelboom, G., Kadri, K., Hassan, F., & Leclerc, X. (2010). Infectious aneurysm of the cavernous carotid artery in a child treated with a new-generation of flow-diverting stent graft: case report. *Neurosurgery,* 66(3), E623–E624. https://doi.org/10.1227/01.NEU.0000365370.82554.08.

[133] Ares, W. J., Tonetti, D. A., Greene, S., Sharma, M. S., Xavier, F., Jankowitz, B. T., & Jadhav, A. (2019). Pipeline Embolization of an Infectious Basilar Artery Aneurysm in a 2-Year-Old Child: Case

Report, Discussion of the Literature and Perioperative Considerations. *Operative neurosurgery (Hagerstown, Md.)*, 17(5), E224–E228. https://doi.org/10.1093/ons/opz002.

[134] Yen, P. S., Teo, B. T., Chen, S. C., & Chiu, T. L. (2007). Endovascular treatment for bilateral mycotic intracavernous carotid aneurysms. Case report and review of the literature. *Journal of neurosurgery*, 107(4), 868–872. https://doi.org/10.3171/JNS-07/10/0868.

[135] Lee, B., Kim, C., & Carrasco, J. (2015). Intracranial Infectious Aneurysm in Orbital Cellulitis. *Orbit (Amsterdam, Netherlands)*, 34(4), 175–178. https://doi.org/10.3109/01676830.2015.1014515.

[136] Aguilar-Perez, M., Hellstern, V., AlMatter, M., Wendl, C., Bäzner, H., Ganslandt, O., & Henkes, H. (2020). The p48 Flow Modulation Device with Hydrophilic Polymer Coating (HPC) for the Treatment of Acutely Ruptured Aneurysms: Early Clinical Experience Using Single Antiplatelet Therapy. *Cardiovascular and interventional radiology*, 43(5), 740–748. https://doi.org/10.1007/s00270-020-02418-4.

[137] Ding, D., Raper, D. M., Carswell, A. J., & Liu, K. C. (2014). Endovascular stenting for treatment of mycotic intracranial aneurysms. *Journal of clinical neuroscience: official journal of the Neurosurgical Society of Australasia*, 21(7), 1163–1168. https://doi.org/10.1016/j.jocn.2013.11.013.

[138] OuYang, M., Huang, X., & Wang, Y. (2019). Endovascular Treatment of Infectious Pseudoaneurysm of Internal Carotid Artery. *World neurosurgery*, *125*, 42–43. https://doi.org/10.1016/j.wneu.2019.01.147.

Chapter 10

Endovascular Treatment of Cerebral Aneurysms

Kirill Orlov*

Federal Center of Brain Research and Neurotechnologies of Federal Medical Biological Agency of Russia, Moscow, Russian Federation

Abstract

This chapter is an overview of the history of the development and current state of endovascular treatment of cerebral aneurysms. It compares embolization and microsurgical clipping of both ruptured and non-ruptured aneurysms of various localizations. It considers in detail indications for invasive intervention and the issues of angiographic diagnostics. It reviews the capabilities of modern endovascular devices such as coils, balloons and stents. The chapter presents an analysis of coiling techniques including balloon-and stent-assisted options. Stent-assistance is discussed in detail starting from the standard technique to complex stenting options, such as Y-stenting, X-stenting, semijailing, transverse stenting, and the waffle-cone technique. The chapter also reviews indications for the use of flow diverters and their implantation techniques. It considers the methods of prevention and treatment of typical complications in endovascular treatment of cerebral aneurysms and describes the techniques of balloon and chemical angioplasty in the complex treatment of aneurysms while acute period hemorrhage accompanied by severe angiospasm.

Keywords: cerebral aneurysms, endovascular treatment, embolization, coils, stents, balloons

Endovascular Aneurysm Repair: History of Development

The search for new methods for the treatment of cerebral aneurysms led to the emergence and development of endovascular surgery, whose principles are to occlude an aneurysm by intravascular injection of agents that cause thrombosis inside the aneurysmal sac. Considering the historical aspect of the development of the endovascular method in reconstructive surgery of cerebral aneurysms, 4 periods can be distinguished:

1. Beginning of the 1970s when balloon catheters became widely used. In this respect, F. A. Serbinenko can rightfully be considered the founder of endovascular neurosurgery, who in

* Corresponding Author's Email: kirill.orlov@rens-russia.org.

In: Understanding and Managing Cerebral Aneurysms
Editor: Xianli Lv
ISBN: 979-8-89113-608-3

1971 developed and proposed the use of a detachable balloon-catheter, which had been originally used for occlusion of carotid-cavernous fistulas, for temporary and permanent occlusion of vessels (Figure 1). Subsequently, he began to use this technique for embolization of cerebral aneurysms, including infraclinoid and posterior-circulation ones that are difficult to access microsurgically. In 1977, Yu. N. Zubkov proposed his own modification of a detachable balloon catheter (Figure 2) and was the first to propose balloon angioplasty for treatment of vasospasm in acute SAH period. The first results obtained using balloon catheters looked impressive, and this technique had been actively applied until the 1990s. However, after accumulating experience and studying long-term results, many shortcomings of the method had become apparent, such as a high risk of intraoperative aneurysm rupture, untimely separation and rupture of the balloon, which led to thromboembolic complications, as well as a high frequency of recanalization and, as a result, the likelihood of recurrent hemorrhages in the late postoperative period due to pressure loss in the occluding balloon [1, 2, 3].

2. In the beginning of the 1990s, G. Guglielmi et al. In 1991 suggested using electrolytically separated coils (Figure 3) to occlude an aneurysmal cavity [4, 5]. The Guglielmi detachable coils (GDC) could be relatively easily delivered through a microcatheter into an aneurysm and separated from the pusher at the right time and place. Later on, various coil separation systems were developed, such as hydraulic and mechanical ones, but the electrolytic separation system, which has been greatly improved to date, remains one of the most reliable and convenient to apply. The optimal dome-to-neck ratio with this technique is 3:1.

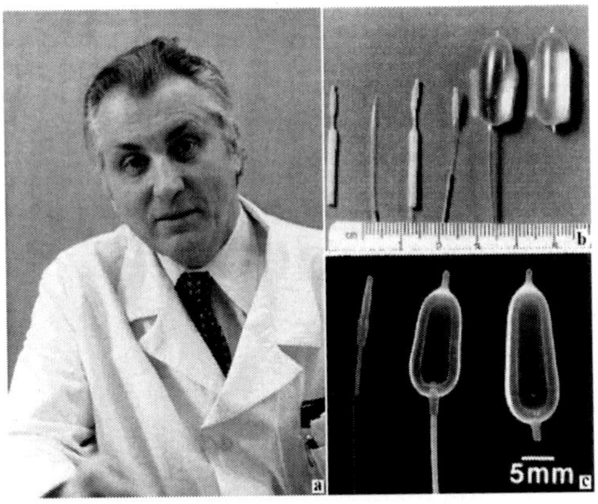

Figure 1. F. A. Serbinenko, the founder of endovascular neurosurgery (a), who was the first to use detachable balloons for aneurysm embolization. Detachable balloons of his design (b).

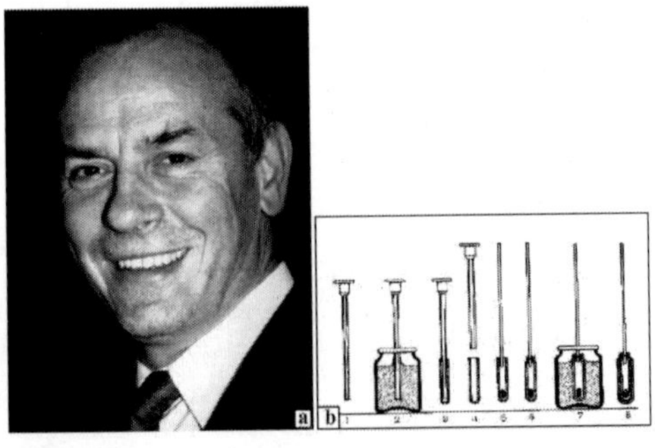

Figure 2. Yu.N. Zubkov who first proposed balloon angioplasty for vasospasm during acute hemorrhage (a); balloon catheter fabrication technique (b).

As the aneurysmal cavity was filled with coils, they created conditions for a blood stasis followed by aneurysm embolization. In a number of cases, it was possible to tightly and reliably embolize the aneurysmal cavity, but in approximately 40–59% of cases, control studies revealed the blood-saturated near-to-neck part, which led to aneurysm recanalization in 2–6 months after surgery [6, 7]. It was noted that the smaller the aneurysm and the more compactly it is filled with coils, the less likely the recanalization to occur and the better the treatment results [8]. In 1998, G. L. Klein et al. achieved a complete occlusion of the bifurcation aneurysm of the basilar artery in 14 out of 21 patients, in the remaining cases the occlusion rate was 90%, in 3 of them an additional procedure was required after 6 months. One patient died from the causes unrelated to the procedure.

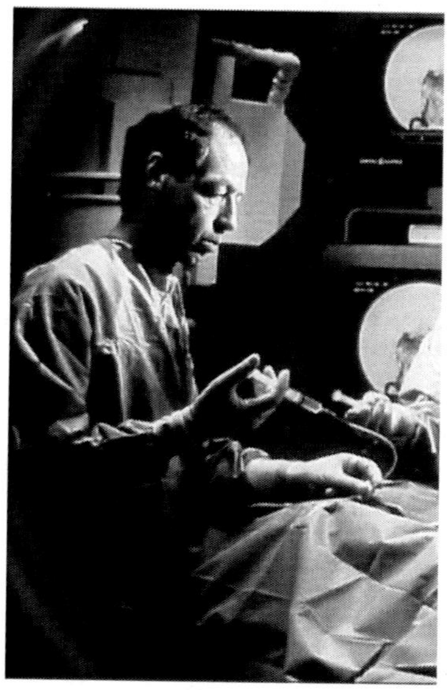

Figure 3. G. Guglielmi who first suggested using coils (GDC) for aneurysm embolization.

In the same year, J. V. Eskrige and J. K. Song demonstrated the advantage of endovascular occlusion of ruptured aneurysms in basilar artery bifurcations in a retrospective multicenter study that included 150 patients, but for unruptured aneurysms, no definite conclusion was made. Accumulation of experience and improvement of the technique contributed to the gradual improvement of treatment results. In 2002, E. Lusseveld et al. in 2002 showed the advantage of the endovascular technique over direct intervention by analyzing the results of treatment of similar groups of 44 patients each. Unsatisfactory results in the first group were observed in 11% of the patients compared with 30% in the second group. In addition, according to angiography data, coils allowed for complete occlusion in 93% of the patients compared with 91% for clips [9].

In 2003, J. N. Valee et al. achieved good results in 86% of observations, the mortality was 6% and disability — 2%. The unsatisfactory results clearly correlated with the initial severe condition of the patients (Hunt-Hess grade IV). In 10 patients, recanalization occurred within 6 months after primary occlusion and required additional coiling. For denser filling of the aneurysmal cavity, the use of so-called 3D coils proved to be optimal [10]. Since the patients with wide-neck cerebral aneurysms are the main problem for endovascular treatment, various techniques have been proposed for remodeling the neck from the side of the carrier vessel while coiling the aneurysmal cavity. These included a temporary occlusion of the neck with a balloon-catheter, using of various devices and even a scheme for double-catheter coil supply [11, 12]. However, neither the use of 3D coils [13] nor the other methods mentioned above fully resolved the issue of reliable occlusion of the near-to-neck part of a wide-neck aneurysm. In 2003–2004, M. Sluzewski et al. summarized the results of endovascular occlusion of 145 aneurysms and concluded that stable and reliable occlusion of small aneurysms (up to 200 mm^3) required a filling density of at least 20%, and for larger aneurysms of 300 mm^3 or more - of at least 24%. Under all other conditions, it was almost impossible to achieve such filling of a wide-neck aneurysm due to the danger of coils migrating into the carrier vessel's lumen. Therefore, the more the aneurysm remains functioning and the wider its neck, the higher the likelihood of recanalization. The attempts to solve the above problem led to the development and creation of stents adapted for implantation in the vessels of the base of the brain.

3. The third development period of endovascular aneurysm surgery is associated with the development of such remodeling techniques as balloon and stent assistance. By that time, the design of the coils had changed significantly, so coils of various softness and thickness became available, including 3D and 360° ones, in which the first two helices had a smaller diameter to simplify their positioning, and reduce the risk of coil migration into the carrier artery, so it became possible to embolize aneurysms of 2:1 dome-to-neck ratio. Currently, various tools are being developed to help one reduce the percentage of aneurysm recanalization, which has resulted in the appearance of next-generation coils such as those with a biodegradable coating to enhance arterial defect covering with endothelium [14]; and hydrocoils containing hydrogel to increase in volume upon contact with blood and enhance thrombosis.

The balloon assistance suggested by J. Moret [15], allows one to embolize wide-neck aneurysms by denser "packing" them with coils, which decreases the likelihood of recanalization, and significantly reduces the risk of coil migration into the carrier-artery lumen.

In 1994, F. Turgman et al. [16] published positive results of the experimental application of stent-assistance in porcine aneurysm models. The use of stents in the surgery of cerebral aneurysms has significantly expanded the indications for endovascular surgery and increased the number of reconstructive procedures [17-22]. The main purpose of a stent is arterial remodeling by setting a metal frame that prevents the coils from leaving the body of the aneurysm. However, in addition to the mechanical support of the coils, stents change the aneurysmal blood flow to enhance thrombosis and create additional conditions for endothelium to cover the arterial defect.

4. The fourth development period of endovascular aneurysm surgery is associated with the appearance of flow diverters (FDs). Giant and fusiform aneurysms are the most challenging ones for endovascular treatment and when embolized with coils, even with stent-assistance, they are characterized by the highest frequency of recanalization and mass effect, which often requires reconstructive operations to occlude the carrier artery.

The experiment demonstrated that implantation of a stent at the aneurysmal neck significantly changed the blood flow in the aneurysm, and this effect began to be used in clinical practice. It was also noted that in a number of cases small aneurysms could thrombose without being coiled, which was especially true for braided stents. To enhance this flow-diversion effect, telescopic stenting was introduced to be sequential implantation of several stents (usually three), a stent into a stent. This technique proved to be effective for treatment of fusiform aneurysms and the aneurysms with near-to-neck recanalization difficult to coil. The effect was used to design self-expanding stents of very dense braiding (Pipeline EV3, Silc Balt), whose main goal was to redirect the blood flow in the lumen, which led to stagnation and stasis of blood in the aneurysm, so it could properly thrombose.

Their application has made it possible to achieve high radicality in the embolization of giant and fusiform aneurysms [23-29]. However, when evaluating the long-term results, it turned out that after implantation of such stents, the risk of the long-term hemorrhagic complications associated with thrombus and aneurysm-wall resorption remains. Although the risk does not exceed 1%, and it is significantly lower than the risk of the natural course of the disease, this problem requires further study and development of methods for the prevention of long-term hemorrhages.

Indications for Endovascular Treatment

Since the advent of the endovascular method, a competition between intravascular surgery and microsurgery has begun, despite the fact both methods have their advantages and disadvantages, so they can perfectly complement each other. In other words, choosing a method for treating an aneurysm depends on many factors, such as the severity of the patient's condition, the anatomical features of the aneurysm and its localization, the presence of a hematoma or ventricular hemorrhage, and the timing of the patient's admission to a dedicated medical center. In addition to the medical factors, it is also necessary to take into account the technical and material capabilities of the clinic, and the presence of microsurgeons and endovascular surgeons, whose qualification in sufficient for performing such procedures. When selecting a treatment tactics, the patient's safety should be a primary consideration, because in the absence of proper experience, equipment and instruments, the risk of endovascular surgery, despite its minimal invasiveness, can be quite high. It is also not recommended to perform endovascular surgeries in a center where there is no emergency neurosurgical service, especially when it comes patients in the acute aneurysmal rupture, since they sometimes require emergency surgery.

When treating aneurysms in the anterior Willis circle, the capabilities of microsurgical and endovascular methods are comparable in terms of radicality, however, the ISAT randomized trial [30, 31] showed the advantage of endovascular surgery in terms of functional outcomes (74.6% of positive outcomes with embolization and 63.6% with clipping). For severe patients with expressed vasospasm, a microsurgical operation is usually contraindicated [32], since its results are comparable, or even worse than the results of the natural course of the disease, where the mortality can reach 30% [33]. Endovascular surgery in such patients (HH III-V), on the contrary, is indicated, since it makes it possible to perform chemical or balloon angioplasty to treat the vasospasm, and to non-traumatically occlude the aneurysm. It has been proven that even a partial occlusion can prevent re-bleeding in acute period, whose risk is 20-30% [34], and subsequently, when the patient's condition is compensated, the aneurysm can be totally occluded endovascularly or microsurgically.

Further development of neuroimaging has increased the number of diagnosed unruptured aneurysms. A large number of studies have been conducted to determine the risk of rupture of unruptured aneurysms [35-38]. One of the largest of these studies is the ISUA first and second study, which examined in detail the risk of hemorrhage from aneurysms of various sizes and locations. In this domain, most authors today prefer the endovascular method, and if in 2001 in the USA, only 20% of patients with ruptured aneurysms were embolized, in 2008 this proportion increased to 63%. In the same year, morbidity rate in patients with clipped aneurysms was 14%, and in patients treated endovascularly it comprised 4.9%. As for the mortality, it comprised 1.2% in the microsurgical group against 0.6% [39-42]. in the endovascular one. The risk of a negative outcome in patients with unruptured aneurysm was 14.8% in 2001, but in 2008 this risk reduced to 7.6%.

Currently, when choosing a tactics for treating patients with posterior-circulation aneurysms accounting for 5–10% of all intracranial aneurysms, most authors also prefer the endovascular method [43-46]. According to ISUIA data, the probability for such an aneurysm to rupture is 1.3-1.5 times higher than the 5-year consolidated figure for patients with anterior-circulation aneurysms. Moreover, the larger the aneurysm, the greater the likelihood of its rupture [47-49].

The relevance of the issue lies with the inaccessibility and complexity of direct interventions for treating the aneurysms of this localization. The first results of such interventions were extremely unsatisfactory: From 30 to 50% of patients died from circulatory disorders in the brain stem or intraoperative aneurysm rupture. For that reason, a number of authors preferred to perform not an open intervention, but to ligate or clip one or both vertebral arteries [50-52]. In the era before the use of microsurgical techniques, favorable outcomes of such operations did not exceed 5-10%.

Further technological advancements in neurosurgery, neuroanesthesiology and neuroreanimatology such as interventions during circulatory arrest, hypothermia, and brain protection with barbiturates [53-56] have significantly improved the situation. According to C. G. Drake et al. who in 1996 analyzed the results of surgical treatment of 1767 patients with posterior-circulation aneurysms, the overall mortality in the group of these patients was 6.6%, unsatisfactory results - 9.6%. The highest number of unsatisfactory results was noted in the group of patients with large and giant aneurysms - 17.2% and 30.5%, respectively, and 9.6% - in the patients with small aneurysms. Despite the improvements of microsurgical techniques, for posterior-circulation aneurysms, as well as for the aneurysms of the para- and infraclinoid ICA sections, endovascular interventions remain less traumatic, allow one to achieve a better functional result and reduce patient morbidity [57].

Until recently, the most difficult problem has been treatment of giant, fusiform and dissecting aneurysms. A significant breakthrough in this domain became introduction of flow-diverters, and considerable experience has now been accumulated in application of this endovascular instrumentation. The very first published clinical series demonstrated the high efficiency of the technique (ref.) that increased the radicality to 95-98% and significantly reduced while the likelihood of immediate (0.1%) and long-term (0.9-1%) complications. It is worth noticing that coiling, even in combination with stent assistance, has never been able to achieve such a result.

The meta-analyses [58] published to date have also shown the high efficiency FD implantation in these types of aneurysms. However, the accumulated clinical experience and investigation of the long-term results have enabled us to identify a new type of long-term hemorrhagic complications: Thrombosis of large and giant aneurysms leads to a large number of proteolytic enzymes released that cause a gradual lysis of both the thrombus and the aneurysmal wall, which, in combination with anticoagulant therapy, can lead to delayed hemorrhages that, in some cases, can be fatal. Currently, the ways to prevent these delayed hemorrhages are currently being investigated along with the effectiveness of the combined coiling/stenting technique, and telescopic stenting with two flow diverters. Analysis of the published data and accumulated experience makes it possible to give the following recommendations for choosing a proper tactics for surgical treatment of cerebral aneurysms.

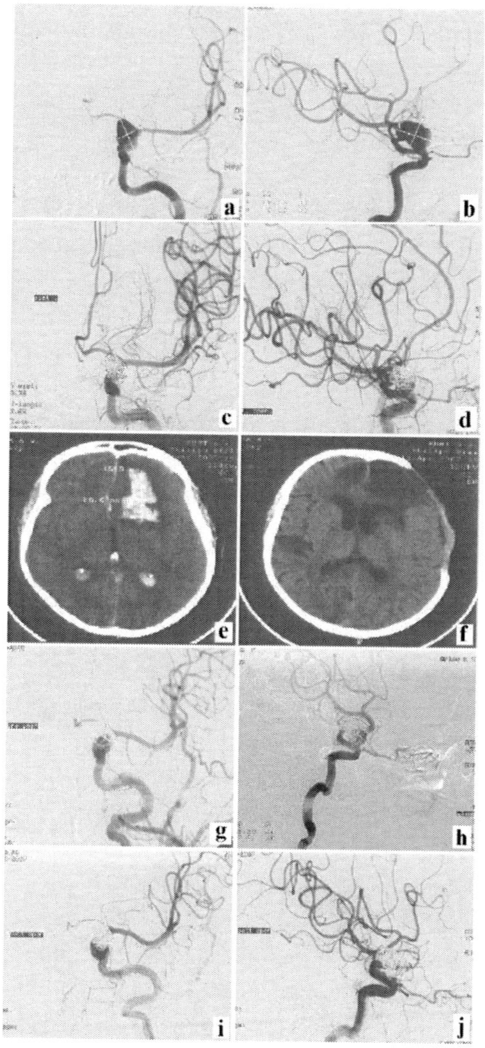

Figure 4. Embolization of the aneurysm of the left internal carotid artery, followed by removal of the intracerebral hematoma: a, b – diagnostic angiography, ICA aneurysm detected; c, d – subtotal aneurysm occlusion on day 2 after hemorrhage;
e - hematoma of the left frontal lobe visualized by CT to be removed immediately after endovascular surgery; f – control CT, 4 weeks after hematoma removal;
g, h - control angiograms 6 months after surgery; residual near-to-neck filling of the aneurysm observed; i, j – control angiography after repeated endovascular surgery in the posthemorrhagic period.

The saccular aneurysms of the anterior Willis circle in compensated patients (HH I-II) in the first 72 hours after a hemorrhage can be operated both microsurgically and endovascularly, while in critical patients (HH III-V) embolization combined with chemical or balloon angioplasty should be preferred; in the presence of a dislocating intracerebral hematoma after endovascular surgery, it has to be removed the hematoma (Figure 4), and ventricular hemorrhage, requires drainage.

Posterior-circulation aneurysms and the aneurysms of the infra- and paraclinoid ICA segments are better to be embolized as well as unruptured aneurysms indicated for surgery.

For giant, fusiform, dissecting and blister-like aneurysms as well as for multiple wide-neck aneurysms located in the same segment, FD implantation is indicated.

Aneurysm Embolization Technique

All endovascular interventions for cerebral aneurysms must be performed under intubation anesthesia. When using different types of coils, the manipulations are approximately identical. The procedure can be divided into several stages.

Performing Angiographic Imaging and Choosing an Approach

After a femoral-artery puncture, one performs selective catheterization of the great cervical artery, in the basin of which the aneurysm is localized. The catheterization is carried out either with an angiographic catheter with subsequent replacement of the latter with a guiding catheter, or directly with a guiding catheter. There are many types of guiding catheters manufactured by various companies. Their main difference from angiographic ones is the presence of a reinforced part and a soft tip, which is necessary for prevention of intraoperative vasoconstrictor reactions. There are both straight and curved guiding catheters. The configuration of the curved ones is usually similar to that of angiographic catheters and the choice of catheter depends on the type of aortic arch and vessel into which the guide catheter is to be inserted. Guide catheters range in size from 5F to 8F, with 5F and 6F catheters being most commonly used. After the catheterization, preoperative angiography is performed, to localize the anatomical features and the size of the aneurysm, and the position of its neck. Then a projection is selected to clearly visualize the neck and the carrier vessel [59-61].

While the angiographic examination, it is necessary to take into account a number of fundamental conditions that are mandatory for implementation:

- In all cases, it is necessary to conduct an angiographic examination of all cerebral vessels (both in the anterior and posterior circulations). Such parameters as difference in vessel size, degree of their physiological bending or pathological deformities in the extracranial brachiocephalic arteries enable one to choose a proper catheterization side for endovascular intervention. In case you have improperly assessed of the diameter of the cerebral artery and selected a guiding catheter of wrong diameter for, e.g., catheterization, this catheter may slow down or stop blood flow in the vessel, which, in turn, will lead to unreliable verification of the vessels above the conduction zone. Moreover, it may provoke catheter thrombosis that may lead to the development of thromboembolic complications.
- When planning an operation on the cerebral arteries, a thorough examination of collateral circulation conditions is required. To do this, it is necessary to examine the anterior communicating and both posterior communicating arteries. Approximate information can be gathered from contrasting one of the carotid or vertebral arteries while alternately clamping the carotid arteries in the neck. A more reliable image is obtained from alternate occlusion of the carotid or vertebral arteries with an

inseparable balloon while a contrast agent is introduced into the right and left carotid or vertebral arteries. The downside of this examination is the need for bilateral transfemoral approach. However, the data obtained can significantly correct the course of the intervention itself, for example, in the case of unforeseen occlusion of the carrier vessel.

- The required contrast agent dose for a single injection in the DSA mode should not exceed 4-5 ml. In case of 3D angiography, it is enough to inject 10 ml of a contrast agent for 5 seconds to obtain a complete reconstruction (2 ml/sec). Increasing the volume and rate of contrast agent administration increases the likelihood of complications, especially in acute SAH patients.
- 3D DSA is the "gold standard" of angiography for aneurysm surgery, because this method makes it possible to comprehensively assess the characteristics of the neck and body of the aneurysm in relation to the carrier vessels; study the geometric parameters of the aneurysm; measure the diameters of the vessels and aneurysms in real mode, which is extremely important for assessing the feasibility of endovascular surgery and correct selection of instruments.

Aneurysm catheterization is performed with a microcatheter selected to match the anatomical features of the aneurysm and carrier vessels, as well as the type of coils used.

Every company manufacturing coils has its own line of microcatheters. As a rule, the catheters can be of straight and pre-shaped configurations, and the same modifications differ in stiffness, diameter and size of the softer distal part. Their internal diameter ranges from 0.010" to 0.021". Coiling microcatheters have at least two radiopaque markers: at the tip of the catheter that enables one to control the position of the catheter; at a distance of 3 cm from the tip to control the positioning of the coil and its separation. The microcatheter is inserted into the aneurysm using a microguide wire. The wires from different manufacturers differ in structure, softness and materials used. All of them have two main parts: a rigid one to pass a microcatheter through, and a distal soft part with a soft or pre-formed tip to insert a guidewire into the aneurysm and catheterize it.

Catheterization of the aneurysmal cavity, as well as of intracranial vessels, especially the basilar artery, should be carried out with the utmost care. Irritation of the basilar artery's intima near the stem branches' ostia can lead to their spasm and the development of transient or persistent neurological disorders. Depending on the localization of the aneurysm and the configuration of the main posterior-circulation branches, in a number of situations, in order to achieve optimal catheterization of the aneurysm, it is necessary to bend the microcatheter's tip in advance. For example, catheterization of an aneurysm in basilar artery bifurcation presents no difficulties, since a microcatheter, when moving along the basilar artery, easily penetrates into the aneurysmal cavity. On the other hand, catheterizing aneurysms in the ostium of the superior cerebellar artery or the orifice of the posterior inferior cerebellar artery can be extremely difficult. Usually, aneurysms of these localizations are located at an angle of 90° (or close to it) relative to the carrier vessel. To perform catheterization and ensure a stable position of the catheter in the aneurysmal cavity, it is necessary to preform the tip of the catheter, giving it a J-shape of about 5 mm in radius, so it to stop against the opposite wall of the carrier vessel. In this situation, the Echelon 14 microcatheters (EV3, USA) of more rigid structure are preferable.

Aneurysm occlusion is achieved using detachable coils. The coils are passed directly into the aneurysm using a microcatheter delivery system. All manipulations related to pushing the coil through the microcatheter and their separation should be carried out while constantly flushing the microcatheter and catheter guide! Ignoring this rule leads either to thromboembolic complications or to problems with passing coils through the catheter, their stretching or premature separation. Often, such technical complications require the extraction of the entire coaxial system including the coil and microcatheter, or the coil, microcatheter and guide catheter, and in some cases, when the coils migrate, make it necessary to use special retrievers to extract the coils.

Different delivery and separation systems enable a coil to be detached in three different ways: electrolytically, hydraulically and mechanically. Electrolytic detachment is a result of electrolysis in the separation zone. Hydraulic detachment occurs when the coils pressed into the delivery system are hydraulically "pushed out" when the pressure in the system is increased. A mechanically detachable coil either detaches spontaneously when the "capture" enters the aneurysmal cavity (this system is the least reliable and is practically not used today), or the coil is rigidly fixed in the delivery system and detached by a special mechanism that shifts the fixing string. The last detachment method is the most reliable and fastest one.

Most modern coils have an anti-stretch protection to prevent them from stretching while they are repositioned in the aneurysm.

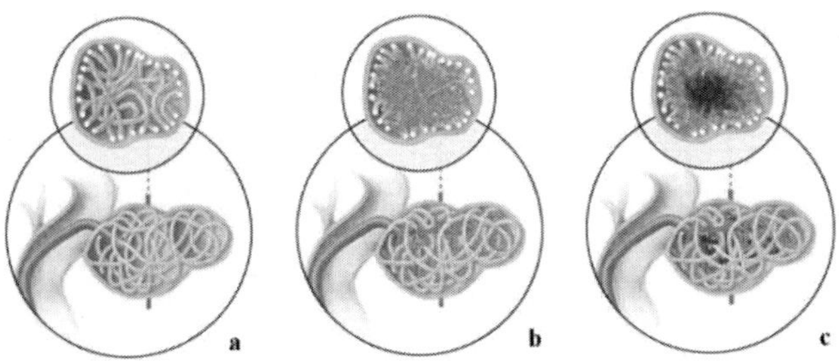

Figure 5. Gradual concentric coiling of the aneurysm (3F): a – framing, b – filling, c – finishing.

When "packing" an aneurysm, its cavity is gradually filled with coils from larger to smaller diameter. Filling the cavity, follow the rule of 3 Fs: Framing for reinforcing of the walls of the aneurysm; Filling for filling the main volume; and Finishing for final "packing" of the neck (Figure 5). For framing, as a rule, 3D coils are used being the largest and most rigid ones. After that the remaining part of the aneurysm is concentrically filled with three-dimensional or two-dimensional, softer coils, whose size gradually decreases while packing. The number and size of the coils is determined by the surgeon during the intervention. It is necessary to continue the packing until a complete occlusion is reached that means no contrasted segments can be seen in control angiographic image. Complete occlusion is usually achieved when 25–30% of the aneurysmal volume is filled with coils (Figure 6).

Manufactures use different materials to produce coils. Basically, it is a platinum thread, whose diameter determines its softness. While platinum coils are most common, there are also bioactive coils (Matrix) having an absorbable PGLA (polylactic-co-glycolic acid) coating, whose effectiveness has been experimentally confirmed [62]. Being absorbed within 10–12 weeks, PGLA causes fibrous tissue formation and enhances neointimal formation in the near-to-neck area of the aneurysm without stenosing the carrier artery.

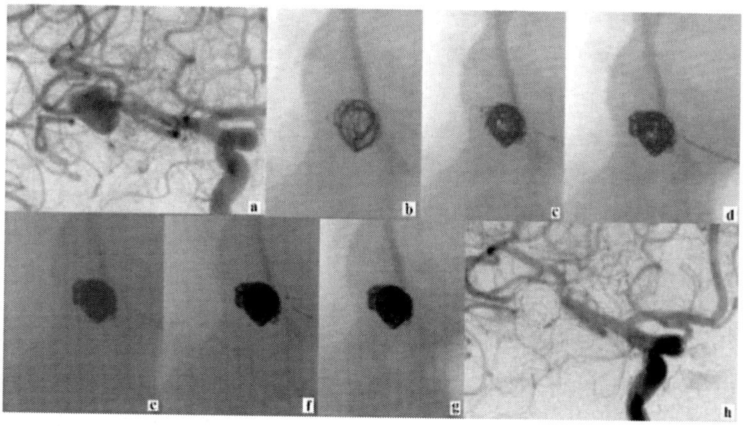

Figure 6. Embolization of an MCA aneurysm using the 3F technique: a - preoperative angiogram, b –placing 1coil, c - 2coils, d - 3coils, e - 4 coils, f –5 coils, g - 6 coils, h –total occlusion of the aneurysm.

Another type of biologically active coils is hydrocoils that contain hydrogel. It swells upon contact with blood and thereby increases the filling volume and reduces the risk of recanalization [63]. In addition, the hydrogel has a porous structure to stimulate thrombosis in the aneurysmal cavity.

Balloon-Assistance

The need for balloon assistance occurs frequently. The use of balloons enables one to significantly increase the radicality of endovascular operations, especially in aneurysms with a wide neck and a complex neck configuration making it possible to pack the aneurysms more tightly and, in the case of intraoperative aneurysm rupture, to stop bleeding in a timely manner.

Only specially designed soft balloons are used for balloon-assistance. Their diameter should be selected to match the size of the carrier artery, and the length should exceed the diameter of the aneurysm neck by at least 5–10 mm. When approaching, it is necessary to implant a wide-lumen guide catheter (at least 6F) to pass through a balloon catheter and a microcatheter. After the guide catheter is delivered, a balloon is brought to the neck of the aneurysm, then the microcatheter is inserted into the aneurysm to deliver the first coil. When the coil's distal part reaches the tip of the microcatheter, it is necessary to inflate the balloon by injecting into it such a volume of contrast agent that does not exceed that specified in the instructions for the balloon, since any excess may lead to the rupture of the balloon, artery or the near-to-neck part of the aneurysm! After the balloon covers the neck, the coil is inserted into the aneurysmal cavity, then, without separating the coil, one deflates the balloon. If, after the deflation, the coil does not move into the arterial lumen, contrast is reintroduced into the balloon, and the coil is separated for the next one to be immediately inserted, but before it is also necessary to check whether it has displaced into the lumen of the carrier artery while the balloon is being deflated. These manipulations are repeated until the aneurysm is totally occluded (Figure 7). After control angiography confirms all parts of the aneurysm are totally occluded, including the near-to-neck one, the microcatheter is removed from the vessel after inflating the balloon.

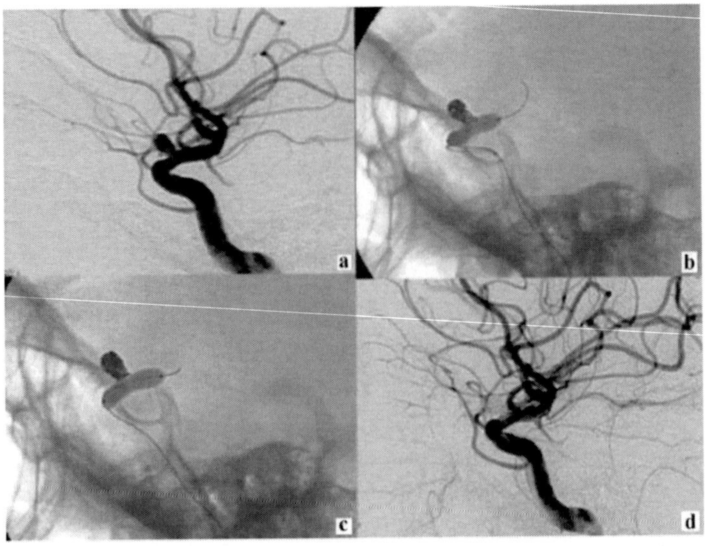

Figure 7. Balloon-assisted embolization of an ICA aneurysm: a - preoperative subtraction angiogram, a native image of an inflated balloon in the ICA that occluded the aneurysmal neck; b - loose coiling of the near-to-neck part; c - dense coiling of the aneurysmal sac; d - the aneurysm was totally occluded.

Stent-Assistance

The use of stents requires medical preparation of the patient, which includes aspirin 100 mg per day and clopidogrel 75 mg per day for at least 3 days, or if it is necessary to perform an operation in an accelerated manner, 300 mg of clopidogrel once 2 hours before the operation. In the postoperative period, it is necessary to carry out anticoagulant therapy to be 100 mg of aspirin and 75 mg of clopidogrel for 6–12 months. During this time, the stent is believed to have been covered with endothelium to exclude the risk of stent thrombosis (Figures 8, 9). The drug therapy is a must for any implanted stent [64-67].

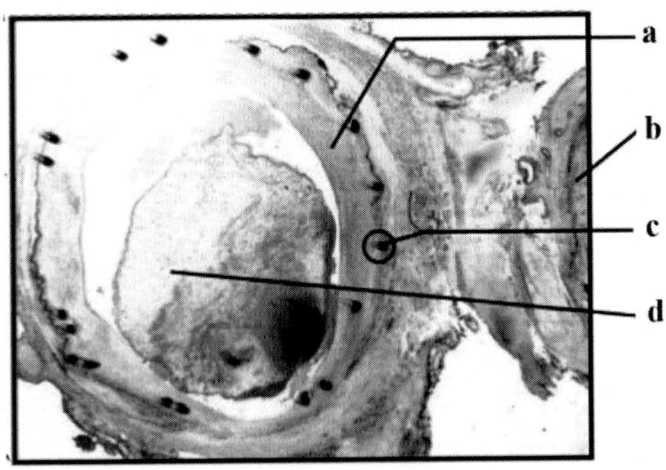

Figure 8. Cross-section of a post-mortem preparation of a previously treated aneurysm, stent endothelialization on day 122 after surgery (death due to causes other than stenting): a - endothelium, b –a thrombus inside the aneurysm, c –stent elements, d - post-mortem thrombus.

There are many options for stent-assistance. The most common technique that is regarded as a standard one and recommended by the manufacturers, is stent implantation followed by insertion of a microcatheter through a stent cell for subsequent coiling. First of all, a microcatheter is inserted distally to the aneurysm, then a stent is inserted into it and the microcatheter is displaced proximally, so its distal mark is at least 5 mm distal to the aneurysmal neck. When the stent is delivered, one first opens its distal part to fix it in the artery, then the whole stent is open to be implanted at the level of the neck and proximal to it. After the stent is implanted, a microcatheter is placed into the aneurysm cavity through one of its cells to embolize the cavity with coils until the aneurysm is totally occluded.

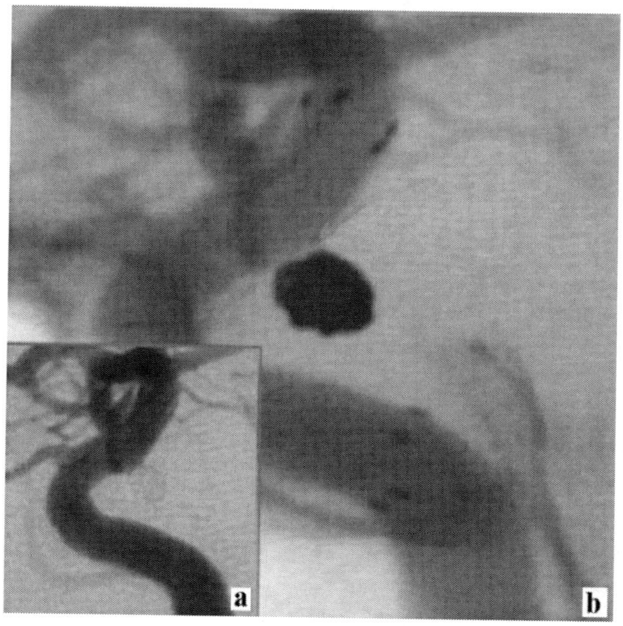

Figure 9. Carotid angiograms demonstrating the conditions of anear-to-neckpart of an aneurysm right after stent-assisted coiling and during the follow-up. Note the endotheliumproliferation (marked with green arrows) in the region of the aneurysmal neck.

Another technique called "jailing" is applied in more difficult situations when additional fixation of the microcatheter is needed. To perform the technique, it is a microcatheter that is first inserted into the aneurysm and followed by another microcatheter placed into the artery. Along the second microcatheter a stent is delivered to be implanted in the neck of the aneurysm. The stent fixes the first microcatheter to the arterial wall and the last is used to embolize the aneurysm with coils and removed when the procedure is over. It should be noted that when using this technique, the risk of stent displacement during removal of the microcatheter is much less than when the microcatheter is passed through a stent cell (Figure 10).

The indications for stent-assistance have expanded significantly with the advent of low-profile stents that are delivered through microcatheters of an internal diameter of 0.017". Being of such a small diameter, they can be safely inserted into more distal vessels to allow for efficient and safe stent-assisted embolization of distal aneurysms. Moreover, low-profile catheters and stents make it possible to carry out rather complex catheterizations and deliver stents into the posterior-circulation vessels using the carotid approach (Figure 11).

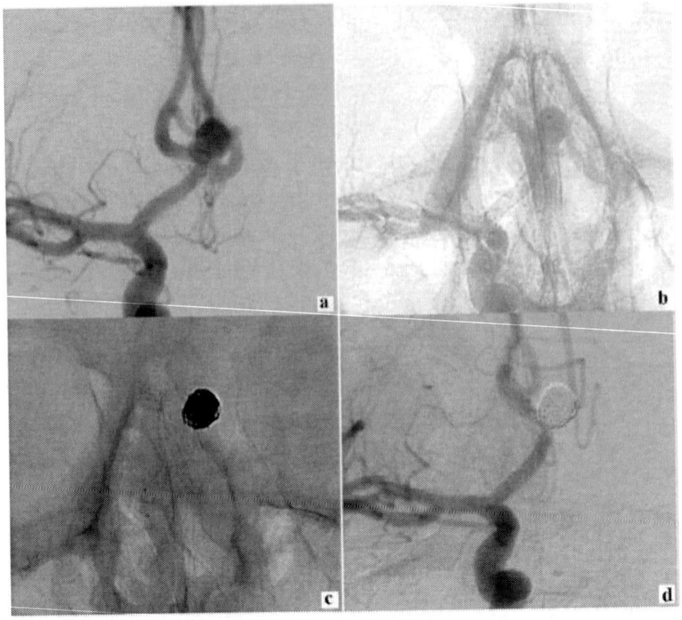

Figure 10. Stent-assisted embolization (Jailing technique) of an Acom aneurysm: a - preoperative angiogram of the right carotid basin in anterior-posterior projection; b - a microcatheter was placed in the aneurysmprecompressed with a stent; c, d –the aneurysm was totally occluded with coils.

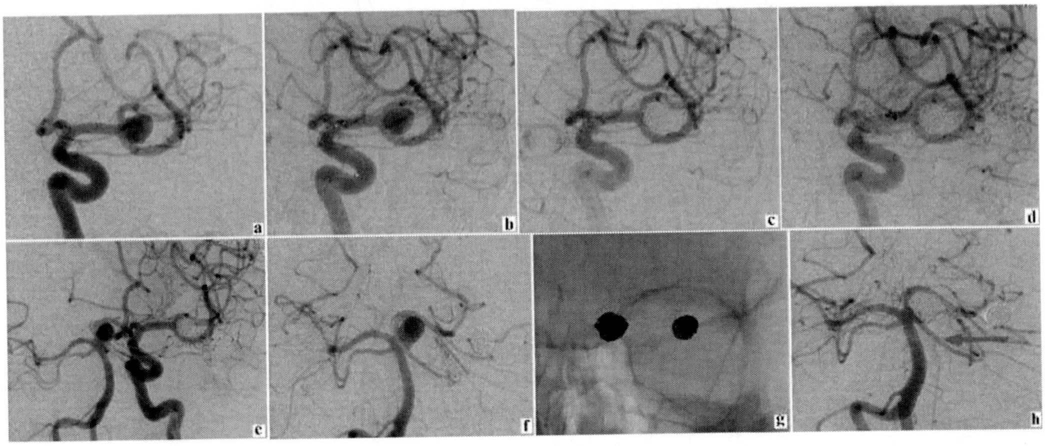

Figure 11. Staged angiograms of LMCA and LSCAaneurysms treated endovascularly in one patient in one procedure: a,b,c,d – total LMCA aneurysm embolization with coils supported with one stent from upper M2 to M1; e,f – visualization of the left Pcom andstentingcatheter path from the LICA to the LSCA through the Pcom (red line); g,h,i,j – the stent implanted, coils placed, the aneurysm was totally occluded.

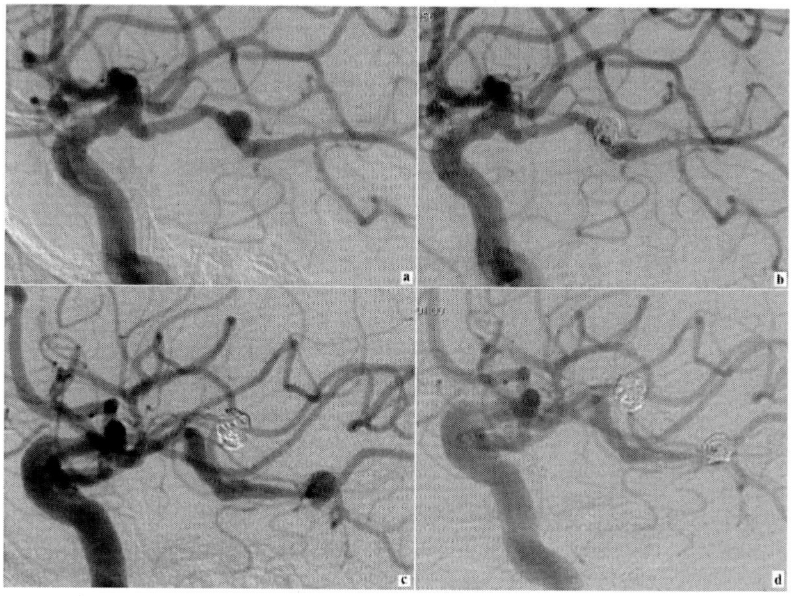

Figure 12. Multiple fusiform aneurysms of both PCAs embolized using the Semijailing technique: a,c - carotid angiograms in lateral projection at the time the treatment of both aneurysms was initiated; b,d – the aneurysms were totally occluded.

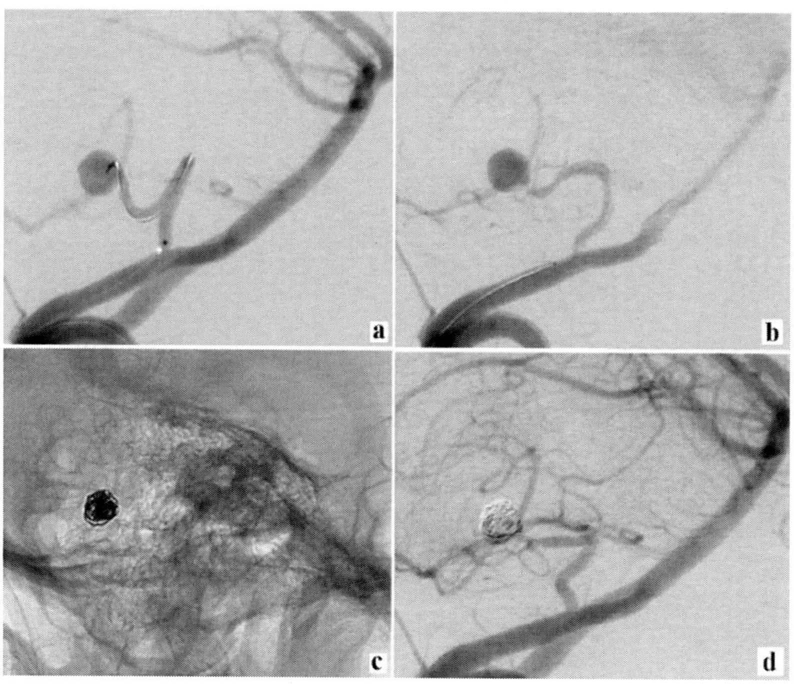

Figure 13. Distal aneurysm of the posterior inferior cerebellar artery totally embolized with stent-assisted coils: a – a coiling microcatheter introduced into the aneurysm; b – a stenting microcatheter delivered posteriorly to the aneurysm, c – a stent was implanted and coils were placed; d – the aneurysm was totally occluded.

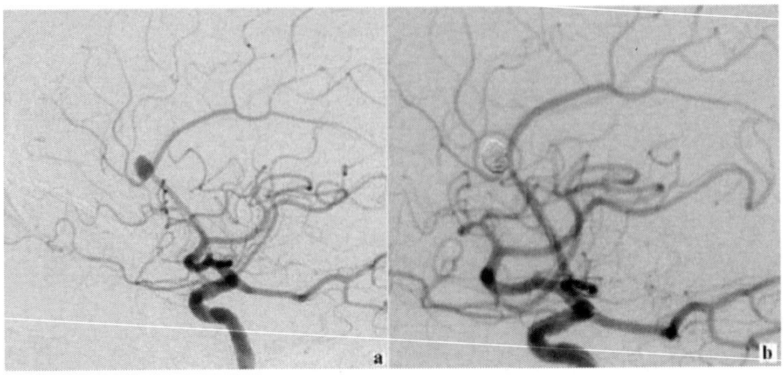

Figure 14. Distal ACA aneurysm: a – the aneurysm before intervention, b – total occlusion after stent-assisted coiling.

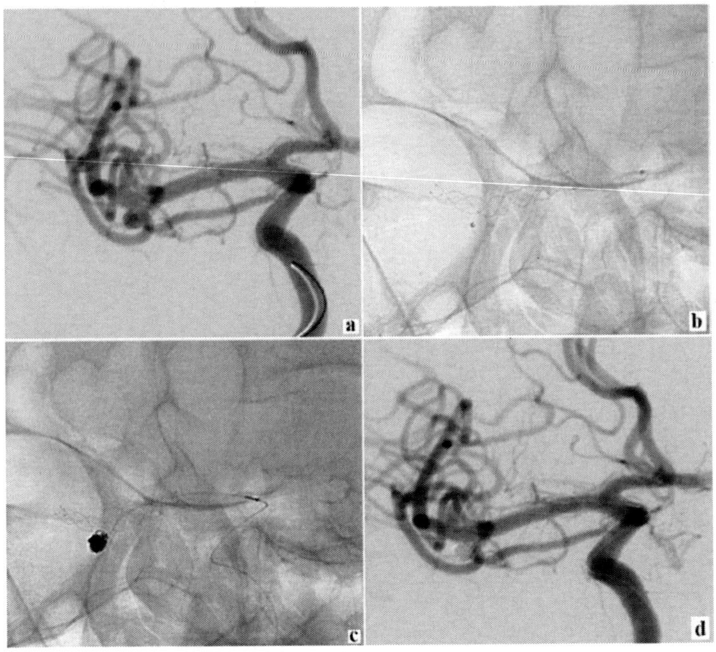

Figure 15. Stent-assisted (1 stent) embolization of a RMCA bifurcation aneurysm:
a – a saccular aneurysm at the M1 bifurcation of the MCA; b - one stent implanted in the M1-M2 segments, a coiling microcatheter was placed into the aneurysm, c - coils were placed in the aneurysmal sac, d - the aneurysm was totally occluded.

To treat fusiform aneurysms, the semijailing technique is applied, when at the first stage, a microcatheter is inserted into the carrier to deliver a stent. Then the aneurysm is catheterized, coils are inserted, and the stent is placed through their tangle to remodel the carrier's lumen. This technique is applicable for the fusiform aneurysms of large (PCA) (Figure 12) and small (PICA) (Figure 13) or pericallosal (Figure 14) arteries. In some cases, when embolizing an aneurysm with a wide neck extending to the bifurcation, it is enough to implant one stent to reduce the width of the neck and then embolize the aneurysm (Figure 15). However, more often than not it is necessary to remodel the bifurcation using two stents. The most common technique applied in this case is Y-stenting that is often used for aneurysms in the MCA and BA bifurcations (Figures 16, 17). For remodeling ACA-Acom bifurcation in presence of an open anterior Willis circle, it is also possible to use Y-stenting, but if the circle is closed, X- or transverse stenting is applied (Figure 18).

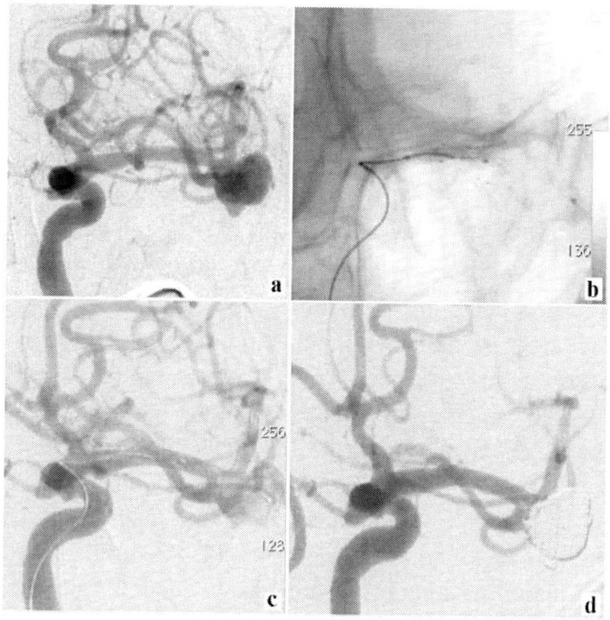

Figure 16. Stent-assisted (2 stents) embolization of an MCA bifurcation aneurysm with detachable coils (Y-stenting, Jailing): a – a saccular aneurysm at the M1 bifurcation of the MCA; b, c – two stents were implanted from different M2 segments into one M1 segment, a coiling microcatheter was delivered into the aneurysm; d – after coiling the sac, the aneurysm was totally occluded.

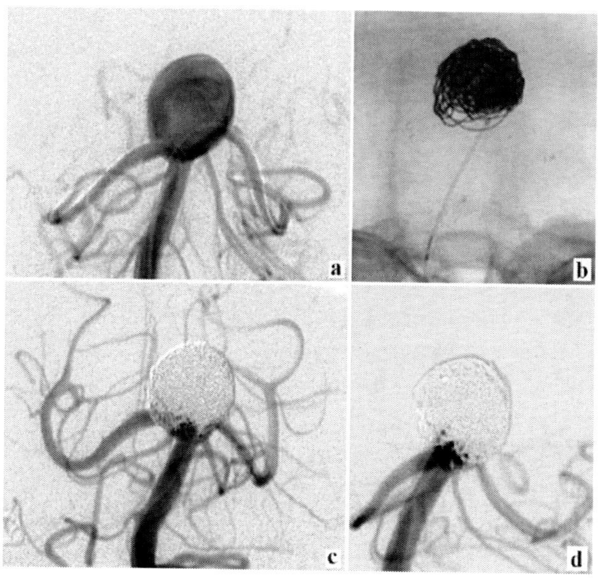

Figure 17. Y-stenting andjailiing for embolization of aBA bifurcation aneurysm:
a – a saccular aneurysm at the BA bifurcation, two microcatheters were placed into both PCAs; b – the stents insertedin the branches intersected in the BA (Y-stenting), coils were delivered; c – the aneurysm was totally occluded; d –the coils clearly visualized in the anterior and posterior overhanging parts of the aneurysmal sac.

Transverse stenting is also effective for treating the aneurysms in the basilar-artery bifurcation, but its application is only possible if the patient has at least one Pcom (Figure 19). F-stenting is an unusual technique that we apply for treating the aneurysms of the superior cerebellar artery (Figure 20). The use of this stenting techniques can be combined with jailing and with introduction of a microcatheter to perform coiling through the cells of the stents. However, if a wide-neck aneurysm is localized in a bifurcation and bifurcation stenting is impossible due to the small size of one of the branches, it is possible to use the waffle-cone technique (Figure 21).

In some cases, if a stent does not fit well to the artery wall, a balloon can be used to expand the stent and ensure its proper adherence. Moreover, a balloon can be used to expand the cells of the first stent during bifurcation stenting. With the advent of double-lumen balloons, a new stenting technique of introducing a stent through a balloon has appeared (link to our article). To perform this technique, first, a double-lumen balloon is placed at the aneurysmal neck, then a microcatheter is delivered into the aneurysm and the standard balloon-assisted embolization is carried out, after which the guide is removed from the lumen of the inflated balloon to be replaced with a low-profile stent. Then, the balloon is gradually deflated and the stent is implanted at the neck of the aneurysm. After that, the balloon is brought back into the stent's lumen through the stent delivery system to the neck of the aneurysm to be inflated and expand the stent, so it adheres better to the artery wall. In addition, if necessary, additional coils are delivered to provide a denser packing of the aneurysm (Figure 22) [68].

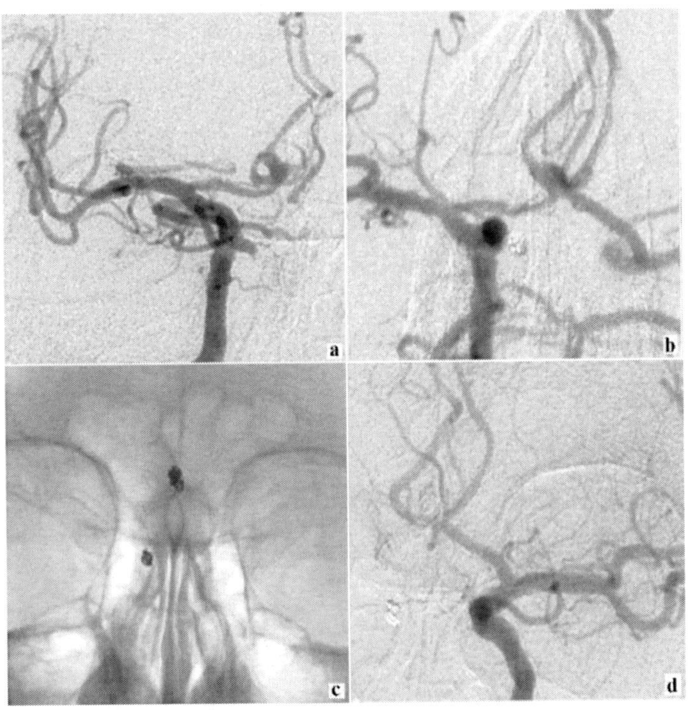

Figure 18. Endovascular treatment of multiple cerebral aneurysms in one stage in one patient suffering from acute SAH: a,b,c – balloon-assisted coiling of RICA aneurysms; d,e,f – stent-assisted coiling of Acom aneurysms, both stents were implanted from the vessels opposite to A2 to the vessels opposite to A1 from different carotid territories, the coils were placed through the primary (jailed) microcatheter (X stenting).

Flow Diverters

A significant breakthrough in the surgery of giant and fusiform aneurysms was the creation of self-expanding FDs with very small cells to reduce the blood flow in aneurysmal sac and set up conditions for the thrombosis and subsequent resorption of the aneurysm, while preserving arterial branches and perforants [69-72].

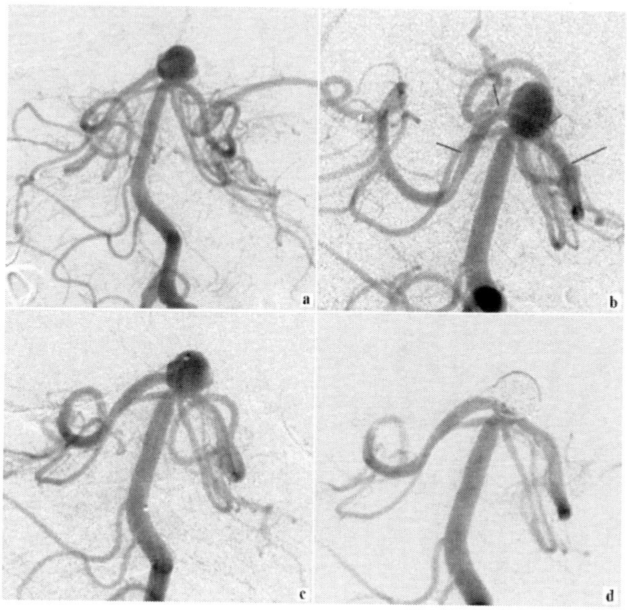

Figure 19. Endovascular treatment of a BAbifurcation aneurysm with stent-assisted detachable coils: a,b– a stenting microcatheter was inserted through the LPcom into the LPCA (red lines); c - the stent was implanted from right P1 to left P2, the microcatheter was fixed in the aneurysm; d – the aneurysm was totally occluded(transverse stenting).

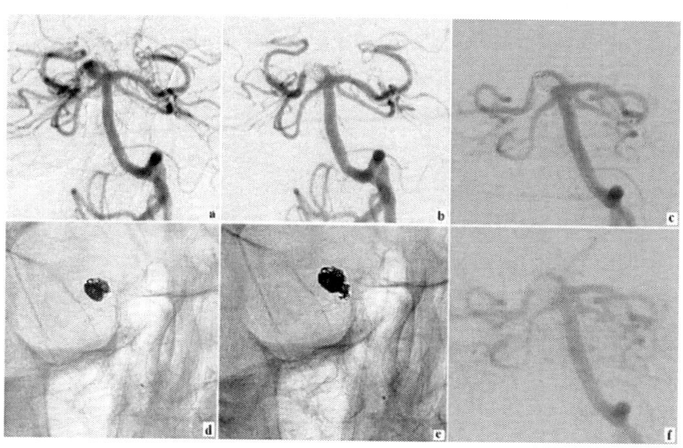

Figure 20. Endovascular treatment of an aneurysm in the ostium of the RSCA with stent-assisted detachable coils: a,b - the first stage of treatment in acute SAH, total embolization with coils; c – near-to-neck recanalization (4-month DSA control); d,e - 2 stents were implanted from right P1 and the SCA into the BA; e, f – the aneurysm was totally occluded (F-stenting).

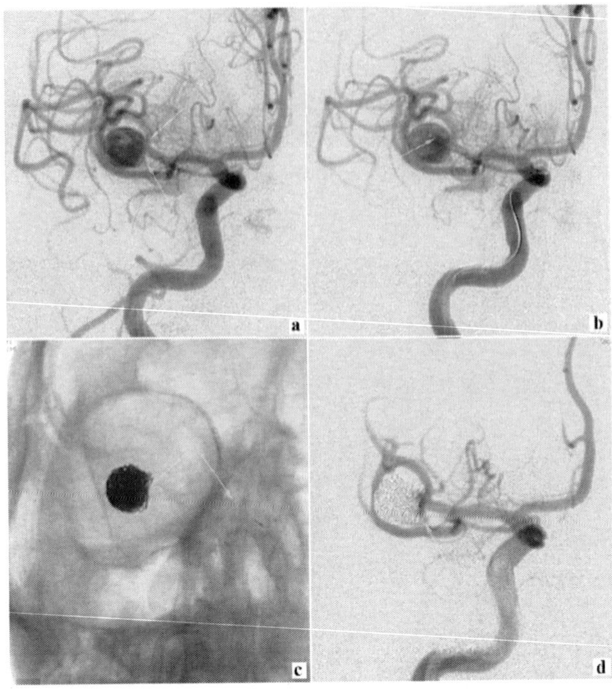

Figure 21. Endovascular treatment of an aneurysm in the bifurcation of the RMCA with stent-assisted detachable coils: a,b - a microcatheter was inserted into the aneurysmal sac; c - a low-profile intracranial stent was implanted from the neck of the aneurysm into the carrier's lumen; d - the aneurysm was totallyoccluded (waffle-cone stenting).

FD implantation technique is similar to that for other intracranial stents, but has its own features. Anticoagulant therapy (75 mg of clopidogrel and 100 mg of aspirin) begins 5-7 days before surgery, or the patient is administered a loading dose of clopidogrel (300 mg in 2 days), after which a test to estimate the effectiveness of dual antiplatelet therapy is performed. If clopidogrel is ineffective, it is replaced with ticagrelor. In the postoperative period, the patient continues to take 75 mg of clopidogrel or ticagrelor for 6-12 months, 100 mg of aspirin for 12 months. However, in giant fusiform aneurysms, the duration of dual antiplatelet therapy can be extended up to life-long. It is necessary to carefully plan the operation thoroughly measuring the diameter of the carrier artery and the size of its defect based digital subtraction or MSCT angiographic images to select a stent of appropriate diameter and length. The diameter of the stent must exactly match that of the artery, the difference to be no more than +0.25 mm, since a smaller stent can migrate distally, and a larger stent will not be able to fully open in the artery, which will lead to stent thrombosis. The length of the stent should be at least 10 mm longer than the length of the arterial defect. The longer the stent, the safer its implantation is, but one has to remember that the arteries have a cone-shaped structure, and the stent is cylindrical, so when implanting a stent of excessive length, its proximal part may not be fixed to the walls of the artery, which can also lead to stent thrombosis, therefore, more experienced surgeons prefer shorter FDs.

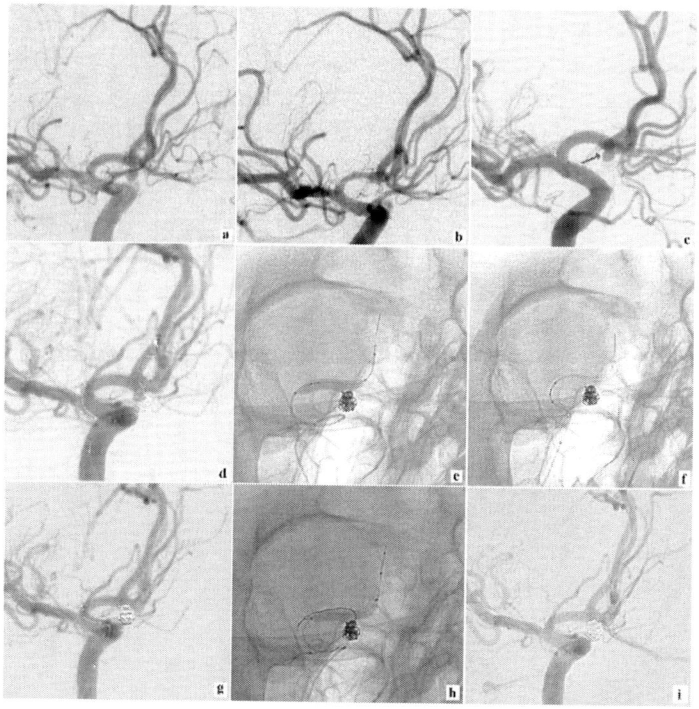

Figure 22. Balloon-and stent-assisted treatment of anAcom aneurysm: a, b – the aneurysm was firsttreatedwhile acute hemorrhage; c –recanalization at follow-up (red arrow); d – coils could not be placed without assistance; e – balloon-assisted coiling; f, g – a low-profile stent implanted through a balloon catheter; h – stent angioplasty performed using the same balloon;i – the aneurysm was totally occluded.

Implantation of an FD typically requires a coaxial distal access delivery system that includes a long sheath and a distal access guiding catheter that is positioned distally enough relative to the cavernous ICA segment (Figure 23) or the V4 segment of the vertebral artery. Then a microcatheter to place a stent is delivered along the guidewire distal to the aneurysm. To deliver these stents one uses larger microcatheters whose distal part size varies from 2.1 to 2.7F. In cases of giant aneurysms, it is not always possible to deliver the microcatheter distal to the aneurysm, so it is necessary to pass the wire through the aneurysm cavity and form a loop in it to bring the microcatheter as distally as possible. When it is done, the guidewire is removed from the catheter and the formed loop is straightened. If the loop cannot be straightened, a thrombextractor is delivered through the microcatheter and used as an anchor (Figure 24). A stent is then inserted into the microcatheter to be delivered as far as the catheter's distal mark. The microcatheter is then displaced proximally, to the position chosen for stent implantation, and the stent is brought 3-5 mm into the lumen after its distal part opens [73-75]. The stent is slowly delivered into the lumen in 3-4 steps, since it takes time to open it. After the stent is implanted and to prevent it from getting caught by the delivery system, the microcatheter is delivered distal to the stent, and the entire delivery system is removed. In case of underexpansion, do not immediately remove the microcatheter, but leave it in the FD's lumen, remove the delivery system and insert a microguidewire to massage the stent with it. If, after these manipulations, the FD remains unexpanded, use a balloon catheter to open it (Figure 25).

In a number of cases, when it was impossible perform antegrade catheterization of an aneurysm and where the anatomy of the cerebral vessels allowed it, we carried out retrograde catheterization inserting a 1.7F microcatheter proximal to the aneurysm to insert a 14F wire of 300 cm through it for delivering an introducer and a 2.7F microcatheter [76-77]. The last was placed distally to the aneurysm and the wire was removed to deliver an FD (Figure 26).

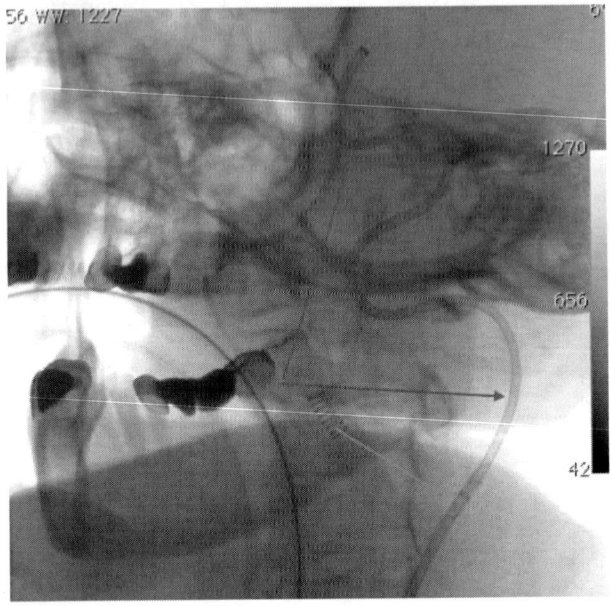

Figure 23. Coaxial system for a distal access in the left carotid territory, consisting of a long sheath (blue line) and a distal guiding catheter (red arrows).

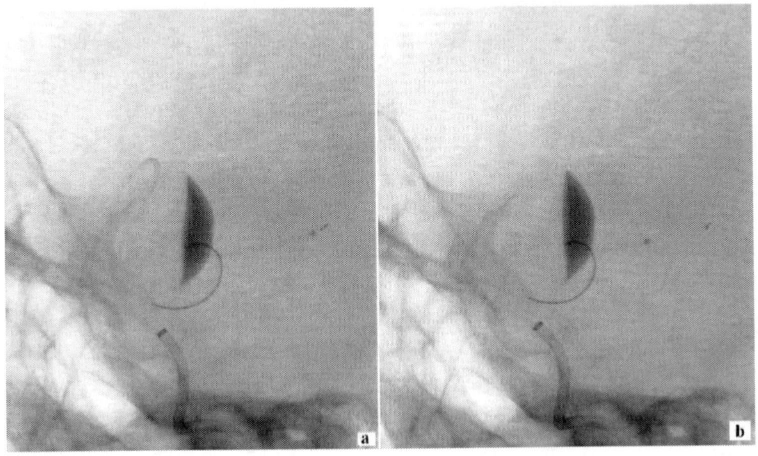

Figure 24. Introducing a microcatheter distal to the aneurysm through the aneurysmal sac (a), followed by loop straightening (b).

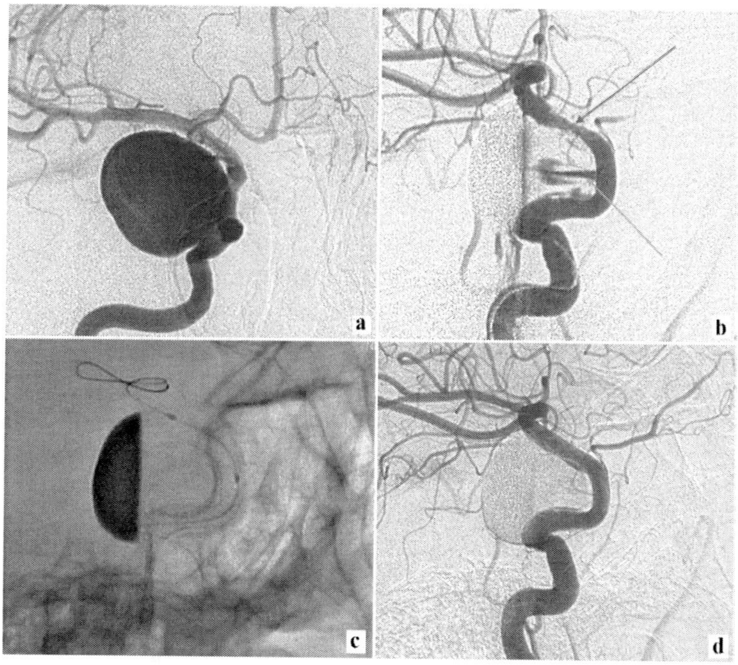

Figure 25. Implanting a Pipeline stent at the neck of a giant aneurysm in the infraclinoid ICA (a, b). After the implantation, a pronounced jet flow (blue arrow) in the aneurysm cavity and underexpansion of the stent's distal part (red arrow) were detected, and balloon angioplasty was performed (c, d).

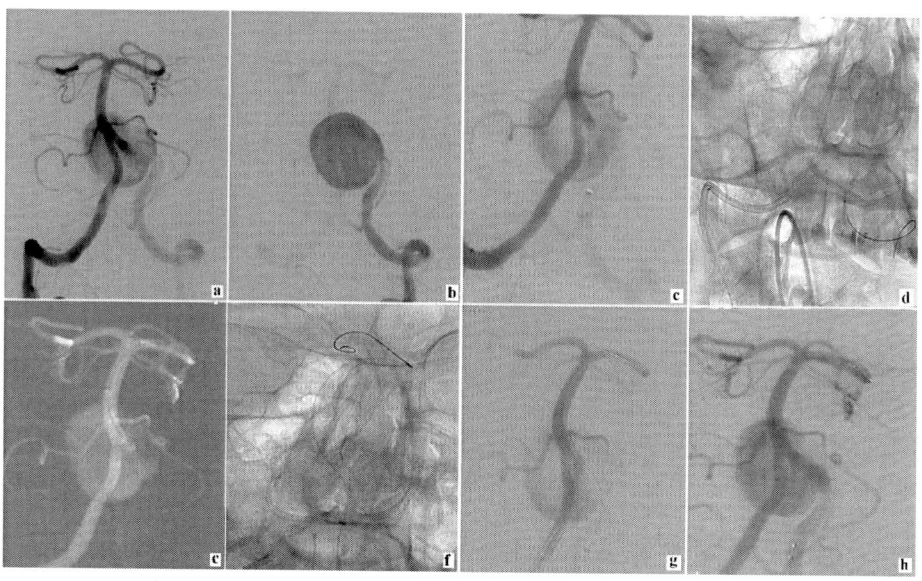

Figure 26. FD treatment of a large aneurysm in the left vertebral artery.
The anatomical features did not allow for antegrade insertion of the 2.7F microcatheter (a, b, c). Therefore, a retrograde delivery of a 1.7F microcatheter from the right vertebral arterythrough the aneurysm into the leftvertebral artery was performed, followed by insertion of a 0.014''-300 cm microguide into the opposite guide catheter and its removal (d). Subsequently, a 2.7F microcatheter (e, f, j) was placed posterior to the aneurysm through this guidewire and an FD was implanted (h).

Post-Embolization Complications

Post-Coiling Complications

These complications are subdivided into three main types to be ischemic, hemorrhagic, and technical ones [78-82].

Intraoperative hemorrhage being the most serious kind that can occur due to improper manipulations with a guidewire or microcatheter. Hemorrhage can occur due to manipulation with a guidewire or microcatheter; in some cases, an aneurysm can rupture when a rigid or improperly sized coil is implanted or when the aneurysm is coiled too tightly (Figure 27); a rupture can also occur while performing aneurysmography (Figure 28) or operating an assistance balloon (Figure 29). Sometimes hemorrhages develop for reasons beyond a surgeon's control, e.g., while diagnostic or staged angiography (Figure 30), or spontaneously, due to an uncontrolled jump in blood pressure.

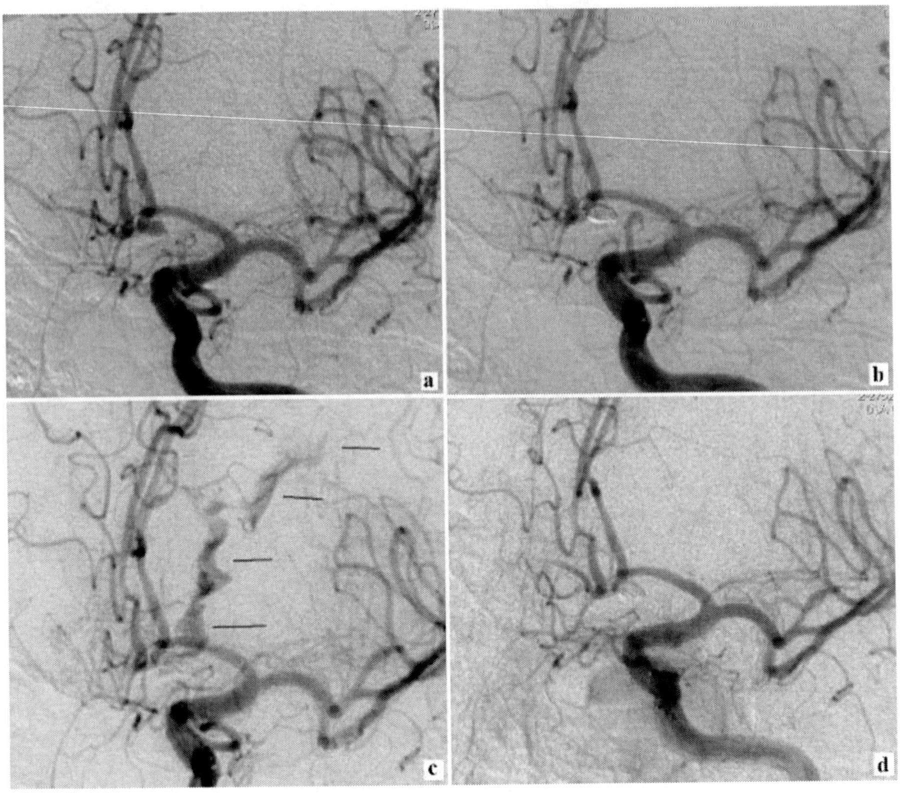

Figure 27. Rupture of anAcom aneurysm:a - diagnostic angiography. b – control angiography before separation of the last coil, the aneurysmwas totally occluded; c, d – near-to-neck rupture, the contrast spread into the cavity of a previously formed hematoma and intraventricularly with the last coil falling into the arterial lumen; e - the bleeding was stopped through controlled hypotension and protamine administration, the aneurysm was totally occluded.

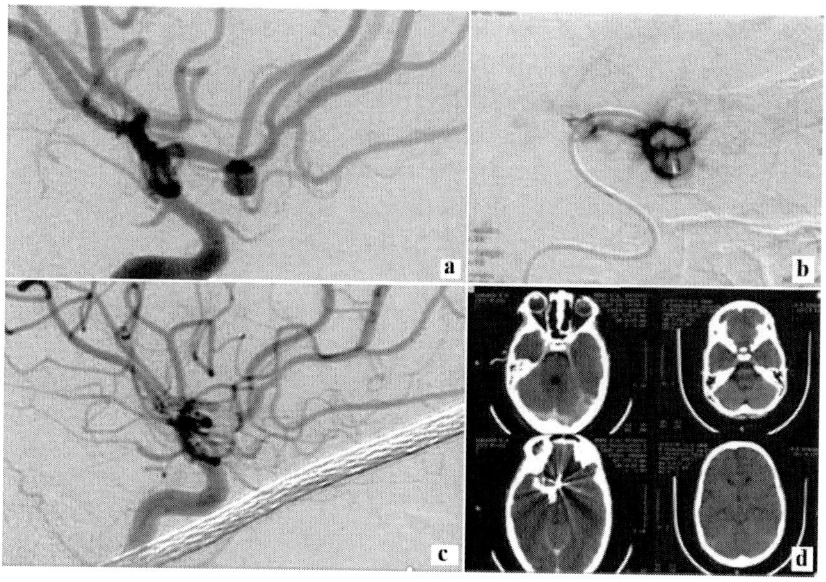

Figure 28. Rupture of anAcom aneurysm:a–an angiographic image before the rupture;b–the aneurysm ruptured during aneurysmography;c - the bleeding stopped after total occlusion of the aneurysm; d - CT scan immediately after the intervention revealed an extravasal contrast spread and SAH; a CT scan 2 weeks later showedSAH regression.

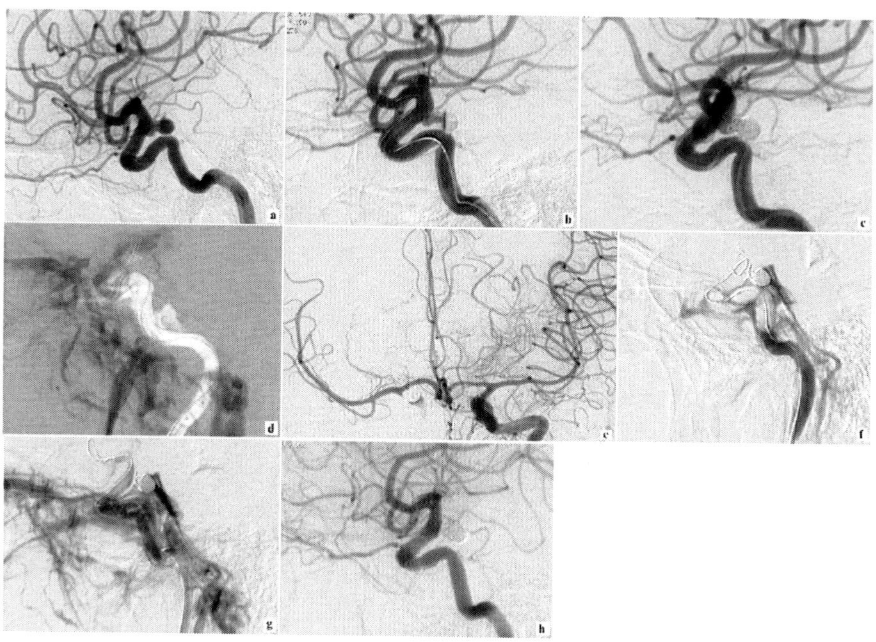

Figure 29. Stent- and balloon-assisted embolization of an ICA aneurysm: a - diagnostic angiography; b - angiography after stent implantation at theaneurysmal neck showed a significant slowdown in blood flow in the aneurysm with contrast stagnation; c– embolization stage, to evacuate theresidual contrast at the neckballoon assistance was performed; d- ICA dissection due to balloon assistance that led to the development of massive SAH and carotid-cavernous fistula; e - the bleeding was temporarily stopped through balloon occlusion of the ICA; f, g - functioning carotid-cavernous fistula in presence balloon occlusion;h–the bleeding stopped after implantation of a graft stent.

Regardless of the causes that have led to an aneurysm rupture, follow this protocol if you have detected contrast media extravasation:

1. Do not panic and do not make unnecessary movements!
2. Even if the manipulation is performed by an experienced surgeon, a colleague should be called in, if possible, a senior one, since one head and two arms are good, but two heads and four arms are always better.
3. Administer protamine to inactivate heparin.
4. Intraoperative rupture is always accompanied by an increase in blood pressure, therefore, in case if such a sudden rise is observed, perform angiography or angioscopy so that the rupture does not go unnoticed, and then ask the anesthesiologist to reduce the blood pressure (down to the average 60–70 mmHg.).

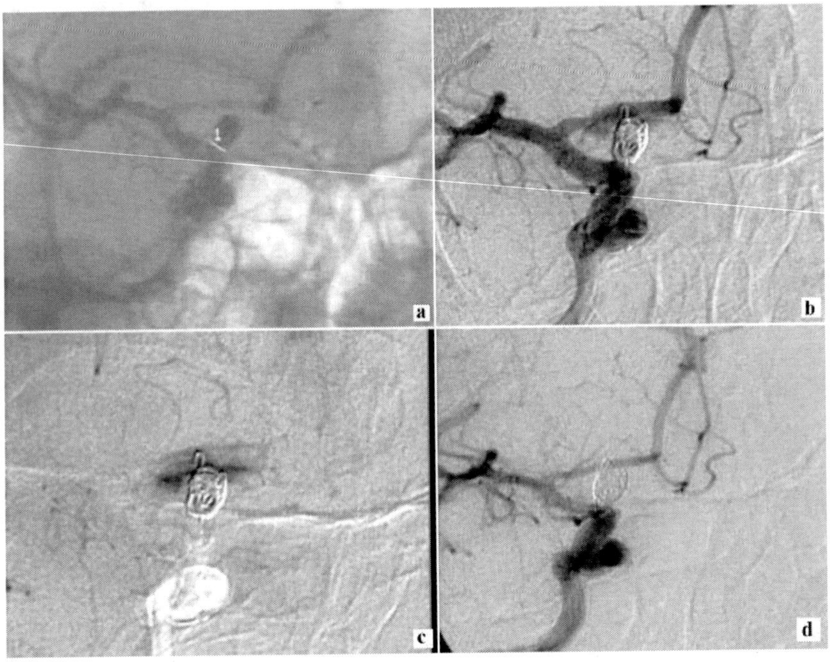

Figure 30. Rupture of an ICA aneurysm while staged angiography: a-diagnostic angiography revealed a wide-neck aneurysm in the ICA; b, c–the aneurysm ruptured during staged angiography after insertion of the second coil into the cavity, the coil prolapsed from the aneurysm and an extravasal contrast spread was detected; d - bleeding stopped after total occlusion of the aneurysm.

5. Do not stop the manipulation and do not remove a microcatheter from the aneurysm, and if the rupture has occurred at the approach stage, insert the microcatheter into the aneurysm as quickly and atraumatically as possible. If the microcatheter has migrated into the aneurysmal defect, do not try to withdraw it from the ruptured area, since sometimes it can cover the perforation and prevent bleeding. In this case, take a coil of maximum length, whose diameter corresponds to that of the aneurysm, and start inserting the coil into the subarachnoid space, gradually moving it into the aneurysmal lumen. Remember that this manipulation is best-performed when using balloon assistance (Figure 31).

6. Start or continue coiling, trying to achieve the total occlusion of the aneurysm as quickly as possible, as this is the only way to reliably stop bleeding (Figure 27-29).
7. When performing balloon assistance, inflate the last at the aneurysmal neck and do not deflate it until the aneurysm is totally occluded (Figure 31).

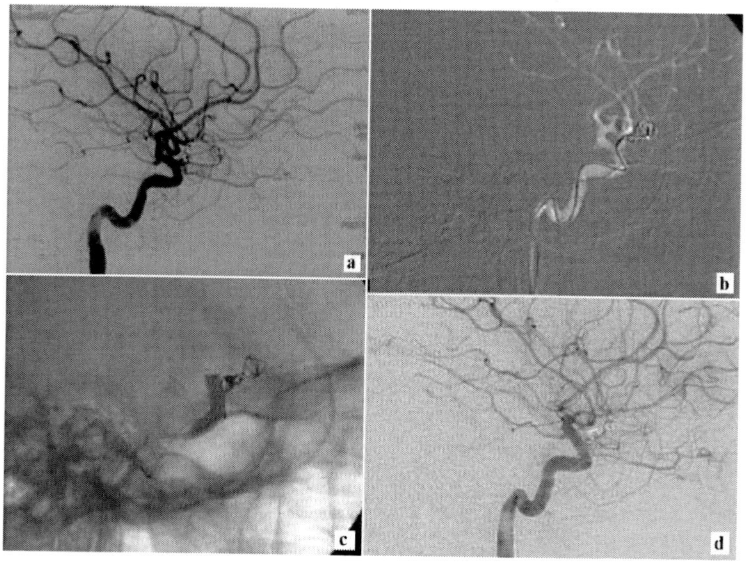

Figure 31. Rupture of an ICA aneurysm: a - diagnostic angiography. b – the coil prolapsed from the aneurysm; c – the bleeding stopped with a balloon; d – the aneurysm was totally occluded.

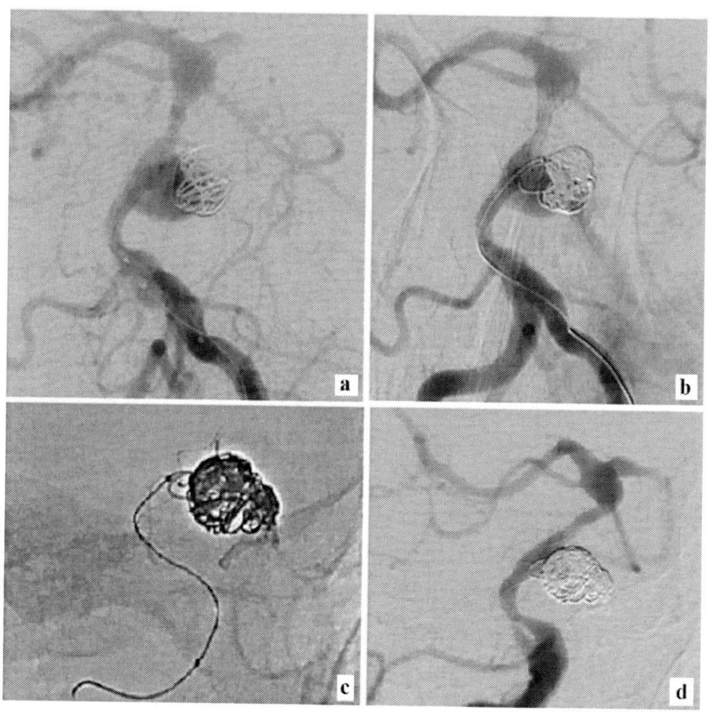

Figure 32. Recanalizationof a BA aneurysmin presence of severe atherosclerosis (a). The aneurysm ruptured while coiling (b). The bleeding was stopped with coils and ONYX (orange arrow) (c, d).

8. If for some reason it is not possible to completely occlude an aneurysm with coils, then hemostasis can be achieved with ONYX injected between the coils (Figure 32)
9. Near-to-neck rupture and carrier-vessel dissection are the most dangerous complications, which, among other reasons, can occur due to total coil occlusion. If such a complication is detected, it is necessary to very carefully occlude the carrier using a balloon. If this manipulation in combination with reduced blood pressure and administration of protamine does not stop bleeding, consider implanting a graft stent (Figure 29). In presence of reliable collaterals, total occlusion in some cases can also be achieved by injecting ONYX between the implanted coils.

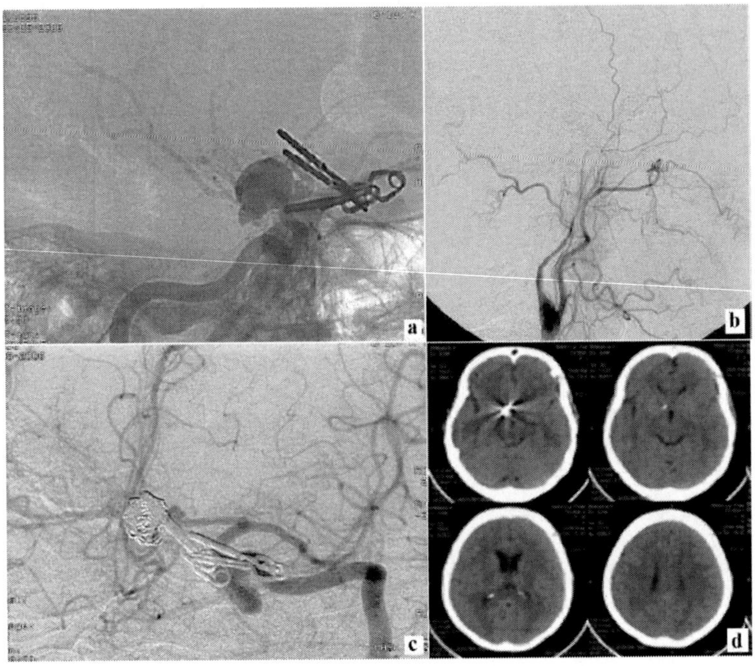

Figure 33. ICA thrombosis while aneurysm embolization: a - diagnostic angiography; b–ICA thrombosis after embolization; c – satisfactory contralateral filling of the thrombosed ICA territory; d - postoperative CT showedno ischemic lesions.

After completion of the operation, do not cancel the anesthesia until performing a control CT to assess the severity of the hemorrhage, and, if necessary, decide on removal of the hematoma, implantation a ventricular drainage and an intracranial pressure sensor. Even if no microsurgical manipulations are required, therapeutic anesthesia is recommended, its duration is determined by hemorrhage severity and the patient's condition. Later, manage the patient following the SAH treatment protocol.

To prevent intraoperative aneurysm rupture, follow these recommendations:

- Use soft atraumatic guidewires of 0.010" (max. 0.014") in diameter with a flexible distal part for aneurysm catheterization;
- Limit guidewire manipulation in the aneurysmal cavity;

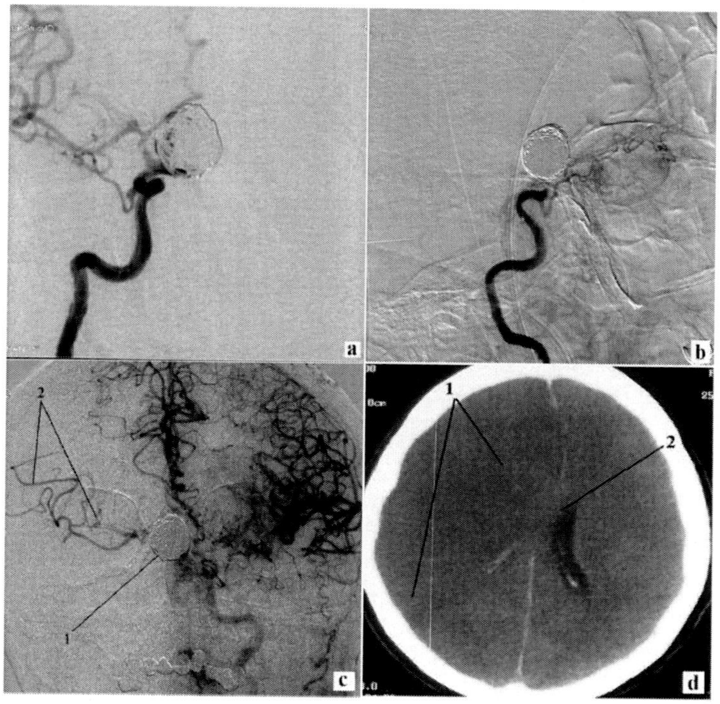

Figure 34. Aneurysm of the ophthalmic RICA segment: a – carotid angiogram in direct projection detected an embolized aneurysm of the right ICA; b – carotid angiogram in oblique projection showedthe ICA lumen thrombosed with a conglomerate of coils with no contrast in the right ACA and MCA; c - control left-sided angiogram:1 - embolized gigantic aneurysm the ophthalmic RICA segment; 2 - filling of the branches of the right MCA from the left carotid basin through the Acom, the RICA was not contrasted; d - CT scan of the brain in axial projection: 1 - total ischemia of the right hemisphere, 2 - transverse dislocation.

- Use soft, atraumatic catheters for catheterization of the cavity; it is desirable to use pre-shaped microcatheters, no larger than 0.017–0. 018" ID;
- Do not perform aneurysmography through a microcatheter if there are other possibilities for visualizing the position of the catheter's distal part, and if it is not possible to assess the position of the catheter otherwise, then it should be performed with a syringe of at least 2 ml, and very carefully;
- Carefully choose the coils to match the size of the aneurysm, do not use rigid coils while acute rupture;
- Perform heparin bolus administration only after the first coil is introduced;
- If it is not possible to introduce a coil into the aneurysm, remove it and take a shorter or smaller one, stop in time when the aneurysm is "packed", especially while acute rupture;
- Always have a balloon ready to perform balloon assistance.

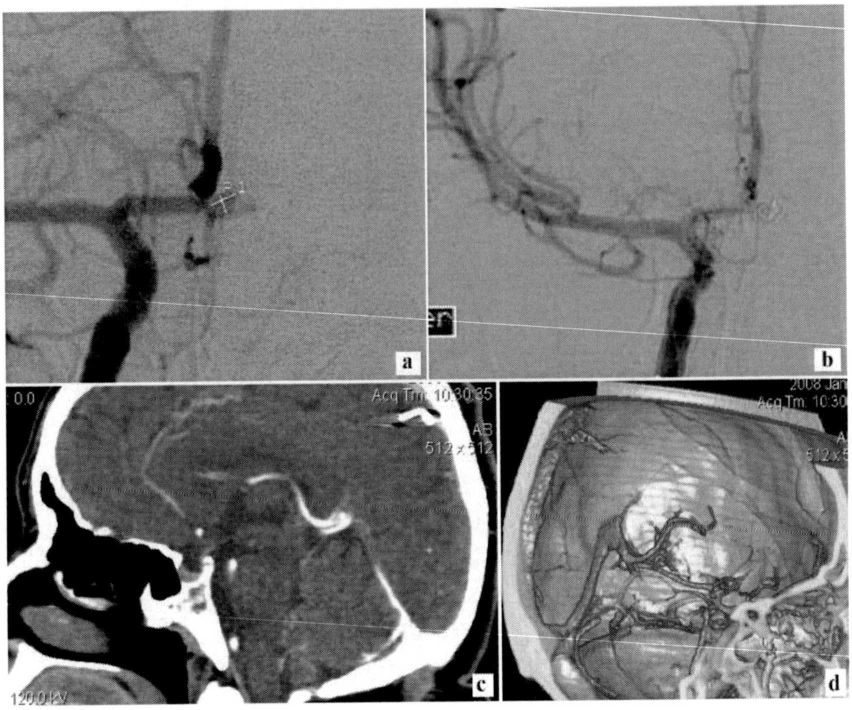

Figure 35. Inadequate embolization of ACA-Acom aneurysm with one coil (a, b). Coil migration to the distal ACA branches in the postoperative period (c, d).

Ischemic complications while endovascular interventions, as a rule, develop for the following reasons:

- Worsening vasospasm while acute rupture;
- Worsening spasm caused by a guide catheter or microcatheter manipulations;
- Thromboembolism from a guide catheter or from the cavity of a partially thrombosed aneurysm, or when an atherosclerotic plaque is torn off by a guide catheter or a microcatheter;
- Stenosis or thrombosis of the carrier artery in case of inadequate aneurysm embolization (Figures 33, 34) or the occlusion of one of the branches while bifurcation aneurysm embolization;
- Migration of a part or even a whole coil into the arterial lumen followed by their further migration into the distal branches (Figure 35);
- Stent thrombosis (Figure 36).

For prevention of ischemic complications, follow these recommendations:

- At all stages, constantly flush the guide catheter and microcatheter;
- Administer a 5000-unit bolus heparin after introduction of the first coil; in case of prolonged manipulations, 1000 units of heparin are to be administered every subsequent hour under ACT control;

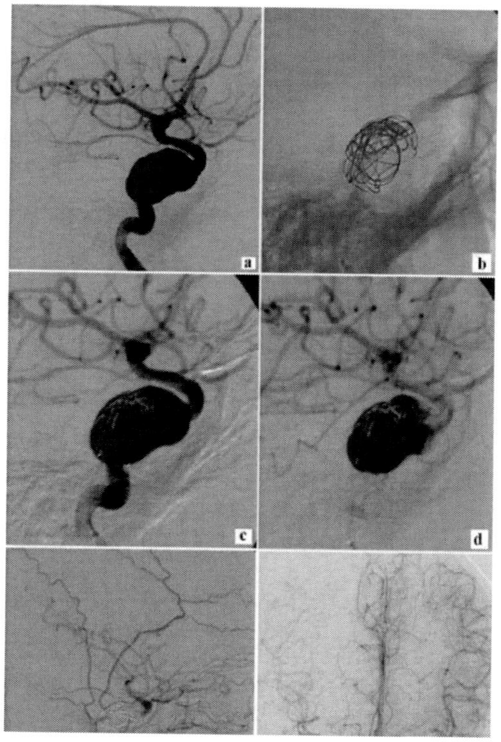

Figure 36. Long-term Silk stent thrombosis in presence of antiplatelet therapy: a - diagnostic angiography, a fusiform aneurysm detected in the right internal carotid artery; b, c, – control angiograms after stent-assisted coiling showed satisfactory contrast stagnation in the aneurysm; d, e - asymptomatic stent thrombosis detected by 6-month control angiography, satisfactory filling of the right internal carotid artery through theECAanastomoses and the Acom.

- Make sure the guide catheter does not block the arterial lumen; there should be no slowdown in blood or contrast flow around the guide catheter;
- In case of a manipulation spasm, move the guide catheter more proximally and slowly inject 0.4–0.8 mg of Nimotop diluted in 20 ml of saline;
- Deliver the microcatheter using the roadmap mode to prevent the dissection of atherosclerotic plaques;
- Balloon or stent assistance is the best way to embolize partially thrombosed aneurysms; for giant partially thrombosed aneurysms an FD should be preferred;
- When coiling an aneurysm, carrier-artery stenosis should be avoided. After introducing each coil, perform staged angiography or angioscopy before its separation, visualizing the patency of all arterial branches around the aneurysm. In a branch not filled with blood, remove the coil to introduce another one of smaller diameter or length;
- Avoid coil migration into the carrier artery; in case of carrier-artery stenosis or uncontrolled coil migration, consider implanting a stent;
- Always strive for dense "packing" of an aneurysm to prevent possible coil migration. Never introduce a single coil in a wide-neck aneurysm. An intervention cannot be limited to reinforcing the walls of the aneurysm;

- Use a retriever to immediately remove a detached coil when the last has migrated into the carrier artery;
- In case of thrombosis or thromboembolism of any of the arteries, thrombus extraction, thromboaspiration or intravenous administration of antiplatelet agents are indicated, if thrombolysis is ineffective.
- If vasospasm is detected while acute aneurysmal rupture, perform chemical angioplasty regardless of hemorrhage duration; if chemical angioplasty is ineffective, consider balloon angioplasty.

Complications After FD Implantation

As with coils, intraoperative complications after FD implantation include hemorrhagic, ischemic, and technical ones; long-term complications should be singled out as a separate group. The hemorrhagic complications usually occur for three main reasons: Perforation of an aneurysm or a small distal vessel by a guidewire when delivering a microcatheter; perforation of a distal vessel by a delivery system's guidewire while implanting an FD; and, being the most formidable one, an aneurysmal rupture due to the microcatheter loop formed when passing it through the cavity. In the case of vessel perforation, coil the artery as soon as possible until the bleeding stops. When an aneurysm ruptures, deconstruct the segment because, as a rule, an FD is implanted to treat the aneurysms that are inaccessible for coil embolization. In addition, given the dual antiplatelet therapy, it is not always possible to stop bleeding using only coils. In such cases, inject ONYX between coils that will occlude the rupture directly and fill the space between coils in the cavity to achieve reliable hemostasis.

Ischemic complications after FD implantation commonly develop either due to stent thrombosis, which can occur even with adequate antiplatelet therapy, or due to thrombosis of perforant vessels. If intraoperative thrombosis is detected, intravenous antiplatelet agents or thrombolytics are to be administered. The use of thrombus extraction or thromboaspiration is undesirable, as this may lead to displacement of the stent.

Technical complications usually occur for two reasons that are improper choice of the size of the stent and its improper implantation. Not only is it important to choose the right length and diameter of the stent, it has to be implanted at least 5 mm distal to the aneurysm and 5 mm proximal to it. A stent that is too short can migrate into the aneurysm, and a stent that is too long may not open properly. A stent that is too long makes it difficult to calculate where its proximal part will end, which can lead to incorrect selection of the stent diameter and an endoleak in the proximal part. The diameter of the stent must exactly match the diameter of the artery, especially in its proximal part. Implanting a stent that is too large in diameter results in its elongation and difficulties with opening. It also changes the stent's cell, which in turn reduces the treatment's radicality. A stent, whose diameter is smaller than that of an artery may provoke an endoleak. Such a stent may also be displaced to the degree it enters into the aneurysm. Another dangerous technical complication is twisting of the stent. In this case, it is preferable not to separate the stent, but to remove it. The most difficult complications, however, are displacements of the stent's distal and proximal parts or of an entire stent into the aneurysm (Figure 37). In such cases, the stents are either removed or telescopic stenting is performed.

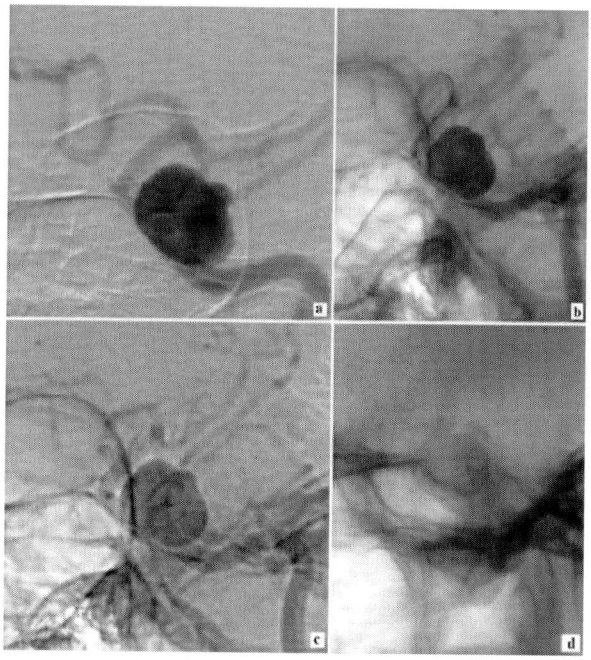

Figure 37. Treatment of a large ICA aneurysm: a –after implantation of a first FD, cerebral angiography detected a reduction of its proximal part, so it prolapsed into the aneurismal sac; b – a loop was used to deliver a microcatheter inside the stent; c, d – a second FD was opened inside the first stent.

Balloon and Chemical Angioplasty

Balloon angioplasty as a technique to treat vasospasm while acute aneurysmal rupture was first proposed by Yu. N. Zubkov et al. (1984). To perform balloon angioplasty, it is necessary to insert a compliance balloon catheter directly into the spasm zone and slowly inflate the balloon until the desired result is achieved. In case of diffuse vasospasm, repeat this manipulation in the vascular territory prone to vasospasm (Figure 38).

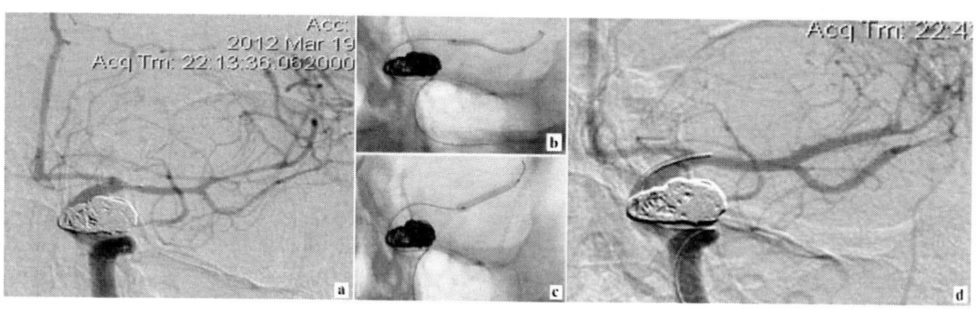

Figure 38. Balloon angioplasty of vasospasm: a – an aneurysm of the left ICA was occluded while acute rupture with detachable coils, pronounced angiographic vasospasm of the MCA was noted; b – balloon angioplasty of the anterior M2 was performed; c – balloon angioplasty of the superior M2 was performed; d – expansion of the M1-M2 segments of the MCA.

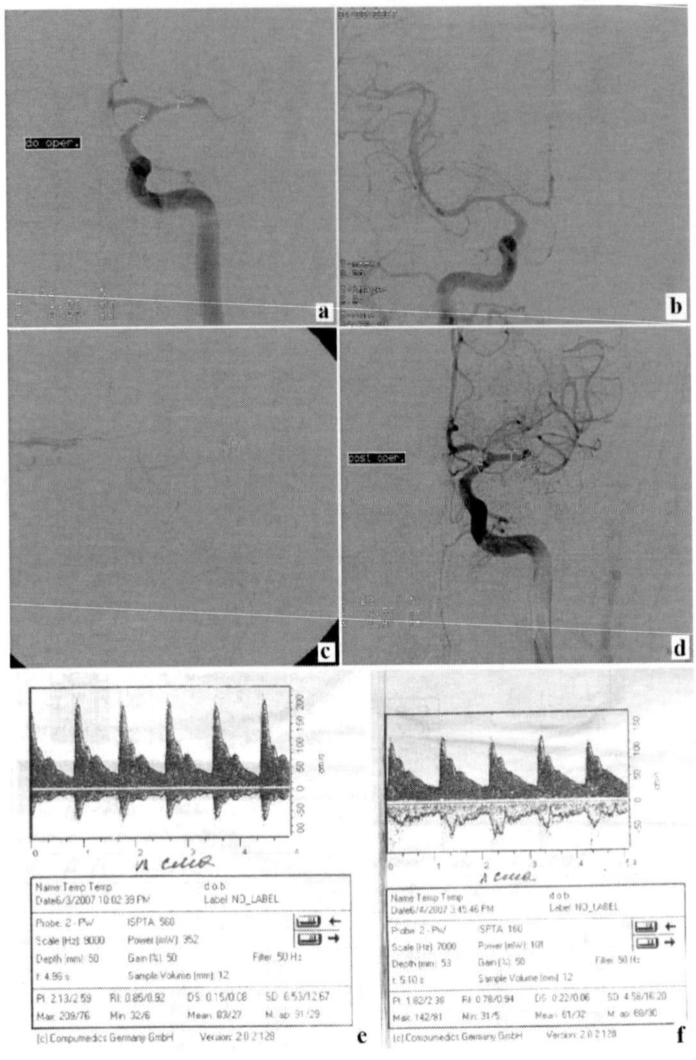

Figure 39. Embolization of an LMCA aneurysm, chemical angioplasty: a, b - diagnostic angiographyrevealed diffuse vasospasm and an aneurysm in the LMCA bifurcation; c - angioplasty in the right carotid territory was performed from the contralateral approach; d – postoperative angiograms demonstrating a total exclusion of the aneurysm, improved filling of the left hemisphere, a significant increase in the diameter of spasmodic arteries after chemical angioplasty; e – transcranial dopplerography of the LMCA before surgery; f – a post-operational image demonstrating a decrease in the linear blood flow velocity.

Later, various options for chemical angioplasty were proposed that included selective and superselective use of antispasmodics, calcium channel blockers, and nitrates. The method that seems to be the most effective is 0.2–0.4 mg of Nimotop diluted in 20 ml of saline. The solution is slowly injected through a guide catheter immediately after it is delivered into the target artery. In presence of an adequate approach to the aneurysm, its embolization is to be performed. If a pronounced vasospasm does not allow delivering a microcatheter through a spasmed vessel or causes a contrast delay in it, then it is necessary to first inject Nimotop into the carrier artery, and then place a microcatheter into the aneurysm cavity to embolize it. After that, the microcatheter is alternately placed in all spasmed arteries for superselective injection of 0.4 mg of Nimotop diluted in 20 ml of saline. The total dose of administered Nimotop should not exceed 2–3 mg, lower doses are usually ineffective, while the overdose and rapid administration can lead to uncontrolled hypotension. In absence of the visible effect, opt for balloon angioplasty. Chemical angioplasty should be performed under intubation anesthesia and radial artery blood pressure control. Blood-flow linear velocity monitoring has shown chemical angioplasty has an unstable effect that lasts no more than a day, but this may be enough to compensate for the patient's condition. In the postoperative period, when the aneurysm is properly occluded, it becomes possible to conduct more intensive therapy aimed at treating vasospasm, including hypertension, hemodilution, and hypervolemia (3H-therapy) (Figure 39).

Conclusion

Being brought into practice more than 50 years ago, embolization has gone a long way from handmade balloons to modern coils, balloon/stent assistance and flow- diverting techniques [83-84]. At the dawn of endovascular surgery, this approach had significant limitations, such as cervical-vessel tortuosity, wide-neck, giant and fusiform aneurysms, but today most of these problems have been successfully resolved. So, nowadays in pronounced tortuosity of bracheocephalic vessels, it has become possible to use coaxial distal access systems that can be delivered up to the cavernous segment of the ICAs and the V4 segment of the vertebral arteries to greatly facilitate manipulations in cerebral arteries. For wide-neck aneurysms, one can apply balloon- and stent-assisted techniques. The advent of low-profile stents has greatly simplified the implementation of complex stenting options, turning them into routine. Introducing FDs has revolutionized the treatment of giant, fusiform and blister-like aneurysms. All these techniques and instrumentation have made endovascular surgery of aneurysms a highly effective method to combine radicality and safety and produce good functional results at a low level of mortality and morbidity, which makes it possible to treat aneurysms of almost any localizations including ruptured and unruptured ones.

References

[1] Zakharov A. G., Suchkov A. A., Krylov V. V. Rupture of arterial cerebral aneurysms being occluded with a microballoon catheter in the early period of subarachnoid hemorrhage. *International Symposium on Cardiovascular and Interventional Radiology*. 1995, 108.

[2] Zubkov Yu. N., Khilko V. A., Yankin V. F. Intravascular interventions for arterial aneurysms. *Intravascular Neurosurgery*. 1982; 1:124-153.

[3] Serbinenko F. A. Catheterization and occlusion of the main vessels of the brain and prospects for vascular neurosurgery development. *Questions of neurosurgery*. 1971; 5:17-27.

[4] Guglielmi G., Vinuela F., Dion J., Duckwiler G. Electrothrombosis of saccular aneurysms via endovascular approach: part 2. Preliminary clinical experience. *J Neurosurg*. 1991, 75:8-14.

[5] Guglielmi G., Vinuela F., Duckwiler G., et al. Endovascular treatment of posterior circulation aneurysms by electrothrombosis using electrically detachable coils. *J Neurosurg*. 1992, 77: p. 515-524.

[6] Groden C., Hagel C., Delling G., Zeumer H. Histological Findings in Ruptured Aneurysms Treated with GDCs: Six Examples at Varying Times after Treatment *AJNR Am. J. Neuroradiol*, 2003. 24:579 - 584.

[7] Halbach V. V., Higashida R. T., Dowd C. F., Barnwell S. L., Fraser K. W., Smith T. P., et al. The efficacy of endosaccular aneurysm occlusion in alleviating neurological deficits produced by mass effect. *J Neurosurg*, 1994, 80:659-666.
[8] Gallas S., Pasco A., Cottier J. P., Gabrillargues J., Drouineau J., Cognard C, and Herbreteau D. A. Multicenter Study of 705 Ruptured Intracranial Aneurysms Treated with Guglielmi Detachable Coils *AJNR Am. J. Neuroradiol*, 2005; 26(7):1723-1731.
[9] Lusseveld E., Brilstra E. H., Nijssen P. C, van Rooij W. J., Sluzewski M., Tulleken C. A., Wijnalda D., Schellens R. L., van der Graaf Y., Rinkel G. J. Endovascular coiling versus neurosurgical clipping in patients with a ruptured basilar tip aneurysm. *J Neurol Neurosurg Psychiatry*, 2002; 73(5): 591-3.
[10] Mordasini P., Schroth G., Guzman R., Barth A., Seiler R. W., Remonda L. Endovascular Treatment of Posterior Circulation Cerebral Aneurysms By Using Guglielmi Detachable Coils: A 10-Year Single-Center Experience with Special Regard to Technical Development. *AJNR Am J Neuroradiol*, 2005; 26:1732-1738.
[11] Kanaan Y., Kaneshiro D., Fraser K., Wang D., Lanzino G. Evolution of endovascular therapy for aneurysm treatment. *Neurosurg Focus*, 2005; 18(2): 128-142.
[12] Malek A. M., Higashida R. T., Phatouros C. C., Dowd C. F., Halbach V. V. Treatment of an intracranial aneurysm using a new three dimensional- shape Guglielmi detachable coil: technical case report. *Neurosurgery*, 1999; 44:1142-1145.
[13] Cloft H. J., Gregory J., Tong F. C., Goldstein J. H., Dion J. E. Use of Three-dimensional Guglielmi Detachable Coils in the Treatment of Wide-necked Cerebral Aneurysms. *AJNR Am. J. Neuroradiol*, 2000; 21:1312-1314.
[14] Molyneux A. J., Cekirge S., Saatci I., Gal G. Cerebral Aneurysm Multicenter European Onyx (CAMEO) Trial: Results of a Prospective Observational Study in 20 European Centers. *AJNR Am. J. Neuroradiol*, 2004; 25:39-51.
[15] Moret J., Cognard C., Weill A, Castaings L., Rey A. Reconstruction technic in the treatment of wide-neck intracranial aneurysms. Long-term angiographic and clinical results. Apropos of 56 cases. *J Neuroradiol*, 1997; Jun;24(1):30-44.
[16] Massoud, T. F, Turgman, F., Ji, C. Endovascular treatment of fusiform aneurysms with stents and coils: technical feasibility in a swine model. *Am. J. Neuroradiol*, 1995; - 16(10):1953–1963.
[17] Alfke K., Straube T., Dorner L., Mehdorn H. M., Jansen O. Endosaccular occlusion of basilar artery bifurcation aneurysms using electrically detachable coils. *AJNR Am. J. Neuroradiol*, 2004; 25:584 - 591.
[18] Brisman J. L., Song J. K., Niimi Y., Berenstein A. Treatment Options for Wide-Necked Intracranial Aneurysms Using a Self-Expandable Hydrophilic Coil and a Self-Expandable Stent Combination. *AJNR Am. J. Neuroradiol*, 2005; 26:1237- 1240.
[19] Chow M. M., Woo H. H., Masaryk T. J., Rasmussen P. A. A novel endovascular treatment of a wide-necked basilar apex aneurysm by using a Y-configuration, double-stent technique. *AJNR Am J Neuroradiol*, 2005; 26(1):198-200.
[20] Islak C., Kocer N., Albayram S., Kizilkilic O., Uzma O., Cokyuksel O. Bare Stent-Graft Technique: A New Method of Endoluminal Vascular Reconstruction for the Treatment of Giant and Fusiform Aneurysms. *AJNR Am. J. Neuroradiol*, 2002; 23: 1589-1595.
[21] Vanninen R., Manninen H., Ronkainen A. Broad-Based Intracranial Aneurysms: Thrombosis Induced by Stent Placement. *AJNR Am. J. Neuroradiol*, 2003; 24:263-266.
[22] Wanke I., Doerfler A., Schoch B., Stolke D., Forsting M. Treatment of Wide-Necked Intracranial Aneurysms with a Self-Expanding Stent System: Initial Clinical Experience. *AJNR Am. J. Neuroradiol*, 2003; 24:1192-1199.
[23] Kan P. Expanding Indications for Flow Diverters: Ruptured Aneurysms, Blister Aneurysms, and Dissecting Aneurysms. *Neurosurgery*, 2020; 86(1):96–103.
[24] Li, Y. L., Roalfe, A., Chu, E. Y., Lee, R. Outcome of Flow Diverters with Surface Modifications in Treatment of Cerebral Aneurysms: Systematic Review and Meta-analysis. *Am. J. Neuroradiol*, 2021; 42(2): 327–333.
[25] Griffin A., Lerner E., Zuchowski A., Zomorodi A., Gonzalez L. F., Hauck E. F. Flow diversion of fusiform intracranial aneurysms. *Neurosurg Rev*, 2021; 44(3):1471-1478.

[26] Orlov K., Kislitsin D., Strelnikov N., Berestov V., Gorbatykh A., Shayakhmetov T., Seleznev P., Tasenko A. Experience using pipeline embolization device with Shield Technology in a patient lacking a full postoperative dual antiplatelet therapy regimen. *Interv Neuroradiol*, 2018; 24(3):270-273.

[27] Li S., Zeng C., Tao W., Huang Z., Yan L., Tian X., Chen F. The Safety and Efficacy of Flow Diversion versus Conventional Endovascular Treatment for Intracranial Aneurysms: A Meta-analysis of Real-world Cohort Studies from the Past 10 Years. *AJNR Am J Neuroradiol*, 2022; 43(7):1004-1011.

[28] Cagnazzo F., di Carlo D. T., Cappucci M., Lefevre P. H., Costalat V., Perrini P. Acutely Ruptured Intracranial Aneurysms Treated with Flow-Diverter Stents: A Systematic Review and Meta-Analysis. *AJNR Am J Neuroradiol*, 2018; 39(9):1669-1675.

[29] Lee J., Kim D. H., Lee S. H., Moon J. H., Yang S. Y., Cho K. T., Kim B. H. Stent-assisted Coiling vs. Flow Diverter for Treating Blood Blister-like Aneurysms: A Proportion Meta-analysis. *Clin Neuroradiol*, 2022; 32(4):889-902.

[30] Molyneux, A., Kerr, R., Yu, Le. International subarachnoid aneurysm trial (ISAT) of neurosurgical clipping versus endovascular coiling in 2143 pts with ruptured intracranial aneurysms: a randomized comparison. *Lancet*, 2005; 366:809–817.

[31] Molyneux, A., Kerr, R., Stratton, I. International Subarachnoid Aneurysm Trial (ISAT) of neurosurgical clipping versus endovascular coiling in 2143 patients with ruptured intracranial aneurysms: a randomised trial. *Lancet,* 2002; 360:1267–1274.

[32] Hemesniemi, J., Koivisto, T. Comments on "The impact of the International Subarachnoid Aneurysm Treatment Trial (ISAT) on neurosurgical practice." *Acta Neurochirgica* (Wien), 2004: 146:203–208.

[33] Shao B., Wang J., Chen Y., He X., Chen H., Peng Y., Yang P., Duan H., Yang F., Teng L. Clipping versus Coiling for Ruptured Intracranial Aneurysms: A Meta-Analysis of Randomized Controlled Trials. *World Neurosurg*, 2019; 127:353-365.

[34] Tang C., Zhang T. S., Zhou L. F. Risk factors for rebleeding of aneurysmal subarachnoid hemorrhage: a meta-analysis. *PLoS One*, 2014; 9;9(6):99536.

[35] Wiebers, D., Whisnant, J., Huston, J. International Study of Unruptured Intracranial Aneurysms Investigators. Unruptured intracranial aneurysms: natural history, clinical outcome, and risks of surgical and endovascular treatment. *Lancet*, 2003; 36:103–110.

[36] Koo, A. B., Elsamadicy, A. A., Lin, I. H. Predictors of Extended Length of Stay Following Treatment of Unruptured Adult Cerebral Aneurysms: A Study of The National Inpatient Sample. *J. stroke Cerebrovasc. Dis*, 2020; 29(11).

[37] Rinaldo, L., Shepherd, D. L., Murphy, M. E. Natural history of untreated unruptured intracranial aneurysms in the elderly. *J. Neurosurg. Sci*, 2020; 64(2):141–146.

[38] Investigators I. S. of U. I. A. International Study of Unruptured Intracranial Aneurysms Investigators: Unruptured Intracranial Aneurysms - risk of rupture and risk of surgical intervention. *N. Engl. J. Med*, 1998; 339:1725–1733.

[39] Konovalov A. N. 1973. *Surgical treatment of cerebral arterial aneurysms*; Moscow, Medicine.

[40] Lazarev V. A. 1983. *Endovasal surgery of arterial aneurysms of the internal carotid artery.* Moscow.

[41] Filatov Yu. M., Eliava Sh. Sh., Myakota A. E. Microsurgical treatment of arterial aneurysms in posterior circulation. In: *Questions of neurosurgery*, 1990; 5: 3-6.

[42] Albayram S., Selcuk H., Kara B., Bozdag E., Uzma O., Kocer N., Islak C. Thromboembolic Events Associated with Balloon-Assisted Coil Embolization: Evaluation with Diffusion-Weighted MR Imaging. *AJNR Am. J. Neuroradiol*, 2004; 25:1768-1777.

[43] Robledo A., Frank T. S., O'Leary S., Kan P. Microsurgical Clipping of a Middle Cerebral Artery Aneurysm After Woven Endobridge Embolization Recurrence. *World Neurosurg*. 2023; 10;177:78.

[44] Batjer H. H., Samson D. S. Causes of morbidity and mortality from surgery of aneurysms of the distal basilar artery. *Neurosurgery*, 1989; 25: 904-916.

[45] Bavinzski G., Killer M., Gruber A., Reinprecht A., Gross C. E., Richling B. Treatment of basilar artery bifurcation aneurysms by using Guglielmi detachable coils: a 6-year experience. *J Neurosurg*, 1999; 90: 843-852.

[46] Drake C. G., Peerless S. J., Herneslielmi U. A. *Surgery of vertebrobasilar aneurysms*. London, Ontario experience on 1767 patients. Springer-Verlag Wein New York, 1996.

[47] Eskridge J. M., Song J. K. Endovascular embolization of 150 basilar tip aneurysms with Guglielmi detachable coils: results of the Food and Drug Administration multicenter clinical trial. *J Neurosurg*, 1998; 89: 81-86.

[48] Gallas S., Pasco A., Cottier J. P., Gabrillargues J., Drouineau J., Cognard C, and Herbreteau D. A. Multicenter Study of 705 Ruptured Intracranial Aneurysms Treated with Guglielmi Detachable Coils *AJNR Am. J. Neuroradiol*, 2005; 26(7): 1723-1731.

[49] Gonzalez N., Murayama Y., Nien Y. L., Martin N., John Frazee, Duckwiler G., Jahan R., Gobin Y. P., Vinuela F. Treatment of Unruptured Aneurysms with GDCs: Clinical Experience with 247 Aneurysms. *AJNR Am. J. Neuroradiol*, 2004; 25: 577-583.

[50] Blanc R., Weill A., Piotin M., Ross L. B., Moret J. Delayed stroke secondary to increasing mass effect after endovascular treatment of a giant aneurysm by parent vessel occlusion. *AJNR Am J Neuroradiol*.,2001; 22: 841-1843.

[51] Brilstra E. H., Rinkel G. J., van der Graaf Y., et al. Treatment of intracranial aneurysms by embolization with coils: a systematic review. *Stroke,* 1999; 30: 470-476.

[52] Chow M. M., Woo H. H., Masaryk T. J., Rasmussen P. A. A novel endovascular treatment of a wide-neckcd basilar apex aneurysm by using a Y-configuration, double-stent technique. *AJNR Am J Neuroradiol*.,2005; 26(1): 198-200.

[53] Tulleken C. A., Streefkerk II. J., van der Zwan A. Construction of a new posterior communicating artery in a patient with poor posterior fossa circulation: technical case report. *Neurosurgery,* 2002; 50: 415-419, 2002.

[54] Sahoo A., Abdalkader M., Saatci I., Raymond J., Qiu Z., Huo X., Sun D., Weyland C. S., Jia B., Zaidat O. O., Hu W., Qureshi A. I., Miao Z., Nguyen T. N. History of Neurointervention. *Semin Neurol*., 2023; 43(3):454-465.

[55] Solomon R. A., Stein B. M. Surgical approaches to aneurysms of the vertebral and basilar arteries. *Neurosurgery,* 1988; 23: 203-208.

[56] Spetzler R. F., Hadley M. N., Rigamonti D. et al. Aneurysms of the basilar artery treated with circulatory arrest, hypothermia, and barbiturate cerebral protection. *J Neurosurg,* 1988; 68: 868-879.

[57] Hulsbergen A. F. C. Long-Term Durability of Open Surgical versus Endovascular Repair of Intracranial Aneurysms: A Systematic Review and Meta-Analysis. *World Neurosurg*. 2019; 132: e820–e833.

[58] Li S., Zeng C., Tao W., Huang Z., Yan L., Tian X., Chen F. The Safety and Efficacy of Flow Diversion versus Conventional Endovascular Treatment for Intracranial Aneurysms: A Meta-analysis of Real-world Cohort Studies from the Past 10 Years. *AJNR Am J Neuroradiol*, 2022; 43(7):1004-1011.

[59] Hallacq P., Piotin M., Moret J. Endovascular occlusion of the posterior cerebral artery for the treatment of P2 segment aneurysms: retrospective review of a 10-year series. *AJNR Am J Neuroradiol*., 2002; 23(7): 1128-36.

[60] Higashida R. T., Smith W., Gress D. et al. Intravascular stent and endovascular coil placement for a ruptured fusiform aneurysm of the basilar artery: case report and review of the literature. *J Neurosurg*., 1997; 87: 944-949.

[61] Horowitz M. B., Purdy P. D., Burns D., Bellotto D. Scanning electron microscopic findings in a basilar tip aneurysm embolized with Guglielmi detachable coils. *AJNR Am. J. Neuroradiol*., 1997; 18: 688 - 690.

[62] Murayama Y., Tateshima S., Gonzalez N. R., Vinuela F. Matrix and Bioabsorbable Polymeric Coils Accelerate Healing of Intracranial Aneurysms: Long-Term Experimental Study. *Stroke,* 2003; 34: 2031-2037.

[63] Xue, T., Chen, Z., Lin, W. et al. Hydrogel coils versus bare platinum coils for the endovascular treatment of intracranial aneurysms: a meta-analysis of randomized controlled trials. *BMC Neurol*., 2018 18(167): 187-197.

[64] Islak C., Kocer N., Albayram S., Kizilkilic O., Uzma O., Cokyuksel O. Bare Stent-Graft Technique: A New Method of Endoluminal Vascular Reconstruction for the Treatment of Giant and Fusiform Aneurysms. *AJNR Am. J. Neuroradiol*., 2002; 23: 1589 - 1595.

[65] Kang H. S, Oh C. W., Han M. H., Byun H. S., Han D. H. Treatment of a sequential giant fusiform aneurysm of the basilar trunk. *Korean J Radiol*., 2005; 6(2): 125-9.

[66] Klein G. E., Szolar D. H., Leber K. A., Karaic R., Hausegger K. A. Basilar tip aneurysm: endovascular treatment with Guglielmi detachable coils-midterm results. *Radiology,* 1997; 205:191-196.
[67] Khurana V. G., Wijdicks E. F. M. et al. Acute deterioration from thrombosis and rerupture of a giant intracranial aneurysm. *Neurology*, 1999; 52: 1697-1699.
[68] Ospel J. M., Brouwer P., Dorn F., Arthur A., Jensen M. E., Nogueira R., Chapot R., Albuquerque F., Majoie C., Jayaraman M., Taylor A., Liu J., Fiehler J., Sakai N., Orlov K., Kallmes D., Fraser J. F., Thibault L., Goyal M. Antiplatelet Management for Stent-Assisted Coiling and Flow Diversion of Ruptured Intracranial Aneurysms: A DELPHI Consensus Statement. *AJNR Am J Neuroradiol.*, 2020; 41(10):1856-1862.
[69] McDougall C. G., Halbach V. V., Dowd C. F., Higashida R. T., Larsen D. W., Hieshima G. B. Endovascular treatment of basilar tip aneurysms using electrolytically detachable coils. *J Neurosurg.*, 1996; 84: 393-399, 1996.
[70] Mehta B., Burke T., Kole M., Bydon A., Seyfried D., Malik G. Stent-within-a-Stent Technique for the Treatment of Dissecting Vertebral Artery Aneurysms. *AJNR Am. J. Neuroradiol.*, 2003; 24: 1814 - 1818.
[71] Gruber D. P., Zimmerman G. A., Tomsick T. A., van Loveren H. R., Link M. J., Tew J. M. Jr. A comparison between endovascular and surgical management of basilar artery apex aneurysms. *J Neurosurg.*, 1999; 90: 868-874.
[72] Kan P. Expanding Indications for Flow Diverters: Ruptured Aneurysms, Blister Aneurysms, and Dissecting Aneurysms. *Neurosurgery*. 2020. 86(1): S96–S103.
[73] Li, Y. L., Roalfe, A., Chu, E. Y, Lee, R. Outcome of Flow Diverters with Surface Modifications in Treatment of Cerebral Aneurysms: Systematic Review and Meta-analysis. *Am. J. Neuroradiol.* 2021. 42(2): 327–333.
[74] Griffin, A., Lerner, E., Zuchowski, A. Flow diversion of fusiform intracranial aneurysms. *Neurosurg. Rev.* 2021. 44(3): 1471–1478.
[75] Shibano A., Sakata J., Fujita A., Harada T., Okino R., Yamamoto D., Miyake S. Stent assisted coil embolization for a dissecting cerebral aneurysm of middle cerebral artery: A case report and the literature review. *Surg Neurol Int*. 2023 20;14:375.
[76] Cagnazzo F., di Carlo D. T., Cappucci M., Lefevre P. H., Costalat V., Perrini P. Acutely Ruptured Intracranial Aneurysms Treated with Flow-Diverter Stents: A Systematic Review and Meta-Analysis. *AJNR Am J Neuroradiol*. 2018;39(9):1669-1675.
[77] Lee J., Kim D. H., Lee S. H., Moon J. H., Yang S. Y., Cho K. T., Kim B. H. Stent-assisted Coiling vs. Flow Diverter for Treating Blood Blister-like Aneurysms: A Proportion Meta-analysis. *Clin Neuroradiol*. 2022;32(4):889-902
[78] Tang C., Zhang T. S., Zhou L. F. Risk factors for rebleeding of aneurysmal subarachnoid hemorrhage: a meta-analysis. *PLoS One*. 2014 9;9(6):e99536..
[79] Tsuji Y., Kuroda Y., Wanibuchi M. Coil embolization for ruptured distal anterior cerebral artery aneurysm at the supracallosal portion: Two case reports. *Surg Neurol Int*. 2023 22;14:444.
[80] Koo, A. B., Elsamadicy, A. A., Lin, I. H. Predictors of Extended Length of Stay Following Treatment of Unruptured Adult Cerebral Aneurysms: A Study of The National Inpatient Sample. *J. stroke Cerebrovasc. Dis.* 2020. 29(11).
[81] Chen C. C., Yi-Chou Wang A., Chen C. T., Hsieh P. C. Coadjuvant Treatment of Vasospasm in Ruptured Unsecured Cerebral Aneurysms with Aggressive Angioplasty, Intra-Arterial Nimodipine, and Aneurysm Embolization. *World Neurosurg*. 2018;116:e452-e459.
[82] Murias Quintana E., Gil García A., Vega Valdés P., Morales Deza E., Escudero Augusto D., Viña Soria L., Gutiérrez Morales J. C. Combined surgery and embolization to treat ruptured cerebral aneurysms with cerebral hematoma and intracranial hypertension: a retrospective analysis and review of the literature. *Radiologia* (Engl Ed). 2019 Jan-Feb;61(1):42-50.
[83] Rabinov J. D., Hellinger F. R., Morris P. P., Ogilvy C. S., Putman C. M. Endovascular Management of Vertebrobasilar Dissecting Aneurysms. *AJNR Am. J. Neuroradiol.,* 2003; 24: 1421 - 1428.

[84] Martínez-Galdámez M., Orlov K, Kadziolka K., Puthuran M., Kalousek V., Pabón B, Escartín J., Rodríguez C., Chandran A., Kislitsin D., Berestov V., Vega P., Diaz C., Dabus G. Safety and efficacy of intracranial aneurysm embolization using the "combined remodeling technique": low-profile stents delivered through double lumen balloons: a multicenter experience. *Neuroradiology*. 2019 Sep;61(9):1067-1072.

Chapter 11

Flow Diversion Treatment on Ruptured Proximal A1 Aneurysms: Three Case Reports and Review of the Literature

Elif Orhun[1]
Yigit Can Senol[1,2]
Atakan Orscelik[3]
Dilara Duman[1]
Recai Kulak[1]
Zeynep Gence Oz[1]
Idris Gurpinar[1]
Musa Onur Ozbakir[1]
Bige Sayin[4]
Ilkay Akmangit[4]
and Ergun Daglioglu[1,*]

[1]Department of Neurological Surgery, Ankara Bilkent City Hospital, Turkey
[2]Department of Neurological Surgery, Mayo Clinic, Rochester, MN, USA
[3]Department of Radiology, Mayo Clinic, Rochester, MN, USA
[4]Department of Radiology, Ankara Bilkent City Hospital, Turkey

Abstract

The treatment of A1 aneurysms through endovascular methods can be difficult. Coiling and assisted coiling are the most commonly used techniques. While flow diverters (FDs) are widely accepted for treating ruptured blister-like and dissecting aneurysms, their efficacy in treating ruptured distal A1 aneurysms requires further investigation. More case studies are needed to determine the safety and effectiveness of using FDs for this purpose. To aim this purpose, we report 3 ruptured A1 aneurysms treated with FDs. Our case series demonstrate FDs' safety and efficacy profile on ruptured distal A1 aneurysms. Ultimately,

* Corresponding Author's Email: edaglioglu@gmail.com.

In: Understanding and Managing Cerebral Aneurysms
Editor: Xianli Lv
ISBN: 979-8-89113-608-3

deciding the most appropriate treatment method for an A1 aneurysm will depend on carefully considering the individual case and the patient's specific needs.

Keywords: A1, distal anterior cerebral artery, flow diverter, ruptured

Introduction

The reported incidence of proximal (A1) segment aneurysms of the anterior cerebral artery (ACA) is relatively low, accounting for approximately 0.5-4% of all intracranial aneurysms [1]. These aneurysms tend to be smaller in size than aneurysms in other locations, but they have a higher risk of rupture due to their proximity to the circle of Willis and the fragile nature of the A1 segment. Due to their location near critical structures such as the optic nerve and chiasm, a ruptured A1 segment aneurysm can cause vision problems and other neurological deficits [2]. Also, rupture can cause bleeding into the interhemispheric fissure, increasing intracranial pressure and potentially life-threatening complications. The complex anatomy of the surrounding blood vessels and proximity to important perforating vessels can also make surgical treatment of these ruptured aneurysms challenging, and although traditional endovascular treatment options, such as coiling or stenting, have been widely used, they may not always provide complete occlusion of the aneurysm or adequate protection of the perforating arteries.

In recent years, a flow diverter (FD) has emerged as a promising alternative for the treatment of intracranial aneurysms (Table 1). Several studies have demonstrated the safety and efficacy of FDs in the treatment of ruptured and unruptured aneurysms in various locations, including the anterior and posterior circulation [3, 4]. FDs have shown promise in previous studies and may be a useful treatment option for A1 segment aneurysms that are not amenable to performing surgical clipping or endovascular coiling. However, there is limited data on the use of FDs specifically for ruptured A1 segment aneurysms, and the existing literature consists mainly of case reports and small case series. This study reported three cases of ruptured A1 aneurysms with wide necks treated with flow diverters.

Case 1

A 66-year-old woman with a medical history of hypertension, diabetes, and hypothyroidism presented to the emergency department with a headache. The patient did not exhibit any neurological deficits during examination, but a CT angiogram revealed a ruptured fusiform dissecting aneurysm measuring 8.5 mm × 6.6 mm in her left A1 artery. The patient was admitted to our hospital, and a DSA procedure was performed. During the procedure, with a nasogastric tube 300mg clopidogrel and 100mg aspirin were started. Moreover, perioperative tirofiban infusion started after deployment of flow diverter.

A flow diverter was placed distal to the aneurysm in the left A1 artery: a Derivo (Acandis, Germany) flow diverter measuring 3.5 mm × 15 mm deployed. Due to a proximal opening problem of flow diverter, a second Neuroform Atlas (Stryker, USA) stent measuring 4 mm × 20 mm deployed telescopically. As a result, stasis in the aneurysm significantly increased, leading to complete thrombosis of the aneurysm. The patient did not experience any complications during or after the procedure, and she was discharged one week with aspirin and clopidogrel postoperatively. Follow-up angiograms on postoperative 6 month showed no residual aneurysmal filling (Figure 1).

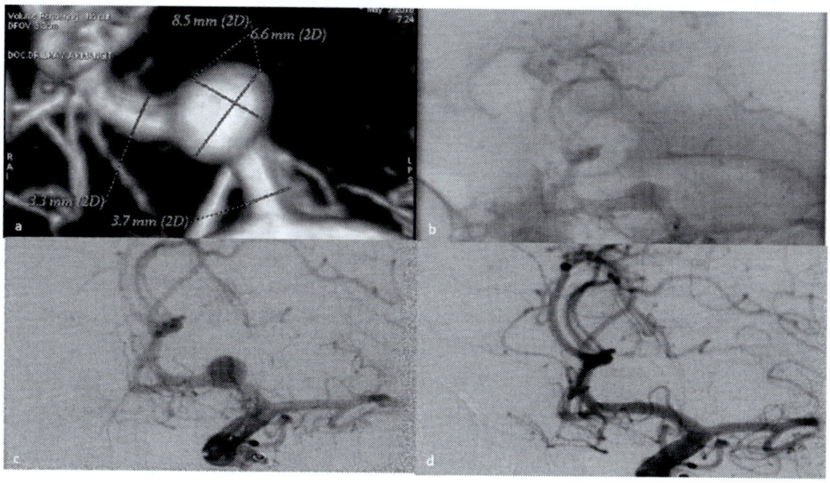

Figure 1. a: A ruptured fusiform aneurysm not suitable for clipping or primary coiling b: A Derivo flow diverter was deployed, but there was a distal opening problem causing decreased distal blood flow (arrow) c: Neuroform Atlas deployed telescopically, and the opening problem was resolved (arrow) d: 6th-month follow-up angiogram showed no residual filling.

Case 2

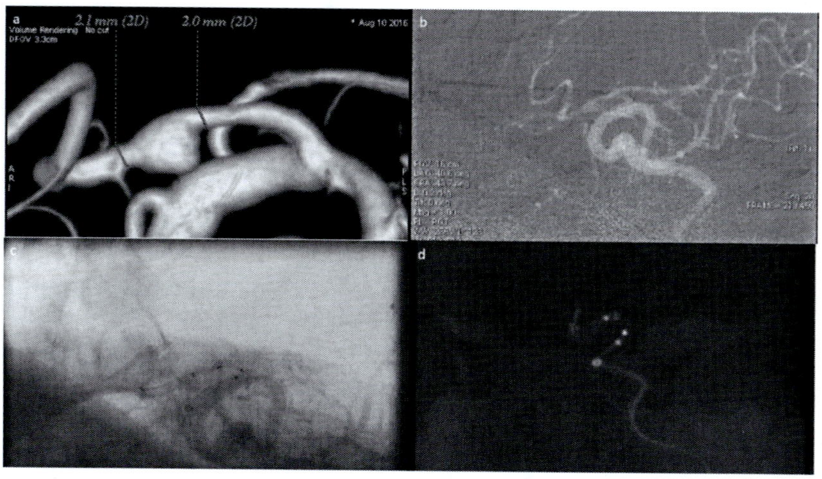

Figure 2. a: Distal A1 aneurysms were seen in 3D reconstructed images b: Perioperative imaging of a 130-degree curve from ICA to A1 c: Perioperative images of flow diverter deployment d: Immediate DSA images after flow diverter deployment, with the flow diverter deployed in the A1 segment.

A 68-year-old male patient with known hypertension presented to another medical center with severe headache and symptoms of drowsiness. A CTA was performed, which revealed a left A1 aneurysm with subarachnoid hemorrhage. The patient was admitted to our clinic. During the DSA procedure, the distal end of the A1 aneurysm was reached, and a Derivo (Acandis,

Germany) 3.5 mm × 15 mm stent was placed at the neck of the aneurysm. 300 mg clopidogrel and 100 mg aspirin was loaded with nasogastric tube. Tirofiban was started perioperatively. During the arterial filling of the distal segments of the left ACA, moderate vasospasm were observed, and capillary and venous filling were weak. The patient was given bilateral intra-arterial nimodipine, and minimal improvement was observed. The patient was continued on aspirin and clopidogrel postoperatively and was followed up with a CT angiography at 45 days and a control DSA at 6 months, which revealed no residual filling (Figure 2).

Case 3

This patient presented to the emergency department with a 5-day history of headache, nausea, vomiting, and drowsiness. A CT scan revealed Fisher grade 3 subarachnoid hemorrhage in the left occipitotemporal sulci, and a subsequent DSA showed a bilobed aneurysm with a diameter of 4 mm ×3 mm at the bifurcation of the left MCA and two aneurysms with a diameter of 2.5 mm on the left A1. Multiple session treatment was planned and Coil embolization was performed on the aneurysm at the left MCA bifurcation. The patient was discharged with medical therapy and a second endovascular treatment was planned for a one month later. A Fred JR(Microvention, USA) 2.5 mm × 13 mm flow-diverting stent was placed at the distal end of the left A1 aneurysm. The patient was discharged three days later with no change in neurological exam. A control angiogram was performed after 6 month of second endovascular treatment and no residual filling was seen both aneurysms (Figure 3).

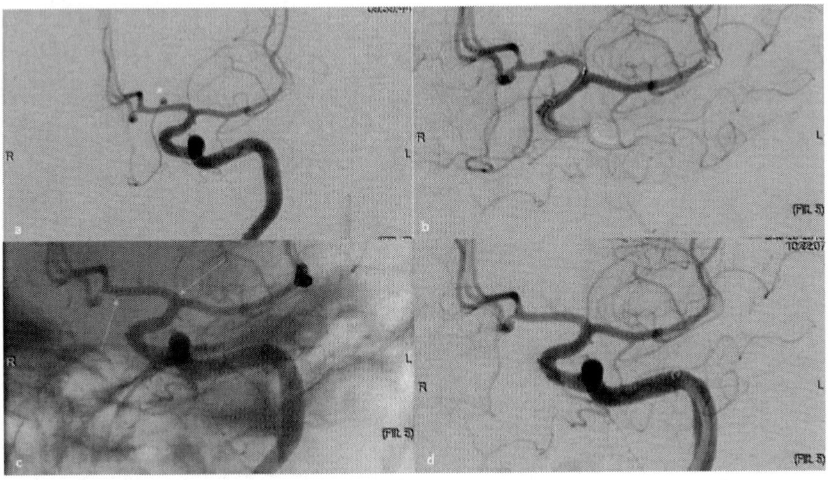

Figure 3. a: A ruptured A1 aneurysm was seen in the middle A1 segment (asterisk) b: The tower of power sheath and microcatheter made the A1 curves easily accessible c: The flow diverter was deployed successfully d: The 6th-month follow-up angiogram showed no residual filling.

Discussion

The choice of treatment for ruptured A1 aneurysms depends on several factors, such as the location, size, and shape of the aneurysm and the patient's age, overall health, and personal preferences. Generally, the first-line treatment options for ruptured A1 aneurysms are surgical clipping and endovascular coiling [5]. Despite several therapeutic modalities, authors have no consensus regarding the optimal management strategy for A1 aneurysms.

A1 aneurysms represent a rare type of intracranial aneurysm that is challenging to treat with surgical clipping due to their location and proximity to important perforating arteries [6]. The primary group of perforating arteries originating from the A1 segment is the medial lenticulostriate arteries which supply critical structures such as the anterior limb of the internal capsule, pallidum, striatum, and anterior hypothalamus. The second subgroup of perforating arteries is the recurrent artery of Heubner, which arises from the A2 segment and supplies structures such as the striatum, anterior limb of the internal capsule, olfactory region, anterior hypothalamus, and frontobasal cortex. Treating A1 aneurysms can be difficult due to the risk of damaging these vital structures. Therefore, the optimal treatment approach should be determined on a case-by-case basis by a team of experienced neurosurgeons and interventional neuroradiologists after carefully evaluating the individual patient's condition.

Treating acutely ruptured aneurysms using flow diverters is still an area of limited understanding. Further investigation and larger studies are necessary to fully assess this treatment approach's long-term effectiveness and safety. Our case reports indicate that in some unique cases, flow diverter deployment alone can be used safely and effectively, while in other cases, a combination of flow diverter deployment and acute coiling may be necessary. Nonetheless, more research is needed to determine the optimal treatment approach for ruptured aneurysms.

Our first case well demonstrated technical complications associated with flow diverter usage in small vessels, prompting the deployment of a second stent to address the issue. However, the development of low-profile flow diverters has led to improved outcomes in similar cases. In a separate case involving a patient with multiple aneurysms and subarachnoid hemorrhage, the order of treatment and the feasibility of treating multiple aneurysms in a single session are important considerations. While our clinic prefers multiple sessions to ensure safe outcomes, there is currently no meta-analysis or clinical trial that indicates multiple sessions are superior to single-session treatments. Most case reports and retrospective cohort studies have suggested positive outcomes for acute coiling following flow diverter treatment [7, 8]. In our case, we initially performed primary coiling on the MCA aneurysms and subsequently deployed a flow diverter for the A1 aneurysms. The development of low-profile flow diverters such as the Silk Vista Baby and Fred JR has increased neurointerventionists' confidence in treating small diameter aneurysms with flow diverters. In a third case involving a patient with delayed subarachnoid hemorrhage, we successfully used a Fred Jr without any complications. However, the off-label use of Fred Jr in ruptured aneurysms still requires further clinical trials to establish its efficacy and safety profile.

It is worth noting that for ruptured A1 aneurysms that are dissecting or cannot be treated with traditional surgical methods, flow diverters may be a viable alternative option. Although only retrospective studies have been conducted on ruptured aneurysms treated with flow diverters, the development of new low-profile flow diverters and the increased experience of neuro-interventionists in the field suggests that the on-label usage of flow diverters should be expanded. To achieve this, larger prospective controlled studies are necessary.

Table 1. Summary of Studies included Literature Review

Authors	Year Publ.	Study Design	Center	Patient Number	Aneurysm Number	Ruptured Rate	Anti-Platelet	Anti-platelet Initiation Time	Anti-platelet Regimen	Flow Diverter Device	Aneurysm Locations
Shüngel et al.	2021	Retrospective	Multicenter	44 patients	47 Aneurysms	21/47 (44.6%)	DAPT	24h prior	ASA + Ticagrelor	Silk Vista Baby (Balt, France)	A1/A2, M1, PICA, V4, BA
Atallah et al.	2019	Retrospective	Single Center	23 Patients	23 Aneurysms	1/23 (5.9%)	DAPT	8h prior	ASA + Clopidogrel	Pipeline (Medtronic, USA)	A1, M1, P1, PICA
Giorgianni et al.	2022	Case Report	Single Center	1 patient	1 aneurysm	1/1 (100%)	DAPT	After the surgery started(24h)	ASA + Clopidogrel	Fred (Microvention, USA)	Proximal A1

DAPT: Dual anti-platelet treatment, ASA: Aspirin, PICA: Posterior inferior cerebellar artery.

Conclusion

This case series demonstrate FDs' safety and efficacy profile on ruptured distal A1 aneurysms. The most appropriate treatment method for an A1 aneurysm depends on carefully considering the individual case and the patient's specific needs.

References

[1] Xu M, Lv N, Sun K, et al. Morphological and Hemodynamic Risk Factors for the Rupture of Proximal Anterior Cerebral Artery Aneurysms (A1 Segment). *Front Aging Neurosci.* 2022;14:835373. doi:10.3389/fnagi.2022.835373.

[2] Campero A, Baldoncini M, Martinez J, Villalonga JF, Lucifero AG, Luzzi S. Microneurosurgical management of aneurysms of the A1 segment of the anterior cerebral artery: Anatomy and surgical technique. *Surg Neurol Int.* 2022;13:310. doi:10.25259/SNI_68_2022.

[3] Brinjikji W, Murad MH, Lanzino G, Cloft HJ, Kallmes DF. Endovascular treatment of intracranial aneurysms with flow diverters: a meta-analysis. *Stroke.* 2013;44(2):442-447. doi:10.1161/STROKEAHA.112.678151.

[4] Kallmes DF, Brinjikji W, Boccardi E, et al. Aneurysm Study of Pipeline in an Observational Registry (ASPIRe). *Interv Neurol.* 2016;5(1-2):89-99. doi:10.1159/000446503.

[5] Hino A, Fujimoto M, Iwamoto Y, Oka H, Echigo T. Surgery of proximal anterior cerebral artery aneurysms. *Acta Neurochir (Wien).* 2002;144(12):1291-1296; discussion 1296. doi:10.1007/s00701-002-1014-6.

[6] Dashti R, Hernesniemi J, Lehto H, et al. Microneurosurgical management of proximal anterior cerebral artery aneurysms. *Surg Neurol.* 2007;68(4):366-377. doi:10.1016/j.surneu.2007.07.084.

[7] Yamazaki H, Fujinaka T, Ozaki T, et al. Staged treatment for ruptured wide-neck intracranial aneurysm with intentional partial coiling in the acute phase followed by definitive treatment. *Surg Neurol Int.* 2022;13:322. doi:10.25259/SNI_529_2022.

[8] Brinjikji W, Piano M, Fang S, et al. Treatment of ruptured complex and large/giant ruptured cerebral aneurysms by acute coiling followed by staged flow diversion. *J Neurosurg.* 2016;125(1):120-127. doi:10.3171/2015.6.JNS151038.

Chapter 12

Reconstructive Endovascular Treatment on Vertebrobasilar Junction Aneurysms: Case Series and Review of the Literature

Afsin Emre Akpinar[1]
Yigit Can Senol[1,2]
Atakan Orscelik[3]
Dilara Duman[1]
Halis Emre Ciftci[1]
Musa Onur Ozbakir[1]
Bige Sayin[4]
Ilkay Akmangit[4]
and Ergun Daglioglu[1,*]

[1]Department of Neurological Surgery, Ankara Bilkent City Hospital, Turkey
[2]Department of Neurological Surgery, Mayo Clinic, Rochester, MN, USA
[3]Department of Radiology, Mayo Clinic, Rochester, MN, USA
[4]Department of Radiology, Ankara Bilkent City Hospital, Turkey

Abstract

Reconstructive treatment for vertebrobasilar junction (VBJ) aneurysms involves repairing or rebuilding the damaged portion of the blood vessel to prevent future rupture or bleeding. These aneurysms are a rare and complex subgroup of saccular aneurysms and require careful consideration when determining the most appropriate treatment method. Endovascular techniques, such as stent placement or flow diverter deployment, are often utilized in reconstructive treatment. The specific technique will depend on various factors, including the size, location, and type of aneurysm as the patient's overall health and medical history. The current study reported three successful cases of VBJ aneurysms treated through combined reconstructive endovascular methods. These case reports demonstrate that endovascular treatment can effectively achieve a curative result and is

* Corresponding Author's Email: edaglioglu@gmail.com.

In: Understanding and Managing Cerebral Aneurysms
Editor: Xianli Lv
ISBN: 979-8-89113-608-3

associated with good clinical outcomes and low mortality rates. It is important to note that these are individual cases, and the results may not represent all patients. Further research and case studies are needed to establish the safety and efficacy of reconstructive treatment for VBJ aneurysms.

Keywords: vertebrobasilar junction aneurysm, endovascular, reconstructive

Introduction

Vertebrobasilar artery junction (VBJ) aneurysms are uncommon posterior circulation aneurysms comprising 2.7% of all aneurysms [1] and are often (40-70%) accompanied by fenestrations [2, 3]. It has also been observed that the increase in the size of these aneurysms becomes more dangerous for patients. Studies have reported that the rate of rupture in VBJ aneurysms increases significantly with the diameter of the lesions. Such aneurysms may present with symptoms related to mass effect, brain stem edema, subarachnoid hemorrhage (SAH), and ischemia, and in case of rupture, they can become fatal due to massive intracranial hemorrhage.

The endovascular approach is at the forefront in such aneurysms because of the complex structure of the brain stem anatomy and the difficulty of reaching the region with microsurgery. Among the endovascular treatments, the most commonly used techniques in the treatment of VBJ aneurysms are reconstructive techniques that protect parent artery formation by using flow diverters, stents, or balloon-assisted coil or primary coiling (Table 1). On the other hand, deconstructive techniques which mainly focus on scarifying the parent artery could be used as a salvage maneuver or primary treatment method for VBJ aneurysms.

This case series will focus on evaluating the clinical and angiographic outcomes and possible complications of EVT methods for VBJ aneurysms. Specifically, the cases will demonstrate differences between both deconstructive and reconstructive treatment modalities.

Treatment with Primary Coiling Case 1

A 45- year-old male patient presented to the emergency department with a severe headache, and a cranial CT revealed a subarachnoid hemorrhage. Further investigation with DSA was conducted to confirm the suspicion of aneurysmal SAH, and a 5.6 mm × 3.4 mm saccular aneurysm was detected in the VBJ. The primary treatment option considered was coiling due to the aneurysm's saccular structure and the subarachnoid hemorrhage. However, a fenestration was observed in the proximal basilar artery, and a suitable angle for treatment was determined using 3D reconstruction. The patient underwent primary coiling treatment without any complications and was transferred to the neurosurgery intensive care unit for postoperative care. The patient had a good recovery and was discharged on the 10th day after the procedure. There were no residual issues in the patient's 6th-month follow-up, and no additional endovascular treatment was required (Figure 1).

Table 1. Summary of Studies

	Years	Study Design	Age	Patient Number	Aneurysm Number	Follow-up Time (month)	Female Gender	Treatment Methods	Country
Islak et al. 2004 [4]	1994-2000	Retrospective	39.9	10	11	29.5	7	PC, BAC	Turkey
Trivelato et al. 2007 [5]	2010-2012	Retrospective	56.5 (9.81)	9	10	16.2	8	PC, SAC, BAC	Brazil
Meckel et al. 2013 [6]	2008-2012	Retrospective	54.2	10	10	16.05	5	FD, FD with coil	Germany
Peluso et al. 2013 [3]	1995-2007	Retrospective	49.5	10	10	17.5	5	PC	Netherlands
Graziano et al. 2014 [7]	2006-2001	Retrospective	57	10	10	24.21	6	PC, SAC, FD	Italy
Zhu et al. 2015 [8]	2007-2014	Retrospective	55.9 (13.9)	10	12	69.5	6	SAC, OS, PC	China
Peng et al. 2022 [9]	2016-2020	Retrospective	-	-	22	12.3	-	FD, SAC	China

BAC: Balloon-assisted coiling, FD: Flow Diverter, OS: Overlapping Stenting, PC: Primary coiling, SAC: Stent-assisted coiling.

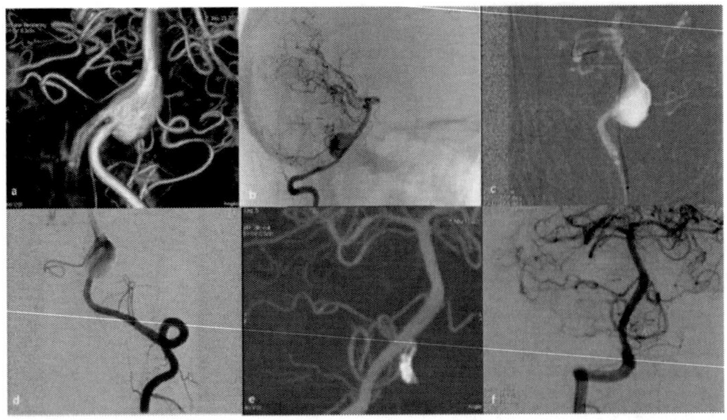

Figure 1. a: A saccular aneurysm seen in the VBJ area (asterisk) b: 3D reconstruction of the aneurysm showing a 3.4x5.6mm aneurysm c: Perioperative primary coiling d-e: Lateral and anterior-posterior control angiograms from the 6th-month follow-up.

Treatment with Flow Diverter Case 2

An 18-year-old male patient presented to the emergency department with neck pain complaints. The cranial MRI revealed a suspicious image of a thrombosed aneurysm in the posterior fossa. The patient was scheduled for elective DSA. During the DSA, a large aneurysm was detected in the VBJ, and flow-diverting treatment was planned. The patient had been started on aspirin 100mg and clopidogrel 75mg five days prior to the procedure. Two overlapping Surpass Evolve (Stryker, Fremont, CA, USA) 4 mm × 30 mm and Surpass Evolve (Stryker, Fremont, CA, USA) 4 mm × 40 mm flow diverters were placed during the operation. Postoperative imaging revealed decreased blood flow, and the patient was started on a tirofiban infusion. No neurological complications were observed in the early postoperative period. The tirofiban infusion was continued for six hours in the postoperative period. During the 6-month follow-up DSA, no residual filling was detected in the patient. The patient's clopidogrel treatment was discontinued at the 6-month mark, and they continued with aspirin 100mg treatment (Figure 2).

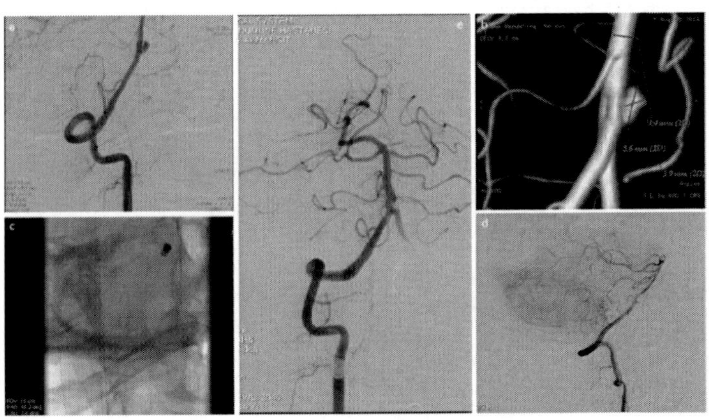

Figure 2. a: A fusiform large aneurysm was seen in the VBJ 3D reconstruction b: Lateral view of the fusiform aneurysm, with a wide neck formation suggesting flow diverter treatment c: A microcatheter was seen perioperatively before flow diverter deployment d: After the deployment of the flow diverter, contrast hanging was seen in the immediate angiogram (OKM C) e-f: 6th-month control angiograms in AP and lateral views.

Treatment with Stent-Assisted Coiling Case 3

A 41-year-old male patient presented to the neurosurgery clinic with complaints of headaches. A cranial MRI was performed, and an elective DSA was scheduled due to suspicion of an aneurysm. During the DSA procedure, two junction aneurysms were identified in the posterior circulation VBJ. Due to fenestration a stent coiling procedure with X configuration was planned. Two Atlas 3 mm × 21 mm stents were placed in an X configuration. Additionally, the aneurysms were filled with coils. There were no intraoperative complications, and a 6-month follow-up DSA showed no residual filling (Figure 3).

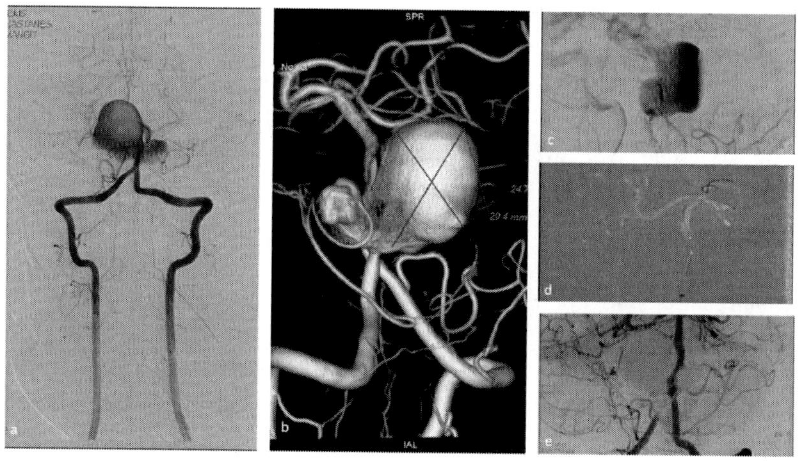

Figure 3. a: Bilateral selective angiogram from both vertebral arteries b: 3D reconstruction of the VBJ aneurysm c-d: Perioperative imaging of stent-assisted coiling e: 6th-month follow-up images showed no residual filling.

Discussion

Our systematic review found that endovascular treatment (EVT) methods for vertebrobasilar junction (VBJ) aneurysms have good occlusion rates with relatively acceptable mortality and complication rates [3-9]. The management of aneurysms in the VBJ is a difficult issue and a decision must be made by considering many factors such as the patient's condition, characteristics of the aneurysm, and vascular structures.

When considering treatment options for VBJ aneurysms, it is worth noting that surgical methods such as trapping, clipping, or cerebral bypass can be viable alternatives. However, the surgical approach to the VBJ zone is challenging and dangerous due to the close proximity of the aneurysm to the brain stem, perforating arteries, and lower cranial nerves. This results in a surgical mortality rate ranging from 8% to 45% [10-12]. Thus, various surgical approaches and techniques have been employed for treating VBJ aneurysms over the years. The high rates of disability and mortality associated with conservative management of VBJ aneurysms also necessitate the development of a safer and more effective treatment method [13].

It is important to note that the first series of primary coiling in VBJ aneurysms was developed by Graves et al. and primary coiling was applied in 3 patients with a 66% complete aneurysm occlusion rate [14]. Despite having a lower rate of complete aneurysm occlusion compared to surgical treatments, the favorable clinical outcomes associated with EVT methods have led to their frequent use. In our case, we used primary coiling for a subarachnoid hemorrhage patient due to the relatively higher risks of using a dual or single antiplatelet regimen. It is important to closely follow primary coiling, despite its conventional and safe nature, due to the significant likelihood of recanalization. While some studies have reported recanalization rates as high as 50%, our case did not exhibit any instances of recanalization [15]. Also, articles showed that the balloon-remodeling technique showed promise for treating wide-neck VBJ aneurysms with high occlusion rates [4-14]. Additionally, a combination of the adjunctive coil, vertebral artery occlusion, and embolizing glue with FD in a study by Meckel et al. suggests that high mortality rates observed in previous studies using FD treatments cannot be entirely attributed to FD treatments [6]. Despite the potential for ischemic complications associated with the use of FDs in posterior circulation aneurysms, the overall ischemic complication rate of combined EVT was lower in our study than in previous studies that used FD treatments. However, it is important to note that the majority of mortality in the literature was associated with EVT treatment with FD treatment [6, 7, 9]. Furthermore, previous studies have reported a high risk of ischemic complications with the use of FDs in posterior circulation aneurysms, particularly when using overlapping FDs or conventional stents [16, 17].

In conclusion, no study in the literature compares deconstructive over reconstructive methods in the treatment of VBJ aneurysms. For the vertebrobasilar dissecting aneurysms, a recent meta-analysis reported that deconstructive techniques were superior to reconstructive methods on long-term angiographic outcomes as predicted but there is no difference between functional outcomes [18]. Although endovascular reconstructive techniques hold promise in treating complex VBJ aneurysms, making an objective assessment would require larger cohort studies to be conducted.

Conclusion

The case reports demonstrate that endovascular treatment can effectively achieve a curative result and is associated with good clinical outcomes and low mortality rates. It is important to note that these are individual cases, and the results may not represent all patients. Further research and case studies are needed to establish the safety and efficacy of reconstructive treatment for VBJ aneurysms.

References

[1] Wiebers DO. Unruptured intracranial aneurysms: natural history, clinical outcome, and risks of surgical and endovascular treatment. *The Lancet*. 2003;362(9378):103-110. doi:10.1016/S0140-6736(03)13860-3.

[2] Kai Y, Hamada J ichiro, Morioka M, Yano S, Fujioka S, Kuratsu J ichi. Endovascular treatment of ruptured aneurysms associated with fenestrated basilar artery. Two case reports. *Neurol Med Chir (Tokyo)*. 2006;46(5):244-247. doi:10.2176/nmc.46.244.

[3] Peluso JPP, van Rooij WJ, Sluzewski M, Beute GN. Aneurysms of the Vertebrobasilar Junction: Incidence, Clinical Presentation, and Outcome of Endovascular Treatment. *American Journal of Neuroradiology*. 2007;28(9):1747-1751. doi:10.3174/ajnr.A0654.

[4] Islak C, Kocer N, Kantarci F, Saatci I, Uzma O, Canbaz B. Endovascular Management of Basilar Artery Aneurysms Associated with Fenestrations. Published online 2002.

[5] Trivelato FP, Abud DG, Nakiri GS, et al. Basilar Artery Fenestration Aneurysms: Endovascular Treatment Strategies Based on 3D Morphology. *Clin Neuroradiol.* 2016;26(1):73-79. doi:10.1007/s00062-014-0336-0.

[6] Meckel S, McAuliffe W, Fiorella D, et al. Endovascular Treatment of Complex Aneurysms at the Vertebrobasilar Junction With Flow-Diverting Stents: Initial Experience. *Neurosurgery.* 2013;73(3): 386-394. doi:10.1227/01.neu.0000431472.71913.07.

[7] Graziano F, Ganau M, Iacopino DG, Boccardi E. Vertebro-Basilar Junction Aneurysms: A Single Centre Experience and Meta-Analysis of Endovascular Treatments. *Neuroradiol J.* 2014;27(6):732-741. doi:10.15274/NRJ-2014-10100.

[8] Zhu DY, Fang YB, Wu YN, et al. Treatment of fenestrated vertebrobasilar junction-related aneurysms with endovascular techniques. *Journal of Clinical Neuroscience.* 2016;28:112-116. doi:10.1016/j.jocn. 2015.09.018.

[9] Peng Q, Zhou Y, Li W, et al. Reconstructive Endovascular Treatment of Basilar Trunk and Vertebrobasilar Junction Aneurysms: A Review of 77 Consecutive Cases. *Front Neurol.* 2022;13: 885776. doi:10.3389/fneur.2022.885776.

[10] Kalani MYS, Zabramski JM, Nakaji P, Spetzler RF. Bypass and Flow Reduction for Complex Basilar and Vertebrobasilar Junction Aneurysms. *Neurosurgery.* 2013;72(5):763-776. doi:10.1227/NEU. 0b013e3182870703.

[11] Seifert V, Raabe A, Stolke D. Management-Related Morbidity and Mortality in Unselected Aneurysms of the Basilar Trunk and Vertebrobasilar Junction. *Acta Neurochirurgica.* 2001;143(4):343-349. doi:10.1007/s007010170088.

[12] Ponce FA, Spetzler RF, Han PP, et al. Cardiac standstill for cerebral aneurysms in 103 patients: an update on the experience at the Barrow Neurological Institute: Clinical article. *JNS.* 2011;114(3):877-884. doi:10.3171/2010.9.JNS091178.

[13] Steinberg GK, Drake CG, Peerless SJ. Deliberate basilar or vertebral artery occlusion in the treatment of intracranial aneurysms. Immediate results and long-term outcome in 201 patients. *J Neurosurg.* 1993;79(2):161-173. doi:10.3171/jns.1993.79.2.0161.

[14] Graves VB, Strother CM, Weir B, Duff TA. Vertebrobasilar Junction Aneurysms Associated with Fenestration: Treatment with Guglielmi Detachable Coils. Published online 1996.

[15] Spetzler RF, Zabramski JM, McDougall CG, et al. Analysis of saccular aneurysms in the Barrow Ruptured Aneurysm Trial. *J Neurosurg.* 2018;128(1):120-125. doi:10.3171/2016.9.JNS161301.

[16] Alwakeal A, Shlobin NA, Golnari P, et al. Flow Diversion of Posterior Circulation Aneurysms: Systematic Review of Disaggregated Individual Patient Data. *AJNR Am J Neuroradiol.* 2021;42(10): 1827-1833. doi:10.3174/ajnr.A7220.

[17] Abdel-Tawab M, Abdeltawab AK, Abdelmonem M, et al. Efficacy and safety of flow diverters in posterior circulation aneurysms and comparison with their efficacy in anterior circulation aneurysms: A systematic review and meta-analysis. *Interv Neuroradiol.* 2021;27(5):609-621. doi:10.1177/15910199 211003017.

[18] Sönmez Ö, Brinjikji W, Murad MH, Lanzino G. Deconstructive and Reconstructive Techniques in Treatment of Vertebrobasilar Dissecting Aneurysms: A Systematic Review and Meta-Analysis. *AJNR Am J Neuroradiol.* 2015;36(7):1293-1298. doi:10.3174/ajnr.A4360.

Chapter 13

Atypical Manifestations of V4 Aneurysms: Persistent Cough May Be an Initial Symptom of an Aneurysm

Naime Dilara Ozkan[1]
Yigit Can Senol[1,2]
Atakan Orscelik[3]
Merve Sakci[1]
Dilara Duman[1]
Batuhan Dereli[1]
Musa Onur Ozbakir[1]
Bige Sayin[4]
Ilkay Akmangit[4]
and Ergun Daglioglu[1,*]
[1]Department of Neurological Surgery, Ankara Bilkent City Hospital, Turkey
[2]Department of Neurological Surgery, Mayo Clinic, Rochester, MN, USA
[3]Department of Radiology, Mayo Clinic, Rochester, MN, USA
[4]Department of Radiology, Ankara Bilkent City Hospital, Turkey

Abstract

V4 aneurysms located in the posterior circulation of the brain can cause uncommon symptoms due to their distinctive position. Although many V4 aneurysms are diagnosed incidentally, there have been case reports of posterior circulation aneurysms causing symptoms due to their anatomic proximity to the brainstem. These symptoms can also be indicative of other medical conditions, so it's important to seek a professional medical evaluation. In some cases, patients with V4 aneurysms may not experience any symptoms at all. The current study reports two cases of V4 aneurysms with uncommon presenting symptoms. The first case was an unruptured V4 aneurysm causing neck pain, and the second one was a V4 aneurysm leading to chronic coughing, which caused a delayed

[*] Corresponding Author's Email: edaglioglu@gmail.com.

In: Understanding and Managing Cerebral Aneurysms
Editor: Xianli Lv
ISBN: 979-8-89113-608-3

diagnosis of a V4 aneurysm. Both aneurysms were treated with endovascular techniques and the patient's symptoms improved after the treatment.

Keywords: V4, aneurysm, neck pain, vertebral artery

Introduction

Vertebral arteries (VA) originate from the subclavian arteries, usually the largest branch. VA supplies blood to the upper part of the spinal cord, the brainstem, and the posterior part of the brain. At the pons level, the vertebral arteries merge to form the basilar artery.

Vertebral artery aneurysms make up 11% of posterior circulation aneurysms and 3-5% of subarachnoid hemorrhages [1]. The intradural part, V4, is adjacent to the pons and medulla. If v4 aneurysms are ruptured, simillar to the other aneurysms, the most common symptoms are, due to the SAH, headache, nausea, vomiting, loss of consciousness, neck pain, and neck stiffness. Unruptured aneurysms are often incidentally detected as their symptoms, which are usually vague, may not be noticeable before rupture. With the development and widespread use of imaging techniques today, the incidence of detecting unruptured aneurysms has increased.

The presenting symptoms of a patient with a brain aneurysm can vary depending on the location and size of the aneurysm and whether it has ruptured or not. Some of the common symptoms of patients with a brain aneurysm include sudden and severe headaches described as the worst headache of a patient's life, vision changes such as double or blurry vision, numbness or weakness on one side of the body, speech problems, seizures, loss of consciousness and cognitive changes. It's important to note that not all patients with a brain aneurysm will experience symptoms. In fact, many aneurysms are found incidentally during brain imaging tests for other conditions [2]. However, both anterior and posterior circulation aneurysms can cause unusual presenting symptoms such as photophobia, olfactory hallucinations[3], Horner's syndrome, hiccups, behavioral changes, hearing loss or tinnitus, facial pain, difficulty swallowing,

These cases highlight the importance of considering the possibility of an aneurysm as a cause of unusual presenting symptoms, as early detection and treatment can significantly improve outcomes. It's important for healthcare providers to be aware of the wide range of presenting symptoms that can be associated with brain aneurysms and to order appropriate diagnostic tests if necessary.

Neck Pain with Vomiting is a Red Flag

A 52-year-old female with a medical history of diabetes mellitus, hypertension, and cardiac valve replacement, and a current smoker, was admitted to the emergency department with sudden onset neck pain radiating to the head, accompanied by nausea, vomiting, and dizziness. She also had an itchy feeling in her left eye and a subconjunctival hemorrhage. A CT scan revealed a Fisher 3 subarachnoid hemorrhage (SAH) in the sylvian fissure and basal cisterns, consistent with a left vertebral artery aneurysm. She was referred to another hospital for further diagnosis and treatment and admitted on the second day of SAH with a Glasgow Coma Scale score of 15. Although she had neck stiffness, her neurological and physical examination was otherwise normal, and the hemorrhage was stable in the follow-up CT scan. Digital subtraction angiography (DSA) showed a dissecting left V4 aneurysm (Figure 1), which was embolized with a flow diverter, resulting in the total obliteration of the aneurysm without any complications. She was then admitted to the neurosurgical intensive care unit, where she received clopidogrel for anticoagulation, and her neurological examination showed no regression. After two days of close monitoring, her presenting symptoms slowly faded away, and she was discharged on the fourth day after the hemorrhage. She was given anti-SAH therapy for 21 days to avoid vasospasm, and a control DSA performed during her one-year follow-up showed no residual filling, but a moderate stenosis of the flow diverter deployed segment. (Figure 2).

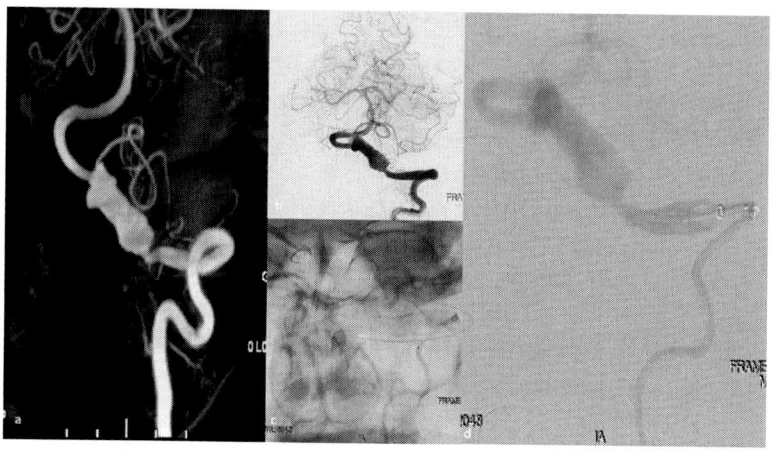

Figure 1. a: Right-sided vertebral artery dissecting aneurysm b: AP images of the vertebral artery aneurysm c: Perioperative images of flow diverter deployment (circle) d: Curves of the vertebral artery make it harder to access the distal basilar artery.

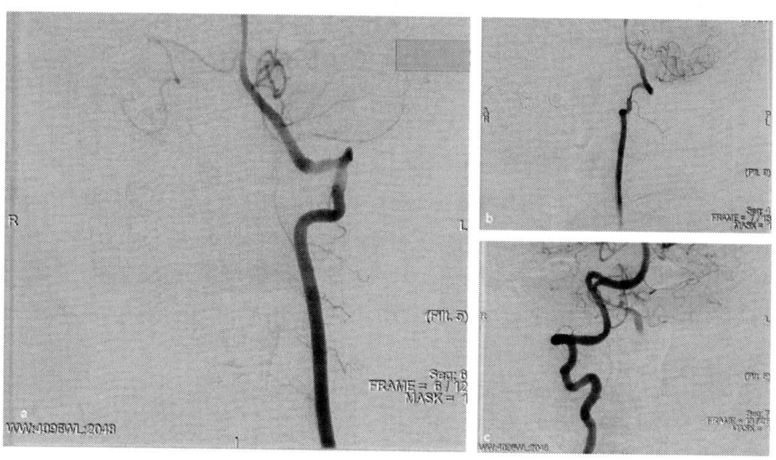

Figure 2. a: Control angiography at the first year showed moderate stenosis of the flow diverter deployed segment b: Lateral view of the stenosis c: The contralateral side of the vertebral artery feeds well; therefore, no additional treatment was planned.

Chronic Cough Could Be Only Symptom of a Vertebral Aneurysm

A 47-year-old female patient was admitted to our hospital in June 2018 due to persistent cough, dyspnea, and hoarseness for a year. Despite being treated with various antibiotics, the patient did not experience any improvement in her condition. In June 2019, the patient's dyspnea worsened, and she was admitted to the emergency department. During the intubation, the emergency room doctor noticed that her left vocal cord was paralyzed. An urgent head and cervical computer tomography angiography was performed, which revealed a large vertebrobasilar aneurysm and compression of the brainstem. The patient was then transferred to the neurosurgery intensive care unit, where she was treated with antibiotics.

After being admitted to the ICU, the patient underwent digital subtraction angiography, which identified a giant spherical aneurysm in the right vertebral V4 segment with a maximum diameter of 30 mm. Informed consent was provided by the patient and her relatives prior to endovascular therapy. A treatment plan was formulated, and the aneurysm was relatively tightly embolized with coils. Clopidogrel was administered, and at 5 days following hospitalization, the giant aneurysm of the V4 segment was embolized with 5mm×35mm Pipeline (Medtronic, USA) flow diverter. After treatment, the patient was transferred to the neuro-ICU and on post-operative day 2 her vitals were improved and extubated. Her chest x-ray revealed improvement. Antibiotics were stopped on the day 10 of the admission. The patient was transferred to the Neurosurgery inpatient service on the day of 12 of her admission.

After 2 months of the operation, the patient had increased white phlegm and her choking cough was continuing. Furthermore, the patient's right limb muscle strength was improved compared with that pre-embolization. Three months after embolization, re-examination of the head MRI and MRA revealed that the aneurysm was completely occluded. At 12 months after endovascular procedure, her phlegm was markedly improved and discontinued with the medical drugs. Cough and hoarseness disappeared. Re-examination of DSA revealed no aneurysm recurrence and no stenosis in the parent artery on MRI and computer tomography angiography. The modified Rankin scale score of the patient is 1 on her last follow-up.

Discussion

Cough and dyspnea can be the only symptoms of these aneurysms, and therefore, vertebral aneurysm should be considered in the differential diagnoses of persistent coughs.

A case report published by Kim et al. describes a patient who presented with pulsatile tinnitus, which is a type of tinnitus that is synchronized with the heartbeat. The patient was found to have an aneurysm in the left internal carotid artery and was successfully treated with coil embolization [4]. Another case report describes a patient who presented with persistent hiccups and was found to have a giant posterior inferior cerebral artery aneurysm that compressed the medulla oblongata. The hiccups were resolved after the surgical removal of the aneurysm and decompression of the medulla oblongata [5]. A study reported the case of giant aneurysm of the vertebrobasilar junction. The patient experienced left-sided walking disability and hoarseness, which were attributed to compression of the brainstem and the posterior cranial nerves. Treatment involved using a Pipeline Flex device with coil embolization, resulting in a modified Rankin scale score of 1 point at 7 months post-embolization [6].

Conclusion

Our cases demonstrated that vertebral artery aneurysms can present with atypical symptoms due to their compression to the brain stem and lower cranial nerves. As a result, a comprehensive evaluation of such symptoms is required. However, a larger set of studies is needed to identify potential warning signs of these unusual presentations.

References

[1] Raper DMS, Caldwell J, Brew S, et al. A comparison of endovascular strategies in the treatment of ruptured vertebral artery aneurysms. *Journal of Clinical Neuroscience*. 2020;75(xxxx):168-175. doi:10.1016/j.jocn.2019.07.018.

[2] Chalouhi N, Hoh BL, Hasan D. Review of cerebral aneurysm formation, growth, and rupture. *Stroke*. 2013;44(12):3613-3622. doi:10.1161/STROKEAHA.113.002390.

[3] Walsh ME. The nose knows: an unusual presentation of a cerebral aneurysm. *J Emerg Med*. 2014;47(5):e113-115. doi:10.1016/j.jemermed.2014.06.023.

[4] Kim DK, Shin YS, Lee JH, Park SN. Pulsatile tinnitus as the sole manifestation of an internal carotid artery aneurysm successfully treated by coil embolization. *Clin Exp Otorhinolaryngol*. 2012;5(3):170-172. doi:10.3342/ceo.2012.5.3.170.

[5] Gambhir S, Singh A, Maindiratta B, Jaeger M, Darwish B, Sheridan M. Giant PICA aneurysm presenting as intractable hiccups. *J Clin Neurosci*. 2010;17(7):945-946. doi:10.1016/j.jocn.2009.09.046.

[6] Zhang CL, Shi ZH, Yan ZZ, et al. Giant aneurysm of the bilateral vertebrobasilar junction treated by pipeline and coils: A case report and literature review. *Exp Ther Med*. 2021;21(1):40. doi:10.3892/etm.2020.9472.

Chapter 14

Intracranial Stents for Cerebral Aneurysms

Huachen Zhang
Shikai Liang
and Xianli Lv*
Department of Neurosurgery, Beijing Tsinghua Changgung Hospital,
School of Clinical Medicine, Tsinghua University, Beijing, China

Abstract

The coil is designed to be tightly packed in the aneurysm cavity, thus blocking the blood flow into the aneurysm and preventing the rupture and growth of the aneurysm. For narrow-neck aneurysms (aneurysm neck<4 mm or body/neck ratio >2), coil embolization is relatively easy to perform. However, when wide-necked aneurysm (aneurysm neck≥4 mm or body/neck ratio ≤2) is encountered, the coil will be easy to protrude from the neck of the aneurysm back to the parent artery, block the blood flow to the distal artery, and increase the risk of thromboembolism complications. Some pioneers began to explore stent-assisted coil embolization, which has become an important technique for the treatment of cerebral aneurysms, and has significantly increased the range of aneurysms that can be treated endovascularly. In this chapter, the stent technique as well as recent new techniques and materials were summarized.

Keywords: wide-neck aneurysm, intracranial aneurysms, stent-assisted coiling

Introduction

In the past 60 years, neurovascular surgery has achieved great success in the treatment of cerebral aneurysms. From the iron-acrylic compound [1], electrocoagulation, detachable balloon in the 1960s to the electrolytic coil in 1991, the endovascular treatment of cerebral aneurysms can be comparable to craniotomy clipping [2]. The early excellent clinical results and experience have promoted the design and technical improvement of the coils for the treatment of cerebral aneurysms. It makes the endovascular coil embolization technique as a safe and effective alternative to surgical clipping, especially in the position related to surgical

* Corresponding Author's Email: lvxianli000@163.com.

In: Understanding and Managing Cerebral Aneurysms
Editor: Xianli Lv
ISBN: 979-8-89113-608-3

complications, such as aneurysm at the posterior circulation (Figure 1). Endovascular treatment is now considered the first line of treatment for cerebral aneurysms; however, wide-neck aneurysms are specifically difficult to treat by endovascular means due to the difficulty in achieving a stable coil mass inside the aneurysm sac [3]. To overcome this problem, stent-assisted coiling techniques provide a scaffold for coil embolization [4]. The concept of the stent-assisted technique inspired creative pioneers to invent new tools like the PulseRider (Pulsar Vascular, Inc. CA, USA) and the pCONUS (Phenox GmbH, Germany), which are a great help in managing wide-neck and bifurcation aneurysms.

The concept of stent within stents and its related hemodynamic effect has led to the novel development of flow diverters for reconstructing the arterial wall and correcting the hemodynamic disturbances. In this article, we review the stents currently in practice for the endovascular management of wide-neck and branch intracranial aneurysms.

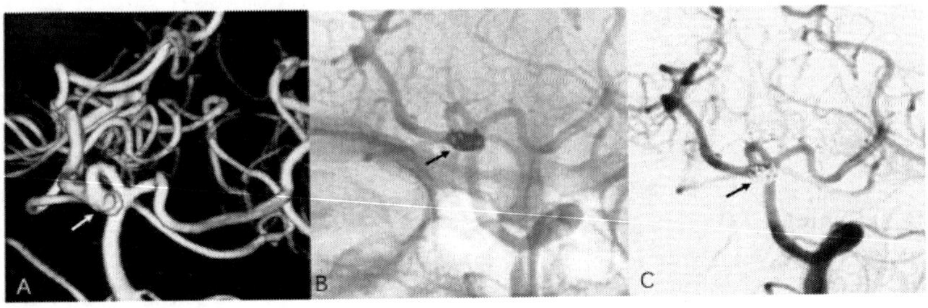

Figure 1. The 55-year-old patient presented with SAH. A, vertebral arteriography, AP view, shows an aneurysm arising from the right P1 segment of the posterior (arrow). B, the fluoroscopic image, AP view, shows the coil mass (arrow). C, vertebral arteriography, AP view, shows near total obliteration of the aneurysm (arrow).

Generations of Neurostents

In intracranial wide-neck aneurysms, simple coil embolization is often not a feasible treatment option. Balloon-assisted coiling comes with the drawback of blood flow impairment (Figure 2). Aneurysmal neck remodeling with stents has recently emerged as an effective treatment option. This method is beneficial for treating aneurysms with wide necks or for situations in which coils protrude into the parent vessel, requiring rescue with a device that can reconstrain the coil within the aneurysm [5]. Currently, various stents specialized for aneurysmal neck remodeling are used during endovascular treatment of intracranial aneurysms. Neuroform stent system (Stryker Neurovascular, Fremont, California, USA) is the first generation of intracranial stent approved for the treatment of wide-necked cerebral aneurysms [5] (Figure 3). Neuroform stent and its subsequent versions (Neuroform EZ, Neuroform EZ3 and Neuroform Atlas) are based on the open-cell design made of laser cutting nickel-titanium alloy (Figure 4) [6].

The second generation of support Enterprise(Codman Neurovascular/Johnson & Johnson) and SolitaireAB (Medtronic, Irvine, CA, USA) abandoned the design of open-cell design, but adopted the closed-cell design, allowing the retrieving of the stent and the repositioning of I t[7-9] (Figures 5 and 6). The third and latest generation of stent LVIS (MicroVention Inc, Aliso Viejo, California, USA) (Figures 7 and 8), LEO+and LEO baby stent series (Balt, Montmorency, France) (Figures 9 and 10) are designed with alloy wire braid to improve the effect of vascular reconstruction and enhance the effect of blood flow diversion, and the effect is excellent so far [10-12].

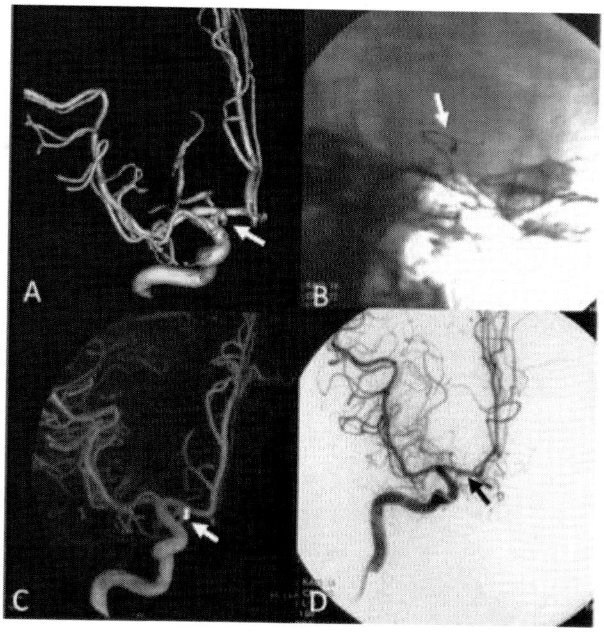

Figure 2. A 49-year-old man presented with Hunt-Hess grade 3 SAH. A, 3-D reconstruction of the right internal carotid artery injection showing an A1 aneurysm of the anterior cerebral artery (arrow). B, unsubtracted image showing the aneurysm was coiled with assistance of a 4 mm × 7 mm Hyperform balloon catheter (Medtronic ev3, USA) (white arrow). C, the right internal carotid artery injection showing the coil mass (arrow). D. oblique view of the right internal carotid artery injection showing the aneurysm was completely occluded (arrow).

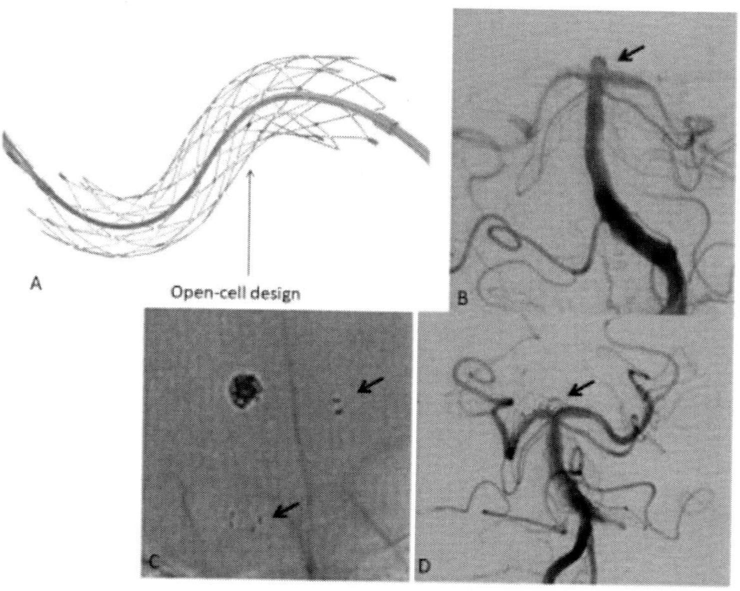

Figure 3. A 53-year-old man presented with Hunt-Hess grade 1 SAH. A, the photograph shows the open-cell design of the Neuroform EZ stent (Stryker Neurovascular, Fremont, California, USA). B, vertebral arteriography, AP view, shows a wide-neck aneurysm arising from the apex of the basilar artery (arrow). C, the fluoroscopic image, AP view, shows the coil mass and marks on both ends of the stent (arrows). D, vertebral arteriography, AP view, shows total obliteration of the aneurysm (arrow).

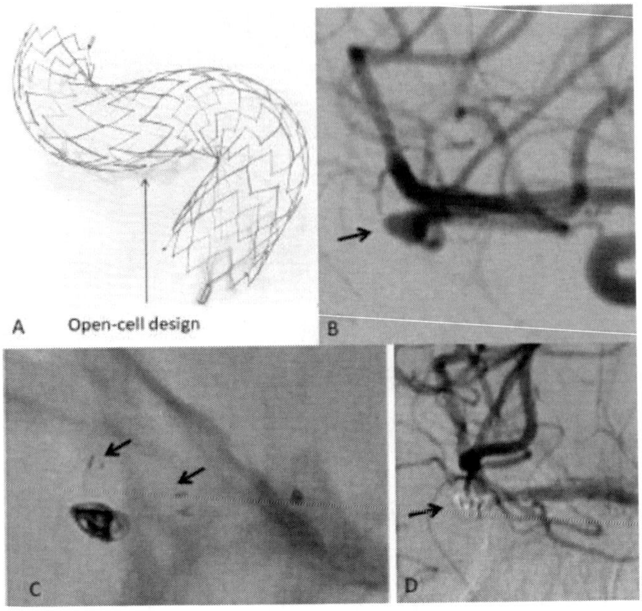

Figure 4. A 46-year-old woman presented with Hunt-Hess grade 3 SAH. A, the photograph shows the open-cell design of the Neuroform Atlas stent (Stryker Neurovascular, Fremont, California, USA). B, the internal carotid artery angiography shows a wide-neck aneurysm arising from the right middle cerebral artery bifurcation (arrow). C, the fluoroscopic image, AP view, shows the coil mass and marks on both ends of the stent (arrows). D, the internal carotid artery angiography shows total obliteration of the aneurysm (arrow).

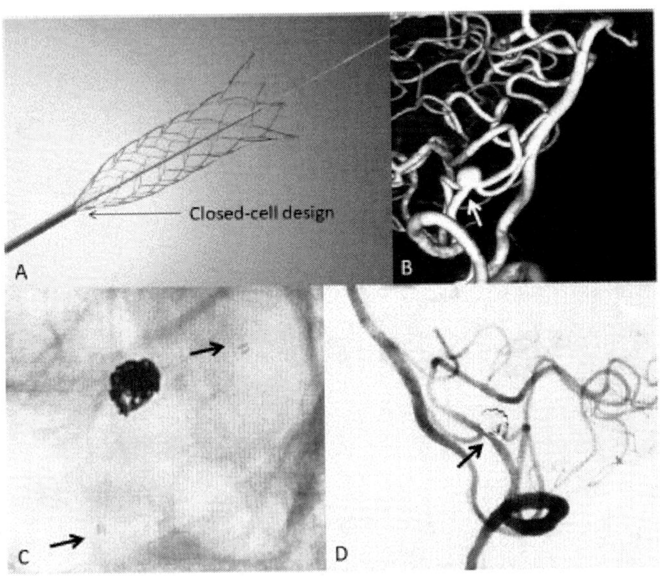

Figure 5. A 62-year-old woman presented with an unruptured aneurysm. A, the photograph shows the Enterprise stent(Codman Neurovascular/Johnson & Johnson) is delivering from the microcatheter, the closed-cell design of the stent allows it to be re-sheathed and placed repeatedly. B, 3-D reconstruction of the vertebral artery injection shows an unruptured aneurysm of the right vertebral artery - posterior inferior cerebellar artery (arrow). C, the fluoroscopic image, AP view, shows the coil mass and marks on both ends of the stent (arrows). D, the vertebral arteriography, lateral view, shows total obliteration of the aneurysm (arrow).

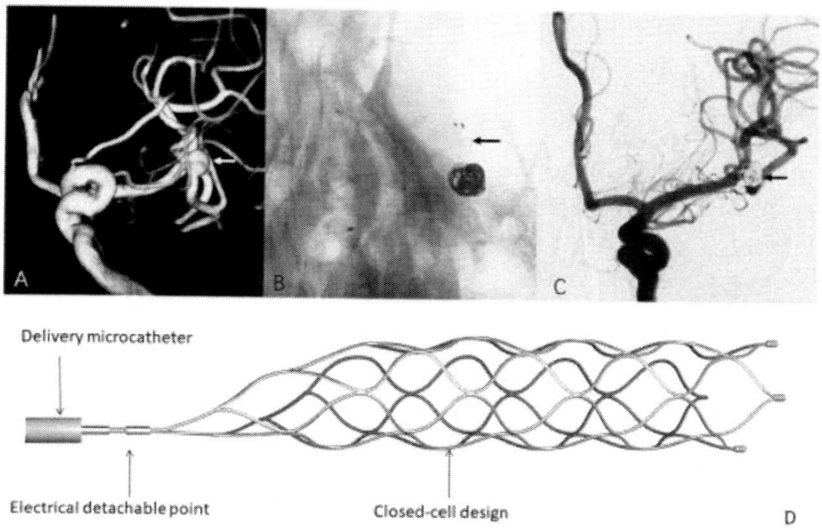

Figure 6. A 68-year-old man presented with an unruptured aneurysm. A, 3-D reconstruction of the internal carotid artery injection shows an unruptured wide-neck aneurysm arising from the left middle cerebral artery bifurcation (arrow). B, the fluoroscopic image, AP view, shows the coil mass and distal marks of the stent (arrow). C, the internal carotid arteriography, AP view, shows total obliteration of the aneurysm (arrow). D, the photograph shows the Solitaire AB stent(Medtronic, Irvine, CA, USA) is delivering from the microcatheter, the closed-cell design of the stent allows it to be re-sheathed and placed repeatedly.

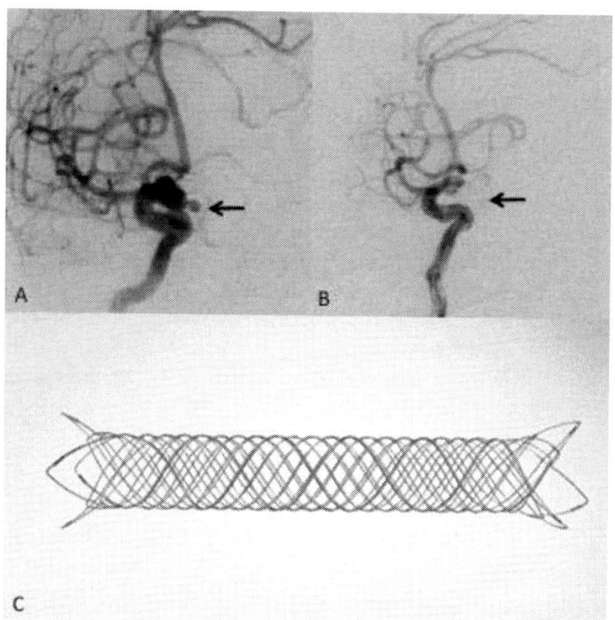

Figure 7. A 66-year-old woman presented with Hunt-Hess grade 3 SAH. A, the internal carotid artery injection shows an ruptured wide-neck aneurysm arising from the left internal carotid artery - posterior communicating artery with a daughter sac (arrow). B, the internal carotid arteriography, working angle, shows total obliteration of the aneurysm after LVIS (MicroVention Inc, Aliso Viejo, California, USA) stent-assisted coiling (arrow). C, the photograph shows the LVIS stent, which is self-expanding stent of braided nickel-titanium alloy structure with closed-cell design. The stent has the best porosity (28%), so it has excellent blood flow guidance characteristics.

Stent-Assisted Coiling Technique

Mesh Piercing Technique

The first step of this technique is to expand the stent at the aneurysm neck. Then the 0.014" microguidewire and microcatheter were inserted into the aneurysm sac through the stent mesh. Place the coil into the aneurysm cavity. Note that the position of the microcatheter should ensure that it is in the aneurysm cavity to avoid the coil entering the parent artery and increase the risk of thromboembolism.

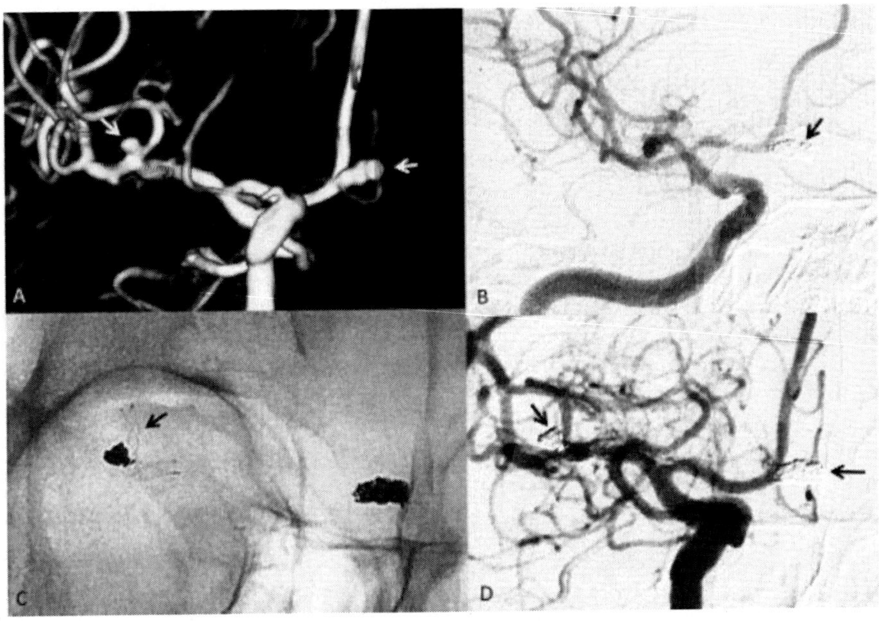

Figure 8. A 73-year-old man presented with two unruptured aneurysms.
A, 3-D reconstruction of the internal carotid artery injection shows two unruptured aneurysms arising from the right middle cerebral artery bifurcation and the right anterior communicating artery of anterior cerebral artery (arrows). B, the internal carotid arteriography, oblique view, shows coil embolization of the aneurysm from the right anterior communicating artery of anterior cerebral artery (arrow).
C, the fluoroscopic image, AP view, shows the coil mass and the LVIS Jr stent for the aneurysms arising from the right middle cerebral artery bifurcation (arrow). D, the internal carotid arteriography, AP view, shows total obliteration of the two aneurysms (arrows).

Jailing Technique

The microcatheter was navigated into the aneurysm cavity prior to the stent placement across the neck of the aneurysm. The stent will squeeze the microcatheter against the nearby vessel wall. Compared with the "mesh piercing" technique, the "jailing" method is conducive to the microcatheter entering the aneurysm cavity, because it may be a difficult task to pass the stent mesh.

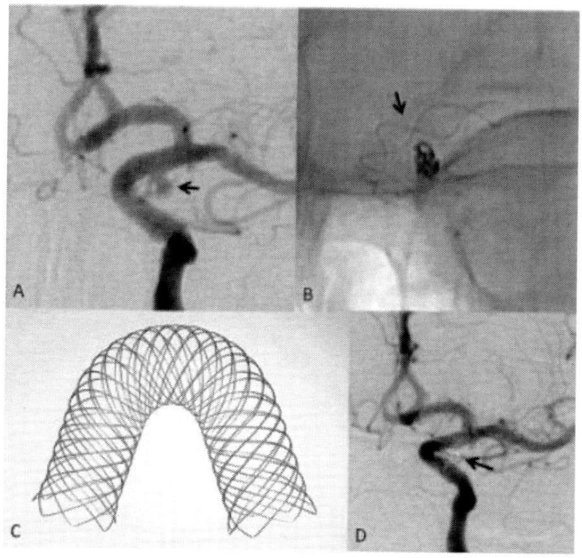

Figure 9. A 57-year-old man presented with an unruptured aneurysm. A, the internal carotid artery injection shows a wide-neck aneurysm arising from the left internal carotid artery - posterior communicating artery (arrow). B, the fluoroscopic image, AP view, shows the coil mass and the LEO+ stent (Balt, Montmorency, France) for the aneurysms (arrow). C, the photograph shows the LEO+ stent, which is a kind of nickel-titanium alloy stent with open holes. Changing the geometric shape of the mesh can reduce the opening area by 39%, increase the radial force, and improve the reconstruction effect of the vascular wall. LEO+has a novel proximal hook, and the stent can be re-sheathed and re-positioned when 90% of the bracket is released. D, the internal carotid arteriography, AP view, shows total obliteration of the aneurysm (arrow).

Stent Technique for Endovascular Treatment of Aneurysms at Bifurcation

Because of their complex morphology and local complex vascular anatomical structure, it is difficult to treat aneurysms at the bifurcation of arteries (such as anterior communicating artery, internal carotid artery bifurcation, middle cerebral artery bifurcation or basilar artery bifurcation). In the process of simple coil, it is difficult to avoid coil herniation into the branch arteries, so sometimes it is necessary to use single stent or multiple stent technique to protect the blood flow of the branch arteries. Two kinds of multi-scaft techniques for bifurcation aneurysms are X stent and Y stent [13]. Y stent technology was described as deploying two stents in the two arterial branches to support the coil [14]. X-stent technology is used for aneurysms at the two parent arteries, such as the anterior communicating artery, in which the stent is sequentially expanded through both arteries [15]. Concerns about potential thromboembolic complications at the intersection of endovascular stents with Y-stent and X-stent technique [13-15]. "Kissing stent" technique is a variant of Y-stent technology, that is, two stents are deployed simultaneously or in sequence side by side without crossing in the proximal artery (Figure 11). The single stent technique can be used for the bifurcation of wide-necked aneurysms with the neck of the aneurysm leaning to the side of the parent artery. T-type double-stent technique can also be used as an alternative to cross-stent technology for the treatment of bifurcation wide-necked aneurysms. T-shaped stent technology is that the proximal end of the second stent terminates at the deployed stent to form a T-shaped configuration. The proximal opening of the second stent should be the neck of the aneurysm (Figure 12).

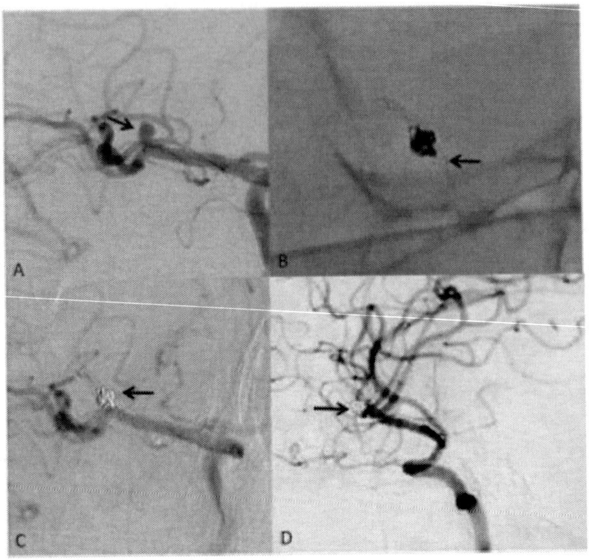

Figure 10. A 54-year-old man presented with an unruptured aneurysm. A, the internal carotid artery angiography shows a wide-neck aneurysm arising from the right middle cerebral artery bifurcation (arrow). B, the fluoroscopic image, working angle, shows the coil mass and marks of the LEO baby stent (Balt, Montmorency, France) (arrow). C, the internal carotid artery angiography shows total obliteration of the aneurysm (arrow). D, 6-month follow-up angiogram confirms the total obliteration of the aneurysm (arrow).

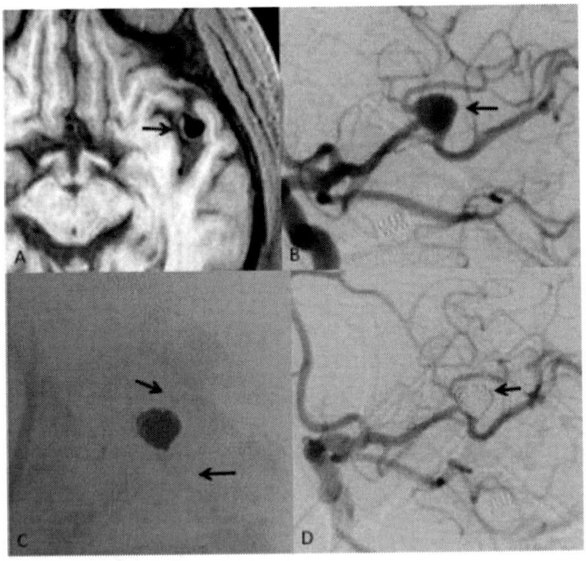

Figure 11. A 78-year-old woman presented with an unruptured aneurysm. A, MRI examination of the head reveals a circular vascular flow void signal in the left Sylvian fissure. B, the internal carotid artery angiography, oblique view, shows a wide-neck aneurysm arising from the right left cerebral artery bifurcation (arrow). C, the fluoroscopic image, working angle, shows the coil mass and distal marks of the two Neuroform Atlas stents (Stryker Neurovascular, Fremont, California, USA) of "Kissing stent" technique (arrows). D, the internal carotid artery angiography shows total obliteration of the aneurysm (arrow).

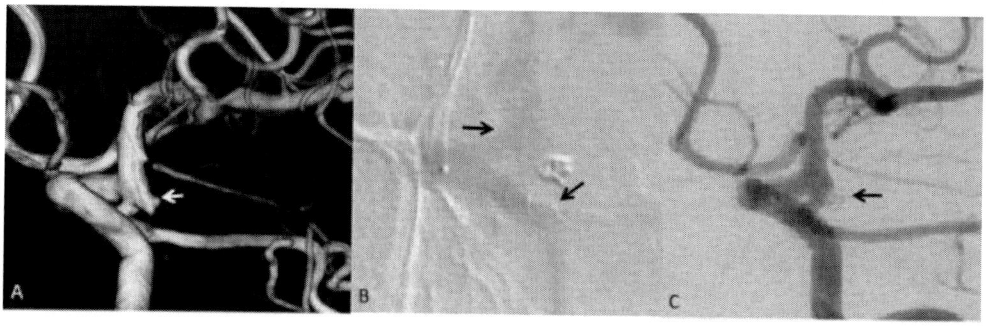

Figure 12. A 64-year-old man presented with Hunt-Hess grade 3 SAH.
A, 3-D reconstruction of the internal carotid artery injection shows a small wide-neck aneurysm arising from the left internal carotid artery - posterior communicating artery (arrow). B, the subtraction image, working angle, shows the LVIS stent in the internal carotid artery and the LEO baby stent in the posterior communicating artery of the T-type double-stent technique (arrows). C, the internal carotid arteriography, working angle, shows total obliteration of the aneurysm (arrow).

The results of mid-term and long-term follow-up have proved that the total occlusion rate of bifurcation aneurysms treated with multi-scaft technique is 90%, and the incidence of thromboembolism complications is 3.9% [16]. Recently, some new devices have been developed to assist in the treatment of these aneurysms and include the pCONus1 and pCONus2 (phenox, Bochum, Germany), the PulseRider® (Pulsar Vascular, Los Gatos, CA, USA), and the eCLIPs™ device (Evasc Neurovascular Enterprises, Vancouver, BC, Canada). These devices share the common feature of providing extra coverage at the aneurysm neck to prevent coil prolapse into the parent vessel [17, 18]. Intrasaccular devices such as the WEB™ (Sequent Medical, Aliso Viejo, CA, USA) represent an alternative technique [19].

Intrasaccular Flow Disruptor

Although coil technique is widely used to treat bifurcation aneurysms, the endovascular technique is complex. This led to the idea of introducing intrasaccular flow disruptor (ISFD) in the treatment of bifurcation aneurysms in 2011 [19]. The Woven EndoBridge (WEB) device (Sequent Medical Inc, Aliso Viejo, CA, USA) is a self-expanding mesh sphere made of braided nickel titanium alloy wire and platinum wire. WEB is the first ISFD to promote thrombosis and aneurysm occlusion. The WEB device was approved by FDA in December 2018 as a safe treatment method for bifurcation wide-necked aneurysms and does not require dual antiplatelet therapy [19]. The first generation of WEB equipment needs to use a micro-catheter with an internal diameter of 0.027-0.033 inches. WEB 21 used 0.021-inch delivery microcatheter in 2015. The latest generation (WEB 17) has a small design for small aneurysms (3-7 mm), suitable for 0.017 inch delivery microcatheters, and its shunt ability is comparable to WEB 21 [20].

Flow-Diversion Devices

The flow-diversion device(FD) emerged in 2007 has fundamentally changed the previous concept of treatment of cerebral aneurysms, from the concept of intra-aneurysm filling, occlusion of the parent artery, clipping of the aneurysm sac, or remodeling of the aneurysm orifice to the concept of pathological arterial wall repair [21]. This is undoubtedly correct, because the basic pathological changes of the occurrence of an aneurysm are the weakness of the intima of the artery wall, atherosclerosis, injury of the artery wall, or infection of the artery wall. Moreover, FD has greatly expanded the scope and elevated the effect of endovascular treatment of cerebral aneurysms, from tiny aneurysms to giant aneurysms, from blister-like aneurysms to fusiform/dissecting aneurysms, from side-wall aneurysms to bifurcation aneurysms (Figure 13) [22]. Flow diversion has become a mainstay of modern endovascular aneurysm treatment. The concept of FD is derived from the experience and lessons learned in the development of stent-assisted coiling. Because stent-assisted coiling directly interrupts the blood flow from the parent artery into the aneurysm and accelerates the thrombosis in the aneurysm, the hemodynamic flow regulation can explain the correlation between the denser coil filling and better angiography and clinical results. The FD of woven mesh device is based on two principles: 1) placing high mesh density device in the parent artery changes the blood flow away from the aneurysm cavity, 2) the device structure provides a scaffold on which endothelial cells can grow. This process is called "new endothelialization," which isolates the aneurysm from the maternal circulation and allows the gradual formation of thrombus in the aneurysm (Figure 14) [23]. The advantage of FD is that it can treat the weakening of the arterial wall (Figure 15). Compared with the high recurrence rate associated with coil embolization, neoendothelialization leads to aneurysm occlusion. In addition, when deploying the FD, the device does not need to enter the aneurysm sac directly, thus eliminating the risk of aneurysm rupture during operation.

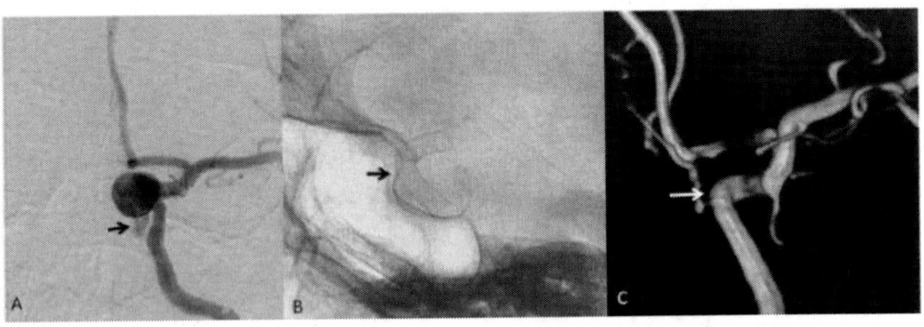

Figure 13. A 48-year-old woman presented with a large aneurysm. A, the internal carotid artery injection shows a large wide-neck aneurysm arising from the ophthalmic segment of the left internal carotid artery with a daughter sac (arrow). B, the subtraction image, lateral view, shows the aneurysm was treated with the pipeline embolization device (PED; Medtronic Neurovascular, Irvine, California, USA) (arrow). C, 2-year follow-up angiogram confirms the total obliteration of the aneurysm (arrow).

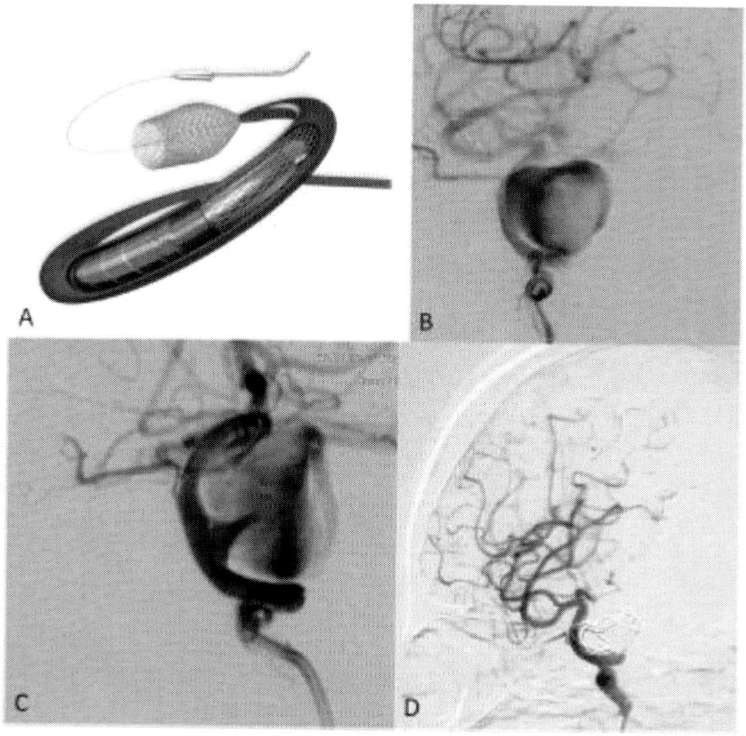

Figure 14. A 60-year-old woman presented with a giant unruptured aneurysm. A, the photograph shows the pipeline embolization device, which is woven from 48 cobalt-chromium-nickel alloy wires, including 12 platinum-tungsten wires as marking wires. The deployment is carried out through 0.027 inch microcatheter combined with push-pull technology. Since its clinical application, PED has shown a high and stable occlusion rate in the treatment of internal carotid artery (ICA) aneurysms. B, the internal carotid artery injection shows a giant wide-neck aneurysm arising from the cavernous segment of the internal carotid artery. C, the internal carotid artery injection shows the contrast retention in the aneurysm immediate after the placement of PED. C, 6-month follow-up angiogram confirms the total obliteration of the aneurysm.

As the first FDA certified FD, the pipeline embolization device (PED; Medtronic Neurovascular, Irvine, California, USA) is still the most popular blood flow modulation device at present. Its off-label clinical application is still a hot topic. Its use has expanded from the treatment of unruptured internal carotid artery aneurysms to the treatment of most cerebral aneurysms, such as anterior cerebral artery, middle cerebral artery and posterior circulation aneurysms (including posterior cerebral artery and posterior inferior cerebellar artery aneurysms) (Figures 16 and 17). Its safety and effectiveness have been widely published. It is a very good choice for aneurysms with accumulated perforating arteries, including ruptured and unruptured aneurysms. For the treatment of blister-like aneurysms, FD has become the first choice [24].

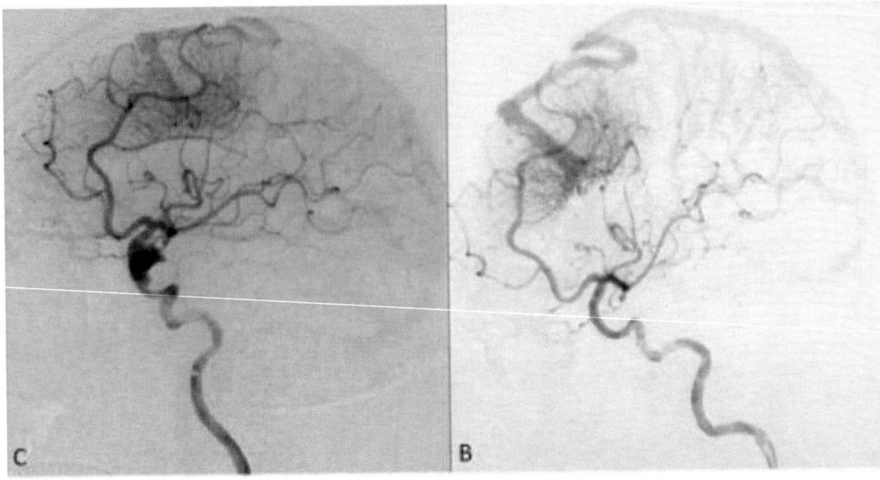

Figure 15. A 52-year-old woman presented with eye swelling and pain. A, the internal carotid artery injection shows a giant wide-neck aneurysm arising from the ophthalmic segment of the internal carotid artery and developmental cenous anomaly of the left frontal lobe. B, 10-month follow-up angiogram confirms the total obliteration of the aneurysm.

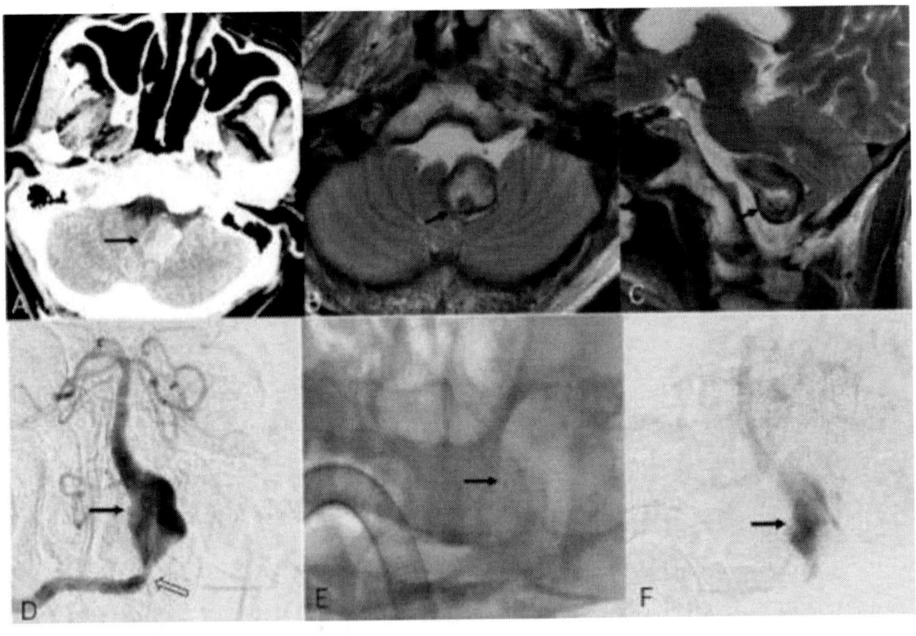

Figure 16. A 61-year-old man presented with brainstem compression. A, cranial CT shows round high-density lesion with calcification on the left side of the brain stem (arrow). B, MRI examination, axial, T2-weighted, shows a round massive lesion on the left side of the brain stem, with low signal around and high signal in the central(arrow). C, MRI examination, sagittal, T2-weighted, shows a round space-occupying lesion on the left side of the brain stem, with low signal around and high signal in the central (arrow). D, the right vertebral artery angiography, AP, shows a giant fusiform aneurysm (arrow) of the right vertebrobasilar artery with proximal stenosis(void arrow). E, the unsubtraction image, AP view, shows the aneurysm was treated with the PED (arrow). F, the vertebral artery injection, AP view, shows the contrast retention in the aneurysm immediate after the placement of PED.

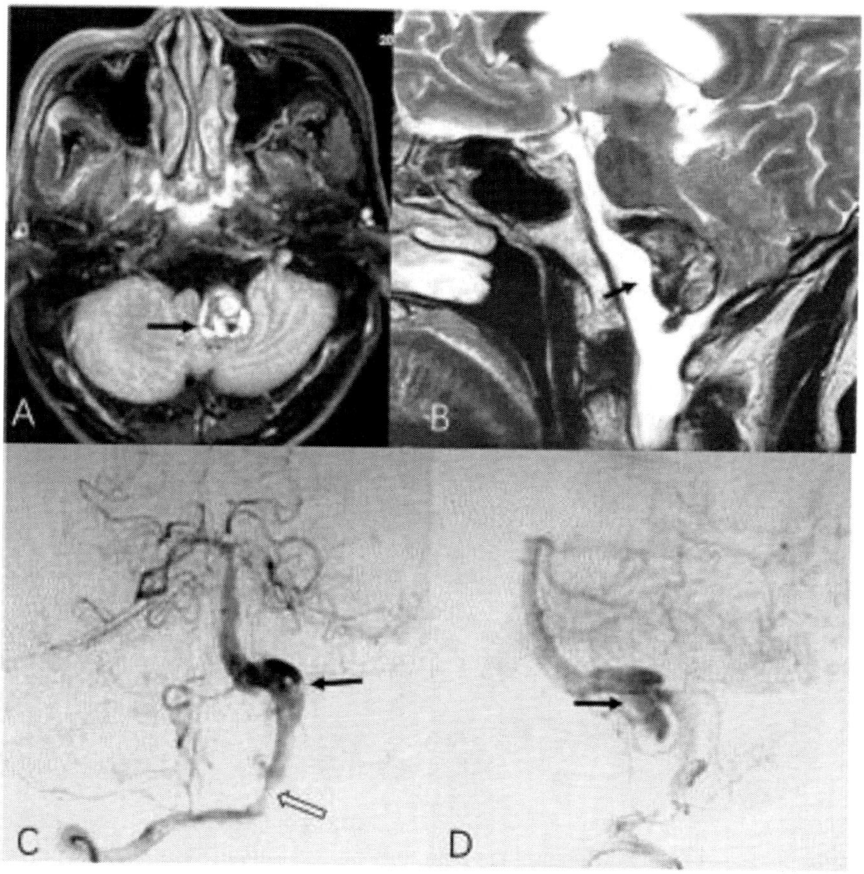

Figure 17. 5 months follow-up images. A, MRI examination, axial, T1-weighted, found that the volume of the lesion on the left side of the brain stem was reduced, and there were mixed signals inside(arrow). B, MRI examination, sagittal, T2-weighted, found that the volume of the lesion on the left side of the brain stem was reduced, and there were mixed signals inside(arrow). C, the right vertebral artery angiography, AP view, showed that the vertebrobasilar aneurysm became smaller, and the proximal stenosis had a tendency to expand compared with the preoperative. D, the right vertebral artery angiography, lateral view, showed that the vertebrobasilar aneurysm became smaller, and the proximal stenosis had a tendency to expand compared with the preoperative.

There are also reports on the treatment of carotid cavernous fistula with FD (Figure 18). In our center, the FD has basically replaced the coil embolization in the treatment of unruptured aneurysms due to its low complication rate, low recurrence rate and high occlusion rate [22]. In a meta-analysis included 11 studies [25], the combined occlusion rates of unruptured intracranial aneurysms at 1 year, 1-2 years, 2 years, 3 years and 5 years follow-up were 77%, 87.4%, 84.5%, 89.4% and 96%, respectively. The rate of in-stent stenosis of long-term follow-up was 5%. No delayed rupture of aneurysm was reported, and there was one delayed ischemic stroke.

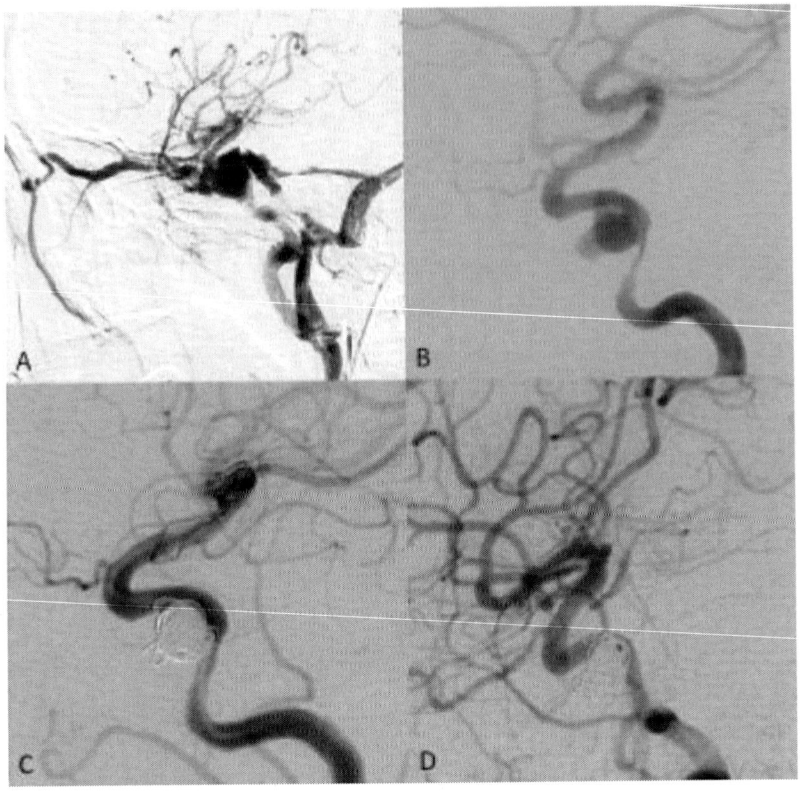

Figure 18. A 62-year-old woman presented with eye protrusion, conjunctival congestion and edema. A, the internal carotid angiography shows that a carotid-cavernous fistula was drained through the ophthalmic vein, the superior petrosal sinus and inferior petrosal sinus. B, One week later, the internal carotid angiography shows carotid-cavernous fistula disappeared and an aneurysm appeared at the cavernous segment of the internal carotid artery, the internal carotid artery proximal to the aneurysm shows stenosis. C, the internal carotid artery angiography, lateral view, shows that the lesion was completely occluded after treatment with PED and coils, and the stenosis of the internal carotid artery had a tendency to expand. D, After 8 months, carotid artery angiography confirms that the aneurysm was occluded and the internal carotid artery stenosis was completely restored to normal.

There are many other FDs with different design concepts on the market [21], such as Silk, Silk+, Silk vista baby (Balt Extrusion; Montmorency, France); Surpass Streamline and Surpass Evolve (Stryker Neurovascular, Fremont, CA); The FRED and FRED Jr (Microvention, Aliso Viejo, California) (Figure 19); p64, p48MW and p48-HPC (Phenox, Bochum, Germany); Derivo Embolization Device (Acandis GmbH, Pforzheim, Germany) (Figure 20) and Tubridge (MicroPort, Shanghai, China); Lattice (Accumedical, Beijing, China) (Figure 21). Therefore, many kinds of devices are available, which may be confusing. At present, the FDA approved PED in 2011, Surpass in 2018 and FRED in 2019, all of which are used to treat large or large wide-necked intracranial aneurysms along the internal carotid artery (FDA. gov). All FDA-approved FDs consist of Nitinol or Co-Cr alloy. If the clinical scenario requires, the endovascular neurosurgeon must be proficient in at least one or two of them. At the same time, if the clinical situation requires, we should maintain a certain understanding and familiarity with the advantages/limitations of these devices.

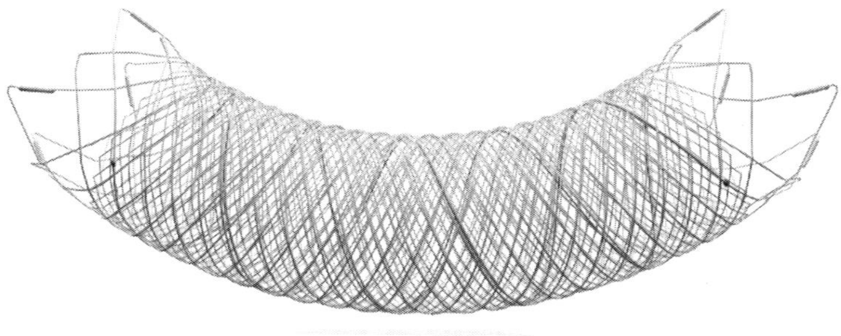

Figure 19. The flow re-direction endoluminal device (FRED) and FRED Jr. flow-diversion devices (MicroVention, Aliso Viejo, California, USA) feature a unique dual-layer construction marked with radio-opaque helix to provide fluoroscopic visibility, distal and proximal markers evenly dispersed on its single layer ends. The FRED Jr. device is the first flow diverter that can be delivered using a 0.021″ microcatheter for safe delivery in distal locations. Both devices may be used with or without embolic coils.

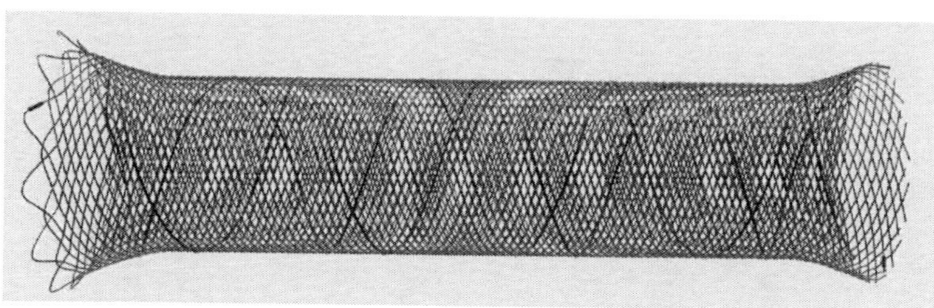

Figure 20. Photograph of the Derivo Embolization Device (Acandis GrmbH & Co KG, Pforzheim, Germany). It is a self-expanding device made up of Nitinol, and it is claimed to be less thrombogenic than other devices owing to its oxide and oxynitride coating. It has a porosity of 60–65% and surface coverage of 33–39%, and the cross-sectional diameter of the wires is 0.003 to 0.009 inches. Its platinum core makes the device radio-opaque with better fluoroscopic visualization, and additional radiopaque markers at each of the 3 flared ends enhance it. Also, the device can be recaptured and repositioned before full deployment.

The main limitation of FD is ischemic stroke associated with stent thrombosis, which requires dual antiplatelet therapy or GP IIb/IIIa inhibitors and their associated bleeding risks [26]. Since 2014, different manufacturers have designed antithrombotic coating FD to reduce its thrombosis. At present, the available antithrombotic coating FDs include Pipeline Flex embolic device with shielding technology (Medtronic Neurovascular, Irvine, California, USA), Derivo embolic device (Acandis GmbH, Pforzheim, Germany) and p48-HPC (Phenox, Bochum, Germany) [27]. Preliminary follow-up data show that these devices are not inferior in terms of angiographic occlusion rate. These data also show that the incidence of stent-related ischemia is low.

The wide use and experience of FDs provide a unique opportunity for its application in the field of cerebrovascular pathology, enabling it to continue to expand to their initial indications of cerebrovascular pathology [28]. Before widespread use of FDs, we should balance the excitement in careful and robust research to prove that FDs is superior to traditional intravascular and surgical methods in terms of safety and effectiveness under off-label conditions. With the increase in the use of FDs in a broader clinical scenario, it is necessary to design and customize the specific aneurysm anatomical structure, location and shape to cover a broader range of clinical indications. Many applications of FD in small vessels (such as anterior communicating artery and the distal artery) have been widely reported [29]. The most common is PED, as well as FRED and SILK series. Few studies support the efficacy of Surpass, p64, Derivo and Tubridge stents in small vessels.

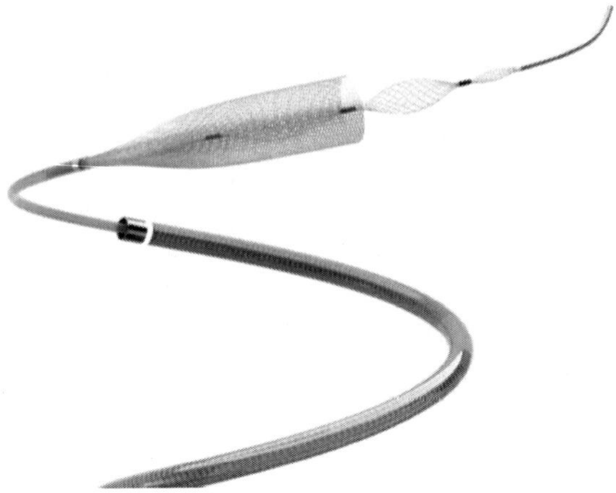

Figure 21. A new type of flow-diversion device made in China (Lattice TM, Accumedical, Beijing, China). It consists of 36 cobalt-chromium alloy wires and 12 platinum-tungsten alloy wires. The design of woven mesh spindle apparatus on the fixed guide wire of the device can make it opening easier.

Conclusion

Stent-assisted coiling and flow-diversion devices have become common endovascular treatments for most cerebral aneurysms. There are many kinds of devices available, which may be confusing. Neurointerventional experts are required to be skilled in them. At the same time, if the clinical situation requires, they should maintain a certain understanding and familiarity of the advantages/limitations of other devices used.

References

[1] Alksne JF, Smith RW. Iron-acrylic compound for steriotaxic aneurysm thrombosis. *J Neurosurg*. 1977 Aug;47(2):137-41.

[2] Wiebers DO, Whisnant JP, Huston J 3rd, Meissner I, Brown RD Jr, Piepgras DG, Forbes GS, Thielen K, Nichols D, O'Fallon WM, Peacock J, Jaeger L, Kassell NF, Kongable-Beckman GL, Torner JC; International Study of Unruptured Intracranial Aneurysms Investigators. Unruptured intracranial aneurysms: natural history, clinical outcome, and risks of surgical and endovascular treatment. *Lancet*. 2003;362(9378):103-10.

[3] Ogilvy CS, Natarajan SK, Jahshan S, Karmon Y, Yang X, Snyder KV, Hopkins LN, Siddiqui AH, Levy EI. Stent-assisted coiling of paraclinoid aneurysms: risks and effectiveness. *J Neurointerv Surg*. 2011;3(1):14-20.

[4] Piotin M, Blanc R, Spelle L, Mounayer C, Piantino R, Schmidt PJ, Moret J. Stent-assisted coiling of intracranial aneurysms clinical and angiographic results in 216 consecutive aneurysms. *Stroke*. 2010;41:110-115.

[5] Maldonado IL, Machi P, Costalat V, Mura T, Bonafé A. Neuroform stent-assisted coiling of unruptured intracranial aneurysms: short- and midterm results from a single-center experience with 68 patients. *AJNR Am J Neuroradiol*. 2011;32(1):131-6.

[6] Ni H, Zhao LB, Liu S, Jia ZY, Cao YZ, Shi HB. Open-cell stent-assisted coiling for the treatment of paraclinoid aneurysms: traditional endovascular treatment is still not out of date. *Neuroradiology*. 2021 Sep;63(9):1521-1530.

[7] Mocco J, Snyder KV, Albuquerque FC, Bendok BR, Alan S B, Carpenter JS, Fiorella DJ, Hoh BL, Howington JU, Jankowitz BT, Liebman KM, Rai AT, Rodriguez-Mercado R, Siddiqui AH, Veznedaroglu E, Hopkins LN, Levy EI. Treatment of intracranial aneurysms with the Enterprise stent: a multicenter registry. *J Neurosurg*. 2009;110(1):35-9.

[8] Lv X, Li Y, Xinjian Y, Jiang C, Wu Z. Results of endovascular treatment for intracranial wide-necked saccular and dissecting aneurysms using the Enterprise stent: a single center experience. *Eur J Radiol*. 2012 Jun;81(6):1179-83.

[9] Lv X, Zhang W, Zhao X, Zhang H, Wang J. Endovascular Treatment of Small Wide-Neck Bifurcation Aneurysms with Single Solitaire AB Stent Technique. *Neurol India* 2021;69:879-82.

[10] Lv X, Jiang C, Liang S. Small ruptured and unruptured complex cerebral aneurysms: Single center experience of low-profile visualized intraluminal support stent. *Journal of Neurorestoratology* 2019;7(4): 235–241.

[11] Lv X, Li Y, Jiang C, Yang X, Wu Z. Potential advantages and limitations of the Leo stent in endovascular treatment of complex cerebral aneurysms. *Eur J Radiol*. 2011;79(2):317-22.

[12] Kim J, Han HJ, Lee W, Park SK, Chung J, Kim YB, Park KY. Safety and Efficacy of Stent-Assisted Coiling of Unruptured Intracranial Aneurysms Using Low-Profile Stents in Small Parent Arteries. *AJNR Am J Neuroradiol*. 2021 Sep;42(9):1621-1626.

[13] Endo H, Mitome-Mishima Y, Suzuki K, Yatomi K, Teranishi K, Oishi H. Long-term outcomes of Y-stent-assisted coil embolization using Low-profile Visualized Intraluminal Support Junior (LVIS Jr) for intracranial bifurcation aneurysms. *Clin Neurol Neurosurg*. 2022 Jun;217:107275.

[14] Cagnazzo F, Limbucci N, Nappini S, Renieri L, Rosi A, Laiso A, Tiziano di Carlo D, Perrini P, Mangiafico S. Y-Stent-Assisted Coiling of Wide-Neck Bifurcation Intracranial Aneurysms: A Meta-Analysis. *AJNR Am J Neuroradiol*. 2019 Jan;40(1):122-128.

[15] Cohen JE, Moscovici S, El Hassan HA, Doron O, Itshayek E. T-microstent-assisted coiling in the management of ruptured wide-necked anterior communicating artery aneurysms: Choosing between Y, X and T. *J Clin Neurosci*. 2016 Dec;34:283-287.

[16] Hagen F, Maurer CJ, Berlis A. Endovascular Treatment of Unruptured MCA Bifurcation Aneurysms Regardless of Aneurysm Morphology: Short- and Long-Term Follow-Up. *AJNR Am J Neuroradiol*. 2019 Mar;40(3):503-509.

[17] Sirakov S, Panayotova A, Sirakov A, Penkov M, Minkin K, Hristov H. Using the pCANvas neck-bridging device in treating a wide-necked aneurysm of the basilar tip. *Neuroradiol J*. 2019 Jun;32(3):193-199.

[18] Lylyk P, Chudyk J, Bleise C, Henkes H, Bhogal P. Treatment of Wide-Necked Bifurcation Aneurysms : Initial Results with the pCANvas Neck Bridging Device. *Clin Neuroradiol*. 2019 Sep;29(3):467-477.

[19] Naamani KE, Chen CJ, Abbas R, Sweid A, Sioutas GS, Badih K, Ramesh S, Tjoumakaris SI, Gooch MR, Herial NA, Zarzour H, Schmidt RF, Rosenwasser RH, Jabbour PM. Woven EndoBridge versus stent-assisted coil embolization of cerebral bifurcation aneurysms. *J Neurosurg*. 2022 Apr 29;137(6):1786-1793.

[20] Iosif C. Neurovascular devices for the treatment of intracranial aneurysms: emerging and future technologies. *Expert Rev Med Devices*. 2020 Mar;17(3):173-188.

[21] Dandapat S, Mendez-Ruiz A, Martínez-Galdámez M, Macho J, Derakhshani S, Foa Torres G, Pereira VM, Arat A, Wakhloo AK, Ortega-Gutierrez S. Review of current intracranial aneurysm flow diversion technology and clinical use. *J Neurointerv Surg*. 2021 Jan; 13(1):54-62.

[22] Zhang H, Ren J, Wang J, Lv X. The off-label uses of pipeline embolization device for complex cerebral aneurysms: Mid-term follow-up in a single center. *Interv Neuroradiol*. 2022 Dec 30:15910199221148800. doi: 10.1177/15910199221148800. Epub ahead of print. PMID: 36583531.

[23] Campos JK, Cheaney Ii B, Lien BV, Zarrin DA, Vo CD, Colby GP, Lin LM, Coon AL. Advances in endovascular aneurysm management: flow modulation techniques with braided mesh devices. *Stroke Vasc Neurol*. 2020 Mar 25;5(1):1-13.

[24] Roy AK, Lekka E, Lee KH, Choi P, Day AL, Roc Chen P. Meta-analysis on the treatment options and outcomes of carotid blood blister aneurysms. *J Clin Neurosci*. 2021 Oct; 92:147-152.

[25] Shehata MA, Ibrahim MK, Ghozy S, Bilgin C, Jabal MS, Kadirvel R, Kallmes DF. Long-term outcomes of flow diversion for unruptured intracranial aneurysms: a systematic review and meta-analysis. *J Neurointerv Surg*. 2022 Sep 23:neurintsurg-2022-019240. doi: 10.1136/jnis-2022-019240. Epub ahead of print. PMID: 36150896.

[26] Hudson JS, Lang MJ, Gross BA. Novel Innovation in Flow Diversion: Surface Modifications. *Neurosurg Clin N Am*. 2022 Apr; 33(2):215-218. doi: 10.1016/j.nec.2021.11.004. Epub 2022 Mar 2. PMID: 35346453.

[27] Akgul E, Onan HB, Akpinar S, Balli HT, Aksungur EH. The DERIVO embolization device in the treatment of intracranial aneurysms: short- and midterm results. *World Neurosurg*. 2016;95:229–240.

[28] Ten Brinck MFM, Shimanskaya VE, Aquarius R, Bartels RHMA, Meijer FJA, Koopmans PC, de Jong G, Wakhloo AK, de Vries J, Boogaarts HD. Outcomes after Flow Diverter Treatment in Subarachnoid Hemorrhage: A Meta-Analysis and Development of a Clinical Prediction Model (OUTFLOW). Brain Sci. 2022 Mar 15; 12(3):394. doi: 10.3390/brainsci12030394. PMID: 35326350; PMCID: PMC8946659.

[29] Dabhi N, Sarathy D, Snyder MH, Kellogg RT, Park MS. Flow Diverter Devices for Treatment of Intracranial Aneurysms in Small Parent Vessels-A Systematic Review of Literature. *World Neurosurg*. 2022 Jun; 162:183-194.e7.

Chapter 15

Stent-Assisted Coiling of Cerebral Aneurysms Using the Laser-Cut Closed-Cell Stents: Enterprise and Solitaire AB Stents

Huachen Zhang
Shikai Liang
and Xianli Lv*
Department of Neurosurgery, Beijing Tsinghua Changgung Hospital,
School of Clinical Medicine, Tsinghua University, Beijing, China

Abstract

Objective: To evaluate the technical feasibility, peri- and post-procedural morbidity and mortality as well as angiographic follow-up of stent-assisted coiling of broad-based cerebral aneurysms using the Enterprise and the Solitaire AB stents.

Methods: Consecutive 77 patients with cerebral aneurysms stented with the Enterprise or Solitaire AB stents were retrospectively studied. Angiographic follow-up (mean 8.25 months) was available in 90.9% of patients.

Results: All stents were successfully deployed. There is a higher acute intra-stent thrombosis complication in Solitaire AB stent placement ($p = 0.012$). However, no significant differences in peri-procedural morbidity and mortality rates ($p = 0.253$), angiographic results ($p = 0.411$), recurrence rate ($p > 0.999$) or long-term neurological deficit ($p = 0.435$), were observed.

Conclusion: Both stents exhibited similar immediate and mid-term results, major neurological morbidities and mortality are low. Thrombogenic complications seems higher in Solitaire AB group.

Keywords: stent-assisted coiling, cerebral aneurysm, Enterprise stent, Solitaire AB stent

Stent-assisted coiling allows endovascular treatment of broad-based cerebral aneurysms, which are challenging for simple coil embolization [1, 2]. In 2002, the first dedicated self-expanding stent Neuroform (Stryker, Karamazu, Michigan, USA) (Figure 1) and in 2003, Leo stent (Balt,

* Corresponding Author's Email: lvxianli000@163.com.

In: Understanding and Managing Cerebral Aneurysms
Editor: Xianli Lv
ISBN: 979-8-89113-608-3

Montmorency, France) (Figure 2) was introduced into the market as open-cell and closed-cell stent [3, 4].

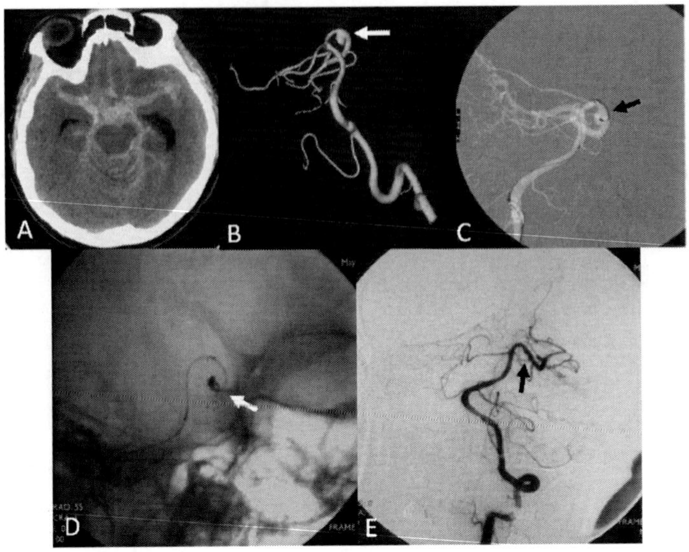

Figure 1. A 41-year-old woman presented with ruptured posterior cerebral artery aneurysm. A, CT scanning showing subarachnoid hemorrhage. B, 3-D reconstruction of the left vertebral artery injection showing a P1 segment aneurysm of the left posterior cerebral artery (arrow). C, under roadmap image a Neuroform stent is deployed as the first step and then a microcatheter is navigated into the aneurysmal lumen via the mesh of the stent (arrow). D, working angle of the unsubtracted image showing the coils are delivered through the microcatheter (arrow). E, frontal view of the left vertebral artery injection after treatment showing the complete occlusion of the aneurysm (arrow).

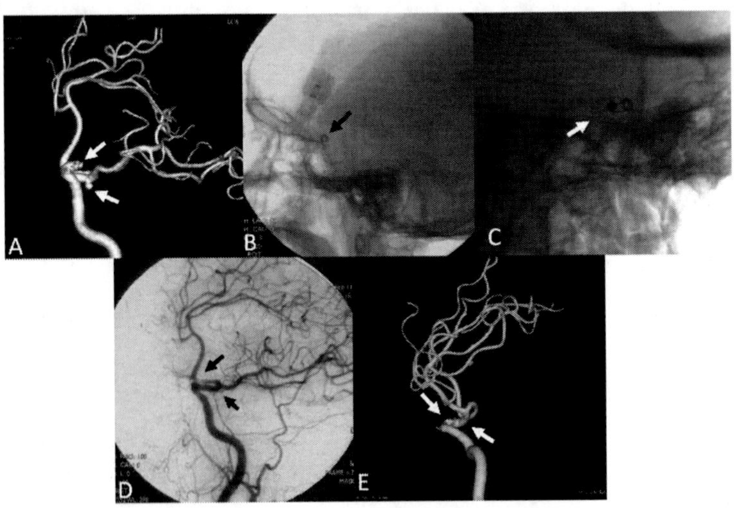

Figure 2. A 66-year-old woman presented with a recurrent aneurysm and a de novo posterior communicating artery aneurysm. A, 3-D reconstruction of the left carotid artery injection showing a recanalized supraclinoid aneurysm and a de novo posterior communicating artery aneurysm of the internal carotid artery (arrows). B, lateral view of the unsubtracted image showing the coil mass of the first treatment. C, unsubtracted image showing the 4.5 mm × 25 mm Leo stent (Balt, France) and coil mass (Microplex, 3 mm × 7 cm, 2 mm × 6 cm, 2 mm × 6 cm, 2 mm × 4 cm; Microvention, USA) after the second treatment. D, oblique view of the left carotid artery injection. E, 3-D reconstruction of the left carotid artery injection. Showing the 2 aneurysms were completely occluded after treatment.

Leo stent is a neurovascular braided stent that can be delivered through microcatheters [4, 5]. Two laser-cut closed-cell stents are available for stent-assisted coiling in the China, the Enterprise stent (Codman Neurovascular/Johnson & Johnson) and the Solitaire AB stent (Medtronic, Irvine, CA, USA) [6, 7]. The goal of this chapter was to report several parameters in the comparison of the Enterprise and Solitaire AB stents in stent-assisted coiling and related mid-term follow-up findings.

Materials and Methods

Patients and Aneurysm Treatment

The imaging and medical charts of 84 consecutive patients with cerebral aneurysms treated with stent-assisted coil embolization between February and September 2020 were retrospectively analyzed. Seven patients harboring 7 aneurysms were treated with Neuroform EZ and flow diverter were excluded. Total 77 patients with 77 aneurysms treated by the Enterprise and Solitaire AB stent-assisted coiling were included in this study.

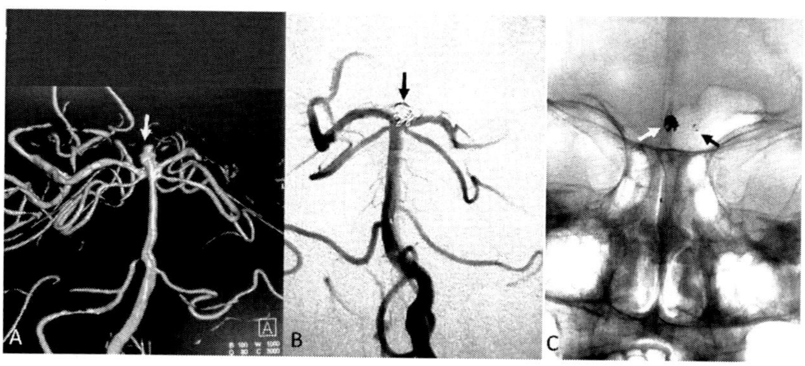

Figure 3. A 52-year-old woman presented with Hunt-Hess grade III subarachnoid hemorrhage. A, 3-D reconstruction of the right vertebral artery injection showing a basilar tip aneurysm (arrow). B, frontal view of the left vertebral artery injection after treatment showing the complete occlusion of the aneurysm (arrow). C, frontal view of the unsubtracted image showing the aneurysm was treated with 4 mm × 15 mm SolitaireAB stent (Medtronic, ev3, USA) (black arrow) and coils (white arrow).

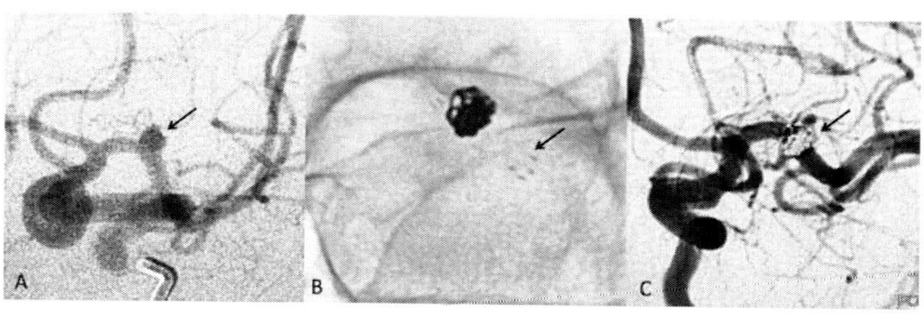

Figure 4. A 67-year-old woman presented with an unruptured M1 aneurysm of the left middle cerebral artery. A, the left internal carotid artery injection showing a M1 aneurysm (arrow). B, frontal view of the unsubtracted image showing the aneurysm was treated with 4.5 mm × 14 mm Enterprise stent (Codman Neurovascular/Johnson & Johnson) (arrow) and coils. C, the left internal carotid artery injection after treatment showing the complete occlusion of the aneurysm (arrow).

Stent-assisted coiling was performed in aneurysms with a dome-to-neck ratio < 2 or a neck diameter > 4 mm and in broad-based aneurysms that were not approachable by simple coil embolization. All aneurysms were coiled with the jailing technique (Figure 3 and 4). All patients was treated under general anesthesia approach in a sterile environment using a common femoral artery approach and anticoagulation with heparin. Patient with unrupture aneurysm was preloaded with the dual antiplatelet agents, 75 mg clopidogrel daily and 100 mg aspirin daily for 3-5 days before treatment. If acute stenting was indicated, patients were preloaded with 300 mg aspirin and 300 mg clopidogrel 2 hours before treatment. Postprocedure, the patients were kept on a dual antiplatelet regimen of 100 mg aspirin/day and 75 mg clopidogrel/day for 3 months and then 100 mg aspirin to 6 months.

Data Collection and Statistical Analysis

In addition to clinical presentation and patient demographics, data was collected for aneurysm size, location, morphology (fusiform vs. saccular), angiographic result, rupture status and periprocedural morbidity and mortality. Pearson's Chi square and Fisher's exact test were determined for demographic, angiographic result, rupture status, periprocedural morbidity and mortality differentiation. Student's t test was used to determine statistical significance in continuous scaled parameters, including age and aneurysm size. A $p < 0.05$ was considered statistically significant.

Clinical and Angiographic Outcome Measures

Clinical evaluations were acquired in conjunction with the follow-up angiography. Technical success was defined by correct placement of the stent. Immediate postprocedure angiography measured aneurysm occlusion using a modification of the Raymond classification scale, which primarily was developed for berry-shaped aneurysms [8]. Intra-stent stenosis, recanalization, and need for retreatment were evaluated on follow-up angiogram. Intra-stent thrombosis was confirmed by on angiography.

Results

Characteristics of Treated Aneurysms

Seventy-seven aneurysms in consecutive 77 patients qualified for treatment by stent-assisted coiling (58 Enterprise and 19 Solitaire AB, respectively). Seventy-five (97.4%) aneurysms were treated with stent and coils, whereas 2 (2.6%) were treated with stent alone (Table 1). Sixty-four (83.1%) of the aneurysms were located in the anterior and 13 (16.9%) in the posterior circulation (Table 2). The mean aneurysm size was 8.31 ± 7.99 mm in the Enterprise group and 8.38 ± 7.67 mm in the Solitaire AB group. Four aneurysms stented by Enterprise had fusiform morphology and 54 were saccular, while 2 were fusiform and 17 were saccular morphology in the Solitaire AB group. A total of 18 ruptured aneurysms (23.4%), 12 in the Enterprise group and 6 in the Solitaire AB group, were treated. In 59 unruptured aneurysms, 33 aneurysms were discovered incidentally, followed by 26 aneurysms were previously discovered, and became clinically apparent, most frequently due to cranial nerve compression symptoms and headache.

Success of Stents

Of the 58 aneurysms intended to be treated with the Enterprise stent, the stent was successfully navigated and deployed in all. In 57 (98.3%) aneurysms, subsequent coiling was performed in the same session. Of the 19 aneurysms intended to be treated with the Solitaire AB stent, the stent was also successfully navigated and deployed in all. In 18 (94.7%) aneurysms, subsequent coiling was performed in the same session.

Procedure Related Morbidity and Mortality

Acute intra-stent thrombosis (one in Enterprise group and 4 in Solitaire AB group) was observed in 5 (7.8%) patients. A significant higher incidence of acute intra-stent thrombosis caused by Solitaire AB stent placement ($P = 0.012$) was observed. However, no difference was observed in peri-procedural morbidity and mortality between both stents ($P = 0.253$).

Procedure-related morbidity with long-term neurological sequela of right paralysis and partial expressive aphasia was 1 (1.7%) in Enterprise group. In the Solitaire AB group, one procedure-related transient paralysis complication was found and resolved to baseline at follow-up. Most minor and major peri-procedural complications observed in this study were related to thrombolysis and thromboembolism (Table 3). There was 1 death in the group of Solitaire AB. The 65-year-old patient was treated for an unruptured anterior communicating artery aneurysm. During coil embolization, both anterior cerebral arteries disappeared on angiogram, the coil embolization was stopped and urokinase was given to thrombolysis until both anterior cerebral arteries were filled with contrast again, but the patient died due to an hemorrhage while on heparin medication 6 hours after thrombolysis treatment. There was no death in the patients treated with the Enterprise.

Initial Angiographic Results

On the immediate post-treatment angiogram, the occlusion grade was as follows: in the Enterprise group: Raymond class 1 in 40 (69.0%) aneurysms, Raymond class 2 in 9 (15.5%) aneurysms and in Raymond class 3 in 9 (15.5%) aneurysms; in the Solitaire AB group, Raymond class 1 in 11 (57.9%) aneurysms, Raymond class 2 in 4 (21.05%) aneurysms and Raymond class 3 in 4(21.05%) aneurysms. Representative cases for each stent are shown in Figure 1 and Figure 2.

Table 1. Baseline Demographics of aneurysms treated using the Enterprise and Solitaire AB stents

	Enterprise	Solitaire AB	p value	OR	95% CI
Age (years ± SD)	53.34 ± 12.69	48.74 ± 11.02	0.161		
Sex (f/m)	36/22	11/8	0.791	0.840	0.293-2.411
Mean max dimension (mm ± SD)	8.3 ± 8.0	8.4 ± 7.7	0.977		
Localization (ant/post)	48/10	16/3	>0.999	0.900	0.220-3.682
Morphology (Saccular/fusiform)	54/4	17/2	0.633	1.588	0.267-9.444
Unruptured/Ruptured	46/12	13/6	0.359	0.585	0.178-1.798
Angiographic results (complete/incomplete)	40/18	11/8	0.411	1.616	0.556-4.698
Acute intra-stent thrombosis complications (yes/no)	1/57	4/15	0.012	15.200	1.580-146.234
Peri-procedural morbidity and mortality(yes/no)	1/57	2/17	0.253	3.294	0.431-25.175
Clinical outcome (with/without new neurological deficits)	1/57	1/18	0.435	3.167	0.188-53.233
Recurrence (present/absent)	5/53	1/17	>0.999	1.247	0.221-7.023

Numbers refer to aneurysms that were eventually treated by stents (n = 58 with Enterprise and n = 19 with Solitaire AB). Abbreviations: F, female; M, male; mm, millimeters; ant, anterior circulation; post, posterior circulation; SD, standard deviation; OR, odds ratio; CI, confidence interval.

Table 2. Location and mean maximum diameter of aneurysms stented using either the Enterprise or Solitaire AB stent

	Total (n)	Enterprise (n)	Mean ± SD (mm)	Solitaire AB(n)	Mean ± SD (mm)
ICA cavernouse segment	13	9	11.7	4	19.0
ICA ophthalmic segment	28	25	5.7	3	6.8
ICA supraclinoid segment	3	3	10.7	0	0
MCA	3	1	25.0	2	4.3
Acoma	2	0	0	2	3.3
Pcoma	15	10	6.6	5	5.7
Basilar apex	3	2	2.7	1	12.0
Basilar trunk	6	6	14.7	0	0
Vertebral artery	4	2	10	2	3.5
Total (n =)	77	58	8.31 ± 7.99	19	8.38 ± 7.67

Abbreviations: n, number of aneurysms; mm, millimeters; ICA, internal carotid artery; MCA, middle cerebral artery; Acoma, anterior communicating artery; Pcoma, posterior communicating artery.

Table 3. Periprocedural mortality and major complications

Patient age, gender	Presentation	Localization	Sac size (mm)	Morphology	Stent	Complication	Treatment	Long-term neurological deficit
59, F	Unruptured	ophthalmic ICA and Pcoma	4 and 6	Saccular	Enterprise	Thromboembolism	Medical	hemiparesis and aphasia
65, M	Unruptured	Acoma	5	Saccular	Solitaire AB	Anti-platelet treatment related ICH		Died
24, F	Unruptured	cavernous ICA	20	Saccular	Solitaire AB	Thromboembolism	Medical	Without neurological deficit
46, F	Ruptured	Pcoma	7	Saccular	Solitaire AB	Thromboembolism	Medical	Transient paralysis and without neurological deficit at follow-up
50, M	Unruptured	M2	6	Saccular	Solitaire AB	Thromboembolism	Medical	Without neurological deficit at follow-up

Abbreviations: F, female; M, male; mm, millimeters; ICA, internal carotid artery; ICH, intracerebral hemorrhage; Pcoma, posterior communicating artery; Acoma, anterior communicating artery; M2, the second segment of middle cerebral artery.

Follow-Up Findings

Follow-up angiogram was available in 70 patients (90.9%) at an average of 8.25 months (range, 3 to 18 months). In 65 patients, treated aneurysms remained stable during the entire observation period. Six aneurysms in 6 patients (8.6%) showed recanalization. No significant intra-stent stenosis
(≥50%) was identified at follow-up angiography. None of the patients experienced aneurysm rupture during the observation period.

Discussion

The endovascular treatment of early cerebral aneurysms is to use a flow-guided detachable balloon catheter to enter the aneurysm cavity (Figure 5) [9]. This method is usually limited by navigation, which makes it difficult to fix the balloon in the aneurysm, and requires injection of curing agent, such as 2-hydroxyethyl methacrylate [9]. Complications related to balloon embolization such as aneurysm rupture and thromboembolism events have led to high morbidity and mortality [9]. Coil embolization is the standard treatment for cerebral aneurysms (Figure 6) [10]. Advances in endovascular technique have allowed the use of coil embolization to treat more challenging aneurysms (Figure 7) [11].

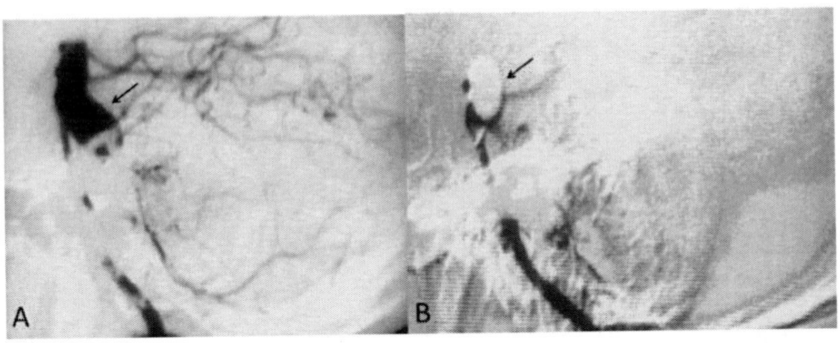

Figure 5. In 1986, Professor Zhongxue Wu successfully embolized cerebral aneurysms with domestic latex balloon. A, the lateral view of vertebral arteriography showed an aneurysm at the top of the basilar artery. B, the lateral view of vertebral arteriography showed that the aneurysm was embolized with detachable balloon.

The appearance of stent combined with coiling technique has greatly improved the ability of endovascular treatment of cerebral aneurysms [11, 12]. Placing the stent on the neck of the aneurysm can fix the coil in the aneurysm cavity and allow the coil to be densely packed (Figure 8) [12]. Stent combined with coiling technique has been developed for more than 20 years [9]. Stents can be divided into two categories: self-expanding or balloon expansion. The balloon expansion stent is made of stainless steel or cobalt, making it have a hard component, such as coronary stents [9]. They are fixed on the balloon and expanded by filling the balloon with contrast agent, and then the stent is expanded. At present, only Willis covered stent is used for the treatment of cerebral aneurysms. In contrast, self-expanding stent is made of nickel-titanium alloy, which is a shape memory nickel-titanium alloy. Choosing appropriate stent size can achieve better vascular wall reconstruction.

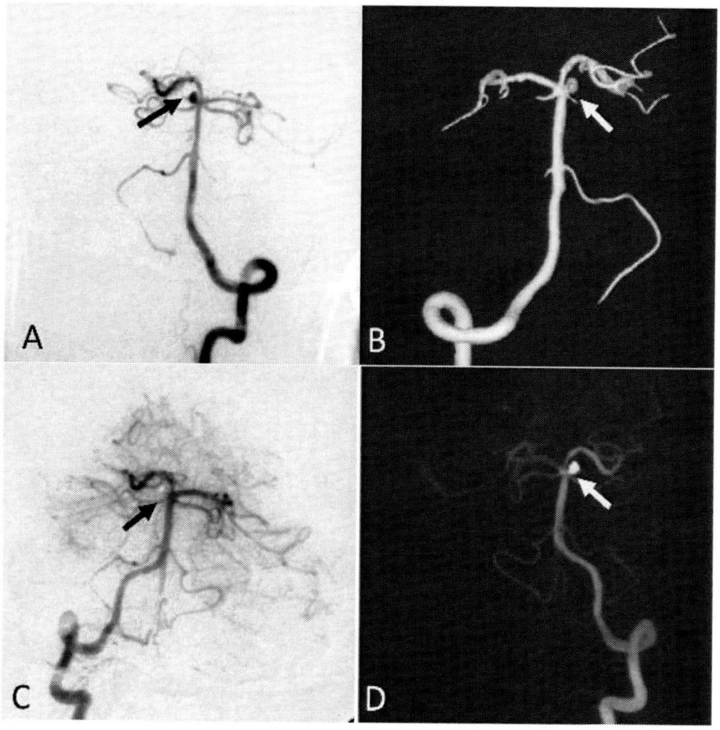

Figure 6. A 56-year-old man with a ruptured aneurysm of the right superior cerebellar artery was coiled with Microplex coils (Microvention, USA). A, frontal view of the left vertebral artery injection showing the aneurysm of the origin of the right superior cerebellar artery (arrow). B, 3-D reconstruction of the left vertebral artery injection showing the aneurysm of the origin of the right superior cerebellar artery (arrow). C, frontal view of the right vertebral artery injection after aneurysm coil embolization. D, 3-D reconstruction of the right vertebral artery injection after aneurysm coil embolization. Showing the aneurysm was completely occluded (arrows).

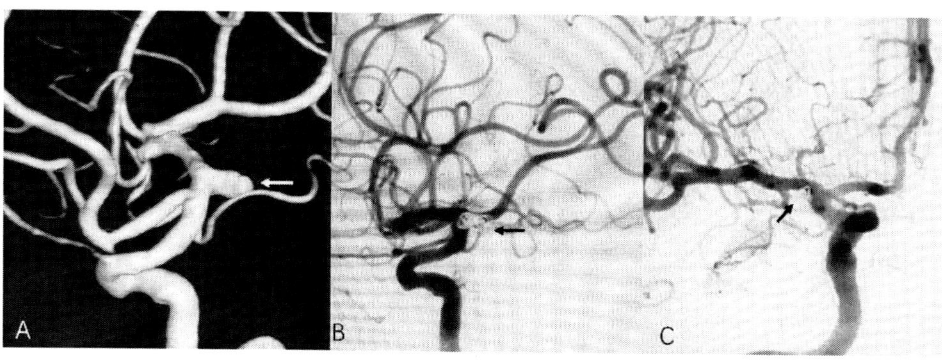

Figure 7. A, the lateral view of internal carotid artery angiography showed M1 segment aneurysm (arrow). B, the lateral view of internal carotid artery angiography. C, the frontal view of internal carotid artery angiography. Showed the M1 segment aneurysm was completely occluded (arrows).

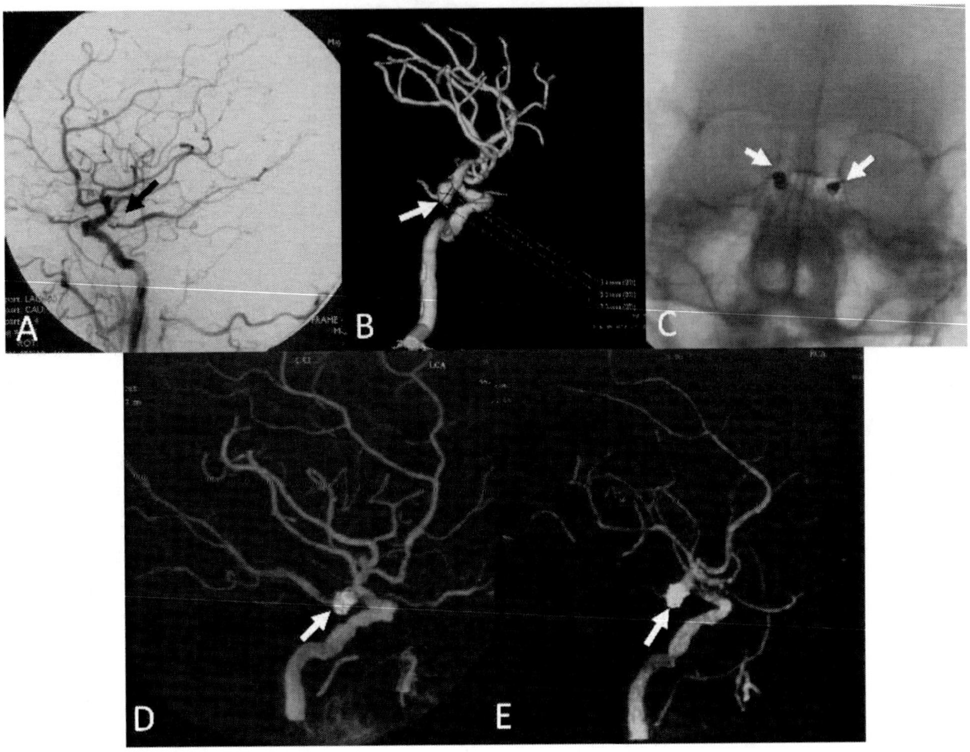

Figure 8. A 71-year-old man presented with left oculomotor nerve palsy. A, lateral view of the left carotid artery injection showing a posterior communicating artery aneurysm was coiled (Microplex, 4 mm × 10 cm, 3 mm × 6 cm, 2 mm × 6 cm, 2 mm × 4 cm, Microvention, USA) after a 4 mm × 20 mm Neuroform stent placement (arrow). B, 3-D reconstruction of the right internal carotid artery injection showing a 5 mm × 7 mm posterior communicating artery aneurysm (arrow), which was treated with 4 mm × 30 mm Neuroform stent and coils (Microplex, 7 mm × 18 cm, 3 mm × 6 cm, 3 mm × 4 cm, 2 mm × 4 cm, 2 mm × 6 cm, 2 mm × 4 cm, 2 mm × 2 cm). C, frontal view of the unsubtracted image showing bilateral aneurysms were all treated with Neuroform stent-assisted coiling (arrows). D, 3-D reconstruction of the left internal carotid artery injection after treatment showing the coil mass in the aneurysm (arrow). E, 3-D reconstruction of the right internal carotid artery injection after treatment showing the coil mass in the aneurysm (arrow).

Laser-cut stents are frequently used in the coiling of wide-necked and fusiform intracranial aneurysms [13]. The procedure related morbidity and mortality of patients treated with stent-assisted coiling was comparable to the matched patient group receiving simple coil embolization [13]. Prior studies have outlined the characteristics of the Neuroform stent, including the stenting success rate, complication rates in ruptured and unruptured aneurysms and intra-stent stenosis rates [1, 2, 14]. One study had showed the success rate was clearly higher in the Enterprise stent than the Neuroform stent and both stents were associated with a comparably low periprocedural complication rate and mortality (4.2% versus 1.9%) [13]. The Solitaire AB stent is the first stent that is fully retractable [15]. The first generation of Solitaire AB stent, the so-called SOLO stent (EV3, Irvine, CA) [16, 17]. The Solitaire AB stent can also be used as a remodeling device to retrieve it at the end of the operation without damaging the blood flow of the parent artery [18]. The microcatheter is placed in the aneurysm, and the Solitaire AB retrievable stent is deployed at the neck of the aneurysm. After embolizing the aneurysm, remove the stent device. Enterprise stent (Codman Neurovascular, Renham,

Massachusetts, USA) is a self-expanding, recyclable nickel-titanium alloy stent with closed cell design and open end [19]. Enterprise support provides a function to reposition the support. The stent was approved by FDA in 2007 for the treatment of wide-necked cerebral aneurysms [19]. The second generation of stent Enterprise 2 still uses obturator design, but compared with the first generation, the vascular reconstruction effect of Enterprise 2 has been significantly improved [20].

In this study, both stents possessed good to excellent procedural feasibility in close agreement with previously reported success rates of 95.9 to 100% for the Solitaire AB and 90 to 100% for the Enterprise [6, 15]. Both stents were associated with a comparably low periprocedural complication rate and mortality than the complication rate of 7.8% in the use of balloon mounted stents [21]. However, the complication rate observed in this study is consistent with other studies ranging from 0 to 16% determined in studies including ruptured as well as unruptured aneurysms and between 4.9 to 24% in studies with ruptured aneurysms only [1-3, 14, 22, 23]. Mortality rates in studies including mainly unruptured aneurysms ranged from 0 to 4.6% and 0 to 20% in reports with a high number of or only ruptured aneurysms [1-3, 10, 22, 23].

In this study, initial angiographic results showed that 83.1% of aneurysms treated with stent-assistance had total flow cessation or only minimal flow into the neck, which is consistent with previous reports [1, 21, 24]. However, 8.8% of followed aneurysms showed major recanalization of the aneurysms. Although Izar et al. reported more than 36% of followed aneurysms showed progressive occlusion [13], a 2-year follow-up study showed the rates of progressive occlusion (stent group, 17/40 [42.5%] versus nonstent group, 34/86 [39.5%]) and recanalization (7/40 [17.5%] versus 18/86 [21.0%]) did not show a statistically significant difference between the 2 groups ($p = 0.895$) [11]. Spontaneous migration of the Enterprise was previously reported [19].

Experience in Using Stents

Laser-cut stents are compressed on themselves within the catheter and are approximately the same length in and outside the catheter, while braided stents are stretched to fit inside the catheter and appear shorter outside [4, 22]. The discontinuous body of an open-cell laser-cut stent makes it impossible to recapture or re-sheath [22].

The mesh design of the stent will affect its radial force, deployment and blood flow characteristics. The main types of intracranial stent mesh design are open-cell and closed-cell stents [23, 24]. The grid of the open-hole bracket is partially open, while the grid of the closed-cell stent is closed. Compared with the open-cell stent, the closed-cell stent has a smaller porosity, which has a better effect on vascular reconstruction, a better blocking effect on the coil, and promotes the formation of aneurysm thrombus. In addition, closed-cell stent has higher radial force, but is not suitable for curved vascular anatomy. Open-cell stent can adapt to tortuous vascular structure. The size of the stent mesh, manufacturing technology and mesh design structure directly affect the ability of blood flow and stent endothelialization. Porosity is the percentage without metal, that is, the ratio of the surface area of the stent to the total surface area of the stent. The third-generation stent uses some functions of blood flow guidance, such as low porosity and fine woven structure, which improves the efficacy of the stent and the ability of blood flow diversion.

Recently, there have been scaffolds that can be delivered through microcatheters with an internal diameter of 0.0165 inches, such as Leo Baby (Bart, France), LVIS Jr (Microvention, USA) and the recently launched small Neuroform Atlas (Karamazu, Michigan, USA) scaffolds [25]. Neuroform Atlas is designed as an open intracranial stent (Figure 1 and 2). For complex aneurysms at the bifurcation of the artery, the use of miniature stent may be a good choice [25]. These micro stents used for nerve and blood vessels can be placed in arterial vessels with diameters ranging from 1.5 mm to 3.0 mm. These micro stents can be delivered through 0.0165 inch microcatheters, which makes them easier to deliver in small blood vessels.

In large vessels (>4 mm), the 6-mm Solitaire AB stent and the Enterprise stent (4.5 mm in diameter) are used to avoid coil protrusion between the stent and the vessel wall. In medium-sized vessels (between 2.5 and 4mm), the Enterprise and the 4 mm Solitaire AB stent are chosen [26]. Pipeline or Silk device is a different concept and have different indications, its navigability, deployment and placement is not easy [25, 27, 28]. Therefore, each stent has different properties that make them more appropriate in different situations. The application of stent technique has improved the cure rate of endovascular embolization of cerebral aneurysms and reduced the recurrence rate [29, 30]. The improvement of intracranial stent technique should continue to focus on the development of new materials and address the limitations of stent technique, that is, aneurysm recurrence and the need for antiplatelet drugs without treatment [31]. At present, it is believed that the recurrence rate of stent combined with coiling technique is not lower than that of flow diversion technique, and flow diversion technique may replace stent combined with coiling technique in the future. Now, a carotid siphon aneurysm is becoming the sole domain of the flow diverter other than indication for using a stent.

Conclusion

This study shows that the Enterprise and Solitaire AB stent are comparably navigatable devices. Both stents exhibited similar immediate and mid-term results, major neurologic morbidities and mortality are low. More thrombogenic complications were found in Solitaire AB group. This technique has greatly expanded the scope of treatable cerebral aneurysms. Stent combined with coiling technique increased thromboembolism complications and bleeding events related to the use of antiplatelet drugs.

References

[1] Biondi A, Janardhan V, Katz JM, Salvaggio K, Riina HA, et al. Neuroform stent-assisted coil embolization of wide-neck intracranial aneurysms: strategies in stent deployment and mid-term follow-up. *Neurosurgery* 2007;61: 460–468.

[2] Tahtinen OI, Vanninen RL, Manninen HI, Rautio R, Haapanen A, et al. Wide-necked intracranial aneurysms: treatment with stent-assisted coil embolization during acute (< 72 hours) subarachnoid hemorrhage–experience in 61 consecutive patients. *Radiology* 2009;253: 199–208.

[3] Akpek S, Arat A, Morsi H, Klucznick RP, Strother CM, et al. Self-expandable stent-assisted coiling of wide-necked intracranial aneurysms: a single-center experience. *AJNR Am J Neuroradiol* 2005;26: 1223–1231.

[4] Lv X, Li Y, Jiang C, Yang X, Wu Z. Potential advantages and limitations of the Leo stent in endovascular treatment of complex cerebral aneurysms. *Eur J Radiol*. 2011;79:317-322.

[5] Luo J, Lv X, Jiang C, Wu Z. Preliminary use of Leo stent in endovascular treatment of wide-necked cerebral aneurysms. *World Neurosurgery* 2010;73:379-384.

[6] Lv X, Li Y, Xinjian Y, Jiang C, Wu Z. Results of endovascular treatment for intracranial wide-necked saccular and dissecting aneurysms using the Enterprise stent: a single center experience. *Eur J Radiol*. 2012 Jun;81(6):1179-83.

[7] Zhang J, Lv X, Yang J, Wu Z. Stent-assisted coil embolization of intracranial aneurysms using Solitaire stent. *Neurol India*. 2012 May-Jun;60(3):278-82. doi: 10.4103/0028-3886.98508. PMID: 22824683.

[8] Raymond J, Guilbert F, Weill A, Georganos SA, Juravsky L, Lambert A, Lamoureux J, Chagnon M, Roy D. Long-term angiographic recurrences after selective endovascular treatment of aneurysms with detachable coils. *Stroke*. 2003;34:1398–1403.

[9] Lv X, Wang G, Wang J, Wu Z. 2021. Frontiers in Clinical Neurosurgery. *IntechOpen*. London, United Kingdom.

[10] Campi A, Ramzi N, Molyneux AJ, Summers PE, Kerr RS, et al. Retreatment of ruptured cerebral aneurysms in patients randomized by coiling or clipping in the International Subarachnoid Aneurysm Trial (ISAT). *Stroke* 2007;38: 1538–1544.

[11] Hwang G, Park H, Bang JS, Jin SC, Kim BC, Oh CW, Kang HS, Han MH, Kwon OK. Comparison of 2-year angiographic outcomes of stent- and nonstent-assisted coil embolization in unruptured aneurysms with an unfavorable configuration for coiling. *AJNR Am J Neuroradiol*. 2011;32:1707-10.

[12] Lubicz B, Bandeira A, Bruneau M., Dewindt A, Balériaux D, De Witte O. Stenting is improving and stabilising anatomical results of coiled intracranial aneurysms *Neuroradiology* 2009; 51 : 419-425.

[13] Izar B, Rai A, Raghuram K, Rotruck J, Carpenter J. Comparison of Devices Used for Stent-Assisted Coiling of Intracranial Aneurysms. *PLoS ONE* 2011;6:e24875.

[14] Maldonado IL, Machi P, Costalat V, Mura T, Bonafe A. Neuroform stent-assisted coiling of unruptured intracranial aneurysms: short- and mid-term results from a single-center experience with 68 patients. *AJNR Am J Neuroradiol* 2011;32: 131–136.

[15] Lubicz B, Collignon L, Raphaeli G, Bandeira A, Bruneau M, De Witte O. Solitaire AB stent for endovascular treatment of intracranial aneurysms: immediate and mid-term results in 15 patients with 17 aneurysms. *J Neuroradiol*. 2010;37:83-8.

[16] Liebig T, Henkes H, Reinartz J, Miloslavski E, Kühne D. A novel self-expanding fully retrievable intracranial stent (SOLO): experience in nine procedures of stent-assisted aneurysmcoil occlusion. *Neuroradiology*. 2006;48:471-8.

[17] Yavuz K, Geyik S, Pamuk AG, Koc O, Saatci I, Cekirge HS. Immediate and midterm follow-up results of using an electrodetachable, fully retrievable SOLO stent system in the endovascular coil occlusion of wide-necked cerebral aneurysms. *J Neurosurg*. 2007;107:49-55.

[18] Almekhlafi MA, Hockley A, Wong JH, Goyal M. Temporary Solitaire stent neck remodeling in the coiling of ruptured aneurysms. *J Neurointerv Surg*. 2013 Nov;5 Suppl 3:iii76-8.

[19] Lavine SD, Meyers PM, Connolly ES, Solomon RS. Spontaneous delayed proximal migration of enterprise stent after staged treatment of wide-necked basilar aneurysm: technical case report. *Neurosurgery* 2009;64: E1012.

[20] Chen L, Zheng C, Wu J, Gong J, Gao Y, Wan S. The Enterprise2 Stent for Endovascular Treatment of Intracranial Aneurysms: Short-Term Results From a Single Center Experience. *Front Neurol*. 2020 Dec 3;11:589689.

[21] Piotin M, Blanc R, Spelle L, Mounayer C, Piantino R, et al. Stent-assisted coiling of intracranial aneurysms: clinical and angiographic results in 216 consecutive aneurysms. *Stroke* 2010;41: 110–115.

[22] Lylyk P, Ferrario A, Pasbon B, Miranda C, Doroszuk G. Buenos Aires experience with the Neuroform self-expanding stent for the treatment of intracranial aneurysms. *J Neurosurg* 2005;102: 235–241.

[23] Wanke I, Doerfler A, Goericke S, Giezeski ER, Sandalcioglu E, et al. Treatment of wide-necked intracranial aneurysms with a self-expanding stent: mid-term results. *Zentralbl Neurochir* 2005;66: 163–169.

[24] Sedat J, Chau Y, Mondot L, Vargas J, Szapiro J, et al. Endovascular occlusion of intracranial wide-necked aneurysms with stenting (Neuroform) and coiling: mid-term and long-term results. *Neuroradiology* 2009;51: 401–409.

[25] Lv X, Wang G, Wang J. 2021. Craniospinal Vascular Diseases and Endovascular Neurosurgery. *Nova Science*, NY, USA.

[26] Lv X, Zhang W, Zhao X, Zhang H, Wang J. Endovascular Treatment of Small Wide-Neck Bifurcation Aneurysms with Single Solitaire AB Stent Technique. *Neurol India*. 2021 Jul-Aug;69(4):879-882.

[27] Byrne JV, Beltechi R, Yarnold JA, Birks J, KamranM. Early experience in the treatment of intra-cranial aneurysms by endovascular flow diversion: a multicentre prospective study. *PLoS One* 2010;5(9): e12492.

[28] Lv X. 2022. Endovascular Surgery of Cerebral Aneurysms. *Springer Nature*, Singapore.

[29] Liu P, Lv X, Li Y, Lv M. Stent-assisted coiling of ruptured wide-necked intracranial aneurysms: A single-center experience of 218 consecutive patients. *Neurol India*. 2016 Mar-Apr;64 Suppl:S70-7.

[30] Ge H, Lv X, Yang X, He H, Jin H, Li Y. LVIS Stent Versus Enterprise Stent for the Treatment of Unruptured Intracranial Aneurysms. *World Neurosurg*. 2016 Jul;91:365-70.

[31] Mocco J, Fargen KM, Albuquerque FC, et al. Delayed thrombosis or stenosis following enterprise-assisted stent-coiling: is it safe? Midterm results of the interstate collaboration of enterprise stent coiling. *Neurosurgery*. 2011;69:908-914.

Chapter 16

Intrasaccular Flow Diverter (WEB) Assisted Cerebral Aneurysm Embolization

Oktay Algin*, **MD**

Interventional MR Clinical R&D Institute, Ankara University, Ankara, Turkey
National MR Research Center (UMRAM), Bilkent University, Ankara, Turkey
Department of Radiology, Faculty of Medicine, Ankara University, Ankara, Turkey

Abstract

Endovascular treatment has lower morbidity and mortality rates than surgical clipping. Woven Endo Bridge (WEB) device (also called an intrasaccular flow diverter) is a new and effective endovascular embolization method primarily used to treat wide-necked or bifurcated cerebral aneurysms. In WEB-assisted embolization, a specially structured scaffold-like metal cage (WEB) is placed within the aneurysm, and the blood flow is redirected to branch arteries. Thus, blood entry into the aneurysm sac is prevented, and the risk of rupture of the aneurysm is reduced. The advantages of WEB embolization are the shorter embolization time and the reduced need for antiaggregant usage and intra-/peri-aneurysmal manipulations compared to coiling with or without stent placement. With the advancing technical developments (e.g., more visible single-layer wires), WEB devices are a safe alternative to other types of aneurysms or unusual locations (e.g., side-wall, PCOM origin, pericallosal, distal, or para-ophthalmic aneurysms. Adequate occlusion rates of the WEB devices were 84% at five years of follow-up. Complex morphology (e.g., the presence of irregular, multilocular, and/or partially thrombosed sac) and a large (>10 mm) neck or width of the aneurysm were found to be associated with recurrences after the WEB placements.

Keywords: intrasaccular flow diverter, Woven Endo Bridge (WEB), cerebral aneurysm, angiography, embolization

Introduction

Aneurysms are local expansion and ballooning because of the loss of mechanical properties in the vessel walls for various reasons. Intracranial aneurysms affect 5% to 8% of the general

* Corresponding Author's Email: oktay.algin@umram.bilkent.edu.tr.

In: Understanding and Managing Cerebral Aneurysms
Editor: Xianli Lv
ISBN: 979-8-89113-608-3

population, according to different sources [1-2]. The greatest risk of cerebral aneurysms is subarachnoid hemorrhage (SAH) due to rupture. It is thought that SAH occurs in 6 out of 100,000 people worldwide each year [3]. Depending on the location of the aneurysm, SAH causes serious consequences for the patient; and it has high mortality (20%) and morbidity (50%) rates [3].

There are two basic methods for treating aneurysms: open surgery and endovascular intervention [2]. Both methods have been used for many years, and their effectiveness has been proven [4]. Open surgery and endovascular intervention have both advantages and disadvantages. Open surgery has a higher risk of complications but a lower risk of aneurysm recurrence [4]. The recovery time of endovascular embolization is shorter and more comfortable, and endovascular treatment of the cerebral aneurysm is the first-line choice [2, 4, 5]. However, the recurrence risk of endovascular embolization is present, and recurrences require regular closer follow-up [3, 5]. Recanalization is the main problem for simple coiling, especially for wide-necked, ruptured, and/or bifurcation aneurysms [4, 5].

To decide on the most appropriate method for treating an aneurysm; many factors, such as the general health status and risk factors of the patient, the location and size of the aneurysm, and its relationship with neighboring vessels, should be evaluated. The main purpose of aneurysm treatments is to restrict or completely stop the blood flow to the aneurysm without obstructing the surrounding arteries [2]. In routine daily practice, microsurgical clipping or endovascular methods are used in aneurysm treatments [3-6].

Wide-Necked and/or Bifurcation Aneurysms (WNBAs)

WNBAs constitute 1/3 of all brain aneurysms [7]. Treatment of these types of aneurysms has challenges for interventionalists due to the need to adequately isolate the aneurysm without affecting the patency of major branches or parent arteries [8]. Embolization of WNBAs is technically difficult and may require the use of complex techniques [6-8]. Conventional stents (with kissing Y-, crossing Y-, T-, or X-stent technique), flow-diverter (FD) stents, or balloon (double or single lumen) assisted coiling techniques have been used to treat WNBAs [5-7]. These treatment options have many individual advantages and disadvantages. For example, the rates of thromboembolic or bleeding complications, in-stent stenosis, branch occlusion, and foreign body reaction are higher with stent-assisted coiling or FD stent placements [5, 6, 9, 10]. FD stents are more feasible in patients with blister-like, side-wall, fusiform, or dissecting-type non-ruptured aneurysms, and they are not indicated for the endovascular treatment of ruptured aneurysms or bifurcation aneurysms [4, 10, 11]. Complications of FD such as remote hematomas or parent artery thrombosis can occur several months after the initial treatment [12]. Additional coil(s) placements and/or percutaneous transluminal angioplasty are required in 50-66% of cases treated with FD [13]. This situation significantly increases the risks associated with interventional procedures (including radiation exposure and contrast-nephropathy) and the total costs of the treatment [4, 13].

The Woven Endo Bridge (WEB) Devices

WEB device is a self-expanding, retrievable, electrothermally detachable device placed within the aneurysm cavity [10]. WEB devices (also called intrasaccular flow diverters/disruptors) have been used first in the Europe market since 2011, and although their effectiveness is higher than traditional methods, more research is ongoing [14-16]. No delayed adverse events from the WEB devices have been reported until now [10, 14, 15]. The latest-generation (EV versions) WEB devices have improved visibility with the aid of drawn-filled tubing technology, and they are made from composite braid nitinol and platinum wires [12]. The WEB devices are manufactured in single-layer spherical (SLS-type) or cylindrical (SL-type) shapes [12]. The SL and SLS versions are available in an expanded range of diameters between 4 and 11 mm and in heights between 3 and 9.6 mm [8, 12, 14]. A scaffold-like infrastructure of the WEB devices reduces intrasaccular flow to the aneurysm neck, and they can support neo-endothelial overgrowth, aneurysm stasis, reendothelialization, and thrombosis [17] (Figure 1).

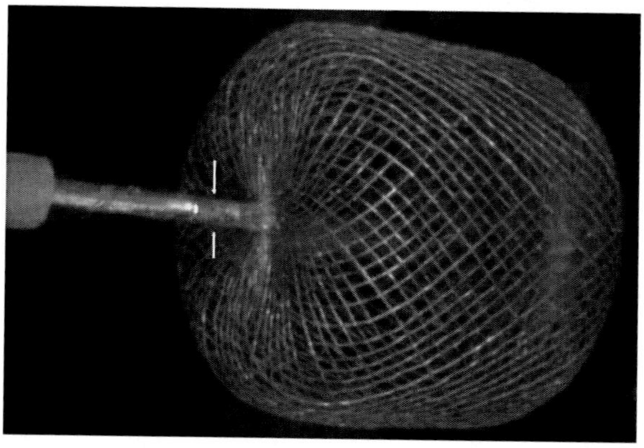

Figure 1. The figure shows the structure and detachment point of the WEB (W5-7-5 SL) device.

Literature data have shown the high safety and efficacy of WEB devices within short- and long-term periods [4, 10, 14, 15]. However, delayed aneurysm ruptures after WEB placement have been reported rarely [18]. Additional techniques (coiling or balloons) may be promising and safe methods, especially for larger side-wall, or irregular aneurysms [17, 18].

The Advantages of the WEB Devices

The advantages of a simple WEB placement are a lower aneurysm rupture risk of post-interventional period or thromboembolism, shorter procedural time, the absence of the need for dual or single antiaggregant(s), the comfortable nature of the intervention with WEB device, and relatively lower cost compared to balloon or stent-assisted coiling techniques [19, 20]. The faster nature of WEB-assisted embolization in experienced hands reduces the risks associated with radiation, iodine-based contrast media, and thromboembolism [14].

Safety and Complication Issues

Short- and long-term efficacy and safety values of the WEB devices are better than coil embolization [21]. The feasibility of the WEB placements in different locations was proved in many reports [10, 14, 15, 20, 22].

The peri-procedural complication rate of WEB-assisted embolization with WEB is approximately 3% and lower than other options [4, 5, 21]. Thromboembolism is the most common complication related to WEB placements; however, the majority of patients remain asymptomatic in the presence of post-WEB thromboembolic imaging findings [21]. Recurrence or complication rates are also higher in large, thrombosed, and/or complex-type WNBAs [4, 20, 22]. Morbidity and mortality rates of WEB placements were reported as less than 3% and 1%, respectively [10, 17, 20]. The performances of the WEB devices are likely improving with the increasing experience of interventionalists, particularly as more aggressive or robust sizing of the device may lead to more durable aneurysm treatment [17]. If the WEB device is markedly oversized, it will frequently not expand symmetrically and instead may take on an intussuscepted comma or crescent shape [8], as observed in 2% of our patients. After complete unsheathing, gentle traction on the system before detachment may allow the WEB device to pop into a fully expanded configuration [8]. However, there is an additional parent artery impingement risk in this condition. After the WEB deployment, the shape memory of the braided structure and friction between the deployed WEB device and the aneurysm wall impede efforts to significantly change the position or configuration of the WEB within the aneurysm sac [8].

Occlusion and Recurrence Assessments

Many scales are used in the evaluation of recurrence or occlusion after treatment. The most used occlusion scores are the WEB occlusion scale (WOS) and Raymond-Roy occlusion classification (RROC) [8, 15, 16, 20-22]. Our most frequently used score is the RROC scoring. The WOS is a 4-point scale using the following grades: complete occlusion, complete occlusion with recess filling, neck remnants, and aneurysm remnants. Scores of RROC are as follows; complete occlusion (RR1), neck remnant (RR2), and aneurysm remnant (RR3) [21]. An adequate occlusion was defined as either complete occlusion or neck remnant without a visible remnant or recurrence on follow-up exams [14]. Complete/adequate occlusion rates were 56%/89% at two years and 47-52%/84-88% at five years of follow-ups, respectively [4, 10, 12, 23]. Even if initial follow-up shows complete occlusion of the aneurysm, there is a 12% chance of aneurysm recurrence being identified later and a 4% retreatment chance [24].

A persistent filling on angiography images appears in 5-16% of cases, and it may be observed within the WEB device, which cannot be accurately assessed using the WOS scale [25]. Therefore, a revised occlusion scale (the Bicètre Occlusion Scale Score: BOSS) specifically for evaluation of the patients within the post-WEB period was introduced [25]: The persistent filling phenomenon (referred to as BOSS 1) may be related to treatment failure, incomplete/ongoing healing process, insufficient fibrosis of the intra-aneurysmal thrombus, and/or partial endothelization at the aneurysmal neck [25]. It has been found that most of the recurrent aneurysms after WEB embolization are stable over long-term periods and generally do not require re-intervention [4, 20].

Compaction or Compression of the WEB Devices

Compaction or compression of the WEB is the decrease in the height of the device. It leads to aneurysm recurrences and these recurrences may be easily treated successfully using the stent-assisted coiling technique or flow diverter placement [18]. Clot organization/retraction or flow dynamics may be associated with morphologic changes in the WEB geometry (e.g., compaction or compression) [20]. It is still unclear if shape changes of the WEB are associated with aneurysm recanalization [10, 20]. WEB compression and aneurysm recurrence rates increased from 18% and 0.6% at one year to 43% and 19% beyond one year of follow-up, respectively [20, 23]. An increase in retreatment rate from 3-4% at one year to 7.15% beyond one year and 15% at two years of follow-up was found [4, 23, 24]. Retreatment rates of the WEB devices at five years were lower than aneurysms treated with simple coiling or stent-assisted coiling [12]. Post-procedural dual antiplatelet therapy and unappropriated device size were independently associated with the BOSS 1 result during follow-up [25]. There is no definite criterion for the retreatment decision [4]. Microsurgical clipping or other endovascular techniques for post-WEB recurrences are safe and effective techniques [26].

Indications for WEB

The WEB device might be considered for every bifurcation aneurysm with a wide neck [20]. More recently, usage of the WEB has expanded to include atypical locations [17] (Figure 2). WEB devices can also be used to treat WNBAs with irregular or complex morphology [8]. The optimal management of antiplatelet therapy before and after WEB implantation is controversial [19, 25].

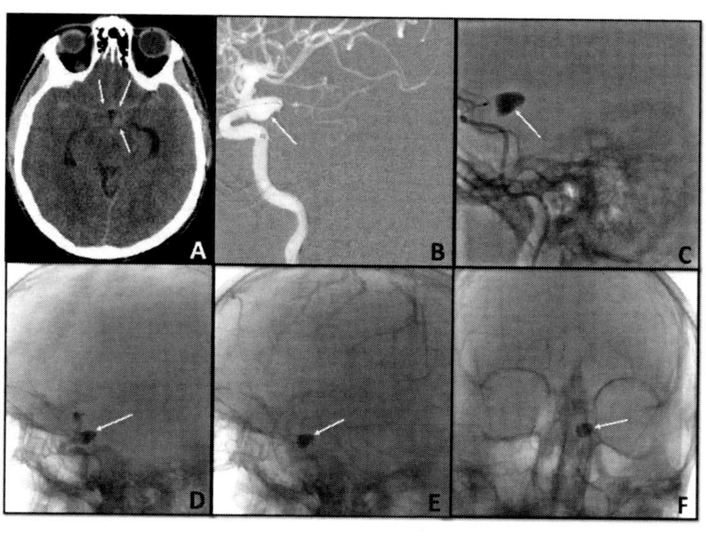

Figure 2. Subarachnoid hemorrhages (arrows) are seen on an axial CT image of a 33-year-old male who applied to the emergency department with a severe headache. A ruptured side-wall left ICA aneurysm is observed on the lateral road map image (B). There was a clearly-visible and permanent contrast media stagnation (C-F) in the aneurysm sac on angiography images during and after the WEB (W2-9-S) placement. In the follow-up examinations performed in the third year after the intervention, no finding of recurrence was observed (not shown here).

Size Selection

Adequate device sizing plays a crucial role in aneurysm treatment, as undersized WEB devices may result in insufficient coverage of the aneurysm neck and cause recurrences [25]. On the 3D time of flight (TOF), CT angiography (CTA), or rotational digital subtraction angiography (DSA), the largest aneurysm size (width and height of the dome outside of additional blebs and daughter aneurysms) can be used to get an accurate size. Average aneurysm width and height were recorded in two separate and perpendicular planes relative to the intended placement of the WEB device [17] (Figure 3). WEB devices were usually selected by adding 1 or 2 mm to the width (to assure good wall apposition) and subtracting 1 mm to the average height of the dome (to adjust for the longitudinal increase caused by transversal compression of the aneurysm walls) to the neck [19, 20]. Device sizing should be calculated based on the expected position of the WEB within the aneurysm sac [8].

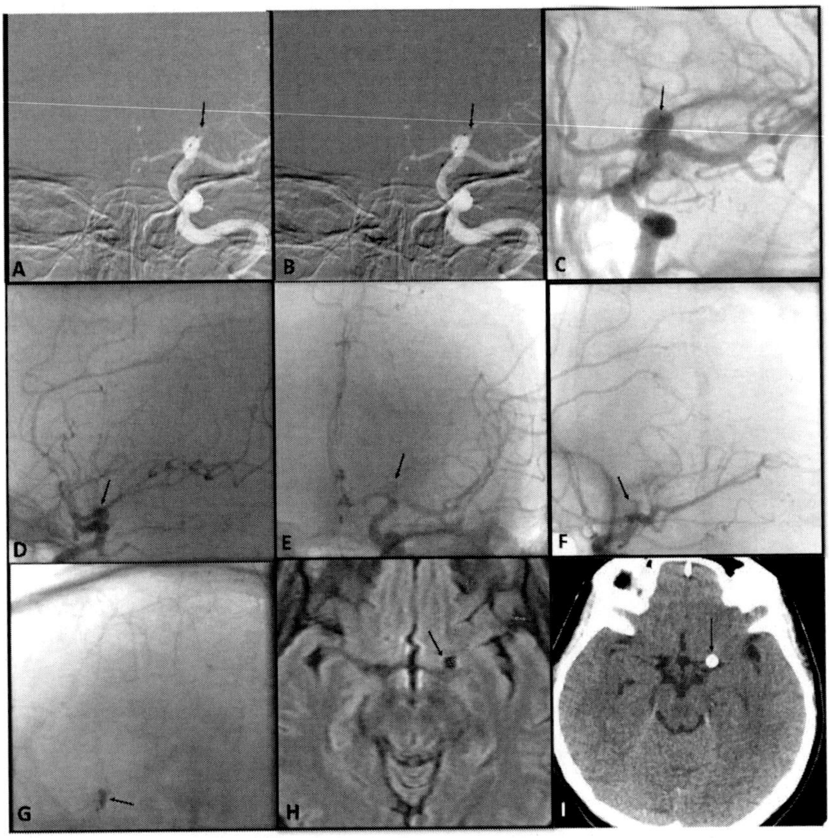

Figure 3. A 39-year-old female patient with left ICA terminus aneurysm and headache. There was no history of rupture. It is observed that the aneurysm also has a baby aneurysm (arrows in A and B). Antero-posterior (C) and lateral (D) angiograms obtained after the WEB device (W5-6-4) placement in the aneurysm show that the position of the device is appropriate. Antero-posterior and lateral angiograms (E-G) obtained in the late phases show that the aneurysm is not filled and there was a stagnation of the contrast agent, especially in the dependent regions of the aneurysm. No complication was found in the MR (axial FLAIR image, H) and CT (axial non-contrast, I) images obtained in the early postoperative period and the clinical evaluation performed during the postoperative 6th month. It is also noteworthy that the WEB device did not cause any artifacts in CT and MR images.

Correct sizing may be more challenging for complex, multi-lobular, and/or partially thrombosed aneurysms [4, 17]. A 'down the barrel' view of branch arteries is essential to visualize and select the best-sized device [8]. A slight rotation or angulation of the WEB device and suboptimal neck coverage immediately after WEB deployment may be seen despite adequate sizing in complex, large, or thrombosed aneurysms [17, 20]. Specifically designed simulators, training platforms, and/or patient-specific models may reduce suboptimal WEB placements [27]. A dual dose 3D rotational DSA may be helpful in further evaluating the WEB in cases where the regional anatomy is complex [8].

Procedural Details of WEB-Assisted Embolization

We mostly use transfemoral access with a 6F sheath introducer (Arrow®, Teleflex, USA) and 5F or 6F soft intermediate guiding catheter (Sofia™, Microvention, Terumo) in a triaxial fashion. The presence of a slim (diameter ≤ 2 mm) radial artery was usually an exclusion criterion for radial access [20]. A 5000 IU intraarterial heparin bolus is typically given at the start of the procedure [17]. The WEB was delivered under roadmap guidance with the aid of a dedicated microcatheter (VIA microcatheter 0.017, 0.027, or 0.033 inches, Sequent Medical, Aliso Viejo, California, USA) [20]. The presence of the proximal surface of the WEB at the aneurysm neck is the goal of the intervention [17] (Figure 4). If there is a crystal-clear contrast-material passage around and on top of the WEB, the device should be removed, and a slightly larger device should be used [8].

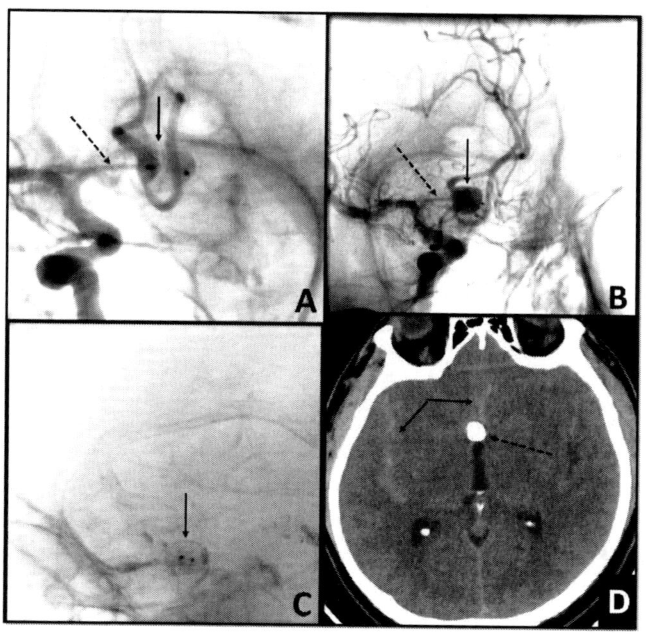

Figure 4. A 52-year-old male with a ruptured and large Acom aneurysm. Antero-posterior (A and B) and lateral (C) angiograms obtained after the WEB device (W2-9-6) placement in the aneurysm sac (arrows) show that the position of the device is appropriate. Also, there is prominent vasospasm in the A1 segment of the right anterior cerebral artery due to subarachnoid hemorrhage (broken arrows in A and B). No complication was found on the axial non-contrast CT image (D) obtained in the early postoperative period. Subarachnoid hemorrhages (arrows) and the WEB (broken arrow) are visible in the CT image due to a previously occurred aneurysm rupture (D).

Since September 2018, the newest fifth-generation WEB devices can be used with the aid of a VIA 17 microcatheter (Sequent Medical, Aliso Viejo, CA, USA) for aneurysms with a diameter of less than 8 mm [21]. According to our experiences and the literature, navigation with the VIA 17 is more comfortable, gentle, and safer than with other VIA microcatheters [8, 14]. Via-17 has two tip markers, and this is an additional advantage for the placement of supplementary or simultaneous coil placements [14]. Also, there are 45° and 90° pre-shaped versions of the Via-17 microcatheters. Balloon-assisted WEB placement may allow for rapid hemostasis in cases of intraprocedural aneurysm rupture [17].

Follow-Up Exams

Isotropic (preferably voxel size ≤ 1x1x1 mm) head CT angiography within the first postoperative day is necessary to evaluate the presence of complications after the WEB procedure. Short-, mid-term, and long-term follow-up findings should be assessed at 6, 12, and 24 months with isotropic CTA or MRA [20]. In the presence of suspected findings on CTA or MRA images for recurrent aneurysms or parent vessel narrowing, a DSA exam is necessary. Stenting after WEB deployment has been reported in approximately 15% of patients [20]. The frequency and type of follow-up exams should be balanced against patient safety, imaging equipment features of the hospital, aneurysm characteristics, embolization types, and cost issues.

Studies showed that high-resolution 3D-TOF images obtained with high tesla MR devices are fast, safe (due to non-invasive, non-contrast, and radiation-free nature), reliable, and effective methods for the management and follow-up of the WEB implantations, and assessment of the circle of Willis [28]. The high-resolution 3D-TOF data easily demonstrated morphological details of the aneurysm and parent vessels, the shortest and safest pathway to achieve the aneurysm for WEB placement, and these features of the 3D-TOF are critical in reducing procedure time and radiation/contrast-media related risks [28]. TOF or contrast-material enhanced MRA should be the first-line modality for follow-up appointments, and it provides a safer and less costly option than catheter-based angiography [24].

Conclusion

WEB has many advantages compared to other aneurysm embolization techniques and promising occlusion rates. WEB indications are increasing. Accurate selection of delivery catheters and the WEB sizes, patient selection, and experience of the intervention team may impact the success or outcomes of WEB implantations. In the future, well-designed and comprehensive studies are necessary to determine the real added value of treating intracranial aneurysms with a WEB device and long-term comparative results.

References

[1] Rinkel GJ, Djibuti M, Algra A, van Gijn J. Prevalence and risk of rupture of intracranial aneurysms: a systematic review. *Stroke* 1998; 29(1): 251-6.

[2] Lee KS, Zhang JJY, Nguyen V, Han J, Johnson JN, Kirollos R, Teo M. The evolution of intracranial aneurysm treatment techniques and future directions. *Neurosurg Rev*. 2022; 45(1): 1-25.
[3] Ran KR, Wang AC, Nair SK, Akça O, Xu R. Acute Multidisciplinary Management of Aneurysmal Subarachnoid Hemorrhage (aSAH). *Balkan Med J*. 2023; 40(2): 74-81.
[4] Alpay K, Nania A, Raj R, Numminen J, Parkkola R, Rautio R, Downer J. Long term WEB results - still going strong at 5 years? *Interv Neuroradiol*. 2022; doi: 10.1177/15910199221139542.
[5] Pierot L. Coated Flow Diverters and Single Antiplatelet Treatment: Where are We? *Cardiovasc Intervent Radiol*. 2022; 45(9): 1375-1376.
[6] Martínez-Galdámez M, Orlov K, Kadziolka K, et al. Safety and efficacy of intracranial aneurysm embolization using the "combined remodeling technique": low-profile stents delivered through double-lumen balloons: a multicenter experience. *Neuroradiology* 2019; 61(9): 1067-1072.
[7] De Leacy R, Yaniv G, Nael K. Cerebral Aneurysm Follow-Up: How Standards Have Changed and Why A perspective on the optimal follow-up frequency and imaging modality type treated cerebral aneurysms. *Endovascular Today* 2019; 18(2): 80-84.
[8] Goyal N, Hoit D, DiNitto J, et al. How to WEB: a practical review of methodology for the use of the Woven EndoBridge. *J Neurointerv Surg*. 2020; 12(5): 512-20.
[9] Bakola E, Papagiannopoulou G, Palaiodimou L, Lagios K, Archontakis E, Theodorou A, Katsanos AH, Triantafyllou S, Zouvelou V, Lachanis S, Tzanetakos D, Tzartos JS, Giannopoulos S, Tsivgoulis G. Delayed Leucoencephalopathy as a Complication after Endovascular Therapy of Intracranial Aneurysms-A Case Series. *J Clin Med*. 2023; 12(2): 496.
[10] Herbreteau D, Bibi R, Narata AP, Janot K, Papagiannaki C, Soize S, Pierot L. Are Anatomic Results Influenced by WEB Shape Modification? Analysis in a prospective, single-center series of 39 patients with aneurysms treated with the WEB. *AJNR Am J Neuroradiol*. 2016; 37(12): 2280-2286.
[11] Saatci I, Yavuz K, Ozer C, Geyik S, Cekirge HS. Treatment of intracranial aneurysms using the pipeline flow-diverter embolization device: a single-center experience with long-term follow-up results. *AJNR Am J Neuroradiol*. 2012; 33: 1436-1446.
[12] Pierot L, Szikora I, Barreau X, Holtmannspoetter M, Spelle L, Klisch J, Herbreteau D, Costalat V, Fiehler J, Januel AC, Liebig T, Stockx L, Weber W, Berkefeld J, Moret J, Molyneux A, Byrne J. Aneurysm treatment with the Woven EndoBridge (WEB) device in the combined population of two prospective, multicenter series: 5-year follow-up. *J Neurointerv Surg*. 2023; 15(6): 552-557.
[13] Oishi H, Fujii T, Suzuki M, et al. Usefulness of silent MR angiography for intracranial aneurysms treated with a flow-diverter device. *AJNR Am J Neuroradiol.* 2019; 40(5): 808-814.
[14] Algin O, Corabay S, Ayberk G. Long-term efficacy and safety of WovenEndoBridge (WEB)-assisted cerebral aneurysm embolization. *Interv Neuroradiol*. 2022; 28(6): 695-701.
[15] Rodriguez-Calienes A, Vivanco-Suarez J, Galecio-Castillo M, et al. Use of the Woven EndoBridge Device for Sidewall Aneurysms: Systematic Review and Meta-analysis. *AJNR Am J Neuroradiol*. 2023; 44(2): 165-170.
[16] Muskens IS, Senders JT, Dasenbrock HH, Smith TR, Broekman ML. The Woven Endobridge Device for Treatment of Intracranial Aneurysms: A Systematic Review. *World Neurosurg*. 2017; 98: 809-817.e1.
[17] Trimboli A, Wenderoth JD, Cheung AK, et al. Balloon assisted Woven endobridge deployment (BAWD): A safety and efficacy study. *Interv Neuroradiol*. 2023; Doi: 10.1177/15910199231185632.
[18] Simgen A, Antes S, Dietrich P, Blumentritt M, Jochum S, von Eckardstein K. Woven Endobridge Device (WEB)-assisted coiling of a large MCA-aneurysm: Case report and technical note. *Interdisciplinary Neurosurgery: Advanced Techniques and Case Management* 2023; doi: 10.1016/j.inat.2023.101785.
[19] Sabuzi F, Cortese J, Da Ros V, Mihalea C, Chalumeau V, Moret J, Caroff J, Spelle L. How a decade of aneurysms embolization with the Woven EndoBridge has changed our understanding and practices? *J Neuroradiol*. 2023: 50(5): 518-522.
[20] Cagnazzo F, Cloft HJ, Lanzino G, Brinjikji W. WEB (Woven EndoBridge) device for intracranial aneurysm treatment: technical, radiological, and clinical findings in a consecutive North American cohort. *Acta Neurochir* (Wien). 2023; 165(8): 2077-2086.

[21] Celik E, Goertz L, Ozpeynirci Y, Schlamann M, Dorn F, Lehnen N, Siebert E, Liebig T, Kabbasch C. Comparative assessment of woven endobridge embolization and standard coil occlusion for the treatment of ruptured basilar tip aneurysms. *Neuroradiology*. 2023; 65(4): 765-773.

[22] van Rooij S, Sprengers ME, Peluso JP, Daams J, Verbaan D, vanRooij WJ, Majoie CB. A systematic review and meta-analysis of Woven EndoBridge single layer for treatment of intracranial aneurysms. *Interv Neuroradiol*. 2020; 26(4): 455-60.

[23] Hassankhani A, Ghozy S, Amoukhteh M, Bilgin C, Kadirvel R, Kallmes DF. Long-term outcomes of the Woven EndoBridge device for treatment of intracranial aneurysms: A systematic review and meta-analysis. *Interv Neuroradiol*. 2023; Doi: 10.1177/15910199231184524.

[24] El Naamani K, Mastorakos P, Adeeb N, et al. Long-Term Follow-Up of Cerebral Aneurysms Completely Occluded at 6 Months After Intervention with the Woven EndoBridge (WEB) Device: A Retrospective Multicenter Observational Study. *Transl Stroke Res*. 2023; doi: 10.1007/s12975-023-01153-5.

[25] Janot K, Charbonnier G, Marnat G, et al. Persistent flow inside the Woven EndoBridge at angiographic follow-up: A multicenter study. *Interv Neuroradiol.* 2023; doi: 10.1177/15910199231185805.

[26] Kranawetter B, Hernández S, Mielke D, Ernst MS, Malinova V, Rohde V. Microsurgical clipping as a retreatment strategy for previously ruptured aneurysms treated with the Woven EndoBridge (WEB) device: a mono-institutional case series. *Acta Neurochir* (Wien). 2023; 165(7): 1881-1889.

[27] Algin O, Keles A, Oto C. Cerebrovascular modelling for the management of aneurysm embolization using an intrasaccular flow diverter made by 3D printing. *Pol J Radiol.* 2022; 87: e557-562.

[28] Algin O, Yuce G, Koc U, Ayberk G. A comparison between the CS-TOF and the CTA/DSA for WEB device management. *Interv Neuroradiol*. 2022; 28(1): 29-42.

Chapter 17

Understanding and Management of Unruptured Intracranial Aneurysms in Elderly Patients

Xianli Lv*
Shikai Liang
and Huachen Zhang
Department of Neurosurgery, Beijing Tsinghua Changgung Hospital,
School of Clinical Medicine, Tsinghua University, Beijing, China

Abstract

The optimal treatment of unruptured aneurysms in elderly patients remains controversial. The variability of life expectancy, comorbidities, and rupture risk, coupled with the heterogeneity of intravascular and surgical treatment, has led to a lack of clear guidelines and current management is highly personalized. Elderly patients exhibit unique considerations, including weakness, cognitive impairment, vascular disease, shortened life expectancy, and overall worsening prognosis at the time of rupture, which determine the risk and success of endovascular and microsurgical treatments. In this chapter, the natural risk of unruptured aneurysms in the elderly and the factors that affect their treatment strategies will be discussed.

Keywords: management, unruptured, cerebral aneurysm, elderly patient

Introduction

With advanced neuroimaging techniques, unruptured intracranial aneurysms (UIAs) are increasingly found in elderly patients [1]. Among the elderly patients with UIA, the prevalence of comorbidities include 4% of congestive heart failure (CHF), 20% of chronic obstructive pulmonary disease (COPD), 15% of diabetes, 70% of hypertension, 7% of peripheral vascular disease and 4% of chronic renal failure (Figure 1) [1]. In clinical practice, the risk-benefit ratio of aneurysm treatment is influenced by these comorbidities. There are conflicting opinions

* Corresponding Author's Email: lvxianli000@163.com.

In: Understanding and Managing Cerebral Aneurysms
Editor: Xianli Lv
ISBN: 979-8-89113-608-3

about embolization or clipping rather than continuing conservative treatment and observation [2]. Elderly patients with UIAs can be given conservative treatment or endovascular treatment under conscious sedation with local anesthetics [3-5], prioritize reducing surgical time and exposure to general anesthesia, and shorten hospital stay [6]. Among patients receiving UIAs treatment, the mortality and morbidity of elderly hospitalized patients were found during surgical clipping and endovascular embolization [1]. Most UIAs are asymptomatic, with a high rate of accidental discovery. Size and location of UIAs are associated with the risk of aneurysm rupture, and the probability of rupture varies depending on its pathology and morphology. Based on the existing literature, it is difficult to determine the long-term risk of UIAs in the elderly.

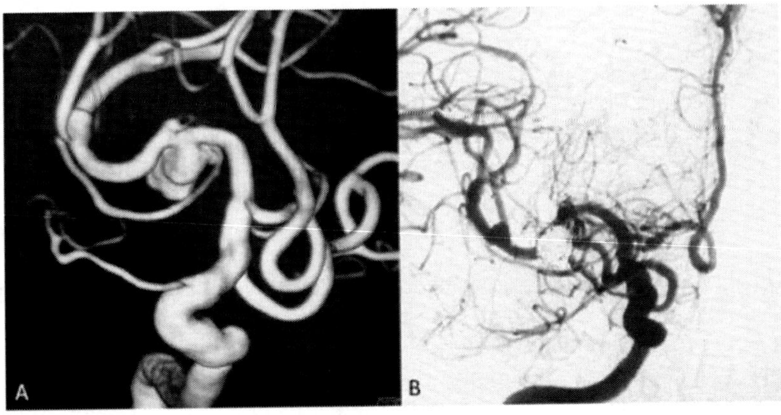

Figure 1. A 66-year-old female presented with Hunt-Hess grade 3 subarachnoid hemorrhage. She has chronic renal insufficiency, polycystic kidney, creatinine 600 μmol/L and platelet 81×10^9/L. A, 3-dimensional reconstruction of the right internal carotid artery angiography showed an aneurysm at the bifurcation of the right middle cerebral artery. B, the right internal carotid artery angiography showed that the aneurysm underwent embolization treatment.

Prognosis of Aneurysm Rupture

Elderly age is considered to be a poor prognostic indicator after subarachnoid hemorrhage (SAH), and the overall poor prognosis of elderly patients after aneurysm rupture is important for patient consultation and management (Figure 2). Lanzino et al. evaluated the relationship between age and prognosis of aneurysmal SAH using data from a randomized trial of multicenter in the treatment of SAH [7]. They reported that levels of consciousness, grading of SAH, and poor imaging features, such as thick clots, hydrocephalus, and intraventricular hemorrhage were worsen with increasing age. Life threatening complications have also increased, and the outcomes of older patients are worse than those of younger patients [7]. Other studies have found that elderly patients were associated with high-level SAH [8, 9]. Even elderly patients with good neurological grading may have a worse prognosis than younger patients. Catapano et al. analyzed the results of stratified patients with aneurysmal SAH in the elderly [10]. They report that patients aged 65 and older are more likely to have poor functional outcomes compared to patients aged 60 to 65 [10]. In patients with good grades during a 6-year follow-up, patients aged 65 or older have poorer outcomes than patients in the 60 to 65 age cohort [10].

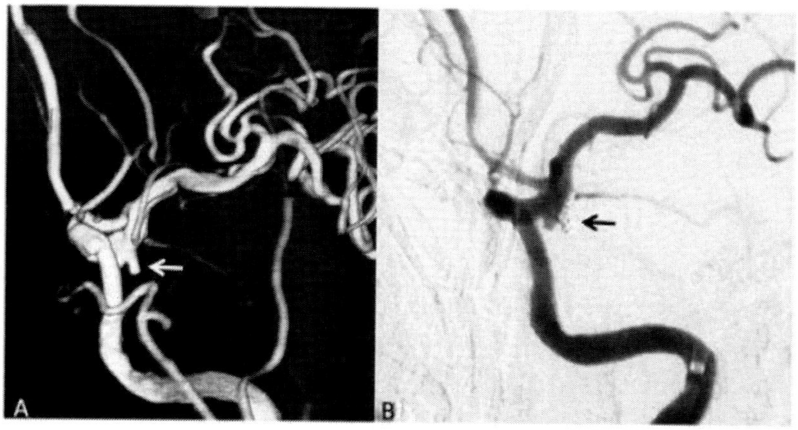

Figure 2. An 87-year-old female with ruptured posterior communicating artery aneurysm and bleeding underwent endovascular embolization treatment. A, 3-dimensional reconstruction of the left internal carotid artery angiography showed an aneurysm at the posterior communicating artery (arrow). B, the left internal carotid artery angiography showed that the aneurysm underwent coil embolization (arrow).

Treatment of UIAs in the Elderly

With the aging of the population, leaving the UIA untreated may not be the most appropriate decision simply because the patient is elderly [11]. Elderly patients over the age of 70 tend to agree to treatment of their UIAs. Patients know that they have a UIA, and most patients experience a decline in their quality of life. Age should not be used solely as an exclusion criterion for the treatment of cerebral aneurysms.

Embolization of UIAs is more popular than clipping in elderly patients. Microsurgical clipping of UIAs is a more invasive option, and older patients are less likely to tolerate general anesthesia than younger patients. The average hospitalization time for elderly patients receiving clipping was 8.0 days, while it was 3.2 days for embolization [1]. The incidence of perioperative stroke in elderly patients receiving clipping therapy was 10.3%, while it was 3.5% in embolization. Elderly patients undergoing clipping have a higher risk of perioperative acute renal failure, while patients with embolism have a higher risk of perioperative deep venous thrombosis and pulmonary embolism. These risks and costs, especially the 2.2% postoperative mortality associated with clipping in the elderly population should be considered between treatment and observation (Figure 1) [1].

Coiling Embolization

Due to different natural histories in literature, the prevalence of vascular curvature, aortic expansion, and intrinsic vascular diseases is high, and the risk-benefit ratio of coiling in the elderly remains highly individualized. Coiling UIAs in the elderly is generally safe and effective (Figure 2). Hwang et al. continuously coiled 122 UIAs in 96 patients over 70 years of age, the aneurysm was successfully occluded without adverse clinical events in 95.9% of cases [12]. A meta-analysis of 21 studies reported 1511 patients aged 65 years or older with ruptured and unruptured aneurysms, reporting long-term occlusion in 79% of patients [13]. The perioperative rates for stroke, intraoperative rupture, and perioperative mortality in patients with UIAs are 4%, 1%, and 1%, respectively. The rate of good 1-year prognosis is 93% [13]. Other reports have highlighted the increased complexity of coiling in elderly patients. Elderly patients may be prone to complications after coiling UIAs. Khosla et al. compared the complications of selective coiling of intracranial aneurysms in elderly and non-elderly patients and reported major complications with and without neurological dysfunction in patients aged 65 and older [14]. Ischemic complications are more likely to develop due to atherosclerosis, vascular stiffness, arterial curvature and decreased vascular reserve in elderly patients. Reducing procedure time, avoiding excessive coil embolization, minimizing coil prolapse, and optimizing management of comorbidities are suggested.

Balloon and Stent Assistance Technique

Among patients aged 70 to 96 years, Gonzalez et al. found that wide-necked aneurysms are more common in patients without SAH [15]. At this time, auxiliary techniques for coil embolization is needed, including balloon and stent assistance. Balloon and stent assistance can "reshape" wide-necked aneurysms, prevent coil prolapse, and expand the ability of coil embolization, including those with unfavorable morphology, or containing branch arteries. In complex aneurysms, the use of assistance techniques often increases risk of thrombosis complication. Benitez et al. have studied the treatment of wide-necked cerebral aneurysms with neurostent, reporting 8.9% of deaths and 7% of thromboembolic events in patients [16]. Elderly patients may be prone to increased complications of endovascular procedures. Stiefel et al. reported on the single center experience of endovascular treatment of UIAs in 77 patients aged 70 years or older, with 66% of patients using stent or balloon assistance [17]. Compared to balloon or stent assistance, coiling alone is significantly safer, with a complication rate of 6%, comparing to 27% and 26% for stent and balloon assistance, respectively. Similar to the general population, with only a 4% permanent rate of neurological morbidity and mortality, endovascular treatment of UIAs can be performed safely in the elderly.

Flow-Diversion Treatment

In elderly patients, the rate of aneurysm occlusion after flow-diversion stent is reduced, but it is acceptable. Kühn et al. evaluated the effect of age on aneurysm occlusion after flow-diversion therapy for UIAs [18]. During a follow-up period of 12 to 18 months, nearly complete to complete occlusion was 100% in patients under the age of 45, 91.4% in patients aged 46 to 64, and 78.4% in patients aged 65 and older (Figure 3). Adeeb et al. reported similar results and found that age 70 and older and non-smoking status were independent risk factors for incomplete aneurysm occlusion [19]. Despite these limitations, the occlusion rate for challenging small, medium, and large wide-necked aneurysms is still very high, and flow-diversion stent is still an effective treatment (Figure 4).

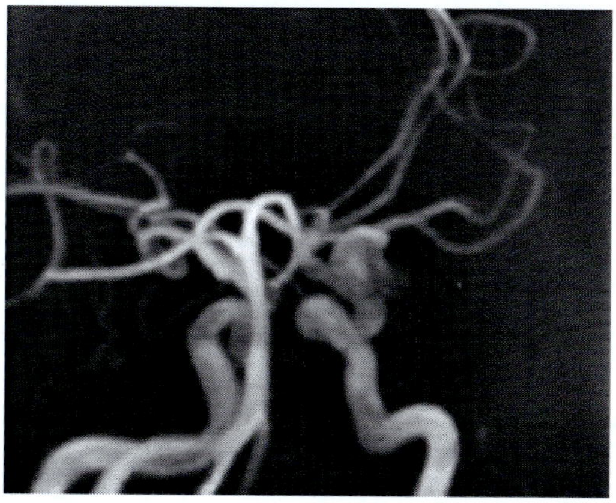

Figure 3. A 68-year-old female presented with kidney stone with a 2 months history of flow diversion treatment for a supra-clinoid segment aneurysm of internal carotid artery. The cranial MRA (non enhanced) showed the aneurysm was not occluded.

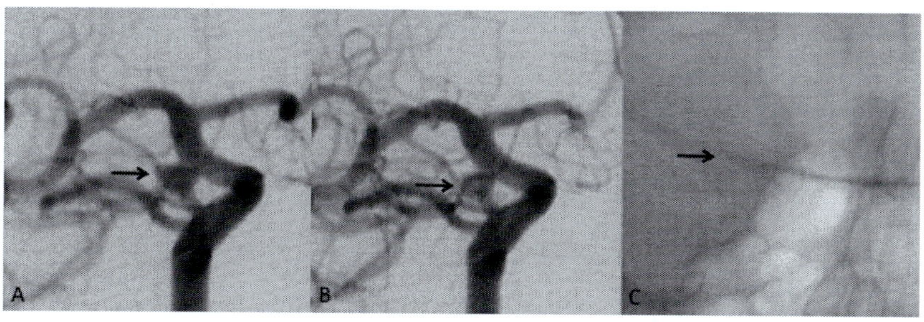

Figure 4. A 66-year-old female had a history of decompensated liver cirrhosis with hepatitis B for 20 years, varicose gastric fundus, 20 years of hypertension and 1 year of diabetes. A, the right internal carotid artery angiography showed an aneurysm at the origin of the posterior communicating artery, which supplies the distal posterior cerebral artery (arrow). B, the aneurysm underwent flow diversion treatment, and the right internal carotid artery angiography immediately after treatment showed partial occlusion of the aneurysm with the patency of the posterior communicating artery (arrow). C, fluoroscopic image showed the flow diversion stent (arrow).

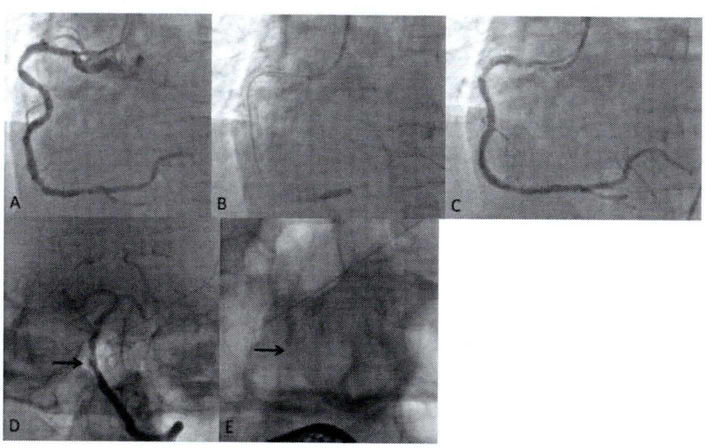

Figure 5. A-C, a 72-year-old male with acute angina underwent coronary angioplasty. D, a dissecting aneurysm of the left vertebral artery was incidentally found by cerebral angiography (arrow) and the flow diversion therapy was performed (E) (arrow).

Compared with young patients, elderly patients receiving flow-diversion treatment are more likely to have aneurysms with large size, complex shape and in the posterior circulation (Figure 5). With the increase of atherosclerosis and artery bending, attention should be paid to the increase of morbidity and mortality. Brinjikji et al. reviewed 711 UIAs after flow-diversion therapy and found that an increase in age was associated with higher morbidity and mortality [20]. The neurological mortality rate for patients aged 70 and older is 7.4%, compared to 3.3% for patients aged 61-70, 2.7% for patients aged 51-60, and 0.5% for patients aged 50 and younger. In different age groups, the incidence of hemorrhage and ischemic stroke is similar, suggesting that elderly patients suffer higher morbidity and mortality due to ischemic or hemorrhagic complications. Meticulous techniques, standardized antiplatelet regimens, and careful patient selection are suggested to maintain low complications.

Factors Affecting the Treatment of Elderly UIAs

Weakness

Weakness is associated with increased intraoperative and postoperative complications, mortality and hospitalization during UIA treatment (Figure 6) [21]. Therefore, understanding baseline frailty levels can adjust conservative or aggressive aneurysm management to match the physiological reserve of elderly patients [21]. Weakness is defined as a decrease in steady-state reserves and is closely related to an increase in age [21]. Weakness is characterized by frail, fatigue, insufficient activity, slow response, and weight loss. Weakness is caused by chronic inflammation involving multiple organ systems, and is due to aging, genetics, disease, lifestyle, and environmental influences that ultimately lead to disability, dependency, and death.

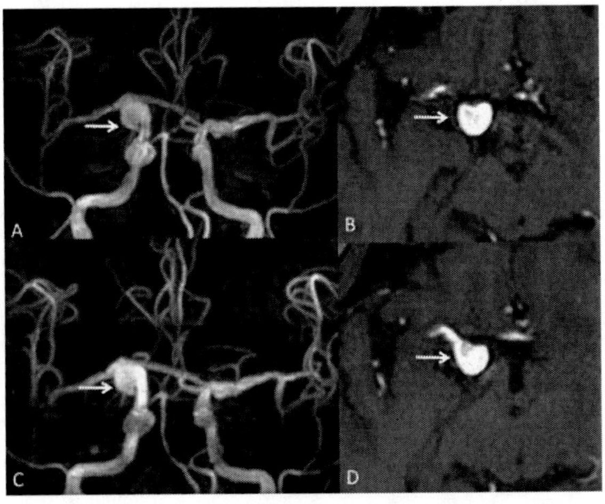

Figure 6. An 81-year-old female was admitted for an unruptured carotid artery aneurysm. She also presented dizziness, nausea, accompanied by tinnitus, night sweats, weakness in both lower limbs, and fever. The cranial MRA (non enhanced) (A) and enhanced T1-weighted MR image (B) showed a fusiform aneurysm in the supra-clinoid segment of the right internal carotid artery(arrow). Due to the patient's weakness, follow-up observation was conducted on the aneurysm. One-year follow-up images, the cranial MRA (non enhanced) (C) and enhanced T1-weighted MR image (D), showed that the morphology of the aneurysm was stable(arrow).

In neurosurgery, brain weakness is the injury of perforating arteries, endothelial dysfunction, rupture of the blood brain barrier, and brain weakness caused by inflammation are signs of poor brain reserve in elderly patients [22, 23]. In advanced imaging, it is evident that white matter has high intensity, micro bleeding, prominent perivascular spaces, lacunar infarction, and brain atrophy [23]. Brain weakness and aging are important risk factors for surgical clipping of UIAs. Matano et al. evaluated 214 patients with UIAs with a mean age of 68 years treated with surgical clipping [24]. They found that severe baseline white matter lesions were significantly associated with poor prognosis and with an increased risk of ischemia, hemorrhage, epilepsy, and hospital stay [24]. The relationship between frailty and prognosis after surgery or endovascular treatment for UIAs are lacking, but a review of 25 studies published between 2015 and 2018 found that frailty is associated with worse outcomes across the neurosurgical subspecialties [25].

Cognitive Function

Patients with UIAs may have cognitive impairment at baseline, which may affect long-term prognosis [8, 9]. Neuropsychological decline, whether due to anxiety about carrying a UIA or as a direct result of treatment, can have a significant impact on quality of life, independence, and overall life expectancy. Cognitive dysfunction may be caused by widespread cerebrovascular disease associated with chronic hypertension and smoking, which is a major risk factor for aneurysm development and chronic ischemic white matter disease. As age increases, limited cerebrovascular reserve becomes more apparent and highly variable, which is associated with heterogeneous cognitive outcomes after treatment of UIAs. The current literature has not established cognitive outcomes after aneurysm treatment. ISUIA reports that 3.2-7.1% of patients receiving clipping or coiling one year after treatment have impaired cognitive function [26]. Postoperative cognitive dysfunction may be related to structural damage to the brain parenchyma. Inoue et al. confirmed that after aneurysm clipping, postoperative T2 imaging changes are positively correlated with a decrease in neurocognitive scores [27]. Patients with baseline chronic ischemic small vessel disease are particularly vulnerable [27]. In a study of 106 patients who underwent surgery of UIAs, Kumon et al. found that preoperative MRI showing moderate to severe deep white matter hyperintensity was independently associated with postoperative neurocognitive impairment [28]. Other reports have described neurocognitive dysfunction related to specific surgical methods, aneurysm location, and age. Ohue et al. reported that among 43 patients with UIAs who underwent surgical treatment, 17 had a deterioration in neurocognitive function [29]. Patients aged 65 years or older, with anterior communicating aneurysms, and requiring an inter hemispheric approach had a greater downward trend in neurocognitive function.

However, other studies have reported no differences in cognitive function between pre- and post-treatment for UIAs. Wagner et al. found that there was no difference in neurocognitive function between baseline and postoperative in 51 patients with UIAs treated with flow-diversion devices [30]. Kubo et al. found that patients aged 70 years or older had no impairment in cognitive function and decreased overall anxiety after microsurgical clipping of UIAs [31]. Patients with the highest preoperative cognitive function score had the greatest reduction in anxiety.

Reduced Life Expectancy

As life expectancy decreases, the possibility of rupture and comorbidities that are more likely to lead to death may raise questions about the benefits of aneurysm treatment. Vindlacheruvu et al. conducted a life expectancy analysis of patients with UIAs based on prospective data from ISUIA to determine whether aneurysm repair would benefit [32]. They found that for patients with aneurysms of 7 mm or larger or with posterior circulation aneurysms, patients aged 45 to 65 years or with a life expectancy greater than 15 to 35 years can receive life years. This makes it uncertain how to treat UIAs in patients aged 65 or older (Figure 7). Pre-existing comorbidities as well as age, can predict the remaining life years after hospitalization. The 1-year survival rates after first admission due to heart failure or initiation of dialysis were 67% and 45.5%, respectively [33, 34].

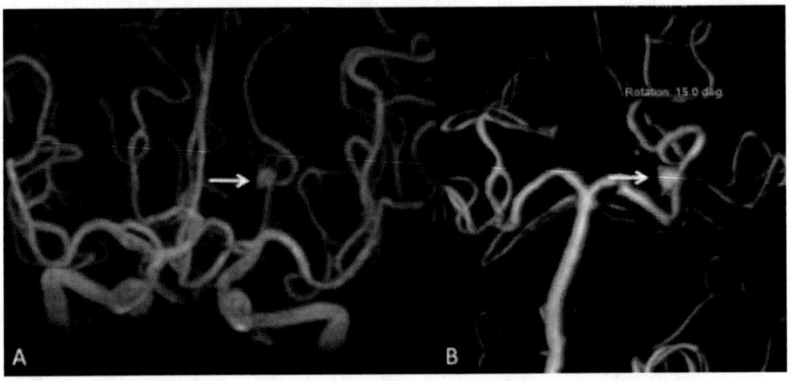

Figure 7. A 71-year-old female had a history of diabetes, coronary heart disease, cardiac insufficiency and renal insufficiency. The MRA (A) and CTA (B) examinations accidentally found a small aneurysm in the P2 segment of the left posterior cerebral artery. The patient was followed.

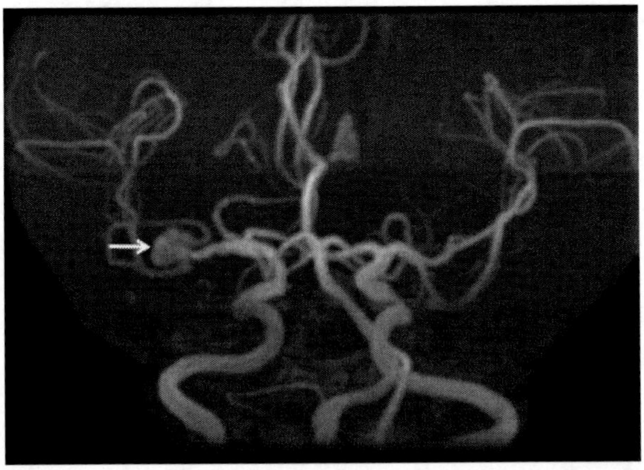

Figure 8. A 72-year-old male with dilated cardiomyopathy underwent coronary artery stent implantation. Cranial MRA examination accidentally discovered an aneurysm at the bifurcation of the right middle cerebral artery (arrow). The aneurysm was not treated and was followed for observation.

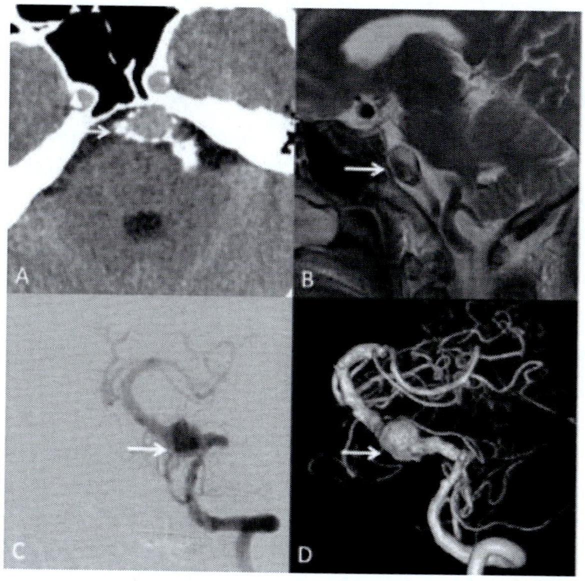

Figure 9. A 39-year-old male had 2 months history of kidney transplantation.
A. CT scan of the head revealed vertebrobasilar artery dilation with arterial wall calcification. B. T2-weighted, sagittal view of MR image showed dilation of the vertebrobasilar artery in front of the brainstem. C. Left vertebral artery angiography, AP position. D. 3D reconstruction of the left vertebral artery angiography showed the left vertebrobasilar aneurysm. The aneurysm was not treated and was followed for observation.

The prevalence of congestive heart failure (Figure 8), chronic obstructive pulmonary disease, diabetes, hypertension, peripheral vascular disease and chronic renal failure (Figure 9) in elderly patients is high. These comorbidities increase the in-hospital mortality after treatment of UIAs. Silva et al. retrospectively studied patients aged 65 years and older with UIAs who were treated with clipping or coiling [35]. They found that perioperative mortality rates were higher in elderly patients receiving microsurgical clipping than in non-elderly patients. In addition, elderly patients is associated with a higher incidence of stroke, cardiac insufficiency, and acute renal failure compared to non-elderly patients after clipping and coiling.

Vascular Pathology

Chronic hypertension and atherosclerosis are common comorbidities that increase with age. They can accelerate calcification of blood vessels or aneurysms, reduce arterial compliance, increase vascular curvature and maternal vascular stenosis, thus complicating treatment. Atherosclerotic aneurysm calcification is more common in larger aneurysms and elderly patients, and is related to the increase of risk after clipping. In a study of 208 patients treated for clipping or wrapping UIAs, the presence of calcification in the aneurysm was the only marker of adverse outcomes [36]. In addition, chronic hypertension can lead to complex aortic arch characteristics and aortic expansion, accompanied by carotid artery curvature and reduced vascular compliance, complicating arterial navigation, increasing technical difficulty, and increasing the risk of ischemic complications during endovascular surgery (Figure 10).

The intracranial atherosclerosis disease adjacent to the cerebral aneurysm also affects the efficacy and complications of endovascular treatment. Gao et al. found that arterial stenosis and tortuous anatomy limit the diffusion of microcatheter tension, which may increase the risk of intraoperative aneurysm rupture and plaque activity, reduce the speed of complete occlusion, and may require the use of stent or balloon assistance, increasing the risk of stent thrombosis and arterial dissection [37]. Although endovascular treatment of intracranial aneurysms with adjacent atherosclerotic stenosis is feasible, it is necessary to carefully evaluate the morphology of aneurysms (Figure 11), the anatomy of the parent artery and collateral circulation before treatment to reduce complications.

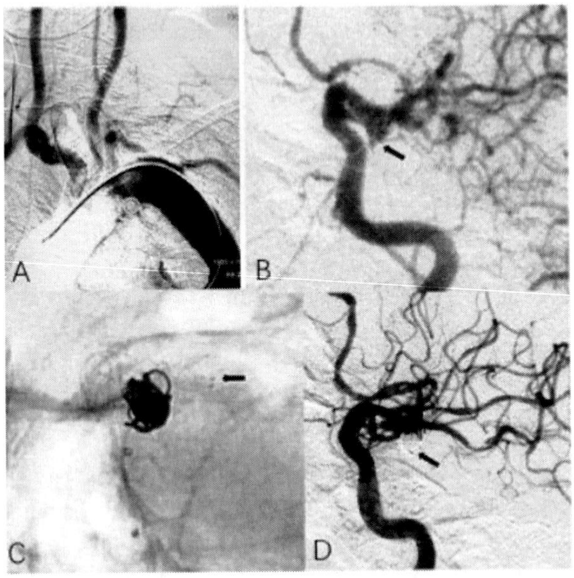

Figure 10. A 74-year-old male presented with subrarachnoid hemorrhage. A, aortic arch angiography showed aortic arch expansion. B. The left internal carotid artery angiography showed the left posterior communicating artery aneurysm. C. Fluoroscopic image showed LVIS stent-assisted coil embolization of aneurysm. D. Postoperative left internal carotid angiography showed complete embolization of the aneurysm.

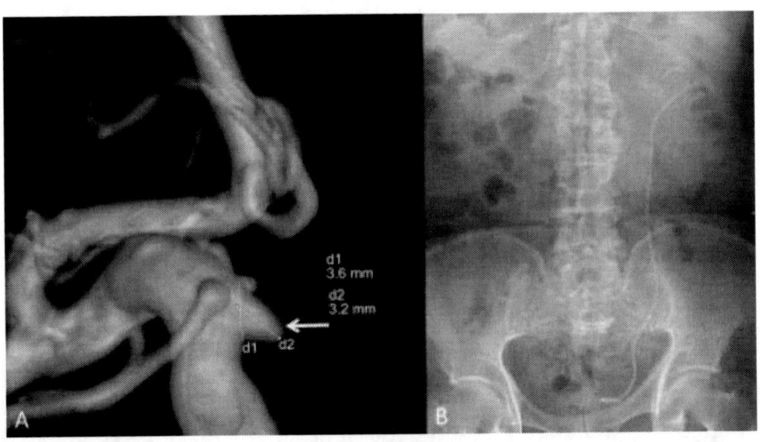

Figure 11. A 69-year-old male had 3 months history of an incidentally discovered small aneurysm of the right internal carotid artery. He presented with left lower back and abdominal pain for 1 day and was treated for kidney stone. The aneurysm was not treated for its small size and conical shape.

Future Direction

In the future, hierarchical treatment decisions for high-risk elderly patients, evaluation of new endovascular devices, and microsurgical innovation will continue to improve the prognosis of elderly patients. It is more common in unstable, growing, and ruptured aneurysms [38], which may improve our understanding of the risk of aneurysm specific rupture in the elderly and help guide treatment. In elderly patients, it is necessary to establish a woven endobridge (WEB) to verify the deployment of an intra-saccular blood flow diversion and the growth of endothelial cells. The continued development of minimally invasive surgical approaches, with priority given to reducing injury, endoscopic assistance to improve visualization, and transcranial nasal approaches for the treatment of high-risk skull base lesions, may be particularly suitable for older patients with higher risk from more traditional surgical strategies. In general, as technological innovation provides more minimally invasive treatment, verification and application in the elderly will be particularly important.

Conclusion

The best treatment for UIAs in elderly patients is unclear. Age should not be the limiting factor when considering endovascular therapy. Current management is personalized and requires an accurate understanding of natural history and rupture risks. It must be weighed against an individual's comorbidity, life expectancy, treatment-related risks, and likelihood of treatment success. These challenges determine the risks, benefits, and possibilities of successful surgery and endovascular treatment, promote innovative surgical techniques, and contribute to the trend of endovascular treatment for elderly patients.

References

[1] Caffes N, Wenger N, Cannarsa G, Oliver J, Onwukwe C, Gandhi D, Simard JM. Unruptured cerebral aneurysms in elderly patients: key challenges and management. *Ann Med.* 2021 Dec;53 (1):1839-1849.

[2] Silva NA, Shao B, Sylvester MJ, Eloy JA, Gandhi CD. Unruptured aneurysms in the elderly: perioperative outcomes and cost analysis of endovascular coiling and surgical clipping. *Neurosurg Focus.* 2018 May;44 (5):E4.

[3] Kan P, Jahshan S, Yashar P, Orion D, Webb S, Siddiqui AH, Hopkins LN, Levy EI. Feasibility, safety, and periprocedural complications associated with endovascular treatment of selected ruptured aneurysms under conscious sedation and local anesthesia. *Neurosurgery.* 2013 Feb;72 (2):216-20.

[4] Xiong J, Wang L, Tian J, Li Y, Gong C, Lv X. Stent-Assisted Coiling of Brain Aneurysms Under Conscious Sedation and Simultaneous Coronary Heart Disease Stenting: A New Concept. *Ann Indian Acad Neurol.* 2020 Jul-Aug;23 (4):572-574.

[5] Xiong J, Tian J, Li Y, Li N, Lv X. Stent-Assisted Coiling of a Ruptured Supraclinoid Internal Carotid Artery Aneurysm in Tetralogy of Fallot Under Conscious Sedation. *Ann Indian Acad Neurol.* 2021 Jan-Feb;24 (1):116-118.

[6] Kandregula S, Savardekar AR, Terrell D, Adeeb N, Whipple S, Beyl R, Birk HS, Newman WC, Kosty J, Cuellar H, Guthikonda B. Microsurgical clipping and endovascular management of unruptured anterior circulation aneurysms: how age, frailty, and comorbidity indexes influence outcomes. *J Neurosurg.* 2022 Sep 30:1-11.

[7] Lanzino G, Kassell NF, Germanson TP, Kongable GL, Truskowski LL, Torner JC, Jane JA. Age and outcome after aneurysmal subarachnoid hemorrhage: why do older patients fare worse? *J Neurosurg*. 1996 Sep;85 (3):410-8.

[8] Cai Y, Spelle L, Wang H, Piotin M, Mounayer C, Vanzin JR, Moret J. Endovascular treatment of intracranial aneurysms in the elderly: single-center experience in 63 consecutive patients. *Neurosurgery*. 2005 Dec;57 (6):1096-102; discussion 1096-102.

[9] Yano S, Hamada J, Kai Y, Todaka T, Hara T, Mizuno T, Morioka M, Ushio Y. Surgical indications to maintain quality of life in elderly patients with ruptured intracranial aneurysms. *Neurosurgery*. 2003 May;52 (5):1010-1016.

[10] Catapano JS, Louie CE, Lang MJ, DiDomenico JD, Whiting AC, Labib MA, Cole TS, Fredrickson VL, Cavalcanti DD, Lawton MT. Outcomes in a Case Series of Elderly Patients with Aneurysmal Subarachnoid Hemorrhages in the Barrow Ruptured Aneurysm Trial (BRAT). *World Neurosurg*. 2020 Jul;139:e406-e411.

[11] Lee SH, Lee SU, Kwon OK, Bang JS, Ban SP, Kim T, Kim YD, Byoun HS, Oh CW. Clinical Outcomes of Clipping and Coiling in Elderly Patients with Unruptured Cerebral Aneurysms: a National Cohort Study in Korea. *J Korean Med Sci*. 2021 Jul 5;36 (26):e178.

[12] Hwang SK, Hwang G, Oh CW, Jin SC, Park H, Bang JS, Kwon OK. Endovascular treatment for unruptured intracranial aneurysms in elderly patients: single-center report. *AJNR Am J Neuroradiol*. 2011 Jun-Jul;32 (6):1087-90.

[13] Sturiale CL, Brinjikji W, Murad MH, Lanzino G. Endovascular treatment of intracranial aneurysms in elderly patients: a systematic review and meta-analysis. *Stroke*. 2013 Jul;44 (7):1897-902.

[14] Khosla A, Brinjikji W, Cloft H, Lanzino G, Kallmes DF. Age-related complications following endovascular treatment of unruptured intracranial aneurysms. *AJNR Am J Neuroradiol*. 2012 May;33 (5):953-7.

[15] Gonzalez NR, Dusick JR, Duckwiler G, Tateshima S, Jahan R, Martin NA, Viñuela F. Endovascular coiling of intracranial aneurysms in elderly patients: report of 205 treated aneurysms. *Neurosurgery*. 2010 Apr;66 (4):714-721.

[16] Benitez RP, Silva MT, Klem J, Veznedaroglu E, Rosenwasser RH. Endovascular occlusion of wide-necked aneurysms with a new intracranial microstent (Neuroform) and detachable coils. *Neurosurgery*. 2004 Jun;54 (6):1359-1368.

[17] Stiefel MF, Park MS, McDougall CG, Albuquerque FC. Endovascular treatment of unruptured intracranial aneurysms in the elderly: analysis of procedure related complications. *J Neurointerv Surg*. 2010 Mar;2 (1):11-5.

[18] Kühn AL, Kan P, Henninger N, Srinivasan V, de Macedo Rodrigues K, Wakhloo AK, Gounis MJ, Puri AS. Impact of age on cerebral aneurysm occlusion after flow diversion. *J Clin Neurosci*. 2019 Jul;65:23-27

[19] Adeeb N, Moore JM, Wirtz M, Griessenauer CJ, Foreman PM, Shallwani H, Gupta R, Dmytriw AA, Motiei-Langroudi R, Alturki A, Harrigan MR, Siddiqui AH, Levy EI, Thomas AJ, Ogilvy CS. Predictors of Incomplete Occlusion following Pipeline Embolization of Intracranial Aneurysms: Is It Less Effective in Older Patients? *AJNR Am J Neuroradiol*. 2017 Dec;38 (12):2295-2300.

[20] Brinjikji W, Kallmes DF, Cloft HJ, Lanzino G. Age-related outcomes following intracranial aneurysm treatment with the Pipeline Embolization Device: a subgroup analysis of the IntrePED registry. *J Neurosurg*. 2016 Jun;124 (6):1726-30.

[21] McIntyre M, Gandhi C, Dragonette J, Schmidt M, Cole C, Santarelli J, Lehrer R, Al-Mufti F, Bowers CA. Increasing Frailty Predicts Worse Outcomes and Increased Complications After Angiogram-Negative Subarachnoid Hemorrhages. *World Neurosurg*. 2020 Feb;134:e181-e188.

[22] Thommen R, Kazim SF, Rumalla K, Kassicieh AJ, Kalakoti P, Schmidt MH, McKee RG, Hall DE, Miskimins RJ, Bowers CA. Preoperative frailty measured by risk analysis index predicts complications and poor discharge outcomes after Brain Tumor Resection in a large multi-center analysis. *J Neurooncol*. 2022 Nov;160 (2):285-297.

[23] Appleton JP, Woodhouse LJ, Adami A, Becker JL, Berge E, Cala LA, Casado AM, Caso V, Christensen HK, Dineen RA, Gommans J, Koumellis P, Szatmari S, Sprigg N, Bath PM, Wardlaw JM; ENOS

Investigators. Imaging markers of small vessel disease and brain frailty, and outcomes in acute stroke. *Neurology*. 2020 Feb 4;94 (5):e439-e452.

[24] Matano F, Mizunari T, Murai Y, Tamaki T, Tateyama K, Suzuki M, Morita A. White Matter Lesions as Brain Frailty and Age are Risk Factors for Surgical Clipping of Unruptured Intracranial Aneurysms in the Elderly. *J Stroke Cerebrovasc Dis*. 2020 Oct;29 (10):105121.

[25] Pazniokas J, Gandhi C, Theriault B, Schmidt M, Cole C, Al-Mufti F, Santarelli J, Bowers CA. The immense heterogeneity of frailty in neurosurgery: a systematic literature review. *Neurosurg Rev*. 2021 Feb;44 (1):189-201.

[26] Wiebers DO, Whisnant JP, Huston J 3rd, Meissner I, Brown RD Jr, Piepgras DG, Forbes GS, Thielen K, Nichols D, O'Fallon WM, Peacock J, Jaeger L, Kassell NF, Kongable-Beckman GL, Torner JC; International Study of Unruptured Intracranial Aneurysms Investigators. Unruptured intracranial aneurysms: natural history, clinical outcome, and risks of surgical and endovascular treatment. *Lancet*. 2003 Jul 12;362 (9378):103-10.

[27] Inoue T, Ohwaki K, Tamura A, Tsutsumi K, Saito I, Saito N. Subtle structural change demonstrated on T2-weighted images after clipping of unruptured intracranial aneurysm: negative effects on cognitive performance. *J Neurosurg*. 2014 Apr;120 (4):937-44.

[28] Kumon Y, Watanabe H, Tagawa M, Inoue A, Ohnishi T, Kunieda T. Relationship between Deep White Matter Hyperintensities on Magnetic Resonance Imaging and Postoperative Cognitive Function Following Clipping of Unruptured Intracranial Aneurysm. *Neurol Med Chir (Tokyo)*. 2021 Feb 15;61 (2):152-161.

[29] Ohue S, Oka Y, Kumon Y, Ohta S, Sakaki S, Hatakeyama T, Shiraishi T, Takeda S, Ohnishi T. Importance of neuropsychological evaluation after surgery in patients with unruptured cerebral aneurysms. *Surg Neurol*. 2003 Apr;59 (4):269-276.

[30] Wagner K, Srivatsan A, Mohanty A, Srinivasan VM, Saleem Y, Cherian J, James RF, Chen S, Burkhardt JK, Johnson J, Kan P. Cognitive outcomes after unruptured intracranial aneurysm treatment with flow diversion. *J Neurosurg*. 2019 Nov 29:1-6.

[31] Kubo Y, Ogasawara K, Kashimura H, Otawara Y, Kakino S, Sugawara A, Ogawa A. Cognitive function and anxiety before and after surgery for asymptomatic unruptured intracranial aneurysms in elderly patients. *World Neurosurg*. 2010 Apr;73 (4):350-3.

[32] Vindlacheruvu RR, Mendelow AD, Mitchell P. Risk-benefit analysis of the treatment of unruptured intracranial aneurysms. *J Neurol Neurosurg Psychiatry*. 2005 Feb;76 (2):234-9.

[33] Jong P, Vowinckel E, Liu PP, Gong Y, Tu JV. Prognosis and determinants of survival in patients newly hospitalized for heart failure: a population-based study. *Arch Intern Med*. 2002 Aug 12-26;162 (15):1689-94.

[34] Wachterman MW, O'Hare AM, Rahman OK, Lorenz KA, Marcantonio ER, Alicante GK, Kelley AS. One-Year Mortality After Dialysis Initiation Among Older Adults. *JAMA Intern Med*. 2019 Jul 1;179 (7):987-990.

[35] Silva NA, Shao B, Sylvester MJ, Eloy JA, Gandhi CD. Unruptured aneurysms in the elderly: perioperative outcomes and cost analysis of endovascular coiling and surgical clipping. *Neurosurg Focus*. 2018 May;44 (5):E4.

[36] Bhatia S, Sekula RF, Quigley MR, Williams R, Ku A. Role of calcification in the outcomes of treated, unruptured, intracerebral aneurysms. *Acta Neurochir (Wien)*. 2011 Apr;153 (4):905-11.

[37] Gao BL, Li ZS, Li TX, Xue JY, Feng G, Wang ZL, Bai WX, Zhao TY, Liang XD. Endovascular Treatment of Intracranial Aneurysms Concomitant with Severe Adjacent Atherosclerotic Stenosis. *World Neurosurg*. 2018 Mar;111:e927-e932.

[38] Matsushige T, Shimonaga K, Ishii D, Sakamoto S, Hosogai M, Hashimoto Y, Kaneko M, Ono C, Mizoue T, Kurisu K. Vessel Wall Imaging of Evolving Unruptured Intracranial Aneurysms. *Stroke*. 2019 Jul;50 (7):1891-1894.

Chapter 18

Understanding and Managing Arterial Aneurysms in AVMs

Huachen Zhang
Shikai Liang
and Xianli Lv*
Department of Neurosurgery, Beijing Tsinghua Changgung Hospital,
School of Clinical Medicine, Tsinghua University, Beijing, China

Abstract

This chapter evaluated whether an arterial aneurysm within an arteriovenous malformation (AVM) angioarchitecture is an indication for endovascular embolization in cases of ruptured and unruptured AVM. 94 patients with AVMs managed between August 2015 and August 2017 were retrospectively reviewed. Nineteen AVM-associated arterial aneurysms were detected in the 17 patients (only one patient had multiple aneurysms). Hemorrhage was the most frequent presenting symptom (11 patients, 64.7%). Ten aneurysms were coiled prior to AVM treatment. The remaining nine were obliterated at the time of AVM treatment, with Onyx embolization used for both procedures. None of the patients developed complications. After a mean 10.4 months (range, 3-25 months) of follow-up, excellent outcomes (modified Rankin Scale score [mRS] = 0 to 1) were recorded for 13 patients (76.5%) and good outcomes (mRS = 2) were noted for four patients (23.5%). Endovascular treatment options of arterial aneurysms in AVMs were comprised coil embolization or parent vessel sacrifice using coils or liquid embolics. Embolization of arterial aneurysms on feeding pedicles should be considered prior to or adjunct AVM embolization.

Keywords: arteriovenous malformation, aneurysm, endovascular treatment

Presence of arterial aneurysms in arteriovenous malformations (AVMs) increases the risk of bleeding, not necessary the AVMs [1-4]. Although the formation of aneurysms is related to hemodynamic changes, only 25% of AVMs have aneurysms, which suggests that potential

---

* Corresponding Author's Email: lvxianli000@163.com.

In: Understanding and Managing Cerebral Aneurysms
Editor: Xianli Lv
ISBN: 979-8-89113-608-3

vascular dysplasia or local vascular malformations play an important role in the formation of aneurysms [1]. Pseudoaneurysms related to vascular rupture or vascular dysplasia near or in the lesion are also common, and sometimes it is difficult to distinguish them from true aneurysms. However, all patients with pseudoaneurysm had bleeding. Especially when the aneurysm is flow-related or infratentorial [1-4]. Even though, there is no consensus on the optimal treatment strategy for arterial aneurysms in AVMs [5]. In this study, clinical application of endovascular treatment strategy for arterial aneurysms in AVMs was evaluated.

Patients and Methods

The cases of 94 consecutive patients diagnosed with AVM between August 2015 and August 2017 were retrospectively reviewed. Seventeen (18.1%) had been diagnosed with AVM accompanied by arterial aneurysm. All 17 patients underwent endovascular treatments performed by the same team. In each of the 17 cases, vascular architecture was evaluated using six-vessel angiography, and the location of the AVM was determined using standard magnetic resonance imaging (MRI). The bleeding focus was determined based on the location and distribution of the hematoma on computed tomography (intracerebral, SAH, intraventricular), and these findings were correlated with angiography results.

Treatment

AVM-related aneurysms were detected during cerebral angiography. The flow-related aneurysms were treated during the same session as the AVM. A superselective microcatheter was placed into the supply artery of each intranidal aneurysm. With the patient under general anesthesia, the intranidal aneurysm and AVM nidus were embolized simultaneously using Onyx (ev3, Medtronic). The intention of the simultaneous procedures was to reduce the risk of hemorrhagic complications during the interval between aneurysm treatment and AVM treatment. Flow-related aneurysms were treated with coil embolization or Onyx embolization. Incidental aneurysms were treated with coiling with or without stent assistance. Each of these techniques was consistent throughout the study period. Neurological outcomes were assessed at each patient's last follow-up visit using the modified Rankin Score Scale (mRS).

Results

Classification of Aneurysms

AVM-related aneurysms were classified as flow-related and incidental (i.e., unrelated to the AVM supply) [6]. Aneurysms within or in the immediate vicinity of the nidus of an AVM were classified as intranidal aneurysms. Aneurysms with infundibular dilation less than 3 mm at greatest diameter were not included.

Patients and Presentation

The patients were seven women (41.2%) and 10 men (58.8%) of mean age 31.1 years (range, 6 to 56 years). Eleven patients (64.7%) initially presented with hemorrhage (the most frequent finding at presentation), and six (35.3%) had presenting symptoms or signs unrelated to hemorrhage. Bleeding was caused by an AVM nidus in 18.2% of the 11 cases (n = 2), and by aneurysm rupture in 81.8% (n = 9). Of the six patients with no history of hemorrhage, two presented with seizure and the other four complained of headaches.

Arteriovenous Malformation Characteristics

Of the 17 AVMs, two (11.8%) of the AVMs were infratentorial and 15 (88.2%) were supratentorial. Two were cerebellar, four were frontal, five were parietal, three were temporal, two were in the basilar ganglion, and one was occipital. Lesion diameter ranged from 1.5 cm to 6 cm (mean, 3.6 cm). Five of the AVMs had deep venous drainage. Seven (41.2%) were Spetzler–Martin grade II, six (35.3%) were grade III, and four (23.5%) were grade IV. One AVM had fistulous component, one received additional external carotid arterial supply.

Aneurysm Characteristics

The 17 patients had 19 AVM-associated arterial aneurysms total (only one patient had multiple lesions). Of the 19 aneurysms, seven were intranidal, seven were flow-related and arose from AVM supply vessels (Figures 1 and 2), four were incidental aneurysms, and one was paraclinoid located in the internal carotid artery associated with AVM supply. All were small (<10 mm diameter) and saccular type.

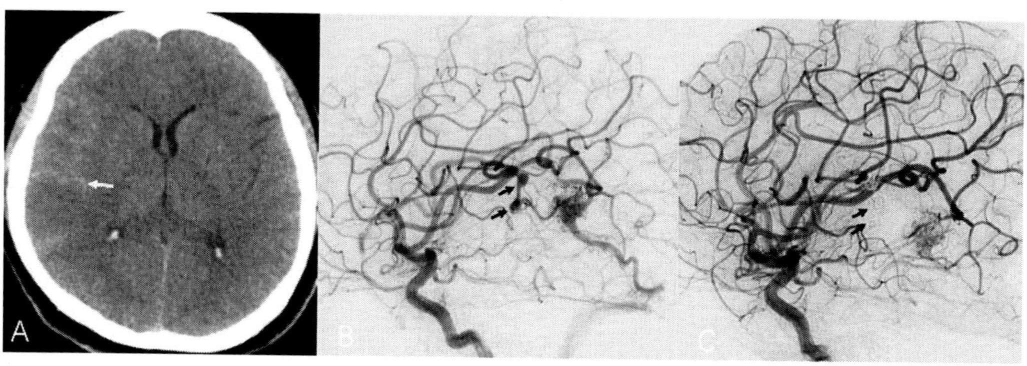

Figure 1. A) Computed tomography scanning shows acute subarachnoid hemorrhage on the right side of the Sylvian fissure (arrow); B) A cerebral arteriogram after contrast injection of the right internal carotid artery, lateral view, shows 2 distal flow-related aneurysms located on the middle cerebral artery and supplying the arteriovenous malformation (AVM) (arrows). The aneurysms were embolized with coils; C) An angiogram of the right internal carotid artery, lateral view, confirms complete obliteration of the aneurysms (arrows).

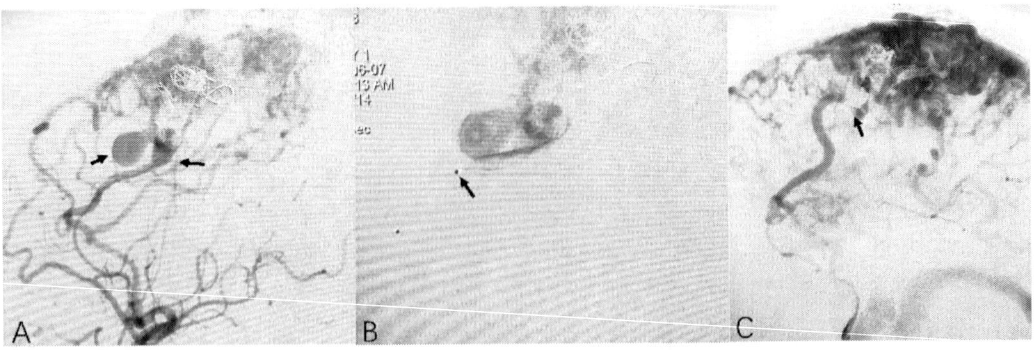

Figure 2. A large unruptured AVM treated previously with coiling and Onyx embolization at the level of the AVM 1 year before. A) An angiogram of the right carotid artery angiogram shows two aneurysms on the anterior cerebral artery that are not presented on the first session (arrows); B) Superselective contrast injection through a Headway 17 soft microcatheter (Microvention, USA) shows the aneurysms and the arteriovenous shunt (arrow); C) A right carotid artery angiogram confirms that the aneurysm was completely occluded after coiling and Onyx injection through the anterior cerebral artery (arrow).

Aneurysm Treatment

All seven intranidal aneurysms were embolized using Onyx18. Of the seven flow-related aneurysms, five that arose from the M2 segment of the middle cerebral artery were treated with coil embolization, one that arose from the posterior inferior cerebellar artery was treated with Onyx embolization, and one that arose from the A4 segment of the anterior cerebral artery was treated with Onyx embolization. The five incidental aneurysms were coiled with stent assisted. All aneurysms were embolized completely.

AVM Treatment

Twenty-three Onyx embolization procedures were performed to treat AVM nidi. Four patients required additional gamma knife radiosurgery. Complete obliteration of the AVM was achieved in six (35.3%) of the 17 cases. There were no complications. During a mean 10.4-month (range, 3-25 months) followed up with DSA or cross-sectional imaging, excellent outcomes (mRS = 0 to 1) were achieved in 13 cases (76.5%) and good outcomes (mRS = 2) in the other four (23.5%).

Discussion

The main finding of our study was that selective endovascular treatment is safe and effective for patients with AVM-associated aneurysms. This is important because it suggests that aneurysm is an indication for selective endovascular embolization in patients with ruptured or unruptured AVMs. Reports in the literature have noted that patients with AVMs and associated aneurysms are more likely to present with hemorrhage than those in the general AVM population [2, 3, 7]. Among patients with AVM-associated aneurysms, the source of hemorrhage was found to be the aneurysm in 50% of cases. Flow-related aneurysms have been identified as the most common source of aneurysmal hemorrhage in patients with AVMs, accounting for nearly 80% of cases [2, 6].

Previous authors found AVM-associated aneurysm to be a significant risk factor for hemorrhage, and reported an association with poor outcome [3]. Such aneurysms appear to develop gradually, as indicated by the more advanced age of most AVM patients who have them [1, 8, 9]. These aneurysms have also been reported to be more frequent in AVMs supplied by the posterior circulation, and this may be explained by a difference in hemodynamic stress [10]. As noted, the presence of an AVM-associated arterial aneurysm is known to increase the risk of AVM bleeding. In one series, the rate of bleeding for AVMs with associated aneurysms was 10% higher than that for AVMs without aneurysms [2]. Awareness of the potential increased hemorrhage risk in patients with AVM-associated aneurysms has important therapeutic implications. Authors have suggested that such aneurysms be treated endovascularly before proceeding with gamma knife radiosurgery [11-13].

Acute, fatal rupture of a feeding artery aneurysm following AVM embolization has been infrequently reported in the literature [14, 15]. While the precise pathobiology of arterial aneurysm rupture following AVM embolization is unknown, it is hypothesized that the risk of feeding artery aneurysm rupture might be higher because the feeding artery pressures increased following AVM embolization (Figure 3) [16, 17]. Reynolds et al. reported a 69-year-old female suffered a fatal feeding artery aneurysm rupture several hours after AVM embolization. They concluded that an increase in AVM feeding artery pressure following endovascular embolization may contribute to the rupture of a feeding artery aneurysm [14]. Even if hemodynamic alterations induced by AVM embolization are unlikely to be significant at a proximal level, other mechanisms, such as retrieval of the microcatheter, may induce rupture of a feeding artery aneurysm [15].

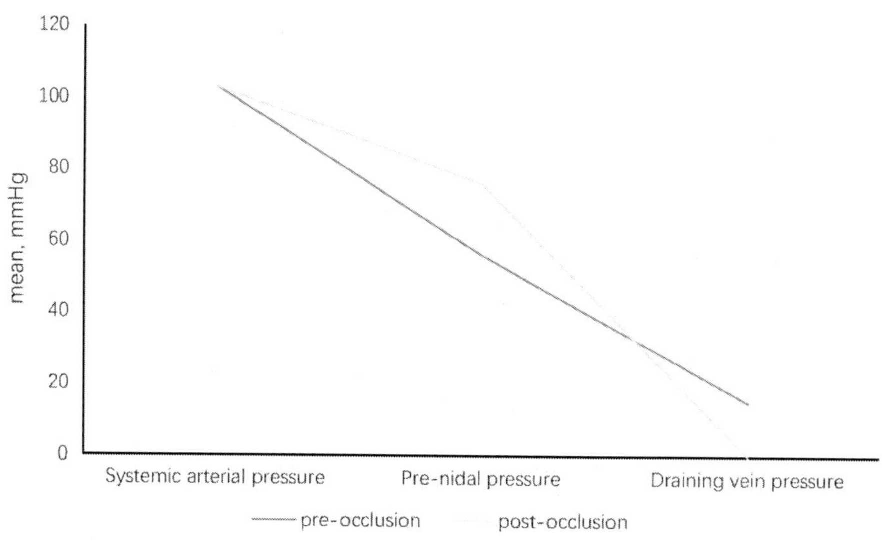

Figure 3. Intravascular pressure data from Handa et al. (1993), showing pressure changes in the AVM before and after AVM embolization. In the arteries feeding the AVM s, the feeding artery pressure rose by about 22 mm Hg after embolization.

Considering the poor outcome after aneurysm rebleeding, endovascular-targeted treatment of the ruptured aneurysm should be performed early using coils or liquid embolic agents, depending on the lesion's location and size [11-13]. The goal of treating with glue, Onyx, or coils is segmental occlusion of the supply vessel that harbors the aneurysm, or the aneurysm itself. Considering the low complication rate for aneurysm occlusion in our series, we recommend treating these aneurysms whenever possible. Aneurysmal bleeding usually causes subarachnoid hemorrhage, and AVM/intranidal aneurysmal hemorrhage results in intraparenchymal hematoma, which can be differentiated diagnostically by combining computed tomography scanning with cerebral angiography. In unruptured cases, the AVM nidus and the coexisting aneurysm can take the hemorrhagic risk simultaneously; thus, we must balance the risks of treatment versus allowing risks to take during their natural course. This issue is of utmost importance, and our experience might be helpful regarding consultation for patients with unruptured AVM.

Conclusion

Endovascular treatment strategies of arterial aneurysms in AVMs are coil embolization or parent vessel sacrifice using coils or liquid embolics. Embolization of arterial aneurysms on feeding pedicles should be considered prior to or adjunct AVM embolization.

Acknowledgment

This work was supported by Tsinghua Precision Medicine Foundation (20219990008), Tsinghua University, Beijing, China & Beijing Municipile Administration of Hospitals Incubating Program (PX2020039), Beijing, China.

References

[1] Lv X, Li Y, Yang X, Jiang C, Wu Z. Characteristics of arteriovenous malformations associated with cerebral aneurysms. *World Neurosurg*. 2011;76(3-4):288-91.

[2] Lv X, Wu Z, Jiang C, Yang X, Li Y, Sun Y, Zhang N. Angioarchitectural characteristics of brain arteriovenous malformations with and without hemorrhage. *World Neurosurg*. 2011;76(1-2):95-9.

[3] Platz J, Berkefeld J, Singer OC, Wolff R, Seifert V, Konczalla J, Güresir E. Frequency, risk of hemorrhage and treatment considerations for cerebral arteriovenous malformations with associated aneurysms. *Acta Neurochir (Wien)*. 2014;156(11):2025-34.

[4] Stein KP, Wanke I, Forsting M, Zhu Y, Moldovan AS, Dammann P, Sandalcioglu IE, Sure U. Associated aneurysms in supratentorial arteriovenous malformations: impact of aneurysm size on haemorrhage. *Cerebrovasc Dis*. 2015;39(2):122-9.

[5] El-Abtah ME, Petitt JC, Kashkoush A, Achey R, Bain MD, Moore NZ. Endovascular Management of Arteriovenous Malformation-Associated Intracranial Aneurysms: A Systematic Literature Review. *World Neurosurg*. 2022 Aug;164:257-269.

[6] Rammos SK, Gardenghi B, Bortolotti C, Cloft HJ, Lanzino G. Aneurysms Associated with Brain Arteriovenous Malformations. *AJNR Am J Neuroradiol*. 2016 Nov;37(11):1966-1971.

[7] Cagnazzo F, Brinjikji W, Lanzino G. Arterial aneurysms associated with arteriovenous malformations of the brain: classification, incidence, risk of hemorrhage, and treatment-a systematic review. *Acta Neurochir (Wien)*. 2016;158(11):2095-2104.

[8] Luo J, Lv X, Jiang C, Wu Z. Brain AVM characteristics and age. *Eur J Radiol*. 2012;81(4):780-3.

[9] Morgan MK, Alsahli K, Wiedmann M, Assaad NN, Heller GZ. Factors Associated With Proximal Intracranial Aneurysms to Brain Arteriovenous Malformations: A Prospective Cohort Study. *Neurosurgery*. 2016;78(6):787-92.

[10] Shakur SF, Amin-Hanjani S, Mostafa H, Charbel FT, Alaraj A. Hemodynamic Characteristics of Cerebral Arteriovenous Malformation Feeder Vessels With and Without Aneurysms. *Stroke*. 2015;46(7):1997-9.

[11] D'Aliberti G, Talamonti G, Cenzato M, La Camera A, Debernardi A, Valvassori L, Mariangela P, Nichelatti M. Arterial and venous aneurysms associated with arteriovenous malformations. *World Neurosurg*. 2015;83(2):188-96.

[12] Li M, Lin N, Wu J, Liang J, He W. Multiple intracranial aneurysms associated with multiple dural arteriovenous fistulas and cerebral arteriovenous malformation. *World Neurosurg*. 2012;77(2):398. E11-5.

[13] Lv X, Wu Z, Li Y, Yang X, Jiang C, Sun Y, Zhang N. Endovascular treatment of cerebral aneurysms associated with arteriovenous malformations. *Eur J Radiol*. 2012;81(6):1296-8.

[14] Reynolds MR, Arias EJ, Chatterjee AR, Chicoine MR, Cross DT 3rd. Acute rupture of a feeding artery aneurysm after embolization of a brain arteriovenous malformation. *Interv Neuroradiol*. 2015 Oct;21(5):613-9.

[15] Gabrieli J, Clarençon F, Di Maria F, Fahed R, Boch AL, Degos V, Chiras J, Sourour NA. Fatal rupture of a brain arteriovenous malformation flow-related aneurysm during microcatheter removal: a rare complication. *J Neurosurg*. 2015 Apr;122(4):929-32.

[16] Zhang H, Liang S, Lv X. Proof-of-Principle for AVM Embolization Complications Caused by the Proximal Occlusion Technique Using Onyx: A Theoretical Basis for Ante-Grade Drifting Technique. *Neurol India*. 2022 Jul-Aug;70(4):1443-1447.

[17] Handa T, Negoro M, Miyachi S, Sugita K. Evaluation of pressure changes in feeding arteries during embolization of intracerebral arteriovenous malformations. *J Neurosurg*. 1993 Sep;79(3):383-9.

Chapter 19

Management of Intracranial Aneurysms with Extracranial Carotid Pathology

Dmitry Usachev, MD, PhD
Vasily Lukshin, MD, PhD
Anna Shulgina*, MD, PhD
Sergey Yakovlev, MD, PhD
Olga Belousova, MD, PhD
and Mark Kondakov, MD
N. N. Burdenko National Medical Research Center for Neurosurgery, Moscow, Russian Federation

Abstract

Reconstructive interventions on the carotid arteries in patients with intracranial aneurysms requires an individual patient-selected approach, in contrast to certain standards based only on the principles of evidence-based medicine. It should be noted that such situations are not uncommon in neurosurgical practice - the incidence of cerebral aneurysms in the population, according to epidemiological studies, varies from 3 to 5%, and in the group of patients with hemodynamically significant stenosis of the carotid arteries, it is 3.2% [1]. In N. N. Burdenko National Medical Research Center for Neurosurgery experience, cerebral aneurysms were diagnosed in 4.1% of all patients who had indications for carotid endarterectomy. At the same time, due to the wider use of CT angiography as a method of primary diagnosis of steno-occlusive pathology, the number of such clinical cases is increasing every year.

Present clinical guidelines classify such patients in a group of increased risk of carotid endarterectomy, pointing out the disagreement in approaches to the treatment of cerebral aneurysms in combination with internal carotid artery (ICA) stenosis and assigning the first role in making a decision the individual characteristics of each individual patient and the capabilities of the surgical hospital. The complexity of determining the tactics of treating such patients is due to the competition of mutually opposite pathogenetic mechanisms that determine the likelihood of ischemic stroke on the one hand and the risk of aneurysm rupture on the other. This, in turn, leads to antagonism of the methods of potential medical and surgical treatment.

* Corresponding Author's Email: ashulgina@nsi.ru.

In: Understanding and Managing Cerebral Aneurysms
Editor: Xianli Lv
ISBN: 979-8-89113-608-3

Taking into account the increased risks of perioperative complications of reconstructive surgery, such patients are often redirected from the departments of vascular surgery to neurosurgical hospitals for the primary treatment of cerebral aneurysms, followed by a decision on the issue of carotid endarterectomy. At the same time, this treatment tactic is not always justified, since it does not take into account the individual risks of aneurysm rupture and possible ischemic cerebrovascular accident.

The aim of this chapter is to determine the algorithm for the treatment of patients with a combination of cerebral aneurysms with carotid stenosis.

Keywords: intracranial aneurysm, carotid stenosis, carotid endarterectomy, ischemic stroke, hemorrhagic stroke, subarachnoid hemorrhage

Introduction

Currently, the following main approaches to the treatment such patients are most often used, which have their own advantages and disadvantages.

1. *Preventive exclusion of the aneurysm from the bloodstream followed by a reconstructive intervention.* This tactic is most common in neurosurgical hospitals [2, 3]. Its main arguments are:
   - Severe clinical course of hemorrhagic stroke and subarachnoid hemorrhage (SAH) in case of aneurysm rupture. According to epidemiological studies, the overall annual risk of hemorrhage is 1-2% [4], while mortality can reach 50% [5].
   - Increased risk of hemorrhage due to changes in cerebral hemodynamics, both during surgery with rises in blood pressure, and after – with an increase in volumetric blood flow in the reconstructed internal carotid artery. Similar changes in cerebral blood flow can be observed for at least 1 month after reconstruction [6], which potentially increases the risk of aneurysm growth and rupture. Studies have shown that the presence of hemodynamically significant stenosis or occlusion of the internal carotid artery can lead to a decrease in the size of distally located intracranial aneurysms [7] and reduce the risk of their rupture [8]. This allows to conclude that the restoration of blood flow in the ICA can contribute to an increase in the size of the aneurysm and the risk of its rupture.
   - The need to prescribe antiplatelet and anticoagulant therapy in the perioperative period of carotid endarterectomy (CEA), which can also potentially affect the risk of cerebral aneurysm rupture. Indeed, studies have shown that taking anticoagulants causes a significantly more severe course of hemorrhage and a worse prognosis [9, 10-12]. Long-term anticoagulant therapy increases the risk of intracranial hemorrhage [13], increases mortality by more than 3 times (OR 3.5) [14] and increases the risks of cerebral hematoma enlargement by more than 6 times (OR 6.2) [14].

Of course, the presence of a cerebral aneurysm complicates the performing of carotid endarterectomy and may increase its risks. There are at least two clinical cases in the literature reporting the development of subarachnoid hemorrhage due to aneurysm rupture after reconstruction of the internal carotid artery [15, 16].

However, not all patients with cerebral aneurysms have equal risk of rupture. There are two large multicenter studies of cerebral aneurysmal disease prognosis - ISUIA (Unruptured intracranial aneurysms - risk of rupture and risks of surgical intervention, 2003, USA and Canada [17] and UCAS (The natural course of unruptured cerebral aneurysms in a Japanese cohort, 2012, Japan [18]. A total of 9383 aneurysms were analyzed in 7412 patients.

It was found that the probability of cerebral aneurysm rupture was significantly determined by its size and location. Aneurysms of the carotid arterial system less than 7 mm had a favorable prognosis of the clinical course - the annual rate of their rupture did not exceed 0.1% in the ISUIA study, 0.36% and 0.5% in the UCAS with sizes up to 4 mm and 7 mm, respectively. Such low risks of hemorrhage in small aneurysms do not differ significantly from the average values in the population, which calls into question the appropriateness of their treatment. Refusal to perform carotid endarterectomy according to indications in such cases seems unreasonable, and priority preventive microsurgical clipping of asymptomatic small aneurysms in the presence of hemodynamically significant stenosis of the ICA increases the risk of severe ischemic complications, which can reach 6.5% [2]. This was the reason for the spread of an alternative approach to the treatment of this group of patients.

2. *Performing carotid endarterectomy as the first stage, followed by a decision on the surgical treatment of cerebral aneurysm.* Such treatment tactics are mainly performed in the departments of vascular surgery, which specialize in the treatment of steno-occlusive pathology of the brachiocephalic arteries.

This approach is based on the findings of the large multicenter study NASCET. When analyzing its results, attention was paid to the issue of the influence of cerebral aneurysms on the outcomes of carotid endarterectomy in patients with symptomatic stenoses [19]. In total, among all patients included in the study, cerebral aneurysms were detected in 90 cases (3.1%), most of them did not exceed 10 mm. Carotid endarterectomy was performed in 32 cases, while only in one case (3%), SAH from an aneurysm located on the side of the stenosis developed immediately after the operation. SAH from aneurysms on the opposite side of carotid endarterectomy was not observed. In 8 cases, microsurgical clipping of the aneurysm was performed as the first stage, while in 2 cases (25%) these interventions were accompanied by the development of ischemic stroke in the early postoperative period.

Based on obtained data, it was recommended that carotid endarterectomy should be performed as the first stage in patients with symptomatic ICA stenoses of more than 70% and intracranial aneurysms of less than 10 mm, since the risk of aneurysm rupture is minimal and does not affect the results of reconstructive intervention [19]. Subsequently, these recommendations were expanded, and began to be used not only for symptomatic, but also for asymptomatic stenoses. At the same time, it was decided to limit the critical size of intracranial aneurysms, allowing for carotid endarterectomy at the first stage, to 6 mm.

In the series presented in the literature, ICA reconstructions in patients with small cerebral aneurysms (up to 6 mm) were also not accompanied by their ruptures either immediately after surgery or during follow-up [8, 20, 21], [22]. This formed a firm opinion that in patients with hemodynamically significant ICA stenoses and concomitant intracranial aneurysms less than 6 mm, the probability of their rupture is indeed extremely low, and the risk of ischemic stroke is high, which makes it possible to perform carotid endarterectomy without exclusion of such aneurysms from the bloodstream even after ICA reconstruction. Moreover, during the follow-up observation of such aneurysms, there were no episodes of SAH and no signs of their increase in most cases (97.6%) [23].

Despite the apparent obviousness of the formulated recommendations confirmed by clinical experience, a significant drawback of the studies was their low representativeness. Indeed, most of the series included no more than 10-15 patients, which significantly reduced the reliability of the conclusions. Therefore, despite the presented optimistic results, a cautious attitude towards carotid endarterectomy in patients with intracranial aneurysms remained among specialists.

The excessive categoricalness of the recommendations formulated in NASCET was also confirmed by meta-analysis of the 27 studies, which included a total of 141 observations [24]. It was found that only carotid endarterectomy in patients with intracranial aneurysms less than 6 mm in 4% of cases was accompanied by their rupture already in the perioperative period: in 2.4% -within 30 days after ICA reconstruction (of which 2 were fatal) and in 1.6% - in the late postoperative period (all fatal). In total, after carotid endarterectomy without a staged exclusion of the aneurysm from the bloodstream, SAH developed in 8% of cases with a mortality rate from hemorrhage of 40%.

These results underline the importance of intracranial aneurysms as an increased risk factor of CEA complications, even if they are small, and the need of more selective approaches to planning staged surgical treatment of such patients.

3. *Simultaneous interventions: exclusion of the aneurysm from the bloodstream and reconstruction of the ICA.* According to the literature, this tactic was chosen in 8% of all described cases of surgical treatment of this comorbidity. The main indications for the use of simultaneous interventions were:
   - The presence of risk factors for aneurysm rupture and unstable complicated atherosclerotic plaque of ICA. In such cases, carotid endarterectomy was performed immediately after clipping of the aneurysm in order to prevent its rupture due to anticoagulants at the main stage of reconstruction and the use of controlled hypertension as a method of protecting the brain from ischemia.
   - Clipping of the aneurysm with the need for proximal control at the level of the extracranial segment of the ICA makes it possible to simultaneously perform carotid endarterectomy [25].
   - Endovascular interventions for ICA stenosis and intracranial aneurysm. The first step is stenting the area of stenosis, followed by intervention for the aneurysm [26].

An example of a single-stage endovascular intervention is shown on Figure 1.

It should be noted that one-stage interventions are technically more complex, require the work of several surgical teams, and are time-consuming. In addition, in case of complications, the question of their differential diagnosis and treatment, taking into account the presence of intracranial and extracranial stages of intervention, sharply arises. Taking into account the low risks of aneurysm rupture or ischemic accidents between staged operations, the simultaneous approach is justified only according to the strong indications. In other cases, it is advisable to perform staged interventions with the period between operations, depending on the individual characteristics of the patient and his condition after the first stage of surgical treatment.

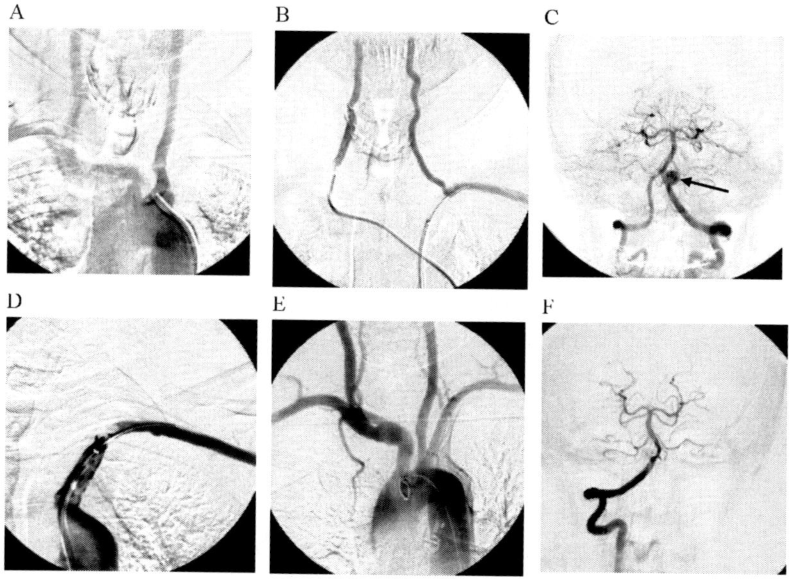

Figure 1. An example of a simultaneous endovascular intervention: recanalization and stenting of the left subclavian artery, followed by embolization of the aneurysm of the left vertebral artery with microcoils: A - occlusion of the first segment of the left subclavian artery; B - steel-syndrome with retrograde flow in the left vertebral artery; C – hemodynamic aneurysm (arrow) of the left vertebral artery; D - recanalization of the first segment of the left subclavian artery; E - stenting with restoration of magistral blood flow; F - result after microcoils embolization of the aneurysm. Occlusion of the aneurysm and no evidence of steel syndrome.

Differentiated Approach to the Choice of Treatment Tactics

So, three main approaches to the surgical treatment of combined aneurysmal and steno-occlusive pathology of cerebral vessels have been described. What is the reason for the contradictions in the conclusions of studies, and what approach is appropriate to choose in a particular clinical situation? An analysis of the presented studies, taking into account the current understanding of the course of ischemic and aneurysmal diseases of the brain, allows us to make the following important observations.

1. It is possible to distinguish groups of patients with extremely high and extremely low risks of aneurysm rupture. In the first case, the primary intervention to exclude the aneurysm from the bloodstream is justified, in the second case the first stage of carotid endarterectomy is justified.
2. Risks of aneurysm rupture or development of ischemic stroke in the territory of a stenotic artery must be assessed taking into account many factors. In abovementioned studies, only the size of the aneurysm was assessed, despite the fact that the risk of SAH is determined, among other things, by location, morphological characteristics, age, gender, and family and somatic anamnestic data. Small aneurysms are also known to rupture. In meta-analysis of literature, 61% of aneurysms ruptured after carotid endarterectomy were less than 6 mm in size [27]. There is also no consensus on the borderline aneurysm size associated with increased risk of SAH. Some authors

consider that this size is 10 mm [17, 28, 29], others - 5 mm [30]. In small series of observations, the influence of other factors on the risks of rupture may not appear, however, in more representative studies, the absence of their consideration is already beginning to affect.

3. Indications for carotid endarterectomy should be compared with the risks of aneurysm rupture. Ignoring intracranial aneurysms as an increased risk factor for carotid endarterectomy, ICA reconstructions can be offered to patients even for relative indications, in which the risks of ischemic accidents are minimal. Such situations should be excluded from clinical practice.
4. After performing reconstructive interventions on the carotid arteries, patients need the appointment of adequate antiaggregant therapy. Despite the fact that studies did not reveal the effect of acetylsalicylic acid preparations on the likelihood of aneurysm rupture, there was a tendency to a more severe course of SAH in cases of completed hemorrhages. This explains the high lethality of SAH in the late postoperative period of carotid endarterectomy.
5. The tactics of treating patients with a combination of steno-occlusive and aneurysmal pathology in the presence of risk factors of both aneurysm rupture and ischemic cerebrovascular accidents seems to be non-obvious. The approaches described earlier do not provide an answer to this problem.

To answer these questions, we analyzed the N. N. Burdenko National Medical Research Center for Neurosurgery experience of surgical treatment of patients with a combination of hemodynamically significant ICA stenosis and cerebral aneurysms operated during the last 5 years. A total of 47 patients were analyzed. Variants of lesions of intracranial and extracranial arteries are presented in Table 1.

Table 1. Variants of lesions of intracranial and extracranial arteries in patients with a combination of ICA stenoses and cerebral aneurysms

CEREBRAL ANEURYSM	RATE
– MCA	39%
– ICA	26%
– ACA-AComA	22%
– Basilar artery	9%
– VA	2%
– PCA	2%
– ACA	2%
Multiple aneurysms	34%
STENOSIS OF THE CAROTID ARTERIES	
– Critical (more than 85%)	93,6%
– Subcritical (60-80%)	6,4%
– Bilateral stenoses	25,5%

A total of 89 surgical interventions were performed: in all cases, carotid endarterectomy was performed on the side of stenosis. 14 patients (30%) with aneurysms were kept under follow-up. In 33 patients (70%), various options for surgical exclusion of aneurysms from the bloodstream were performed - aneurysm clipping (26 cases - 55%), flow diversion stents (4 cases - 9%), occlusion of the aneurysm with microcoils (3 cases - 6%). There were no complications after surgical treatment. The interval between interventions was chosen individually and started from 1 week (when risk factors for aneurysm rupture or ischemic accident were identified) - in 18% of cases. In most cases, the second surgical intervention was performed 2-3 months after the first one. Based on the results, it was concluded that differentiated approach based on a comparison of the possible risks of hemorrhage, on the one hand, and ischemic accident on the other is the most optimal. Depending on this, indications for surgical interventions, their sequence and the time between them were determined.

Based on this approach, the algorithm for determining the tactics of surgical treatment is schematically shown on Figure 2.

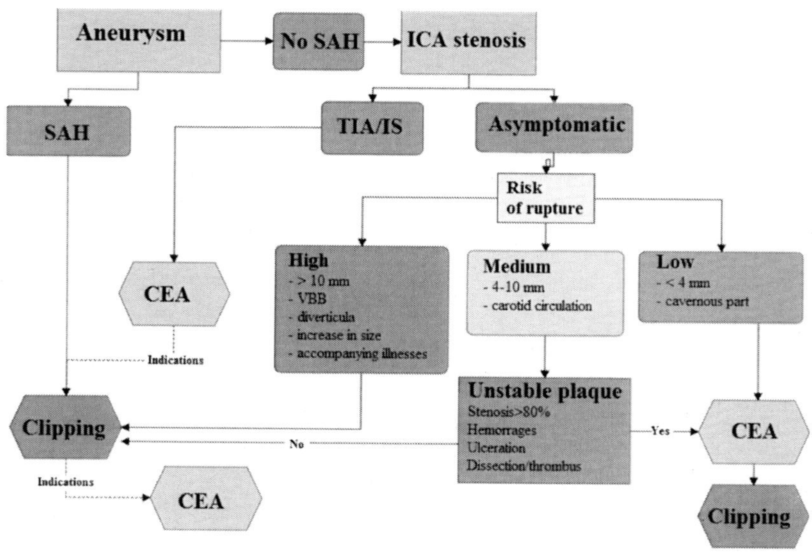

Figure 2. Algorithm for determining the tactics of staged surgical treatment of patients with cerebral aneurysms in combination with ICA stenosis.

It is obvious that the greatest danger in patients with a combination of ICA stenosis and intracranial aneurysms is the rupture of the aneurysm with the development of subarachnoid hemorrhage, therefore, the group with an increased risk of SAH should be identified first. To do this, it is necessary to assess the risks of aneurysm rupture based on epidemiological studies.

Risk Assessment for Aneurysm Rupture

When planning staged surgical treatment, patients with a history of SAH are identified first of all - they are the ones who have the highest risk of re-bleeding, which justify the need for priority aneurysm clipping. In the first 2 weeks after aneurysm rupture, rebleeding occurs in 6-22% of patients [31-34]. The maximum risk of rebleeding occurs on 4-9 days [32]. The risk of death in case of re-rupture of the aneurysm during the first week after hemorrhage is 32-50% [35], in the second week - 43%. In the first 6 months after aneurysm rupture, rebleeding develops in 50% of patients with a mortality rate of up to 60%. Since then, the risk of rebleeding is 3% per year with a mortality rate of 2% per year [33].

The most dangerous are aneurysms of the vertebrobasilar system, in which the frequency of repeated hemorrhages reaches 71.4% within 1 week after SAH with a mortality of 46.7% [36]. In patients with multiple intracranial aneurysms, mortality from rebleeding during follow-up is 11.5% [37].

In order to reduce the risk of aneurysm rupture in patients with anamnesis of SAH, the first step is to exclude the aneurysm from the bloodstream. Concomitant stenosis of the ICA complicates manipulations at the level of the aneurysm, so the priority method of surgical treatment is microsurgical clipping of the aneurysm. When cerebral aneurysms are localized in the vertebrobasilar system, endovascular interventions are the methods of choice.

Carotid endarterectomy is performed as the second stage when the indications for reconstructive intervention are confirmed. It should be noted that even in the presence of clinical symptoms due to stenosis, carotid endarterectomy is not performed at the first stage due to the high probability of severe hemorrhagic complications.

The timing between interventions is determined individually, depending on the time of hemorrhage, the patient's condition, the degree of stenosis and signs of atherosclerotic plaque instability. In the early stages after SAH or with subcritical stenoses of the ICA in the absence of signs of atherosclerotic plaque instability, it is advisable to perform the second stage after 1-3 months. The presence of critical embologenic stenosis of the carotid arteries, on the contrary, is an indication for accelerated carotid endarterectomy, which is usually performed in such cases within one inpatient stay of the patient - usually on 3-7 days after clipping the aneurysm. To illustrate this treatment strategy, we present a typical clinical case.

Clinical Case

Patient M, 72 years old. Complaints of headaches, unsteady gait. Anamnesis: a month and a half ago he developed SAH, which manifested with severe headaches and dizziness (Hunt-Hess 1-2).

The patient underwent selective angiography (Figure 3 A-B), which revealed the source of hemorrhage - a saccular aneurysm of the left vertebral artery (VA) at the level of the posterior inferior cerebellar artery (PICA) up to 5 mm in diameter. Additionally, a critical stenosis of the left ICA was diagnosed with the narrowing of lumen artery up to 90%.

After conservative therapy the patient's condition was stabilized, and he was referred to Burdenko Neurosurgical Center for the treatment.

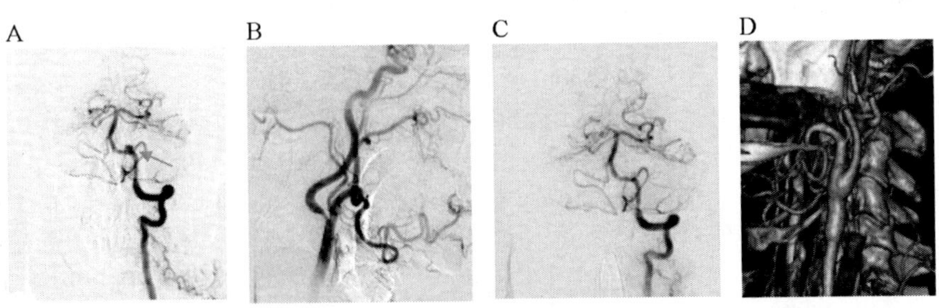

Figure 3. Angiographic examination: A – aneurysm of the left VA in the area of PICA origin (arrow); B - critical stenosis of the left internal carotid artery; C – angiographic control after aneurysm embolization with microcoils; D – CT angiographic control after carotid endarterectomy on the left.

Upon admission, the patient was in a satisfactory condition. There were no focal neurological symptoms except partial left-sided homonymous hemianopia.

Anamnesis of SAH, as well as the size and location of the aneurysm, indicate a higher risk of its re-rupture, compared with the likelihood of ischemic stroke due to asymptomatic stenosis of the left ICA. This justified the need to exclude the aneurysm from the bloodstream. At the first stage, the patient underwent endovascular occlusion of the cavity of the aneurysm of the left vertebral artery with microcoils. There were no complications after endovascular intervention. Given the presence of critical stenosis of the left ICA, a decision was made to perform an accelerated reconstructive intervention. When choosing a technique for surgical intervention, the patient's age (over 70 years), the critical degree of stenosis, and the presence of a pronounced C-shaped tortuosity of the left ICA were taken into account. According to the CREST multicenter study, carotid angioplasty and stenting are associated with higher risks of embolic and cardiac complications, and placement of a stent in the proximal third of the extracranial segment of the left ICA against the background of its deformation could lead to the formation of septal stenosis in this area. Therefore, carotid endarterectomy was chosen as the reconstruction method. For the same reason, it was decided to refrain from simultaneous endovascular interventions on the carotid and vertebral arteries.

On the 7th day after the first stage, left carotid endarterectomy was performed. The main stage of reconstruction was performed without the use of a temporary intraluminal shunt due to signs of cerebral blood flow compensation during the clamping. There were no complications during the postoperative period. The patient was discharged in a satisfactory condition. At follow-up examinations, there were no signs of cerebral aneurysm and ICA restenosis (Figure 3 C-D).

The choice of tactics for the treatment of patients with unruptured aneurysms appears to be more difficult. In such situations, it depends on the risks of possible hemorrhage. Based on the results of ISUIA and UCAS cooperative studies, it is possible to identify factors that affect the likelihood of rupture of an asymptomatic intracranial aneurysm, among which the most significant are its size and localization (Table 2). It was found that the risk of rupture of intracranial aneurysms increases with their size [19]. Carotid aneurysms less than 7 mm in diameter have the lowest risk of hemorrhage. Thus, according to ISUIA, there were no signs of SAH for 5 years with aneurysms of this size [29]. According to a large Japanese UCAS trial, the annual rate of aneurysm rupture less than 4 mm did not exceed 0.36% and did not differ from the average rate of SAH in the population [18]. Indications for their surgical treatment are extremely limited and are associated primarily with the presence of SAH in history. The influence of carotid reconstructions on the probability of rupture of such aneurysms may not be taken into account when planning surgical treatment of patients with concomitant hemodynamically significant stenoses.

Aneurysms larger than 7 mm in diameter have higher risks of rupture - the average annual incidence of SAH in such cases exceeds 1.7% and significantly depends on the localization. The lowest risks of rupture are observed with aneurysms of the cavernous and petrosal segments of the ICA. Such aneurysms often slowly increase in size and present with a pseudotumorous course. Even in the event of a rupture, they clinically manifest as symptoms of a carotid-cavernous fistula and are rarely accompanied by intracranial hemorrhage. Only when the size is more than 2-2.5 cm, aneurysms of this localization become more dangerous - spreading beyond the cavernous sinus, they can lead to the development of SAH in case of rupture with a frequency of more than 6.4% per year (Table 3).

Table 2. Annual rate of rupture of asymptomatic aneurysms by size according to cooperative studies

Trial	Size of aneurysm, mm	Rupture risk	
		Carotid aneurysms	Basilar aneurysms
International Study of Unruptured Intracranial Aneurysms Investigators, (ISUIA) 2003 [29]	< 7 7-12 13-24 >25	0,1% 2,6% 14,5% 40%	2,5% 14,5% 18,4% 50%
The natural course of unruptured cerebral aneurysms in a Japanese cohort (UCAS) [18]	3-4 5-6 7-9 10-24 >25	0,36% 0,50% 1,69% 4,37% 33,4%	

Table 3. Annual rate of asymptomatic aneurysm rupture by size and location according to ISUIA [29]

Localization	Size		
	7-12 mm	13-24 mm	>25 mm
Cavernous part of ICA	0	3%	6,4%
Intracranial part of ICA	2,6%	14,5%	40%
Vertebrobasilar circulation	14,5%	18,4%	50%

Carotid aneurysms with intracranial localization larger than 7 mm have a medium risk of rupture, their annual frequency varies from 2.6% (<12 mm) to 40% (>25 mm).

Regardless of size, aneurysms of the vertebrobasilar arterial basin are the most dangerous. The risk of their rupture even with small sizes (less than 7 mm) exceeds 2.5%, reaching 50% annually (more than 25 mm).

In addition to size, the probability of aneurysm rupture is influenced by its morphological characteristics [38]. The factors that increase the risk of developing SAH include the irregular shape of the aneurysm, the presence of diverticula, the narrow neck of the aneurysm, the predominance of the maximum size of the aneurysm to the diameter of the artery by more than 2 times, hemodynamic features in aneurysms [39-41]. Signs of aneurysm growth during follow-up increase the risk of aneurysm rupture by more than 2.4 times [42]. Meta-analysis of 19 of the largest series of observations identified the risk factors for the development of SAH, among which, in addition to those previously given, include female sex and age over 60 years [38].

Given the variety of factors that determine the risks of rupture of asymptomatic intracranial aneurysms, it is reasonable to divide them into 3 main groups depending on the expected risk of developing intracranial hemorrhage.

Aneurysms with *high risk* of hemorrhage *(more than 3% annually):*

- anamnesis of SAH;
- aneurysms of the vertebrobasilar arterial system more than 7 mm;
- giant intracranial aneurysms of the carotid system more than 25 mm;
- aneurysms of the carotid system more than 7 mm with diverticula, signs of enlargement during dynamic observation.

Aneurysms with *medium risk* of hemorrhage *(no more than 3% per year):*

- intracranial aneurysms of the ICA, MCA and ACA more than 7 mm;
- cavernous aneurysms over 13 mm;
- small aneurysms of the vertebrobasilar arterial system (up to 7 mm);
- complicated aneurysms of the carotid system (diverticula, signs of growth during follow-up, heredity, somatic risk factors)

Aneurysms with *low risk* of hemorrhage *(less than 1% per year):*

- Carotid aneurysms less than 7 mm, especially less than 4 mm, without concomitant risk factors;
- Aneurysms of the cavernous or petrosal ICA segments less than 13 mm.

Depending on whether the aneurysm belongs to a certain risk group, the choice of further tactics for staged surgical treatment is determined, taking into account the risks of ischemic stroke (Figure 1).

In patients with a low-risk intracranial aneurysm, the surgical interventions is usually limited to the ICA reconstruction, followed by dynamic observation of the aneurysm. If signs of an increase in size or the appearance of additional risk factors is detected, a decision is made to exclude it from the bloodstream. The reconstructive intervention itself in this group of patients, its anesthetic management and management of patients in the early postoperative period usually does not differ from conventional carotid endarterectomy.

Performing carotid endarterectomy in patients with medium-risk aneurysms is already associated with an increased risk of perioperative complications, so it is advisable to treat such patients in neurosurgical hospitals with the possibility of performing surgery on both extra- and intracranial arteries. Considering the relatively low risks of aneurysm rupture, it is advisable to perform carotid endarterectomy as the first stage, followed by planned clipping or embolization of the aneurysm. Usually, in the practice of Burdenko Center for Neurosurgery, the second stage of surgical treatment was performed within 1 to 3 months after the first operation.

Patients with subcritical stenoses from 60 to 75% without gross hemodynamic significance and signs of plaque instability can be considered an exception to this tactic of surgical treatment. As will be shown below, in such cases, the risks of ischemic stroke are minimal, which allows firstly to routinely exclude the aneurysm from the bloodstream.

The most difficult is the choice of tactics of surgical treatment in patients with hemodynamically significant stenoses and aneurysms with an increased risk of rupture. In such cases, the decision is made individually after a detailed assessment of the clinical course of the disease and the risks of developing cerebrovascular accident in the territory of the stenotic internal carotid artery. Primary reconstructive surgery is justified only in the group of patients with an increased risk of ischemic stroke.

Patients with Increased Risk of Ischemic Stroke

As was noted above, in patients with asymptomatic aneurysms without anamnesis of SAH, the choice of tactics for staged surgical treatment is influenced by the presence of signs of "instability" of the atherosclerotic plaque, which determines the risk of developing ischemic cerebrovascular accident in the territory of the stenotic artery.

Numerous studies have made it possible to assess the risk of ischemic cerebrovascular accident in patients with hemodynamically significant stenoses, depending on its degree, the presence of clinical symptoms and additional risk factors (Table 4).

Table 4. Risk of ischemic stroke due to ICA stenosis

Factors	Risks	Reference
Symptomatic stenosis	For 1 year / 3 years	ECST [43, 44]
70-79%	6% / 17%	
80-89%	11% / 20%	
90-99%	18% / 35%	
Symptomatic stenosis	For 2 years	NASCET [45-47]
70-99%	26,0% (mortality 12%)	
Retinal TIA	17%	
Hemispheric TIA	44%	
Signs on CT + TIA	26%	
Contralateral ICA occlusion	54,6%	
Asymptomatic stenosis >70%	Total stroke risk 11%	ACAS [48, 49], 1995
Asymptomatic stenosis		
Stable stenosis 70-99%	Annually up to 1%	[50-52]
Unstable plaque	Increase by 2.6 times	Gupta, 2015 [53]
Hemorrhage in plaque	Increase by 3.6 times	ESVS Guidelines [54]
Silent ischemic foci on CT	Increase by 3 times	ESVS Guidelines [54]
Increased stenosis during observation	Increase by 4.6 times	ESVS Guidelines [54]

The greatest risk of ischemic stroke is observed in patients with transient ischemic attacks (TIA) or the presence of ischemic symptoms. Thus, in patients with TIA, caused by an "unstable" atherosclerotic plaque with more than 90% ICA stenosis, the probability of developing an ischemic stroke within a year reaches 44% [45]. In such cases, in the presence of hemodynamically significant stenosis, it is advisable to perform carotid endarterectomy as the first stage. Further treatment tactics are determined by risk factors for aneurysm rupture - patients from the low-risk SAH group can be dynamically observed with an assessment of the size and morphology of the aneurysm.

A more difficult issue is the choice of tactics for the treatment of patients with no obvious focal clinical symptoms and anamnesis of SAH. This group of patients is very heterogeneous, which dictates the need for an individual approach to the choice of surgical treatment tactics based on the identification of signs of atherosclerotic plaque instability. The main signs of instability of ICA stenosis include:

- *Degree of stenosis.* Regression analysis (Rothwell, 2005 [55]) found that the risk of ischemic stroke increased with a greater narrowing of the lumen of the internal carotid artery - an increase in the degree of stenosis by each 10% increases the risk of ischemic stroke by 18% of the initial values. So, if the risk of cerebrovascular accident (CVA) is estimated as 2% annually, an increase in the degree of stenosis by 10% leads to 2.36% risk.

- *Morphological signs of "instability" of an atherosclerotic plaque.* They are one of the most important predictors of probable ischemic stroke. The most important signs of a "complicated" atherosclerotic plaque include: ulceration of the surface of the plaque, the presence of intramural hemorrhage, heterogeneity of the structure with a predominance of the soft tissue component due to atheromatosis and a thin fibrous layer. The detection of such changes increases the risk of cerebrovascular accident by more than 3.6 times.
- *The presence of silent foci of ischemia on CT/MRI.* When evaluating data from computed tomography and magnetic resonance imaging, small lacunar foci of ischemia can be detected, located in functionally insignificant areas of the brain and not manifesting by clinical symptoms. Their predominance on the side of stenosis indicates the instability of the atherosclerotic process due to a possible cerebral embolism from the plaque.

Patients with subcritical asymptomatic stenoses of no more than 80% narrowing of the ICA lumen without signs of "instability" of atherosclerotic plaque have a low risk of ischemic stroke, less than 2% per year (0.7-1.7%) [50, 51, 56]. Therefore, primary reconstructive surgery on the carotid arteries in such cases is justified only in patients with a low risk of aneurysm rupture that does not need its surgical treatment. In other cases, the first step should be surgical exclusion of the aneurysm from the bloodstream (Figure 4).

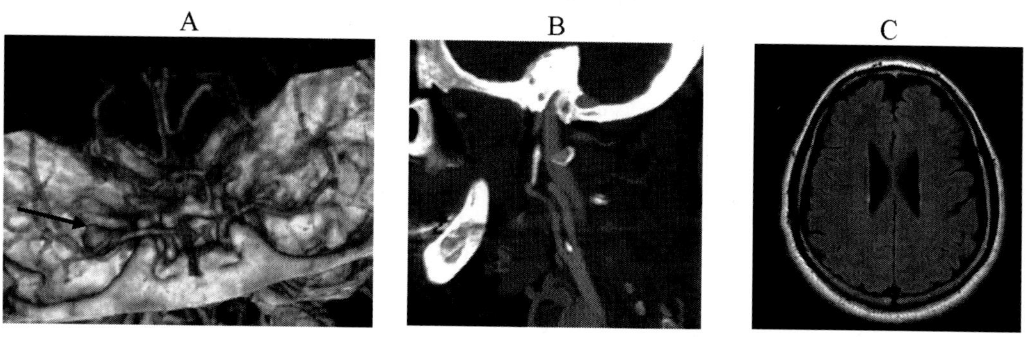

Figure 4. Indications for first step clipping of an asymptomatic aneurysm: A - large aneurysm of the right MCA with an increased risk of rupture; B - subcritical stenosis of the right internal carotid artery up to 70% due to uncomplicated plaque (low risk of ischemic stroke); C – no foci of cerebral ischemia on MRI of the brain (T2-FLAIR mode).

In the clinical case shown in Figure 4, the patient was diagnosed with an asymptomatic bifurcation aneurysm of the right MCA up to 1 cm in size with a risk of rupture of more than 3% per year, in combination with an asymptomatic uncomplicated atherosclerotic plaque of the right ICA, which stenosed the arterial lumen by 70%. The annual risk of ischemic stroke in such a case is estimated at 1-2%. Thus, in the above clinical case, a cerebral aneurysm posed a greater risk to the patient, so its primary clipping was the most justified. CEA could be performed already at the second stage after 1-3 months. There were no indications for accelerated reconstructive intervention.

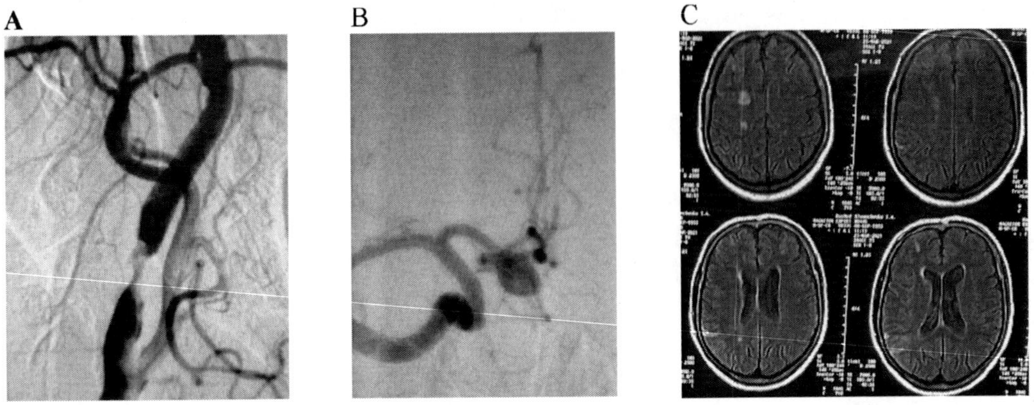

Figure 5. Indications for first step CEA: A - critical stenosis of the right ICA; B – large AComA aneurysm; C - ischemic foci in the territory of the right MCA.

It should be noted that the presence of medium risk aneurysm in a patient does not always indicate the need for its priority surgical exclusion from the bloodstream. An example is a patient with complicated atherosclerotic plaque and silent foci of cerebral ischemia (Figure 5). In such cases, the risk of ischemic stroke can reach 10-15% (see Table 4) per year, which significantly exceeds the estimated annual rate of aneurysm rupture based on data from multicenter studies (no more than 3% per year). In such cases, carotid endarterectomy should be performed firstly (Figure 5).

Effect of Antiplatelet Therapy on the Risk of Hemorrhage

During the treatment of patients with severe carotid stenosis and intracranial aneurysms, there is an actual question about the eligibility of rheological therapy, the appointment of which is indicated in all protocols and clinical guidelines for the treatment of cerebral ischemia. Based on the experience of treating such patients, one often encounters a widespread opinion of specialists that advocates an unequivocal refusal of antiplatelet and anticoagulant therapy in patients with cerebral aneurysms, even if they do not have a history of SAH. Given the need to prescribe rheological therapy during and after carotid endarterectomy, such an approach calls into question the very possibility of performing a priority carotid reconstruction. How justified are such fears from the standpoint of evidence-based medicine, and should we be afraid of priority reconstructive interventions in this group of patients?

Indeed, a number of publications indicate that all anticoagulants/antiplatelet agents are associated with an increased risk of intracranial hemorrhage. In particular, in a large national study that included 729,818 patients, the annual risk of hemorrhagic manifestations in patients not receiving rheological therapy was 0.076% versus 0.3% in those who taking [57]. A more detailed analysis of the study group, however, reveals its pronounced heterogeneity - some of the patients already had a history of intracranial hemorrhage, and the majority of them received dual antiplatelet and anticoagulant therapy. Thus, the question of the effect of rheological monotherapy in patients with cerebral aneurysms without rupture remained open.

The meta-analyses of large studies devoted to this problem suggest that the degree of influence of rheological therapy on the risk of cerebral hemorrhage depends on the group of drugs used, the duration of their use, and anamnesis of SAH.

Thus, long-term administration (more than 3 months) of antiplatelet monotherapy with aspirin (or clopidogrel) to patients with asymptomatic cerebral aneurysms did not significantly increase the incidence of intracranial hemorrhages [58], [59], [60], but even contributed to its decline. Aspirin was found to almost halve the risk of aneurysm rupture (40% vs 28%; P = 0.016) [61]. Analyzing the results of the randomized multicenter study ISUIA, we can also conclude that the probability of SAH decreases depending on the regularity of taking antiplatelet agents - when taking aspirin daily, the probability of SAH decreased by 3.7 times, when taken 3 times a week - by 2.5 times, and once per month - only 25% of the initial values [62]. These observations were pathophysiologically substantiated in biological models - it was shown that the reduction in the risk of SAH from asymptomatic aneurysms occurs due to the blocking of inflammatory reactions [63], that provoke their formation and rupture [64, 65].

At the same time, it was found that antiplatelet therapy has a more aggressive effect on the clinical course of patients with a history of hemorrhagic stroke. Thus, in a number of studies, it was found that taking aspirin by patients with a history of SAH more than 8 times increases the risk of rebleeding [66]. In addition, taking antiplatelet agents at the time of the development of a hemorrhage may worsen the prognosis of its clinical course, increase the size of the hematoma and the likelihood of an unfavorable outcome [60].

Recent publications devoted to this problem point to the anti-inflammatory and rheological properties of aspirin and its analogues, which can improve the prognosis of the clinical course of patients after subarachnoid hemorrhage - their administration is justified after the aneurysm has been removed from the bloodstream. Studies have shown a positive effect of antiplatelet therapy on the outcome of hemorrhage - more than two-fold reduction in the risk of cerebral ischemia (odds ratio 0.41) [67]. According to Nagahama, dual antiplatelet therapy after SAH reduces the risk of vasospasm (OR 0.244, p = 0.003) and delayed ischemia (OR 0.056, p = 0.001) with no significant difference in the risk of recurrent intracranial hemorrhage. Saber et al. found a significant reduction in the risk of vasospasm (OR 0.31 P < 0.001), stroke (OR 0.32; P < 0.001) and worse outcome (OR 0.40) [68].

In contrast to antiplatelet therapy, long-term use of anticoagulant therapy with warfarin, heparin, or factor Xa inhibitors is significantly associated with an increased risk of hemorrhage and worse clinical outcomes. Thus, taking warfarin more than 2.8 times increases the risk of intracranial hemorrhage and 1.6 times increases the risk of SAH. With INR values greater than 3, the probability of hemorrhagic complications increases by 7 times [60]. First of all, the negative effect of anticoagulant therapy is manifested when it is taken for a long time or is prescribed directly in the acute period of hemorrhage. At the same time, a single or short-term administration of heparin or its low molecular weight derivatives under the control of INR does not have a significant effect on the risks of intracranial hemorrhage [59]. According to Burdenko Center for Neurosurgery experience, a single use of 2500-5000 IU of heparin at the main stage of carotid reconstruction in 145 patients with cerebral aneurysms was not accompanied by any hemorrhagic complications in any case.

Summarizing the above facts, we can draw the following conclusions:

1. Antiplatelet therapy *does not increase the risk* of asymptomatic aneurysm rupture.
2. Antiplatelet therapy at the time of hemorrhage aggravates its clinical course and increases the volume of the hematoma.
3. Long-term anticoagulant therapy increases the risk of aneurysm rupture and worsens the clinical outcome of hemorrhagic stroke.
4. Single or short-term administration of heparin in patients with functioning asymptomatic aneurysms has a negligible effect on the risk of hemorrhage.

Thus, it is possible to partially dispel the myths regarding the use of rheological therapy in patients with intracranial aneurysms requiring carotid endarterectomy. Prescribing aspirin or its analogues to patients after CEA before exclusion of cerebral aneurysms from the bloodstream is justified and is not associated with an increased risk of intracranial hemorrhage, especially in patients with low- and moderate-risk aneurysms.

When diagnosing an aneurysm with a high risk of rupture, one should be cautious about prescribing antiplatelet therapy due to its negative effect on the severity of possible intracranial hemorrhage and contraindications to surgical treatment (high risk of hemorrhagic complications of direct surgical interventions). In such cases, it is advisable to first exclude the aneurysm from the bloodstream, followed by reconstructive intervention, which requires the appointment of concomitant rheological therapy.

The use of flow-diversion stents or stent-assistance techniques to exclude an aneurysm from the bloodstream also makes its own adjustments to the choice of tactics for staged surgical treatment. The need for aggressive antiplatelet therapy aimed at preventing stent thrombosis dictates the need for simultaneous endovascular reconstruction of the carotid arteries or open surgery as the first stage, followed by intravascular intervention in a short time after the first operation.

Conclusion

This chapter presents only the basic principles of the choice of surgical and conservative treatment tactics. In a real clinical situation, a differentiated approach should be used, requiring justification for the choice of surgical options, their sequence, timing of interventions, as well as the features of peri- and postoperative management, including concomitant rheological therapy. Undoubtedly, the treatment of patients with a combination of steno-occlusive pathology of the main cerebral arteries and intracranial aneurysms is associated with higher perioperative risks and requires an individual approach. The main goal is to reduce the risks of adverse outcomes of treatment at each stage. Often this requires the use of additional diagnostic methods and an vast opportunities of direct and endovascular surgical interventions on the extra- and intracranial arteries of the brain. Therefore, the treatment of patients with this comorbidity, especially in the presence of aneurysms of medium and high risk of rupture, is justified in specialized neurosurgical hospitals.

References

[1] Héman, L. M., Jongen, L. M., Van Der Worp, H. B., Rinkel, G. J. E., & Hendrikse, J., Incidental intracranial aneurysms in patients with internal carotid artery stenosis: a CT angiography study and a metaanalysis. *Stroke*, 2009. **40**(4): p. 1341-6.

[2] Zheng, Y. and C. Wu, Surgical treatment and perioperative management of intracranial aneurysms in Chinese patients with ischemic cerebrovascular diseases: a case series. *BMC Neurol*, 2018. **18**(1): p. 142.

[3] Krylov, V. V., Chernyavsky, M., Komakha, B., & Artemova, A. Treatment of patients with atherosclerotic lesions of the brachiocephalic arteries in combination with intracranial aneurysms. *Neurosurgery.*, 2013. (2): 80-85. (In Russ)

[4] Khanna, R. K., G. M. Malik, and N. Qureshi, Predicting outcome following surgical treatment of unruptured intracranial aneurysms: a proposed grading system. *J Neurosurg*, 1996. **84**(1): p. 49-54.

[5] Heros, R. C. and J. P. Kistler, Intracranial arterial aneurysm--an update. *Stroke*, 1983. **14**(4): p. 628-31.

[6] van Laar, P. J., Van Der Grond, J., Moll, F. L., Mali, W. P. Th. M., & Hendrikse, J. Hemodynamic effect of carotid stenting and carotid endarterectomy. *J Vasc Surg*, 2006. **44**(1): p. 73-8.

[7] Cronqvist, S., N. Lundberg, and H. Troupp, Temporary or Incomplete Occlusion of The Carotid Artery in the Neck for the Treatment of Intracranial Arterial Aneurysms. *Neurochirurgia (Stuttg)*, 1964. **7**: p. 146-51.

[8] Ladowski, J. S., Webster, M. W., Yonas, H. O., & Steed, D. L. Carotid endarterectomy in patients with asymptomatic intracranial aneurysm. *Ann Surg*, 1984. **200**(1): p. 70-3.

[9] Schuss, P., Hadjiathanasiou, A., Brandecker, S., Güresir, Á., Borger, V., Wispel, C., Vatter, H., & Güresir, E. Anticoagulation Therapy in Patients Suffering from Aneurysmal Subarachnoid Hemorrhage: Influence on Functional Outcome-a Single-Center Series and Multivariate Analysis. *World Neurosurg*, 2017. **99**: p. 348-352.

[10] Franke, C.L., De Jonge, J., Van Swieten, J. C., Op De Coul, A. A., & Van Gijn, J. Intracerebral hematomas during anticoagulant treatment. *Stroke*, 1990. **21**(5): p. 726-30.

[11] Ma, M., Meretoja, A., Churilov, L., Sharma, G. J., Christensen, S., Liu, X., Weir, L., Davis, S. M., & Yan, B. Warfarin-associated intracerebral hemorrhage: volume, anticoagulation intensity and location. *J Neurol Sci*, 2013. **332**(1-2): p. 75-9.

[12] Rosand, J., Eckman, M. H., Knudsen, K. A., Singer, D. E., & Greenberg, S. M. The effect of warfarin and intensity of anticoagulation on outcome of intracerebral hemorrhage. *Arch Intern Med*, 2004. **164**(8): p. 880-4.

[13] Frontera, J. A., John J. Lewin, Alejandro A Rabinstein, Imo P Aisiku, et al. Guideline for Reversal of Antithrombotics in Intracranial Hemorrhage: A Statement for Healthcare Professionals from the Neurocritical Care Society and Society of Critical Care Medicine. *Neurocrit Care*, 2016. **24**(1): p. 6-46.

[14] Flibotte, J. J., Hagan, N., O'Donnell, J., Greenberg, S. M., & Rosand, J. Warfarin, hematoma expansion, and outcome of intracerebral hemorrhage. *Neurology*, 2004. **63**(6): p. 1059-64.

[15] Adams, H. P., Jr., Carotid stenosis and coexisting ipsilateral intracranial aneurysm. A problem in management. *Arch Neurol*, 1977. **34**(8): p. 515-6.

[16] Riphagen, J. H. and H. J. Bernsen, Rupture of an intracerebral aneurysm after carotid endarterectomy: a case report. *Acta Neurol Belg*, 2009. **109**(4): p. 314-6.

[17] Антонов Г. И. Хирургическое лечение церебро-васкулярной патологии, обусловленной заболеванием ветвей дуги аорты. 1998: *С-Петербург.*

[18] Morita, A., Takaaki Kirino, Kazuo Hashi, Noriaki Aoki, Shunichi Fukuhara, Nobuo Hashimoto, Takeo Nakayama, Michi Sakai, Akira Teramoto, Shinjiro Tominari, Takashi Yoshimoto. The natural course of unruptured cerebral aneurysms in a Japanese cohort. *N Engl J Med*, 2012. **366**(26): p. 2474-82.

[19] Kappelle, L. J., M. Eliasziw, A. J. Fox, H. J. Barnett. *Small,* unruptured intracranial aneurysms and management of symptomatic carotid artery stenosis. North American Symptomatic Carotid Endarterectomy Trial Group. *Neurology*, 2000. **55**(2): p. 307-9.

[20] Stern, J., Whelan, M., Brisman, R., & Correll, J. W. Management of extracranial carotid stenosis and intracranial aneurysms. *J Neurosurg*, 1979. **51**(2): p. 147-50.

[21] Kann, B. R., T. Matsumoto, and M. D. Kerstein, Safety of carotid endarterectomy associated with small intracranial aneurysms. *South Med J*, 1997. **90**(12): p. 1213-6.

[22] Suh, B. Y., W. S. Yun, and W. H. Kwun, Carotid artery revascularization in patients with concomitant carotid artery stenosis and asymptomatic unruptured intracranial artery aneurysm. *Ann Vasc Surg*, 2011. **25**(5): p. 651-5.

[23] Cho, Y. D., D., Jung, K.-H., Roh, J.-K., Kang, H.-S., Han, M. H., & Lim, J. W. Characteristics of intracranial aneurysms associated with extracranial carotid artery disease in South Korea. *Clin Neurol Neurosurg*, 2013. **115**(9): p. 1677-81.

[24] Khan, U. A., Thapar, A., Shalhoub, J., & Davies, A. H. Risk of intracerebral aneurysm rupture during carotid revascularization. *J Vasc Surg*, 2012. **56**(6): p. 1739-47.

[25] Shumann, M. U., Mirzai, Sh., Samil, M., & Vorkapic, P. Xenon/CT CBF measurements as valuable diagnostic tool in a case of bilateral occlusive cerebrovascular disease associated with intracranial aneurysm. *Acta Neurol Scand Suppl*, 1996. **166**: p. 104-9.

[26] Badruddin, A., Teleb, M. S., Abraham, M. G., Taqi, M. A., & Zaidat, O. O. Safety and feasibility of simultaneous ipsilateral proximal carotid artery stenting and cerebral aneurysm coiling. *Front Neurol*, 2010. **1**: p. 120.

[27] Jeong, Y. G., Jung, Y. T., Kim, M. S., Eun, C. K., & Jang, S. H. Size and location of ruptured intracranial aneurysms. *J Korean Neurosurg Soc*, 2009. **45**(1): p. 11-5.

[28] Bederson, J. B., I. A. Awad, D. O. Wiebers, D. Piepgras, E. C. Haley Jr, T. Brott, G. Hademenos, D. Chyatte, R. Rosenwasser, C. Caroselli. Recommendations for the management of patients with unruptured intracranial aneurysms: A statement for healthcare professionals from the Stroke Council of the American Heart Association. *Circulation*, 2000. **102**(18): p. 2300-8.

[29] Wiebers, D. O., J. P. Whisnant, J. Huston, I. Meissner, R. D. Brown Jr, D. G. Piepgras, G. S. Forbes, K. Thielen, D. Nichols, W. M. O'Fallon, J. Peacock, L. Jaeger, N. F. Kassell, G. L. Kongable-Beckman, J. C. Torner, Unruptured intracranial aneurysms: natural history, clinical outcome, and risks of surgical and endovascular treatment. *Lancet*, 2003. **362**(9378): p. 103-10.

[30] Lai, H. P., K. M. Cheng, Simon C. H. Yu, K. M. Au Yeung, Y. L. Cheung, C. M. Chan, W. S. Poon, W. M. Lui. Size, location, and multiplicity of ruptured intracranial aneurysms in the Hong Kong Chinese population with subarachnoid haemorrhage. *Hong Kong Med J*, 2009. **15**(4): p. 262-6.

[31] Liu, Q., Jiang, P., Wu, J., Li, M., Gao, B., Zhang, Y., Ning, B., Cao, Y., & Wang, S. Intracranial aneurysm rupture score may correlate to the risk of rebleeding before treatment of ruptured intracranial aneurysms. *Neurol Sci*, 2019. **40**(8): p. 1683-1693.

[32] Rosenørn, J., Eskesen, V., Schmidt, K., & Rønde, F. The risk of rebleeding from ruptured intracranial aneurysms. *J Neurosurg*, 1987. **67**(3): p. 329-32.

[33] Konovalov, A. N., et al. Recommended protocol for the management of patients with subarachnoid hemorrhage due to ruptured cerebral aneurysms. *Clinical guidelines*, 2012. (In Russ).

[34] Inagawa, T., Kamiya, K., Ogasawara, H., & Yano, T. Rebleeding of ruptured intracranial aneurysms in the acute stage. *Surg Neurol*, 1987. **28**(2): p. 93-9.

[35] Wu, T. C., Tsui, Y. K., Chen, T. Y., Lin, C. J., Wu, T. C., & Tzeng, W. S. Rebleeding of aneurysmal subarachnoid hemorrhage in computed tomography angiography: risk factor, rebleeding pattern, and outcome analysis. *J Comput Assist Tomogr*, 2012. **36**(1): p. 103-8.

[36] Mizutani, T., Aruga, T., Kirino, T., Miki, Y., Saito, I., & Tsuchida, T. Recurrent subarachnoid hemorrhage from untreated ruptured vertebrobasilar dissecting aneurysms. *Neurosurgery*, 1995. **36**(5): p. 905-11; discussion 912-3.

[37] Heiskanen, O., Risk of bleeding from unruptured aneurysm in cases with multiple intracranial aneurysms. *J Neurosurg*, 1981. **55**(4): p. 524-6.

[38] Wermer, M. J., Van Der Schaaf, I. C., Algra, A., & Rinkel, G. J. E. Risk of rupture of unruptured intracranial aneurysms in relation to patient and aneurysm characteristics: an updated meta-analysis. *Stroke*, 2007. **38**(4): p. 1404-10.

[39] Lall, R. R., Christopher S Eddleman, Bernard R. Bendok, H. Hunt Batjer. Unruptured intracranial aneurysms and the assessment of rupture risk based on anatomical and morphological factors: sifting through the sands of data. *Neurosurg Focus*, 2009. **26**(5): p. E2.

[40] You, S. H., Kong, D. S., Kim, J. S., Jeon, P., Kim, K. H., Roh, H. K., Kim, G. M., Lee, K. H., & Hong, S. C. Characteristic features of unruptured intracranial aneurysms: predictive risk factors for aneurysm rupture. *J Neurol Neurosurg Psychiatry*, 2010. **81**(5): p. 479-84.

[41] Krylov, V. V., et al. Clinical guidelines for the treatment of unruptured asymptomatic cerebral aneurysms. *"Issues of Neurosurgery" named after N.N. Burdenko*, 2016. 80(5): p. 124-135. (In Russ).

[42] Rahman, M., Smietana, J., Hauck, E., Hoh, B., Hopkins, N., Siddiqui, A., Levy, E. I., Meng, H., & Mocco, J. Size ratio correlates with intracranial aneurysm rupture status: a prospective study. *Stroke*, 2010. **41**(5): p. 916-20.

[43] Endarterectomy for moderate symptomatic carotid stenosis: interim results from the MRC European Carotid Surgery Trial. *Lancet*, 1996. **347**(9015): p. 1591-3.

[44] Randomised trial of endarterectomy for recently symptomatic carotid stenosis: final results of the MRC European Carotid Surgery Trial (ECST). *Lancet*, 1998. **351**(9113): p. 1379-87.

[45] Barnett, H. J., Barnett, H. J. M., Taylor, D. W., Eliasziw, M., Fox, A. J., Ferguson, G. G., Haynes, R. B., Rankin, R. N., Clagett, G. P., Hachinski, V. C., Sackett, D. L., Thorpe, K. E., Meldrum, H. E., & Spence, J. D. Benefit of carotid endarterectomy in patients with symptomatic moderate or severe stenosis. North American Symptomatic Carotid Endarterectomy Trial Collaborators. *N Engl J Med*, 1998. **339**(20): p. 1415-25.

[46] Barnett, H. J. M., D. W. Taylor, R. B. Haynes, D. L. Sackett, S. J. Peerless, G. G. Ferguson, A. J. Fox, R. N. Rankin, V. C. Hachinski, D. O. Wiebers, M. Eliasziw. Beneficial effect of carotid endarterectomy in symptomatic patients with high-grade carotid stenosis. *N Engl J Med*, 1991. **325**(7): p. 445-53.

[47] Eliasziw, M., J. Y. Streifler, A. J. Fox, V. C. Hachinski, G. G. Ferguson, H. J. Barnett. Significance of plaque ulceration in symptomatic patients with high-grade carotid stenosis. North American Symptomatic Carotid Endarterectomy Trial. *Stroke*, 1994. **25**(2): p. 304-8.

[48] Barnett, H. J., Eliasziw, M., Meldrum, H. E., & Taylor, D. W. Do the facts and figures warrant a 10-fold increase in the performance of carotid endarterectomy on asymptomatic patients? *Neurology*, 1996. **46**(3): p. 603-8.

[49] Endarterectomy for asymptomatic carotid artery stenosis. Executive Committee for the Asymptomatic Carotid Atherosclerosis Study. *Jama*, 1995. **273**(18): p. 1421-8.

[50] Abbott, A. L., Medical (nonsurgical) intervention alone is now best for prevention of stroke associated with asymptomatic severe carotid stenosis: results of a systematic review and analysis. *Stroke*, 2009. **40**(10): p. e573-83.

[51] Marquardt, L., Olivia C Geraghty, Ziyah Mehta, Peter M Rothwell. Low risk of ipsilateral stroke in patients with asymptomatic carotid stenosis on best medical treatment: a prospective, population-based study. *Stroke*, 2010. **41**(1): p. e11-7.

[52] Spence, J. D., Management of asymptomatic carotid stenosis. *Neurol Clin*, 2015. **33**(2): p. 443-57.

[53] Gupta, A., Kesavabhotla, K., Baradaran, H., Kamel, H., Pandya, A., Giambrone, A. E., Wright, D., Pain, K. J., Mtui, E. E., Suri, J. S., Sanelli, P. C., & Mushlin, A. I. Plaque echolucency and stroke risk in asymptomatic carotid stenosis: a systematic review and meta-analysis. *Stroke*, 2015. **46**(1): p. 91-7.

[54] Naylor, A. R., A R Naylor, J. B. Ricco, G. J. de Borst, et al. Editor's Choice - Management of Atherosclerotic Carotid and Vertebral Artery Disease: 2017 Clinical Practice Guidelines of the European Society for Vascular Surgery (ESVS). *Eur J Vasc Endovasc Surg*, 2018. **55**(1): p. 3-81.

[55] Rothwell, P. M., Mehta, Z., Howard, S., Gutnikov, S., & Warlow, C. Treating individuals 3: from subgroups to individuals: general principles and the example of carotid endarterectomy. *Lancet*, 2005. **365**(9455): p. 256-65.

[56] Murray, C. J. L., Theo Vos, Rafael Lozano, Mohsen Naghavi, et al. Disability-adjusted life years (DALYs) for 291 diseases and injuries in 21 regions, 1990-2010: a systematic analysis for the Global Burden of Disease Study 2010. *Lancet*, 2012. **380**(9859): p. 2197-2223.

[57] Gulati, S., Solheim, O., Carlsen, S. M., Øie, L. R., Jensberg, H., Gulati, A. M., Madsbu, M. A., Giannadakis, C., Jakola, A. S., & Salvesen, Ø. Risk of intracranial hemorrhage (RICH) in users of oral antithrombotic drugs: Nationwide pharmacoepidemiological study. *PLoS One*, 2018. **13**(8): p. e0202575.

[58] Phan, K., Moore, J. M., Griessenauer, C. J., Ogilvy, C. S., & Thomas, A. J. Aspirin and Risk of Subarachnoid Hemorrhage: Systematic Review and Meta-Analysis. *Stroke*, 2017. **48**(5): p. 1210-1217.

[59] Qian, C., He, Y., Li, Y., Chen, C., & Zhang, B. Association Between Aspirin Use and Risk of Aneurysmal Subarachnoid Hemorrhage: A Meta-analysis. *World Neurosurg*, 2020. **138**: p. 299-308.

[60] García-Rodríguez, L. A., Gaist, D., Morton, J., Cookson, C., & González-Pérez, A. Antithrombotic drugs and risk of hemorrhagic stroke in the general population. *Neurology*, 2013. **81**(6): p. 566-74.

[61] Gross, B. A., Rosalind Lai, P. M., Frerichs, K. U., & Du, R. Aspirin and aneurysmal subarachnoid hemorrhage. *World Neurosurg*, 2014. **82**(6): p. 1127-30.

[62] Hasan, D. M., Mahaney, K. B., Brown, R. D., Meissner, I., Piepgras, D. G., Huston, J., Capuano, A. W., Torner, J. C., & for the International Study of Unruptured Intracranial Aneurysms Investigators. Aspirin as a promising agent for decreasing incidence of cerebral aneurysm rupture. *Stroke*, 2011. **42**(11): p. 3156-62.

[63] Starke, R. M., Chalouhi, N., Ding, D., & Hasan, D. M. Potential role of aspirin in the prevention of aneurysmal subarachnoid hemorrhage. *Cerebrovasc Dis*, 2015. **39**(5-6): p. 332-42.

[64] Chyatte, D., Bruno, G., Desai, S., & Todor, D. R. Inflammation and intracranial aneurysms. *Neurosurgery*, 1999. **45**(5): p. 1137-46; discussion 1146-7.

[65] Frösen, J., Piippo, A., Paetau, A., Kangasniemi, M., Niemelä, M., Hernesniemi, J., & Jääskeläinen, J. Growth factor receptor expression and remodeling of saccular cerebral artery aneurysm walls: implications for biological therapy preventing rupture. *Neurosurgery*, 2006. **58**(3): p. 534-41; discussion 534-41.

[66] Can, A., Robert F. Rudy, B. S., Victor M. Castro, M. S., Sheng Yu, PhD, Dmitriy Dligach, PhD, et al. Association between aspirin dose and subarachnoid hemorrhage from saccular aneurysms: A case-control study. *Neurology*, 2018. **91**(12): p. e1175-e1181.

[67] Darkwah Oppong, M., Oliver Gembruch, Daniela Pierscianek, Martin Köhrmann, Christoph Kleinschnitz, Cornelius Deuschl, Christoph Mönninghoff, Klaus Kaier, Michael Forsting, Ulrich Sure, Ramazan Jabbarli. Post-treatment Antiplatelet Therapy Reduces Risk for Delayed Cerebral Ischemia due to Aneurysmal Subarachnoid Hemorrhage. *Neurosurgery*, 2019. **85**(6): p. 827-833.

[68] Saber, H., Aaron Desai, Mohan Palla, Wazim Mohamed, Navid Seraji-Bozorgzad, Muhammed Ibrahim. Efficacy of Cilostazol in Prevention of Delayed Cerebral Ischemia after Aneurysmal Subarachnoid Hemorrhage: A Meta-Analysis. *J Stroke Cerebrovasc Dis*, 2018. **27**(11): p. 2979-2985.

Chaper 20

Exoscope Digital Systems: The Present and Future of Visual Aid Devices for Neurovascular Surgery

Iype Cherian[1,*]
and Pablo Villanueva[2]
[1]Krishna Institute of Medical Science. Karad, Maharashtra, India
[2]Hospital Público Dr. Guillermo Rawson. San Juan, Argentina

Introduction

Preface

Surgery has not always been well tuned to technology. While concepts such as "surgical skill," "anatomical basis," or "aptitude and attitude" played a role in the usual surgeon's parlance, technology was diversely understood.

Now, the times are changing, and technology has arrived to play a leading role. Oversight of this situation could lead to a compromise in surgical results and may result in not giving the patient the best of what is available.

Neurosurgery and many other surgical fields have been brought to a new level since the microscope was introduced more than five decades ago [1, 2].

Books were written, instruments were built, and the neurosurgical universe is now measured in small parts of a millimetre because of the microscope. Microsurgical anatomy has become the norm.

Training hand skills and system-related handling *is mandatory* for microscopic surgeons nowadays. The starting point for this goal should be related to visual aid systems, new tools, their benefits and limitations, and scientific methods to gain proper confidence and dexterity using them.

* Corresponding Author's Email: drrajucherian@gmail.com.

In: Understanding and Managing Cerebral Aneurysms
Editor: Xianli Lv
ISBN: 979-8-89113-608-3

Basic Concepts [3, 4]

Visual aid systems (VAS) are defined as optical, digital, robotic, and any other technical features added to improve the surgeon's visual capabilities. Loupes and microscopes could be considered the beginning of this era.

Visual magnification is achieved by the use of lenses and mathematical calculations following the main formula:

$$m = \frac{h_i}{h_0} = \frac{d_i}{d_0}$$

m = magnification, h = height, d = distance, i = image, o = object

Magnification level is the relationship between the size of the object and the size of the image generated by a given lens system.

As well as magnification, some other optics/physics concepts should be properly understood.

Focus refers to the point where different light rays meet the optimum adjustment of an imaging system. A "focused" image allows the surgeon to be capable of sharply separating two different points, as in the real object.

Depth of Field refers to the distance between two planes (background and foreground) that has acceptable image sharpness. It allows the surgeon to properly define the points of an image (and the real object) that are placed at different distances from the lens and the observer. Without a proper 3D perception of the image, this feature is only "simulated" by lights and shadows in a 2D image.

Most of the optical performance of a lens (or group of lenses) depends on the most intrinsic lens property: focal length (f). This relationship is expressed mathematically as follow:

$$\frac{1}{f} = \frac{1}{s} + \frac{1}{d}$$

f = lens focal lenght, s = object-lens distance, d = lens-retina distance

This formula helps us to appreciate that the lens (or group of lenses) will be responsible for allowing useful ranges at the object-lens distance (working distance) and the lens-observer distance (observer-device distance).

Also, as much the lens is capable to open, the more light rays it will be allowed to form the image (luminosity). Sadly, as much the lens open, it will be also configuring a shallow depth of field (Figure 1).

The depth of field, then, could be referred as *shallow* (small distance between background and foreground with a proper focus), or *deep* (long distance between background and foreground with a proper focus).

As we can infer, small *working distance* means that the lens must be placed too close to the object (this could be a problem for properly work between the lens and the object). On the other hand, huge distances could also pose difficulties since the ocular of the microscope needs to be attached to the operator's eyes.

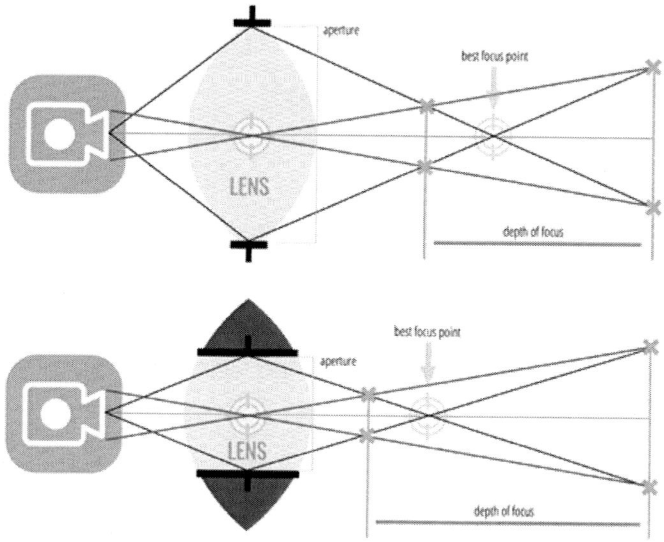

Figure 1. Lens aperture, focus and working distance.

An appropriate lens for a surgical device should be one that allows the lens and the observer to be set at comfortable working distances with optimal optical features.

The *circle of confusion* is a useful term regularly used by photographers to describe how depth of focus and definition interact. This term describes the range of distances for a specific point that can be sharply perceived by the human eye. Obviously, it also depends on that particular human eye's capabilities. The standard value for this will be 5 lpmm (lines per millimeter), which means a 0.2 circle of confusion value (CoC). (1 mm/5 lines).

Magnification, depth of field and circle of confusion will be mathematically and practically related: if we need a certain magnification level, lens capabilities should be able to present good working distances and acceptable CoC ranges. This will be interpreted by the surgeon as the capability to work with sharp images at different distances and magnifications.

While working at high magnification levels, the CoC values change. This new magnification level sets direct proportional requirements. If we plan to enlarge the image by x10, then our CoC value will be 0.2/10 = 0.02.

Digitalization means that the image is obtained by a lens, and then it is digitally transformed by a central processing unit to finally be displayed on a screen. This digitalization method could be measured in terms of the quality of the resulting image (HD, 4K) and dimension capabilities (2D, 3D). To be able to perceive 3D images using a screen, special glasses should be used by the surgeon.

Digital improvement is a feature available in hybrid and fully digital systems. It allows the surgeon to see real-time digital modifications of the surgical field (e.g., contrast, brightness, and colour modifications; different lights applied to the object; fluorescence; dynamic flow-vessels aid assistance; etc.). It can also be referred to as "augmented reality" when a surgical field is added by landmark navigation devices or pre-operative image fusion (magnetic resonance, CT scans).

Robotic assistance means that a particular VAS has the possibility to modify its position and/or angle by using electronic commands. The last allows the surgeon to control these parameters without taking his or her sight out of the surgical field or modifying his or her working position by using hand controls, foot controls, and others [5][6]; thus, improving time, attention field, and effectiveness of the procedure.

Visual Aid Systems

The Need for Details

> "Those working with their souls, are artists. Those working with their minds, are scientists. Those working with their hands, are handicraftsmen... Those working with soul, mind and hands are surgeons."

Surgery is a multi-skilled, demanding field. Those skills must be mixed in a unique balanced manner to get the most from the surgeon each time they are requested.

There is a logical path to follow while planning a surgical procedure:

Anatomy knowledge > Pathological changes (clinical findings and images) > Pre-op planning > Visual recognition (visual-aid requirements) > Hand manipulation (instruments requirements).

These steps mentioned above allow us to understand that the same relationship exists between the need for a very fine jeweler forceps to manipulate an M4 vessel and the need to previously identify this vessel with a proper magnification or definition level.

Only then can actions be taken confidently and safely. A narrow and extremely direct correlation exists between the surgical results and the variables just mentioned. The skill level of the surgeon is the common denominator for every single item in this plan.

Table 1. VAS main features

PROPIERTY	MEANING
Light source	It allows the correct level of intensity, shadowing, and chromatic differentiation in the small details of a desired surgical field. It also has a role in times of continuous use and source-object dispersion.
Magnification	The level of details that the user will be able to identify properly. Just as an example, x35 should be enough for small details (e.g., 3 mm diameter vessels). Levels of x100 can be reached by some VAS.
Depth of field	Major importance while working at high magnification levels. A good depth allows to see focused images at different levels of depth. Shallow depth means that the tip of your instrument could be focus, but not the element immediately underneath.
Work distance	The distance that lenses should be away from the object. Distances less than 200 mm are hardly compatible with any instrument length.
Operators	Eye pieces for the surgeon and 1 or 2 assistants (at HLM, the field of vision could vary due to optical angle differences between the surgeon and assistants). For VAS using a screen, the same view and angle are available for all the team members.
Movement range	How much the optical centre of the VAS can be displaced over the surgical field without changing the base position.
Angle range	How much the angle can be tilted from the optical center of the VAS and the object. A small size VAS, allows wider variations in angling the device.
Robotic aids	Electronic control of the VAS optical center positioning (free moves) and angles (lock on target).
Costs	The cost of purchase and maintenance will determine the VAS's affordability.

Visual, without any doubt, comes first. Proper and thorough identification of our landmarks will guide our approach to the surgical field, and, once there, the more details that the surgeon is capable to see, the more precise and effective the procedure can get [7, 8].

Anatomy recognition in a surgical scenario is not always an easy task. Human anatomy could be really challenging to explore, even more so in some particular regions where bony surfaces or soft tissues mimic a valley-hill landscape, places where light and vision are not frequent guests.

At this particular condition, some requirements start to be of major importance (Table 1).

From the Microscope to Novel Options

The microscope is nowadays the gold-standard system as a VAS. All neurosurgical departments around the world now have a whole set of devices and instruments that were thought to be used with microscope assistance and from a microscope surgical field perspective.

Not only infrastructure, but the training and skill level of a neurosurgery unit staff also needed to improve because of VAS inclusion. The experiences of many surgeons through these decades have written the "surgical microscope history" [9, 10, 11]. Following them, we can affirm:

1. Anatomy should be understood in a closer and micro-detailed way (literally speaking).
2. The essential need to understand this new device (microscope), it's optical and mechanical features.
3. Thinking, developing, and starting to use new instruments that are adapted for this new magnification level and working distances.
4. Review all procedures and surgical goals, aiming to take the most of all these new tools.

The microscope is defined as a VAS who mix:

1. optical
2. lightning
3. mechanical
4. digital features (optional)

A basic diagram is now proposed for optical features and mechanical features (Figure 2 and 3):

1. Optical features: they are provided by a set of lenses involved in generating the final image for the surgeon. For microscopes, this system is binocular, giving a true tri-dimensional image obtained by the physiological mixing of each eye's perception. A main difficulty should be taken into account: optical aberrations [12], which tend to increase proportionally with increasing magnification levels.

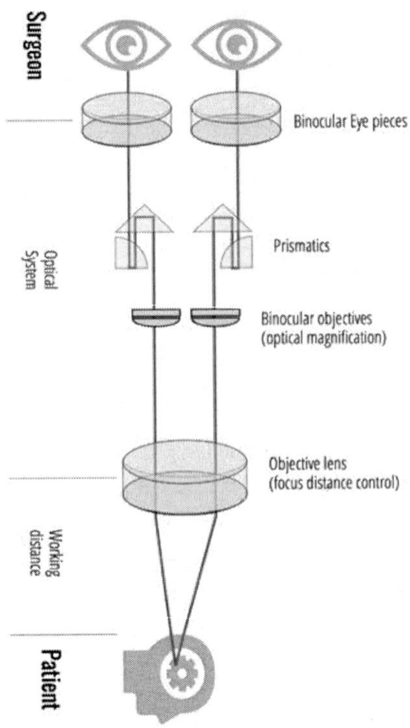

Figure 2. Optical pieces diagram (modified, Cordero I [4]).

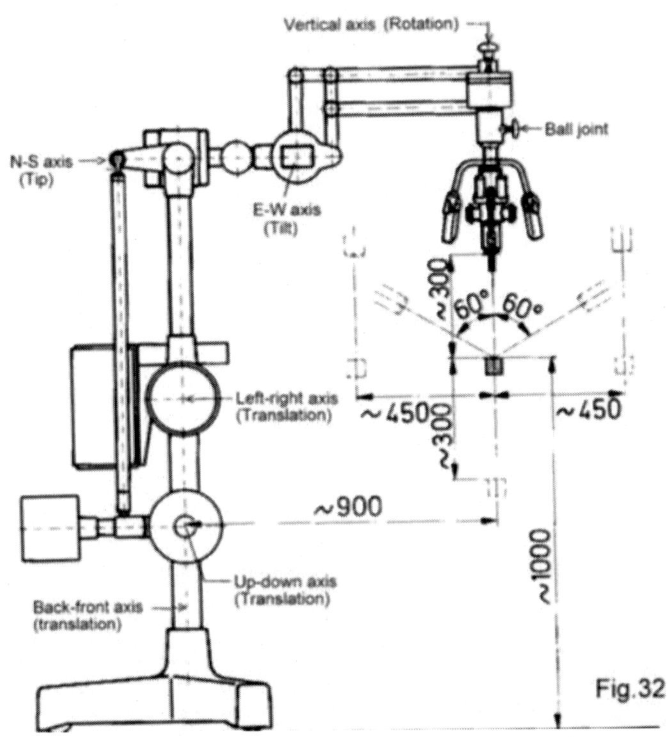

Figure 3. Mechanical parts diagram (from Shultz F [2]).

2. Light features: different kinds of light have been tested for surgical microscopes, such as light temperature, light intensity, light sharpness, multiple or single sources, and many other variations. Nowadays, Xenon light, automatic iris adaptation, and focus distance-related intensity are mainly used.
3. Mechanical features: all the parts involved in holding and moving the optical and lightning pieces. The mechanics involved in a VAS, including the range of angles and the easiest ways to change positions, could be essential. In the present time, mechanical aids represent fully or partially robotic aids, giving extra comfort, precision, and friendly interaction with the system.
4. Digital features: as a part of the process, the image obtained can be digitalized and shown in real time using a screen. This process can add some precious features while understanding anatomy, even more so when this anatomy is modified by pathology (tumours, vessels, and trauma).

Microscope evolution has been developing for many years. Today's microscopes are smaller, handy, efficient, and bring extremely high image quality; but also, limits were found: certain angles for illumination are very hard to obtain (when possible); certain positions are not possible due to patient or surgeon positions; other positions are possible to get but impossible to use by the operator; among others.

Looking forward to pushing those limits further, technological advances promote:

- The use of robotics to get precise and smooth changes of position and angles.
- Getting smaller and more efficient optics systems to get access to new positions.
- Creating options for digital image manipulation, so the same surgical field could be displayed on a screen with a whole pack of digital features (image effects, hypervision, fusion, endoscope split view, etc).

Binocular eyepieces are the best way to assure a real 3D depth sensation, but not without some issues[12]. These problems are partially solved by special corrective lenses. Even so, working in this scenario also needs training and time to get used to.

Another problem with binocular sight is that, at the moment, the surgeon's head is almost sentenced to be attached to the eye pieces. Thus, the surgeon's position, comfort, and capability to safely maneuver can be compromised.

The evolution of certain types of cameras with incredible small sizes and great magnification power is being used for manipulation at HML (from 40x and further). Some of those new cameras are being used for hand-repairing circuits or electronic small parts. But the idea of starting to use them in surgical scenarios is not feasible if there is no 100%-free misrepresentation of the third dimension on a screen.

Since several years ago, many users of optical devices (including microscope users, film makers, and photographers all around the world) have been making efforts to bring real 3D to the flat screen. After many decades of evolution, this volumetric effect can be efficiently achieved on a monitor by using, for example, polarized goggles.

In conclusion, this pack of technological advances has brought the possibility to diminish optical structure dimensions, offer a real 3D image, and use all the potential of digital images to improve the visualization and mechanisms that are used to move and angle the point of view. At present day hybrid microscopes are one of the best examples as final product in this field.

Exoscope. The External-Scope Solution

Basics of an External-Scope VAS

> Ethimology. Greek root: exo (ἐξω) "outside" and skopeúō (σκοπεύω) "to observe." To observe from the outside

If, well, both VAS (microscope and exoscope) are "observing from the outside" and both are meant to show "microscopic details," a way to differentiate one from the other is to emphasize (when using the prefix "exo") that the point of view from the exoscope is different: is external, is not attached to the surgeon.

When analysing a surgical microscope in action (even the more advanced ones) a main situation is observed: there is a need for close proximity between the surgeon's eyes and the microscope eye pieces. This situation mimics the relationship between a surgeon's hand and their instruments.

Following this sequence, we can notice that the eyes are intimately linked to the head movements, and the last mentioned modifies the entire body's positioning while adjusting.

On the contrary, hand position has a wonderful physiological adaptation mechanism: shoulders, elbow, and wrist provide an extremely efficient manner to properly work in diverse conditions without big body movements.

Even more details can be suggested to better understand this observation (e.g., the physiological need to maintain a "zero-horizontal level" to better conjugate vision; cervical reflexes acting over eye positioning control while the head is tilted or rotated, etc.). The information regarding this paragraph is huge and thrilling, but it certainly exceeds the scope of this chapter. We propose, however, some lectures about it [13, 14, 15].

It is not difficult to see that (after detecting this "eye-to-eye-piece" dependence) if somehow this problem is solved, new features, freedom, and comfort could be gained.

Following this way of thought, the idea of an external camera directly pointed to the surgical field, allowing the surgeon to see and handle the structures while watching at a screen, reminds a familiar situation: endoscopic procedures (being aware of all the differences in this regard).

With great experiences in this area and some novelties introduced, this external camera could also be precise enough in definition and depth perception, so the surgeon will be confident in the operating field.

As a final result, a 3D real-time screenplay, robotic assistance for finest movements and wider ranges, a 4K-definition image, enhanced magnification power, and extra digital benefits will offer a complete set of features for this new system.

Exoscope could be technically defined as a complete set of lenses and cameras, handled by a robotically assisted full-motion capabilities arm, adding complete digital image assistance for hypervision features, which bring the surgeon's special visual aid to work at mircoscopic levels of magnification.

In a simplified manner, the Exoscope is a novel VAS that brings the possibility of showing the surgical field with powerful magnification, extra handling, angling, and positioning possibilities in order to build a safe and more comfortable surgical scenario.

Table 2. VAS main differences

Feature	Microscope	Exoscope
Vision	Direct view under Binocular-individual eye pieces.	Googles assisted screen play for a 3D visualization.
Surgeon	Device movements are directly linked to surgeon's position.	The lens-camera set moves independently from the surgeon.
Optic set	Bigger optical set is needed, hindering some positions and angles.	Smaller optical structure allow wider ranges of free movements for angles and positions.
Mechanic arm	Robotic assistance in modern models. Bigger and stronger arms are needed.	Robotic fully commands. Smaller pieces for every element.
Comfort levels	It depends on anatomy, patient position, and the need for changes while operating.	The system facilitates the surgeon's ability to preserve ergonomics and a comfortable operating posture.
Magnification	Through optical parts. Most recent hybrid models can reach x45-60 levels of magnification.	True optical + Digital assited magnification levels can reach up to near x100 levels.
Digital assistance and modes	Only available in most advanced hybrid models.	A full digital image makes it simple and faster to acquire the digital transformation of the image and to present it in real time.

In the same way that the microscope was defined at the beginning of this chapter, now we apply this criteria to the exoscope description:

a. *Optical*: a powerful set of lenses and cameras gives the possibility for optical and digital combination for zoom levels without the need of being attached to any kind of eyepiece. The surgical field is now displayed in a true 3D and fully digitally processed image. Special glasses must be used for this purpose. The digital source of the image also makes it possible to correct some optical aberrations. A very small lens-camera set makes this device versatile and easy to use in the operating room.
b. *Light:* a fully adaptive (intensity, sharpness, color temperature) LED light source is offered for a complete scene homogenous illumination.
c. *Mechanical*: multiple robotized articulations make it possible to set proper angulations and positions, which can be controlled by electronic commands or by hand freely. Robotic assistance makes it possible to save positions and switch "fixed to point" on and off.
d. *Digital features:* being the source a fully digital one, image can be processed to offer the surgeon real time alternatives. Digital images also provide extra definition, lens correction and zoom capabilities.

It is essential to clearly see similarities and differences from the microscope-based and the exoscope-based devices (Table 2).

VAS Correct Choosing

A thorough description of technical features can be reached with the above-mentioned paragraphs and the alternative lectures proposed. Extra care must be given to other, not less important, topics in this decision: costs, effectiveness, and personal goals should also be carefully revised.

Costs are nowadays an "always-to-include" subject. How much our budget changes will also affect how much our target is moving about selecting cases, pathologies, and the number of patients.

VAS should be precisely selected because not every pathology needs high levels of magnification to be treated. Otherwise, some cases will be greatly benefited if some extra features are added (like working at very high zoom levels with added definition and lighting). Vascular, skull base, and minimally invasive strategies for surgery could benefit from these features.

Because we are always talking about a procedure (surgical procedures), effectiveness is always a key term to be evaluated. Not only the whole procedure's effectiveness but also each step's and every tool's effectiveness could and should be analysed at this level.

The procedure's effectiveness depends, among others, on surgeon's skill level [21], specific training, tools, and devices used during the procedure.

Exoscope, for sure, will be subject to a learning curve effect. Dedicated training methods will be necessary, as with any other technological novelty. This device's particularities (being thought of specially to facilitate surgeons' posture, vision, and hands work) can be a reason to think that this curve could be affordable and even enjoyable. Some experience could be reached in different publications at this respect [16, 17, 18].

It is the author's opinion that every surgical procedure should constantly look for better results. To include those procedures in a continuous improvement situation seems like a suitable and precise way to reach new goals [7, 8, 19, 20].

Surgeons' preferences should always be part of the surgical equation. Personal interest does not have to be cast aside. Technology inclusion, the willingness to learn, and research should be considered while exoscope enlightens a whole new field: new vision, challenges, instruments, and strategies.

Limitations and Areas to Further Develop

Some disadvantages of exoscopic visualization were reported, especially in the early 2D exoscope, such as a limited applicability in deep seated cranial pathologies and tissue identification in case of bleeding.

All of these disadvantages seem to be solved with new 3D exoscopes, which however led to headache and nausea in very few cases due to the use of polarized glasses [16, 21, 22, 23, 24].

Microvascular Neurosurgery: Exoscope Accepted the Challenge

Among the different challenging scenarios in neurosurgery practice, aneurysm surgery represents a special one. Approach, dissection, thorough details about lesion understanding, and many other extremely important details should be not only understood but also perfectly seen during the surgical procedure.

For a very long time, surgical clipping was the gold standard treatment, but nowadays endovascular techniques appear to be winning yards in this field. Less invasiveness and good results promote the use of catheters instead of clips.

Although a surgical approach to this pathology remains a valid option, it is sometimes also the only one in many situations, like anatomical particularities (dome/neck relations, proximity to vital branches, kinking, dysplasia or narrowing, etc.), endovascular team availability, and cost-benefit evaluation at a particular health system scenario.

In those cases when clipping represents the best option for the patient, microsurgical approaches should be taken properly. Classical descriptions mention several kinds of approaches. Anterior circulation accounts for most of the cases due to epidemiological characteristic and development-anatomical facts [25].

All of them represents different situations and needs, but a common denominator could be also applied: positioning and angles should be thoroughly managed to get into the microscopic aneurysm scenario.

Once there, the level of magnification should be such that very thin arachnoid adhesions and millimeter vessel branches could be perfectly identified and dissected out of the dome and neck.

This level of detail also requires top standards for image definition, focus depth, light conditions, and digital options, which help the surgeon achieve clipping and posterior perfusion/patency proofs.

Small changes in angles, positioning, and digitally provided image assistance will be of precious value and should be precisely and smoothly capable of being modified.

This micrometric exploration is perfectly achieved using Exoscope as the selected VAS. The robotic arm allows us to reach every angle and position requested in a more quick, efficient, and comfortable manner than our previous experiences using a hybrid microscope.

In addition, it is possible to affirm that the surgeon's position remained unchanged during entire procedures. Comfort becomes essential when patience and smooth maneuvers are combined with more than 2 hours of the finest dissection we can offer.

Extra magnification capabilities without any loss in quality directly mean being aware of more details. Hand skills should be trained properly for this goal, but once achieved, they could represent a significant increase in our surgical results.

Surgical Examples

Complex Aneurysms

A young female was admitted to our emergency room with an intense and abrupt headache. Following the corresponding protocols for this situation, a spontaneous subdural hemorrhage was diagnosed, and further studies revealed a complex vascular lesion (an aneurysm) in the anterior circulation (Figure 4).

It was possible to observe a dominant right A1 segment and a hypoplastic left A1 segment. Following right A1, a first fenestration is noticed. After the fenestration rejoins the same pathway, a second small fenestration appears, with an aneurysm present at the proximal aspect. The lesion was localized at the bottom end of the interhemispheric region.

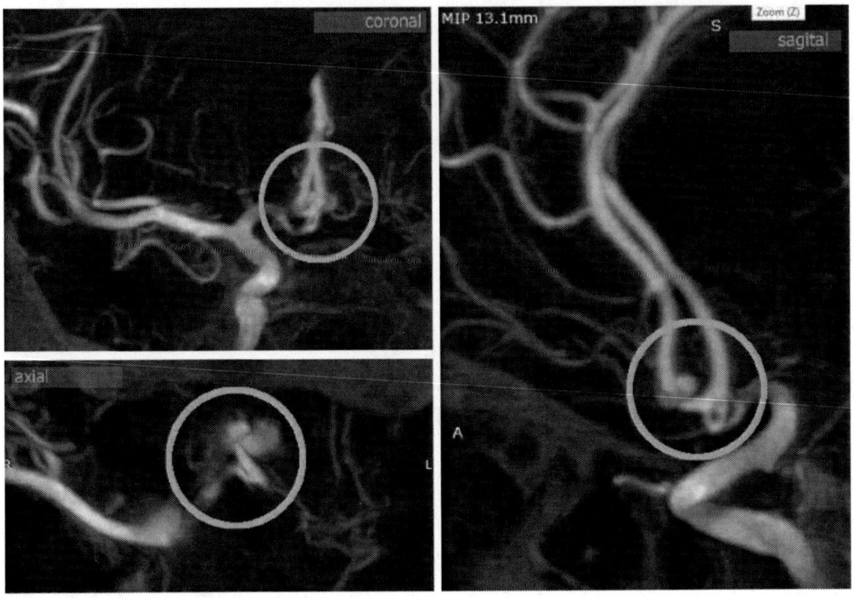

Figure 4. CTangio reconstruction using MPR.

Treatment options for the acute phase were considered, and an exoscope clipping surgery was proposed.

The main reasons for this selection were:

- Achieving good light and view conditions at the anterior skull base.
- The need for a thorough dissection of the interhemispheric region
- Possibility to small and smooth changes in position and angles while dissecting the lesion, in order to gain complete domus and neck exposure, in the safest possible conditions.
- Being able to perform patency comprobation once clipping was done, including small branch preservation.

Before 48 hours, the patient arrived at the OR, presenting a Fisher IV and Hunt-Hess 3 score. A slightly modified pterional approach was performed to reach an entire anterior middle-right skull base exposure.

The optic nerve and clinoid carotid segment serve as the main landmarks. Then the A1 segment was followed medially up to the interhemispheric region. Dissection progressed following the main vessel, and the aneurysm was finally discovered.

Optic chiasm and the proximal contralateral optic nerve were also seen. Interhemispheric dissection was mandatory to complete the task and reveal the aneurysm (Figure 5).

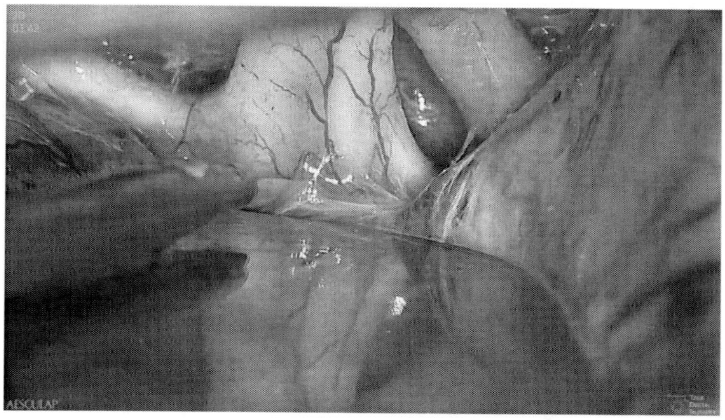

Figure 5. Right ICA and optic chiasm.

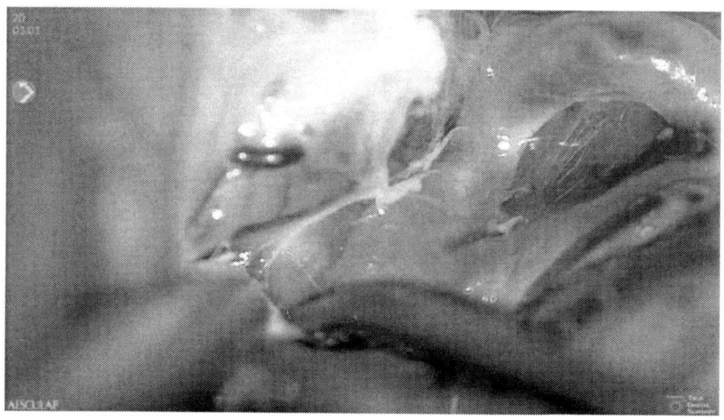

Figure 6. High magnification level at the neck (over the right hand dissector) of the aneurysm.

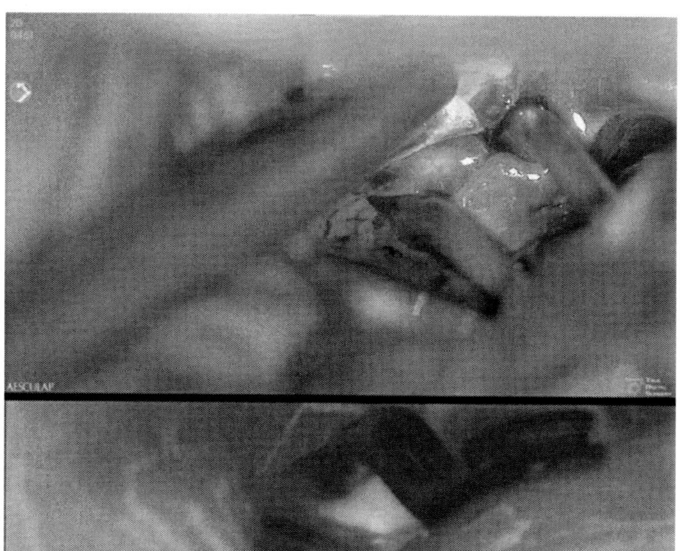

Figure 7. Clipping of the aneurysm and posterior revision using IV fluorescence methods.

Once situated at the final landmark, the dome and the neck of the aneurysm were dissected. The complexity of the lesion and the numerous small branches in this particular region presented a challenging situation (Figure 6).

Exoscope's visual and robotic capabilities offered a quality solution for this demanding scenario. The aneurysm was clipped without any immediate complications, and patency was tested with good results after clipping (Figure 7).

After a 3-hour surgery, the patient left the operating room and was extubated after 24 hours. No symptoms, nor neurological deficit were present at the moment of evaluation. Control images presented also good results.

Microanastomosis

A female patient with 3-year headache records was admitted because of left side arm and leg numbness, and a mild sense of losing strength.

After going for brain and brain-vessel images, the diagnosis of a partially thrombosed giant cavernous segment aneurysm was made (Figure 8).

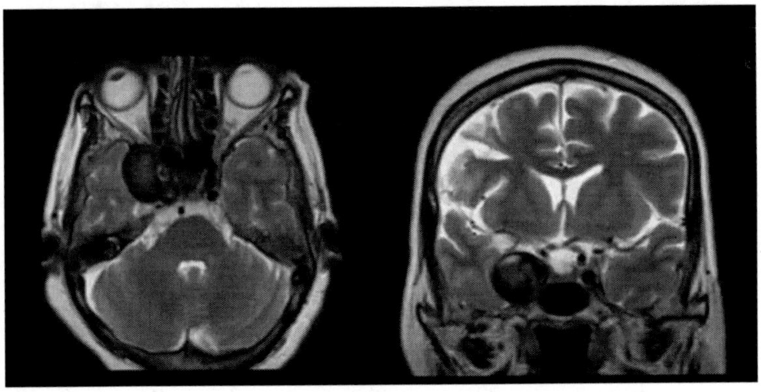

Figure 8. Giant partially thrombosed right cavernous segment aneurysm.

Due to anatomical facts and surgical preferences, an exoscope approach is selected. It was considered the best option for our surgical team because:

- The clinoid region presents special features in its surface and volumetrical characteristics, requiring extremely smooth and wide-ranging angles and position control.
- Details of the lesion should be especially considered while dissecting and mobilizing structures. Extreme sensibility and the precious anatomical details of this region will be of vital importance for achieving good results.
- Vascular suture with a 10/0 element requires high levels of magnification and precise dexterity for instrument manipulation. Visual aids, magnification level, the surgeon's comfort, and digital aberration correction will all impact the quality and timeliness of the final results.
- Need for image-assisted verification testing using real-time flow confirmation [27].

The patient arrived in the OR, and a modified pterional approach was made. Soft tissues were kindly treated in order to preserve the superficial temporal artery (STA, external carotid terminal branch). The use of the exoscope was also beneficial at superficial stages because of its high image quality at high levels of magnification (near x100). In the hands of a specifically trained surgeon, dissection of the STA could be performed easier and faster (Figure 9).

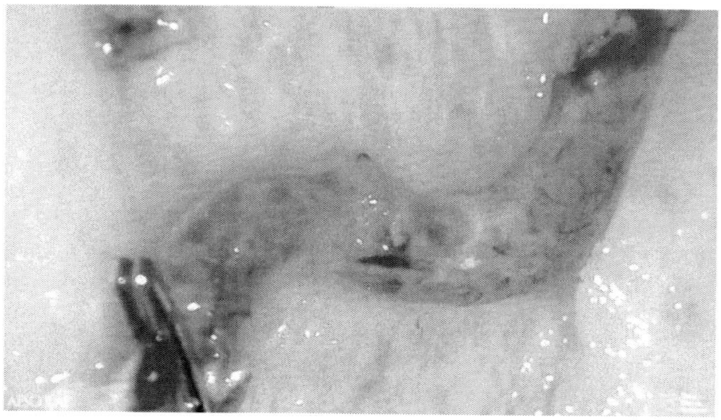

Figure 9. STA fully dissected. Details of the vasa-vasorum could be noticed.

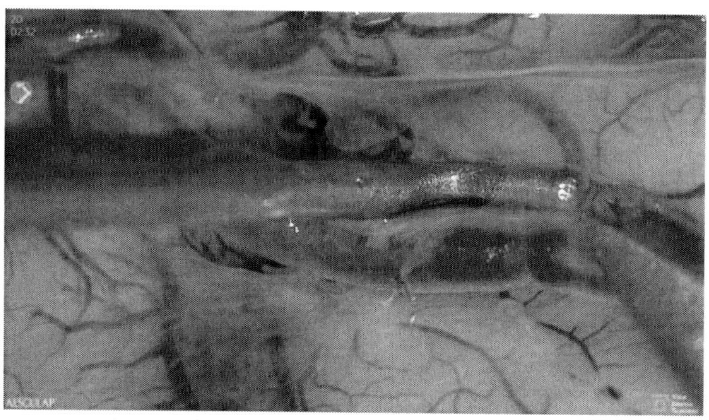

Figure 10. MCA being dissected from arachnoid and pia. Brain surface small vessels could be noticed and preserved.

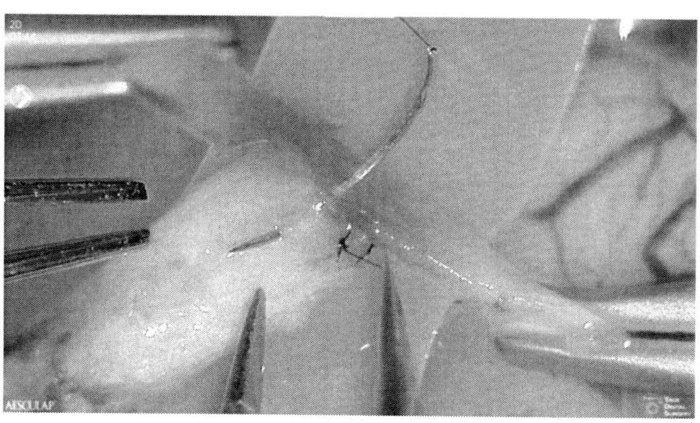

Figure 11. STA-MCA latero-terminal suture using 10/0 at near x90.

After STA dissection and clipping, the dura was opened in a wide manner to completely expose superficial branches of the middle cerebral artery (MCA, internal carotid artery terminal branch). The emergence point was dissected; the artery freed from any arachnoid and pia attachments, and then properly mobilised to expose the anastomotic site (Figure 10).

A 10/0 suture and a termino-lateral STA-MCA anastomosis were performed under high magnification. Verification tests using IV-fluorescein (and appropriate exoscope filters for this mode) showed proximal and distal patency. No leaks were observed at the suture line (Figure 11).

Skull Base and Other Fields

For all mentioned above, Exoscope rejoins all desirable features for a VAS, working at the skull base.

Easier and wider modifications of angles and/or positions (while the surgeon is comfortably placed in the surgical room) allow proper visualization, which should be considered of main importance in the search for better results.

Extra abilities, using its fully digital processing capabilities, open the door for a vast number of options.

Exoscope surgery brings new possibilities but also a whole new challenge to use this technology in multiple fields. Research and training will be the main engines to start moving forward in this matter.

References

[1] Yaşargil MG, *Microsurgery*, Academic Press, 1969, ISBN 9781483227566, doi: 10.1016/B978-1-4832-2756-6.50003-3.

[2] Fritz Schulze. How the Humble Stereomicroscope Found its Way into Modern Surgery: The Zeiss Operating Microscope. *Miscape Magazine*. doi: https://www.microscopy-uk.org.uk/mag/artdec12/fs-Zeiss-Operating-Microscopes-1.pdf.

[3] Ray, Sidney F. (2002). *Applied Photographic Optics* (3rd ed.). Oxford: Focal. ISBN 0-240-51540-4.

[4] Cordero I. Understanding and caring for an operating microscope. *Community Eye Health*. 2014;27(85):17. PMID: 24966460; PMCID: PMC4069782.

[5] Cherian et all. *Innovations in neurosurgery: hypervision and robotic assistance*. Teaching video from Krishna Vishwa Vidiapeeth. Institute of medical science. Karad, Maharashtra, India. 03-2023.

[6] Villanueva P, Cherian I. *Head and Eye commands for robotic-controlled surgical visual assistance*. Teaching video from Krisna Vishwa Vidiapeeth, India & Salta National University. 03-2023.

[7] Villanueva P, Villanueva B, Sanmarco C, Rodriguez H, Arciénaga A, Lagier M, Cherian I, Formento H. *Kaizen: Engineering tools for development, evaluation, certification and continuous improvement of microsurgical abilities and procedures*. Medicina em foco explorando os avanços e as fronteiras do conhecimento. Chapter 49. Seven Editorial. 2023. 10.56238/medfocoexplconheci-049.

[8] Villanueva P, Villanueva B, Arcienaga A. *Improving effectiveness of microsurgical procedures*. Sociedad Argentina de Mejora Continua & Salta National University. Argentina. 2023 (project still in procces).

[9] Ma L, Fei B. Comprehensive review of surgical microscopes: technology development and medical applications. *J Biomed Opt*. 2021 Jan;26(1):010901. doi: 10.1117/1.JBO.26.1.010901. PMID: 33398948; PMCID: PMC7780882.

[10] Uluç K, Kujoth GC, Başkaya MK. Operating microscopes: past, present, and future. *Neurosurg Focus.* 2009 Sep;27(3):E4. doi: 10.3171/2009.6.FOCUS09120. PMID: 19722819.

[11] Kriss TC, Kriss VM. History of the operating microscope: from magnifying glass to microneurosurgery. *Neurosurgery.* 1998 Apr;42(4):899-907; discussion 907-8. doi: 10.1097/00006123-199804000-00116. PMID: 9574655.

[12] Mortimer A, Davidson M. *Anatomy of a Microscope - Optical Aberrations.* Olympus LS. (n.d.). doi: https://www.olympus-lifescience.com/en/microscope-resource/primer/anatomy/aberrations/

[13] Somisetty S, M Das J. *Neuroanatomy, Vestibulo-ocular Reflex.* [Updated 2022 Jul 25]. In: StatPearls [Internet]. Treasure Island (FL): StatPearls Publishing; 2023 Jan- Available from: https://www.ncbi.nlm.nih.gov/books/NBK545297/

[14] Hunyor AP. *Reflexes and the eye.* Aust N Z J Ophthalmol. 1994 Aug;22(3):155-9; discussion 153. doi: 10.1111/j.1442-9071.1994.tb01710.x. PMID: 7818872.

[15] Baloh RW. Vestibulo-ocular, cervico-ocular, and visuo-ocular reflexes. *Bull Soc Belge Ophtalmol.* 1989;237:35-66. PMID: 2486114.

[16] Montemurro N, Scerrati A, Ricciardi L, Trevisi G. The exoscope in neurosurgery: an overview of the current literature of intraoperative use in brain and spine surgery. *J Clin Med.* 2021 Dec 31;11(1):223. doi: 10.3390/jcm11010223. PMID: 35011964; PMCID: PMC8745525.

[17] Villanueva P, Cherian I, Amayta S, Parmar H, Bhore E, Saatova N, Koniev T, Chaurasia R, Salve V, Parmar I. *Visual aid systems: Microscope and exoscope performances at different levels of magnification.* Krishna institute of medical science – Karad, Maharashtra, India (in process to be published).

[18] Hafez A, Haeren RHL, Dillmann J, Laakso A, Niemelä M, Lehecka M. *Comparison of Operating Microscope and Exoscope in a Highly Challenging Experimental Setting. World Neurosurg.* 2021 Mar; 147:e468-e475. doi: 10.1016/j.wneu.2020.12.093. Epub 2020 Dec 29. PMID: 33385603.

[19] Formento, HR, Chiodi, FJ, Cusolito, FJ, Altube, LA, & Gatti, SP. (2013). *Key factors for a continuous improvement process. Independent Journal of Management & Production*, 4(2), 391-415. doi: 10.14807/ijmp.v4i2.76.

[20] Parenti A. [et al.]; coordinación general de Marcos Ignacio Rodríguez. *Emprendiendo Kaizen* - 1a ed. - General San Martín: Instituto Nacional de Tecnología Industrial - INTI, 2019. Digital book. ISBN 978-950-532-415-6. CDD 658.5. doi: https://www.inti.gob.ar/assets/uploads/files/tecnologia-de-gestion/emprendiendo-kaizen.pdf.

[21] Shirzadi, A, Mukherjee, D, Drazin, DG, Paff, M, Perri, B, Mamelak, AN, Siddique, K. *Use of the video telescope operating monitor (VITOM) as an alternative to the operating microscope in spine surgery.* Spine 2012, 37, E1517–E1523. [CrossRef].

[22] Parihar, V, Yadav, YR, Kher, Y, Ratre, S, Sethi, A, Sharma, D. *Learning neuroendoscopy with an exoscope system (video telescopic operating monitor): Early clinical results.* Asian J. Neurosurg. 2016, 11, 421–426. [CrossRef].

[23] Oertel, JM, Burkhardt, BW. Vitom-3D for exoscopic neurosurgery: Initial experience in cranial and spinal procedures. *World Neurosurg.* 2017, 105, 153–162. [CrossRef] [PubMed].

[24] Rossini, Z, Cardia, A, Milani, D, Lasio, GB, Fornari, M, D'Angelo, V. *VITOM 3D: Preliminary experience in cranial surgery.* World Neurosurg. 2017, 107, 663–668. [CrossRef] [PubMed].

[25] Iwamoto H, Kiyohara Y, Fujishima M, Kato I, Nakayama K, Sueishi K, Tsuneyoshi M. *Prevalence of intracranial saccular aneurysms in a Japanese community based on a consecutive autopsy series during a 30-year observation period.* The Hisayama study. *Stroke.* 1999 Jul;30(7):1390-5. doi: 10.1161/01.str.30.7.1390. PMID: 10390312.

[26] Zhao X, Belykh E, Cavallo C, Valli D, Gandhi S, Preul MC, Vajkoczy P, Lawton MT, Nakaji P. *Application of Fluorescein Fluorescence in Vascular Neurosurgery.* Front Surg. 2019 Sep 18;6:52. doi: 10.3389/fsurg.2019.00052. PMID: 31620443; PMCID: PMC6759993.

Chapter 21

High-Resolution Vessel Wall Magnetic Resonance Imaging in Intracranial Aneurysm: A Review

Shambaditya Das*
Souvik Dubey
and Biman Kanti Ray
Department of Neurology, Institute of Post Graduate Medical Education and Research, Bangur Institute of Neurosciences, Kolkata, India

Abstract

High resolution Intracranial vessel wall imaging (HR-IVWI) has emerged in recent years as an adjunct to conventional imaging. Although, not studied as extensively as in intracranial atherosclerotic diseases, experiences with HR-IVWI in cerebral aneurysms are growing. HR-IVWI has been found to be helpful in differentiation of a stable from an unstable aneurysm in cases of unruptured cerebral aneurysms. Circumferential aneurysmal wall enhancement (CAWE) has been found to be the only independent predictor of instability of an aneurysm. HR-IVWI might also be used to identify the culprit lesion in subarachnoid hemorrhage (SAH) with multiple aneurysms. Furthermore, HR-IVWI might also be used to determine the source of hemorrhage in patients with angiogram negative non-perimesencephalic SAH. Thus, to conclude, HR-IVWI may serve as an important additional tool in the diagnostic armamentarium of cerebral aneurysms that can guide neurointerventionist regarding the selection and timing of appropriate treatment strategies.

Keywords: magnetic resonance imaging, MR vessel wall imaging, intracranial aneurysm

Introduction

The prevalence of intracranial aneurysm is 3-5% in the general population [1]. However, the incidence of its rupture leading to a SAH is significantly low. This suggests that a large proportion of intracranial aneurysm remains asymptomatic and does not rupture in the lifetime [2]. This, it becomes imperative to have ways to anticipate the behaviour of these intracranial

* Corresponding Author's Email: drshambadityadas@gmail.com.

In: Understanding and Managing Cerebral Aneurysms
Editor: Xianli Lv
ISBN: 979-8-89113-608-3

aneurysms and predict the future risk of rupture. The existing classification systems encompassing the characteristics of intracranial aneurysm and demographic profile of the patient (PHASES score) have not found wide acceptability as a predictive model for future risk of aneurysm rupture [2, 3]. High resolution intracranial vessel wall imaging (HR-IVWI) has emerged as a novel non-invasive imaging modality which might be useful in evaluation of intracranial aneurysm [4]. Although HR-IVWI has been maximally used in the context of ischemic stroke, the experiences of HR-IVWI with intracranial aneurysm have been increasing. Aneurysm wall enhancement (AWE) on HR-IVWI as a marker of rupture of intracranial aneurysm has drawn a lot of attention in recent times. In this article, we reviewed the role of HR-IVWI in the evaluation of intracranial aneurysm and its implications [2, 5].

Pathophysiology of Aneurysmal Wall Enhancement

The conventional angiography images the lumen, although the actual pathology lies in the wall of the vessel [6]. Thus, it is expected that an imaging modality that visualizes the vessel wall architecture will yield more information regarding the pathophysiological changes [4, 6]. The application of HR-IVWI can thus be extended to evaluation of intracranial aneurysm in an attempt to delineate the underlying structural changes in the aneurysm wall that leads to rupture or increases the future risk of rupture [4, 7]. Matouk et al., in their initial studies demonstrated that the presence of AWE in HR-IVWI might be helpful to pinpoint the intracranial aneurysm that might have ruptured in a patient with multiple aneurysm presenting with SAH [8]. Since then, AWE in the HR-IVWI of intracranial aneurysms has been a topic of great interest and research [4]. Previous studies have revealed that AWE in the aneurysmal wall is frequently associated with acute and chronic inflammatory cell infiltration, presence of vasa vasorum and intra-luminal thrombus formation. Vasa vasorum, which is normally absent intracranially, appears in the diseased state later in life, and is probably responsible for conveying inflammatory cells into the aneurysmal wall. Furthermore, due to its fragile nature, there is leakage of blood constituents and microhemorrhages. And this becomes instrumental in upregulating the inflammatory cascade within the aneurysmal wall. The lack of intact endothelial layer in the wall of intracranial aneurysm potentiates thrombus formation due to the exposure of the thrombogenic milieu. The thrombus with its trapped blood constituents then exacerbates the chronic inflammatory changes within the walls of intracranial aneurysm. Besides, it has also been noted that intra-luminal thrombus is essential for the formation of vasa vasorum. Chronic inflammation within the walls of intracranial aneurysm is already known to cause wall degeneration leading to aneurysmal instability and subsequent rupture. Atherosclerosis is also not uncommonly associated with intracranial aneurysm. AWE is significantly associated with the presence of atherosclerotic changes in the intracranial aneurysm. Atherosclerosis in itself is a result of chronic inflammation and it further perpetuates the chronic inflammatory process by recruitment of macrophages and leukocytes and subsequent release of cytokines. All these factors ultimately through enhanced oxidative stress and weakened aneurysmal wall architecture, subsequently leads to aneurysmal instability and future risk of rupture [2, 5, 9].

Current Applications of Vessel Wall Imaging of Intracranial Aneurysms

1. Acute SAH in patients with multiple aneurysms: HR-IVWI may be useful in determination of the particular aneurysm that might have ruptured in a patient harboring multiple intracranial aneurysms presenting with SAH. Several studies have shown that the ruptured aneurysms demonstrated thick peripheral enhancement as compared to those unruptured aneurysms. So, lack of enhancement will likely suggest a more stable, unruptured intracranial aneurysm [2, 4, 10].
2. Determination of source of hemorrhage in angiogram negative SAH patients: HR-IVWI has also been evaluated to identify the source of hemorrhage in angiogram negative peri-mesencephalic SAH. However, the initial reports are not promising [4, 11].
3. Predicting the future risk of rupture of saccular aneurysm: Inflammation is instrumental in aneurysmal growth in size and precedes the rupture of aneurysm. Naturally the role of HR-IVWI in detecting this aneurysmal wall inflammation as AWE has become an area of interest in predicting the future risk of rupture of intracranial aneurysms. Several studies have supported the notion of AWE on HR-IVWI as a possible marker for unstable aneurysm and future risk of rupture. However, these studies are mostly cross-sectional or include a limited follow-up period. So, prospective longitudinal studies with a longer duration of follow-up might be the way forward to either refute or confirm the correlation of AWE with unstable aneurysm [2, 4, 5, 7, 10].
4. Vasospasm: HR-IVWI may be used to predict vasospasm following SAH and aneurysm treatment by occurrence of early vessel wall contrast enhancement in the second and third order intracranial arteries. However, it is only backed by a handful of observational studies and requires dedicated future research to be of clinical significance [9, 12].

Pitfalls in Interpretation of Aneurysmal Wall Enhancement

There are several factors to consider while interpreting the contrast enhancement of the aneurysmal vessel wall. “Pseudo-enhancement” can occur due to incomplete suppression of the slow flowing blood along the walls of aneurysm. This leads to over-estimation of AWE as distinction between the two by the current principles of HR-IVWI is difficult. The presence of dura or veins (which usually enhances avidly) in close proximity to aneurysmal walls can also similarly lead to misinterpretation of AWE. Insufficient suppression of blood by the current techniques of HR-IVWI can further complicate the determination of AWE. During the acquisition of HR-IVWI, the orthogonal planes must be preferred, as tangential views can frequently lead to over-estimation of AWE. Lastly, the distinction between dissecting aneurysm and a thrombosed saccular aneurysm must be made due to their differences in pathogenesis and clinical implications. While dissecting aneurysm has presence of intimal flap, often with an intra-mural hemorrhage, seen as a crescent shaped region of spontaneous high T1 signal; thrombosed saccular aneurysm has an eccentric filing defect on post-contrast imaging with a corresponding iso-hyperintense signal changes on pre-contrast T1 sequence on HR-IVWI [2, 4, 11, 13].

Research Gap

While the last several years have seen a surge of research pertaining to HR-IVWI in intracranial aneurysm, still there is a dearth in prospective studies with long-term follow-up. Our experiences of HR-IVWI in intracranial aneurysm are limited to observational studies with either cross-sectional design or limited follow-up [2, 11]. Future studies directed to these research gaps are needed to have robust evidence regarding the utility of HR-IVWI in intracranial aneurysm. Also, the techniques and protocols of HR-IVWI used and the definitions used for AWE have varied considerably in the previous studies, making comparison difficult. HR-IVWI of smaller aneurysms that are usually treated conservatively, have not been studied well previously and remain an area of future interest. Also, there are only a handful of studies that have histologically correlated with HR-IVWI characteristics. Thus, several theories regarding the pathophysiological basis of AWE are still speculative and need further dedicated future research [2, 10, 11, 13-15].

Conclusion

HR-IVWI is a novel non-invasive imaging modality that might provide new insights regarding the evolution of intracranial aneurysm and its management strategies. It can greatly aid in identification of ruptured intracranial aneurysm as well as in the prediction of future risk of rupture. AWE in HR-IVWI is considered as the most prominent feature underpinning the instability; however, it is believed to have a stronger negative predictive value. Future studies with prospective designs and uniform techniques will further help to standardize the clinical applications of HR-IVWI in intracranial aneurysm.

References

[1] Etminan N, Rinkel GJ. Unruptured intracranial aneurysms: development, rupture and preventive management. *Nat Rev Neurol* 2016 1212. 2016 Nov 3;12(12):699–713.

[2] Matsushige T, Shimonaga K, Mizoue T, Hosogai M, Hashimoto Y, Takahashi H, et al. Lessons from Vessel Wall Imaging of Intracranial Aneurysms: New Era of Aneurysm Evaluation beyond Morphology. *Neurol Med Chir (Tokyo)*. 2019;59(11):407.

[3] Greving JP, Wermer MJH, Brown RD, Morita A, Juvela S, Yonekura M, et al. Development of the PHASES score for prediction of risk of rupture of intracranial aneurysms: A pooled analysis of six prospective cohort studies. *Lancet Neurol*. 2014 Jan 1;13(1):59–66.

[4] Mikulis DJ, Edjlali M, Saloner D, Ansari SA, Wasserman BA, Matouk C, et al. Intracranial Vessel Wall MRI: Principles and Expert Consensus Recommendations of the American Society of Neuroradiology. *Am J Neuroradiol*. 2017 Feb 1;38(2):218–29.

[5] Santarosa C, Cord B, Koo A, Bhogal P, Malhotra A, Payabvash S, et al. Vessel wall magnetic resonance imaging in intracranial aneurysms: Principles and emerging clinical applications. *Interv Neuroradiol*. 2020 Apr 1;26(2):135.

[6] Das S, Mossa-Basha M, Dey M, Hazra A, Pandit A, Das G, et al. High-resolution vessel wall magnetic resonance imaging in intracranial vasculopathies: an experience from eastern India. *Br J Radiol.* 2023 Apr 17;96(1145):20230114.

[7] Mossa-Basha M, Alexander M, Gaddikeri S, Yuan C, Gandhi D. Vessel wall imaging for intracranial vascular disease evaluation. *J Neurointerv Surg*. 2016 Nov 1;8(11):1154–9.

[8] Matouk CC, Mandell DM, Günel M, Bulsara KR, Malhotra A, Hebert R, et al. Vessel wall magnetic resonance imaging identifies the site of rupture in patients with multiple intracranial aneurysms: Proof of principle. *Neurosurgery*. 2013 Mar;72(3):492–6.

[9] Young CC, Bonow RH, Barros G, Mossa-Basha M, Kim LJ, Levitt MR. Magnetic resonance vessel wall imaging in cerebrovascular diseases. *Neurosurg Focus*. 2019 Dec 1;47(6):E4.

[10] de Havenon A, Chung L, Park M, Mossa-Basha M. Intracranial vessel wall MRI: a review of current indications and future applications. *Neurovascular Imaging* 2016 21. 2016 Jun 2;2(1):1–13.

[11] Coutinho JM, Sacho RH, Schaafsma JD, Agid R, Krings T, Radovanovic I, et al. High-Resolution Vessel Wall Magnetic Resonance Imaging in Angiogram-Negative Non-Perimesencephalic Subarachnoid Hemorrhage. *Clin Neuroradiol.* 2017 Jun 1;27(2):175–83.

[12] Mossa-Basha M, Huynh TJ, Hippe DS, Fata P, Morton RP, Levitt MR. Vessel wall MRI characteristics of endovascularly treated aneurysms: association with angiographic vasospasm. *J Neurosurg*. 2018 Sep 21;131(3):859–67.

[13] Choi YJ, Jung SC, Lee DH. Vessel Wall Imaging of the Intracranial and Cervical Carotid Arteries. *J Stroke*. 2015 Sep 1;17(3):238–55.

[14] Adhithyan R, Kesav P, Thomas B, Sylaja P, Kesavadas C. High-resolution magnetic resonance vessel wall imaging in cerebrovascular diseases. *Neurol India*. 2018 Jul 1;66(4):1124.

[15] Edjlali M, Guédon A, Hassen W Ben, Boulouis G, Benzakoun J, Rodriguez-RéGent C, et al. Circumferential Thick Enhancement at Vessel Wall MRI Has High Specificity for Intracranial Aneurysm Instability. *Radiology.* 2018 Jul 3;289(1):181–7.

Chapter 22

Procedural Complications in Endovascular Surgery of Cerebral Aneurysms

Huachen Zhang
Shikai Liang
and Xianli Lv*
Department of Neurosurgery, Beijing Tsinghua Changgung Hospital,
School of Clinical Medicine, Tsinghua University, Beijing, China.

Abstract

Although endovascular devices and treatment techniques are continuously developing, these minimally invasive procedures still carry treatment-specific risks. Before entering the era of flow diverter stents, the standard stent-assisted coiling technique has become a well-established treatment option for most cerebral aneurysms. The placement of permanent stents during coiling is associated with greater durability and higher risk of thromboembolic complications. In addition, permanent stents require platelet inhibition, increasing the risk of haemorrhagic complications. Awareness of complications, their predisposing factors, and their prevention and management can further reduce morbidity and mortality.

Keywords: complication, endovascular, surgery, cerebral aneurysms, procedure

Introduction

A Little Error May Lead to a Large Discrepancy — Yi Jing

Endovascular surgery of cerebral aneurysms is a rapidly evolving and complex field practiced by clinicians with backgrounds ranging from radiology to neurosurgery [1-3]. Endovascular coil embolisation continues to evolve a valid modality in managing ruptured and unruptured cerebral aneurysms (Figures 1 and 2) [4]. Technological advances in coil properties, adjunctive

* Corresponding Author's Email: lvxianli000@163.com.

In: Understanding and Managing Cerebral Aneurysms
Editor: Xianli Lv
ISBN: 979-8-89113-608-3

devices and interventional techniques continue to improve clinical results of cerebral aneurysms (Figures 3-6) [5-9], but also carry the potential for new iatrogenic injuries [10]. Every step of every endovascular procedure carries risk, and a thorough understand of potential complications is fundamental to maximizing safety. This chapter presents the most frequent and dangerous iatrogenic injuries, their presentation, identification, prevention, and management.

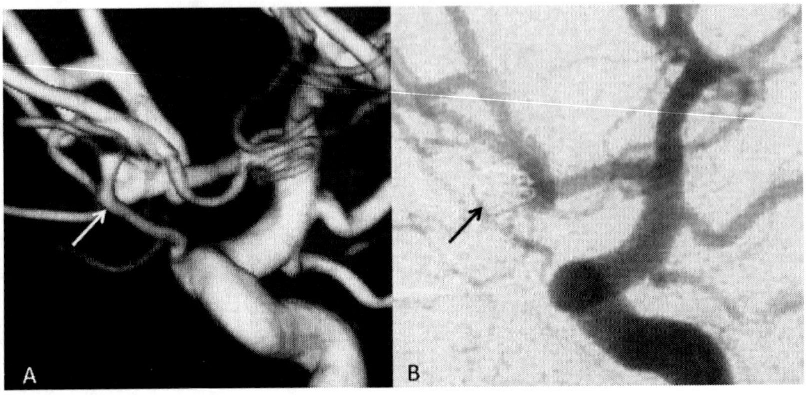

Figure 1. A ruptured anterior communicating artery aneurysm was treated with endovascular coil embolization. A. Preoperative 3-dimensional reconstruction of the left internal carotid artery injection revealed a left anterior communicating artery aneurysm (arrow) B. Postoperative angiography revealed complete embolization of the aneurysm (arrow).

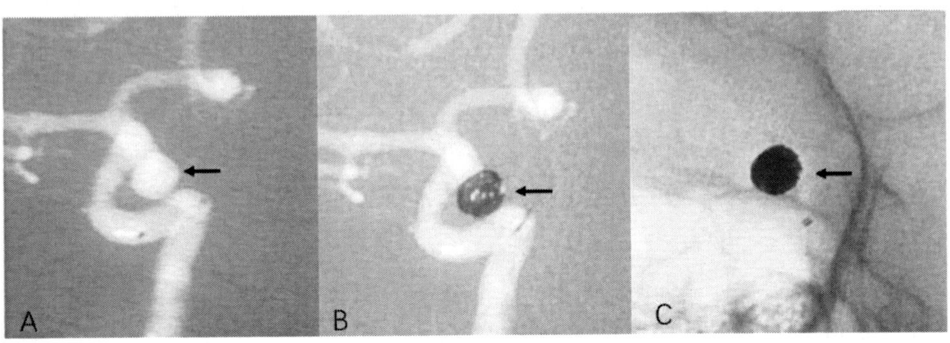

Figure 2. An unruptured internal carotid aneurysm was treated with endovascular coil embolization. A. The preoperative roadmap of the internal carotid artery showed an aneurysm in the clinoid segment of the internal carotid artery (arrow) B. The roadmap of the internal carotid artery showed a 3-dimensional coil embolization via a microcatheter (arrow). C. Postoperative unsubtraction image revealed complete embolization of the aneurysm (arrow).

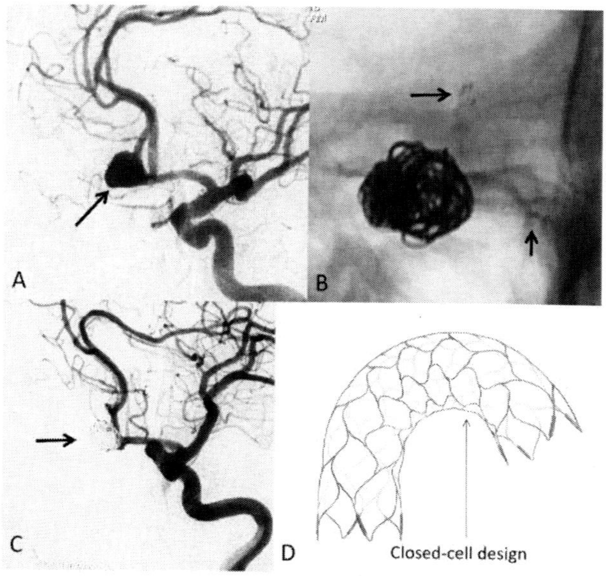

Figure 3. A 67-year-old male patient had an unruptured anterior communicating artery aneurysm treated with endovascular coil embolization. A. Preoperative left internal carotid artery angiography showed a large wide-necked aneurysm at the left anterior communicating artery (arrow) B. The non-subtracted image showed that the aneurysm was treated with Enterprise stent-assisted coil embolization (arrows showed X-ray markers on both ends of the stent). C. Postoperative angiography revealed complete embolization of the aneurysm (arrow). D. The Enterprise stent(Codman Neurovascular/ Johnson & Johnson) picture shows the laser-cut and closed-hole design of the stent.

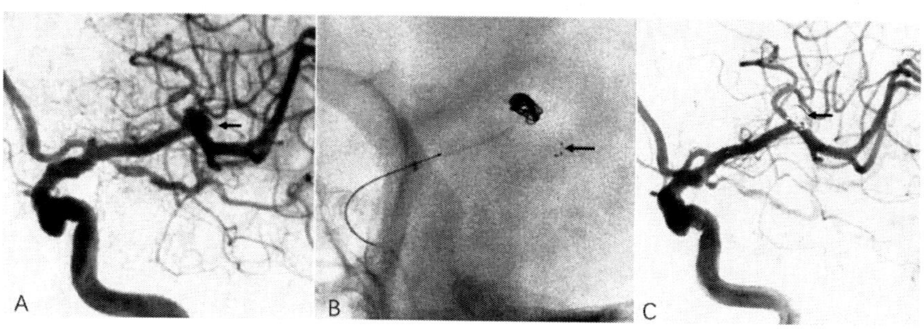

Figure 4. A 78-year-old female patient had an unruptured aneurysm at the left middle cerebral artery bifurcation treated with endovascular coil embolization. A. The preoperative left internal carotid artery angiography showed a wide-necked aneurysm of the left middle cerebral artery (arrow) B. The non-subtracted image showed that the aneurysm was treated with Solitaire AB (Medtronic, Irvine, CA, USA) stent-assisted coil embolization (arrow showed the X-ray markers at the distal end of the stent). C. Postoperative angiography revealed complete embolization of the aneurysm (arrow).

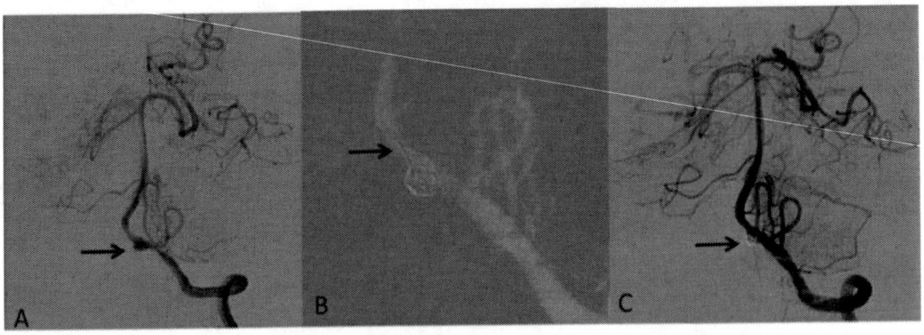

Figure 5. A 60-year-old male patient presented with Hunt-Hess grade 1 subarachnoid hemorrhage. A. The preoperative left vertebral artery angiography showed a fusiform aneurysm of the V4 segment of the left vertebral artery (arrow), and the left posterior inferior cerebellar artery arose from the proximal side of the aneurysm. B. The image of the left vertebral artery roadmap showed that the aneurysm was treated with Leo+ (Balt, Montmorency, France) stent assisted coil embolization (arrow shows two spiral markers under X-ray of the stent). C. Postoperative left vertebral artery angiography revealed complete embolization of the aneurysm (arrow).

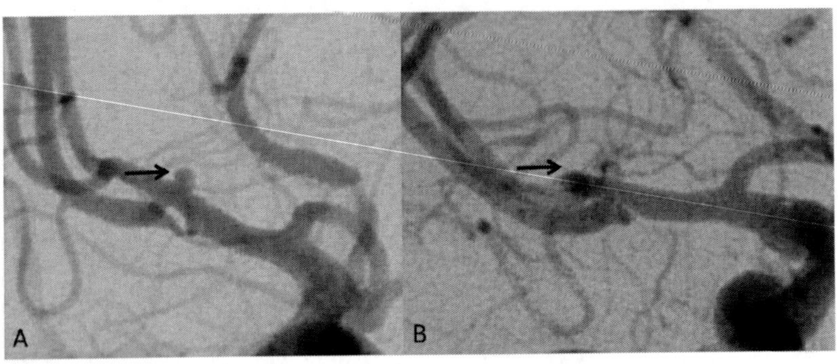

Figure 6. A 63-year-old female patient with an unruptured microaneurysm underwent sole stent placement treatment. A. Preoperative right internal carotid artery angiography revealed an unruptured microaneurysm at the bifurcation of the left middle cerebral artery (arrow). Considering that the aneurysm is not ruptured and is a small wide-necked aneurysm, there is a greater risk of coil embolization. Therefore, only one Neuroform Atlas (Stryker Neurovascular, Fremont, California, USA) stent was placed in the middle cerebral artery for hemodynamic remodeling treatment. B. The right internal carotid angiography at 9-month follow-up showed the aneurysm completely disappeared.

Procedural Complications

Overall complication rates for coiling of intracranial aneurysms range from 11.3%-19.4% [11-13]. Predictors of complications related to endovascular aneurysm embolization were: size of aneurysm, aneurysm location, atherosclerotic disease, treatment volume, endovascular modality and age [14]. Risk is increased in patients with subarachnoid hemorrhage (SAH), with the middle cerebral artery and posterior circulation aneurysms, with the use of balloon- and stent-assisted coiling or flow diverter, treatment of very small and very large aneurysms, and performance by inexperienced operators [10]. The associated complications were listed according to the probability and severity of their occurrence.

Thromboembolic Events

Thromboembolic events are considered one of the most serious complications in endovascular aneurysm treatment. Therefore, neurointerventional physicians must be very familiar with the prevention and treatment of thrombotic complications during the treatment of cerebral aneurysms. Thromboembolic events cause symptomatic stroke. Symptomatic thromboembolism occurs in 2 to 8% of patients during aneurysm coiling [15-18]. The thrombus formation is usually associated with the introduction of the stents and flow diverter stents (Figure 7) [19]. In a systematic review, the incidence of clinically significant thromboembolic events in stent-assisted coiling of ruptured aneurysms was 6%, which was higher than the complication rates that have been previously reported in the coil embolization of ruptured aneurysms [20]. Other identified risk factors for thromboembolic events are endovascular treatment more than 36 h after SAH, balloon-assisted coiling, the use of fiber coils and manipulation of catheters, wires, coils [10, 21]. Fiber coils were thrombogenic in order to induce rapid thrombosis of the aneurysm (Figure 8) [10]. However, in case of coil loop protrusion or coil dislodgement, the risk of thrombus formation is even higher [10].

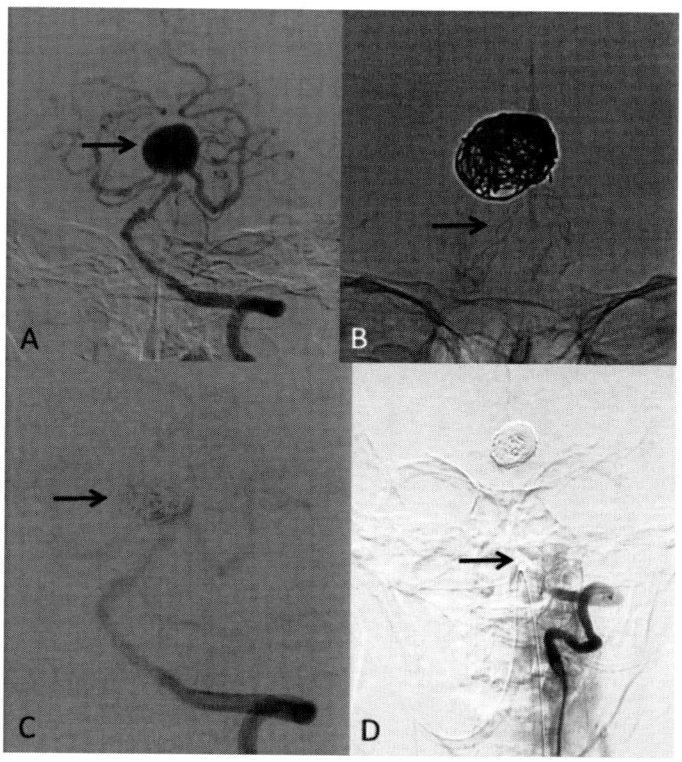

Figure 7. A 63-year-old female patient died of delayed thrombosis of flow diverter. A. Preoperative left vertebral artery angiography revealed a giant aneurysm at the top bifurcation of the basilar artery that was unruptured (arrow). Considering that the aneurysm is not ruptured and is a giant wide-necked aneurysm, coil embolization and flow diverter stent implantation should be performed. B. The non-subtracted image showed a partial coil embolization of the aneurysm, with a Tubridge (MicroPort, Shanghai, China) flow diverter stent placed from the left posterior cerebral artery to the basilar artery (arrow showed two spiral markers of the stent developed under X-ray). C. Postoperative left vertebral artery angiography showed partial embolization of the aneurysm, and good blood filling of both posterior cerebral and basilar arteries (arrow). D. One week later, the patient suddenly fell into a coma and the left vertebral artery angiography showed complete occlusion of the basilar and distal arteries due to stent thrombosis. Tirofiban treatment failed and the patient died.

Using heparinized saline flush is mandatory on each line continuously during endovascular aneurysm treatment, including guide catheter, distal access catheter, and microcatheter to avoid thrombus formation [23]. Empty or turned-off flush lines can be the cause of thrombus formation and present a frequent and serious risk to the patient. All flush lines should be monitored continuously and carefully. The guide catheter should not be placed directly against a bend in order to limit guide-catheter induced vasospasm.

Thrombus formation during coiling and stenting is primarily mediated by platelet aggregation [24]. In cases of acute thrombus formation, the thrombus will continuously grow. It is advisable to compare angiographic runs with a preprocedural angiographic run to detect filling defects at an early stage. Thrombus may be directly visualized with guide catheter angiogram as a filling defect within the parent vessel, or as a distal vessel occlusion.

Following the appearance of antiplatelet agents as inhibitors of the glycoprotein IIb/IIIa receptor, lytic agents as Urokinase or tPA are no longer used as first-line therapy by most teams facing an acute thromboembolic complication [25]. Depending on the occlusion of the aneurysm, a glycoprotein IIb/IIIa receptor antagonist that inhibits platelet aggregation, can be administered either intravenously or intraarterially. Abciximab, eptifibatide, and tirofiban are the GpIIb/IIIa inhibitors that prevent platelet cross linking and aggregation, while inducing disintegration of newly formed platelet clusters [26]. The treatment of thromboembolic events was performed via a bolus of intra-arterial Abciximab (0.25 mg/kg) through guiding catheter followed by a 12-h intravenous infusion (0.125 mg/kg/min) when judged necessary and/or when neurological deficits were present immediately after the procedure and not related to hemorrhage by emergency computed tomography (CT) [27].

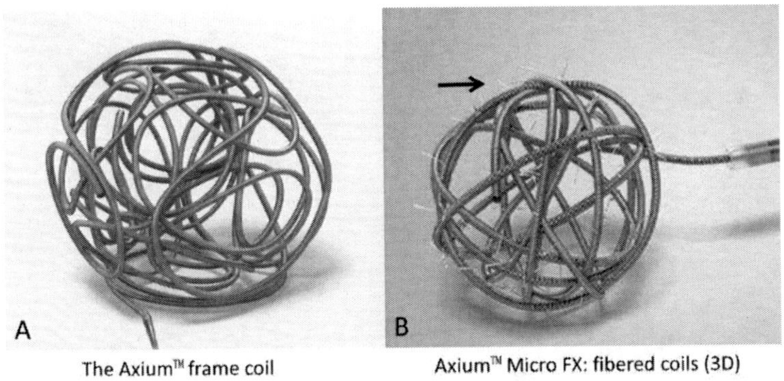

Figure 8. Fibered coils are standard bare-platinum coils with additional polymer microfilament threads protruding from the primary coil. For example, the Axium coil (Medtronic Neurovascular, Irvine, California, USA) is available as a bare-platinum coil (A) and as a fibered coil (B) with either polymer polyglycolic-lactic acid or nylon microfilament (arrow).

Tirofiban/eptifibatide resulted in significantly higher recanalization rates compared with abciximab [26]. Tirofiban showed a low risk of symptomatic hemorrhagic or thromboembolic complications. Reports on the use of intra-arterial tirofiban or intravenous infusion of tirofiban (a low dose of intravenous administration of tirofiban 5 μg/kg over 1 min, followed by a maintenance dose of 0.1 μg/kg/min) for 24 h in ruptured and unruptured aneurysms indicate that such treatment is relatively safe and effective (Figure 9) [28]. Mechanical thrombectomy is necessary in some cases of large vessel occlusion [29]. Interventional techniques like the

Penumbra aspiration catheter (Penumbra, Inc) or stent-trievers can also be used to re-open an occluded vessel.

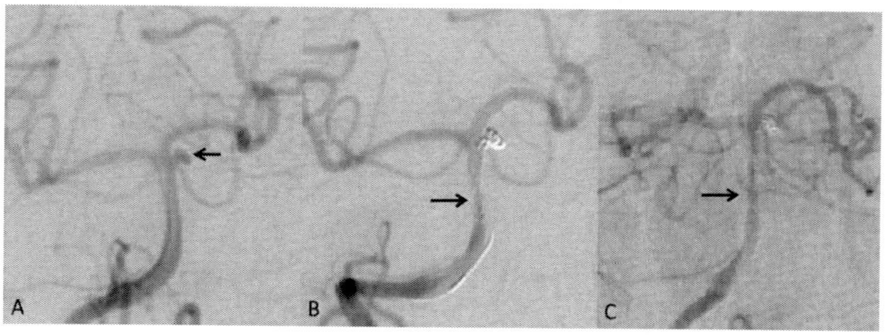

Figure 9. A 54-year-old male patient presented with Hunt-Hess grade 1 subarachnoid hemorrhage. A. Preoperative vertebral artery angiography revealed a left basilar artery-superior cerebellar artery aneurysm (arrow). During coil embolization, a coil loop protruded into the basilar artery. Therefore, a LVIS Jr (MicroVention Inc, Aliso Viejo, California, USA) stent was inserted from the left posterior cerebral artery to the basilar artery for salvage treatment. B. Vertebral artery arteriography revealed a thrombus at the proximal end of the stent (arrow). C. Postoperative vertebral artery arteriography showed that the thrombus disappeared after treatment with tirofiban(arrow), the aneurysm was completely obliterated, and both posterior cerebral and basilar arteries were well filled with blood.

The occlusion of the retinal artery may be related to the endovascular treatment of ophthalmic artery segment aneurysms, especially the use of balloon catheters to block blood flow during the embolization of the aneurysm. Since 2009, the use of balloon catheters in endovascular treatment of ruptured and unruptured aneurysms has been decreased because of the appearance of better intracranial stent and flow diversion systems. The retina is very sensitive to ischemia, and the retinal artery is the terminal artery without collateral artery anastomosis. From this perspective, the retina is more susceptible to ischemic damage than the brain. The occlusion of the retinal artery during the treatment of unruptured intracranial aneurysms using stent and flow diversion techniques without the use of balloon catheters is very rare.

Periprocedural Hemorrhage

Aneurysm Perforation

The overall risk of aneurysm perforation is 4.1% during treatment of ruptured aneurysms and 0.5% with treatment of unruptured aneurysms [30]. Risk of perforation is higher during the treatment of aneurysms smaller than 4 mm [31]. Aneurysm perforation during embolization is obvious on fluoroscopy or angiography associated with a sudden elevation in blood pressure (Figure 10). Whenever a perforation is identified or suspected, the perforating wire, catheter, or coil should be left in position and a prompt guide catheter angiogram should be done.

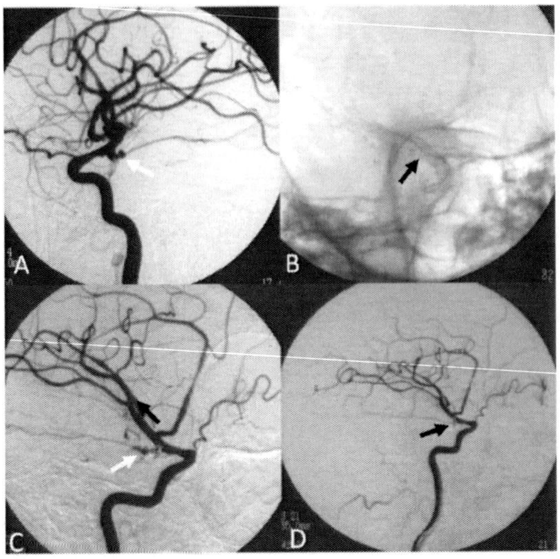

Figure 10. Intraoperative rupture during aneurysm coiling. A 25-year-old female patient presenting with subarachnoid hemorrhage from an anterior choroidal artery aneurysm. A, a digital subtraction angiogram showing a 3mm×6mm ruptured anterior choroidal artery aneurysm (arrow). B, unsubtracted image showing a 4.5 mm × 25 mm Leo stent (Balt, Montmorency, France) was placed (arrow). C, intra-operative angiogram image showing contrast extravasation during coiling (arrow). D, final angiography image showing no contrast extravasation after 4 coils were introduced (Microplex, 2 mm × 4 cm, 2 mm × 3 cm, 2 mm × 1 cm, 2 mm × 2 cm; Microvention, Aliso Viejo, CA, USA).

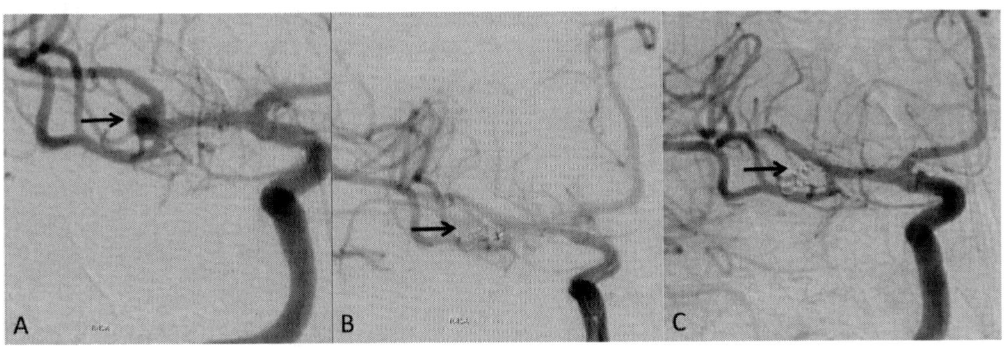

Figure 11. Intraoperative rupture during aneurysm coiling. A 68-year-old female patient presented with Hunt-Hess grade 1 subarachnoid hemorrhage. A. Preoperative right carotid artery angiography revealed an aneurysm at the bifurcation of the right middle cerebral artery (arrow). During coil embolization, a coil loop pierced the aneurysm. An assistant doctor compressed the right carotid artery while continuing to fill the coil for embolization. B. Intraoperative angiography of the right internal carotid artery showed that the contrast agent overflowed from the aneurysm, indicating that there was still bleeding (arrow) and coil embolization was continued. C. Postoperative right internal carotid artery angiography showed complete embolization of the aneurysm (arrow), no contrast agent continued to overflow, and the distal end of the middle cerebral artery was well filled with blood.

Following aneurysm perforation, coils must be deployed to treat the perforation. Alternatively, a second microcatheter can be used to continue coiling the aneurysm while the first microcatheter is left in place [32]. Another strategy is to compress the carotid artery to reduce the bleeding by an assistant doctor (Figure 11). In some cases, parent vessel sacrifice by embolization may be necessary to stop the hemorrhage.

A CT scan performed postperforation will appear to show more subarachnoid blood than is actually present due to the presence of contrast material in the subarachnoid space. According to the indications of neurosurgery, it is decided whether to perform craniotomy to remove hematoma or decompress with bone flap (Figure 12).

Delayed Aneurysmal Hemorrhage

Delayed aneurysmal hemorrhage after coiling of ruptured aneurysms occurs in 0.9% of cases within 30 days after the procedure [33]. In the CARAT study, half of the ruptures occurred during the first 3 days after treatment [34]. Early rehemorrhage usually occurs in aneurysms that were incompletely occluded after initial treatment. Certain factors contribute to aneurysm bleeding post treatment are aneurysm large or giant size, dissecting pathology (Figure13) [35-37]. Therefore, in aneurysm treatment, it is important to achieve adequate obliteration of aneurysm no matter what treatment modality is taken. Late rehemorrhage typically occurs in aneurysms with recanalization, underscoring the need for routine surveillance of coiled aneurysms [34].

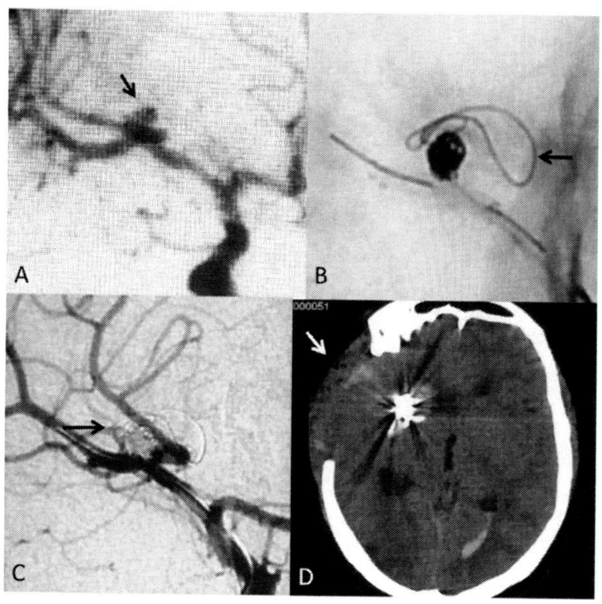

Figure 12. Intraoperative rupture during aneurysm coiling. A 47-year-old female patient had an unruptured aneurysm. A. Preoperative right internal carotid artery angiography revealed a wide-necked aneurysm at the bifurcation of the right middle cerebral artery (arrow). B. The non-subtractive image shows a coil loop puncturing the aneurysm during Enterprise(Codman Neurovascular/Johnson & Johnson) stent assisted coil embolization (arrow). Continue filling the coils for embolization until the aneurysm is completely embolized. C. Postoperative right internal carotid artery angiography showed complete embolization of the aneurysm (arrow), no contrast agent continued to overflow, and the distal end of the middle cerebral artery was well filled with blood. D. Cranial CT scanning showed that the patient had undergone decompressive bone flap removal treatment(arrow).

Device Failure

Coil Stretching

The reported rate of coil stretching during embolization is decreasing because most coils now have stretching-resistance design, which is tiny filaments extend between the two ends of the coil to prevent it from unravelling unintentionally when pulled on (Figure 14). But, some coils do not have stretching-resistance design, such as Microplex (MicroVention Inc, Aliso Viejo, California, USA) (Figure 15). When the distal portion of a coil becomes trapped inside an aneurysm, attempted withdrawal of the coil can lead to stretching or unraveling [38]. Coil stretching is usually caused by adjusting the position of the coil many times, so it is necessary to avoid repeatedly adjusting the coil many times. The stretched coil will herniated into the parent artery led to a large stroke or without any clinical complications. A slightly stretched coil may still be deployed using stent or balloon assistance [39, 40]. If the stretched coil was entrapped with previous coils, it should not be retrieved by a microsnare or stent, which will not be effective and may take the coil mass dislogement [38]. Alternatively, the coil can be partially withdrawn, redirected, and released into an extracranial artery, such as the external carotid artery or subclavian artery [41].

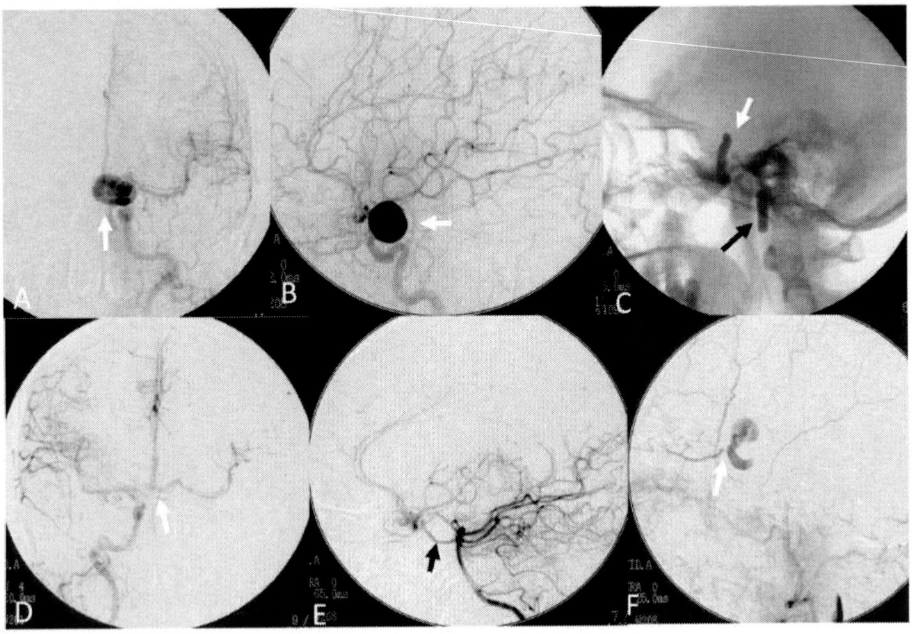

Figure 13. Delayed aneurysm rupture caused by arterial anastomosis. A 55-year-old woman presented with blurred vision of the left eye. A, frontal view of the left carotid artery injection. B, lateral view of the left carotid artery injection. Showing a giant aneurysm of the supraclinoid segment of the internal carotid artery (arrow). C, unsubtracted image, lateral projection, showing the left internal carotid artery was occluded using 2 detachable balloons (arrows). D, frontal view of the right carotid artery. E, lateral view of the left vertebral artery injection. Showing the left anterior cerebral artery and the left middle cerebral artery were filled through the anterior communicating artery (white arrow) and the posterior communicating artery (black arrow). F, lateral view of the late phase of the left external carotid artery injection showing the aneurysm was refilled through the ophthalmic artery. The patient died of aneurysm rupture 7 days after treatment.

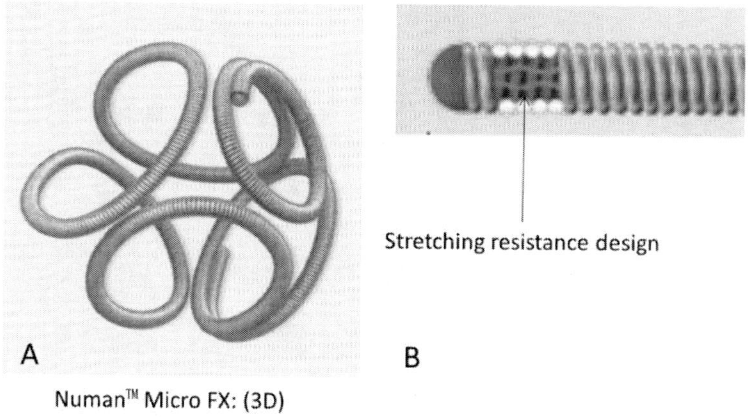

Figure 14. The pictures showed a frame coil (Numan™, MicroPort, Shanghai, China) (A) has stretching-resistance design, which is tiny filaments extend between the two ends of the coil to prevent it from stretching (B).

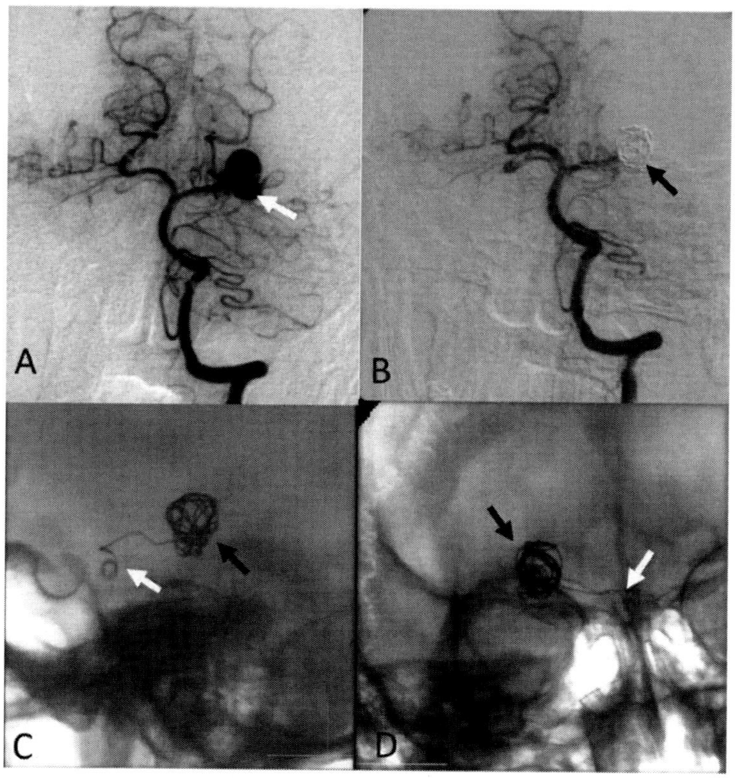

Figure 15. Coil stretching. A, frontal view of the left vertebral artery injection showing a large aneurysm of the P2 segment of the left posterior cerebral artery (arrow). The aneurysm was embolized with Microplex coils (MicroVention Inc, Aliso Viejo, California, USA). B, intra-operative angiography showing the aneurysm was completely thrombosed (arrow). Unsubtracted images, lateral projection (C) and frontal projection (D), showing the stretching of the coil. The white arrow indicates the stretching coil in the basilar artery. The black arrow indicates the coils in the aneurysm sac.

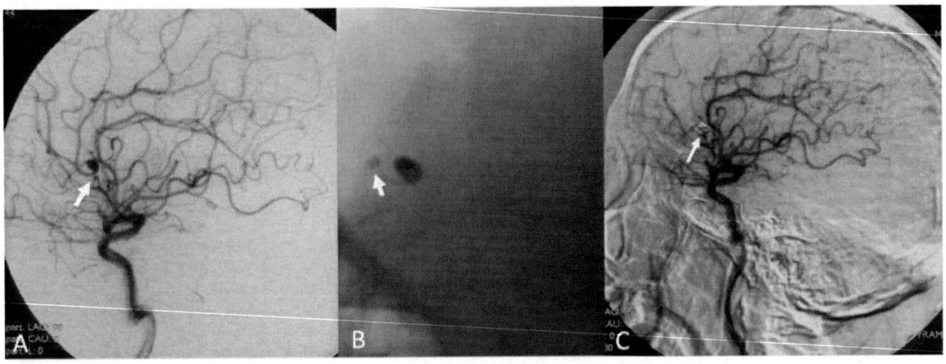

Figure 16. Coil dislodgement. A 44-year-old man presenting with subarachnoid hemorrhage from a distal anterior cerebral artery aneurysm. A, later view of the left internal carotid artery angiogram showing a 3 mm × 4 mm aneurysm at the origin of the marginal callosal artery. B, Unsubtracted image, lateral projection, demonstrating the dislodged coil in the marginal callosal artery (arrow). C, lateral view of the left internal carotid artery angiogram showing the complete occlusion of the aneurysm and thrombosis of the marginal callosal artery (arrow).

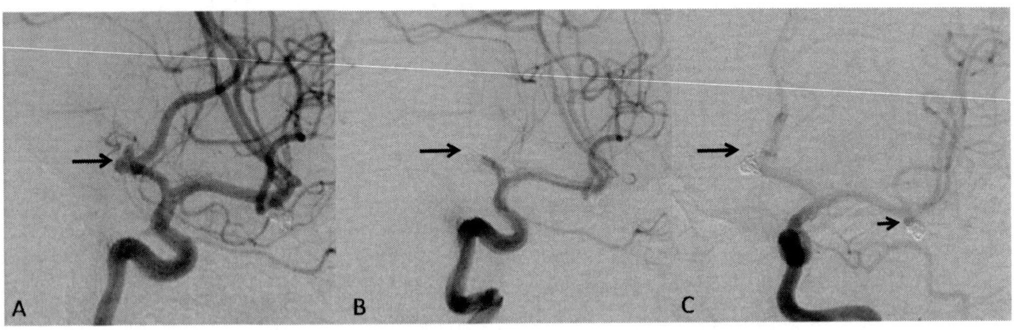

Figure 17. A 50-year-old female patient presented with Hunt-Hess grade 1 subarachnoid hemorrhage at 8 years after embolization of a left middle cerebral artery aneurysm. A. Preoperative left internal carotid artery angiography revealed a left anterior communicating artery aneurysm with two lobes (arrow). B. The left internal carotid artery angiography showed that the anterior cerebral artery was occluded due to the protruding coil (arrow). A Neuroform Atlas stent was placed in the anterior cerebral artery for salvage treatment. C. Postoperative left internal carotid angiography showed that the aneurysm was completely embolized (arrow), no contrast agent continued to overflow, and the distal end of the left anterior cerebral artery was well filled with blood. There is a slight recurrence at the neck of the embolized middle cerebral aneurysm(short arrow), and follow-up observation is recommended.

Failure to Detach

Failure of the coil to detach is a known complication, but this topic has not been explored in more detail. Ideally, the coil can still be retrieved without dislodging the coil package. Failure to detach is a very rare condition, and it can only be seen in electrolytic coil. It can be resolved by replacing the electrolytic device or battery.

Coil Dislodgement

Coil dislodgement is infrequent and can occurred in simple coiling, balloon-assisted coiling and laser-cut stent-assisted coiling embolization (Figure 16). It can cause occlusion of the parent artery or other arterial branches, carrying a high risk to induce ischemic complications when compromising blood flow [39, 42]. An appropriately sized initial framing coil is essential for successful embolization. An unstable or malpositioned coil can herniate into the parent vessel or embolize distally. Overpacking of an aneurysm can also dislodge previously released coils. If coil dislodgement occurs, the protruding loop can be fixed to the vessel wall by placement of an intracranial stent (Figure 17).

Wide-necked aneurysms are at greatest risk of coil dislodgement, with an overall incidence of 0.5% [43]. Stent-assisted coiling can reduce the risk of coil dislodgement. If aneurysm is very small, a braided stent is recommended because of its smaller mesh holes. Due to the large mesh hole of the laser-cut stent, the displacement of the small coil may occur.

Coil dislodgement increases risk of flow compromise or thrombus formation in the parent vessel, while coil migration can result in distal ischemia. Stent may be used to reinsert herniated coils into the aneurysm [40, 42]. There have been several reports of successful coil extraction with endovascular devices, such as the Amplatz goose-neck microsnare (Medtronic, Irvine, CA, USA) or the Alligator retrieval device (Medtronic, Irvine, CA, USA); recently, stent-trievers have also been utilized for ischemic stroke treatment [44]. If the coil cannot be safely retrieved or repacked into the aneurysm, straighten the coil in the vessel and long-term antiplatelet therapy is recommended.

Failure of Flow Diverter Treatment

Flow diversion failure in the long term (incomplete or nonocclusion) has been reported to occur in up to 5% of cases at 5 years follow-up in clinical trials of the pipeline for uncoilable or failed aneurysm [45]. It should be noted, however, that these results are in the setting of ideal conditions of a clinical trial. When examining meta-analyses that also include retrospective observational studies evaluating FD efficacy, the rate of incomplete occlusion increases to approximately 15% at last followup [46]. There have been several factors as described in the review article include the presence of branch vessel from the aneurysm dome or body, fusiform morphology, bifurcation aneurysms (Figure 18), parent vessel geometry, and inadequate coverage of the aneurysm neck (Figure 19) [46, 47]. Other factors such as age older than 70 yr and aneurysm size greater than 15 mm have been reported in other studies [46]. It is important to mention that older age may be related to inadequate endothelialization [46]. The main approach as mentioned by the authors is the placement of an additional flow diverter covering the aneurysm neck (Figure 20).

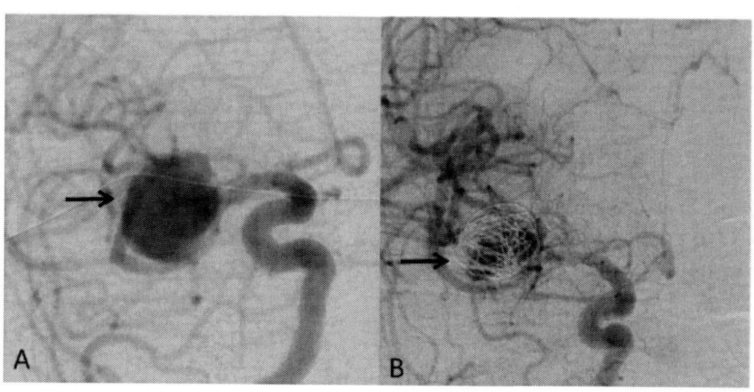

Figure 18. A 62-year-old female patient had a large aneurysm of the right middle cerebral artery bifurcation. A. Preoperative right internal carotid artery angiography revealed a large aneurysm at the bifurcation of the right middle cerebral artery. Partial coil embolization and the pipeline embolization device (PED; Medtronic Neurovascular, Irvine, California, USA) treatment were performed.
B. The 2-year follow-up of the right internal carotid artery angiography revealed that the aneurysm was mostly occluded (arrow). It is recommended to continue follow-up observation.

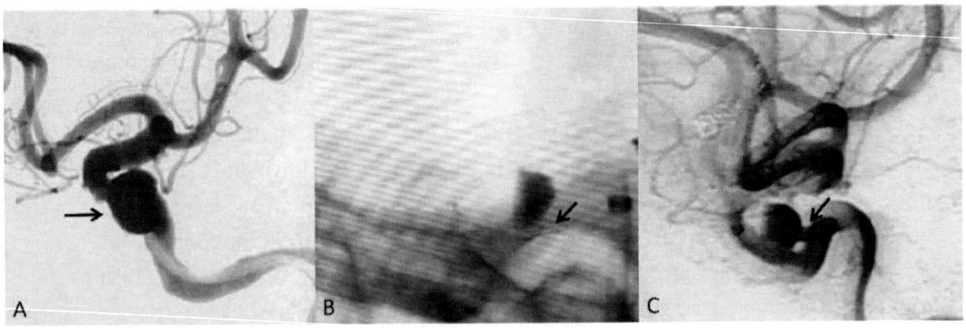

Figure 19. A 64-year-old female patient had an unruptured aneurysm of the left internal carotid artery. A. Preoperative angiography of the left internal carotid artery, oblique view, revealed a cavernous segment aneurysm of the left internal carotid artery (arrow). A PED treatment was performed. B. The non-subtracted image showed that the end of the flow diverter stent does not completely cover the aneurysm orifice (arrow). C. An 8-month follow-up angiography of the right internal carotid artery revealed that the aneurysm orifice was not completely occluded (arrow). It is recommended to place an additional PED covering the aneurysm neck.

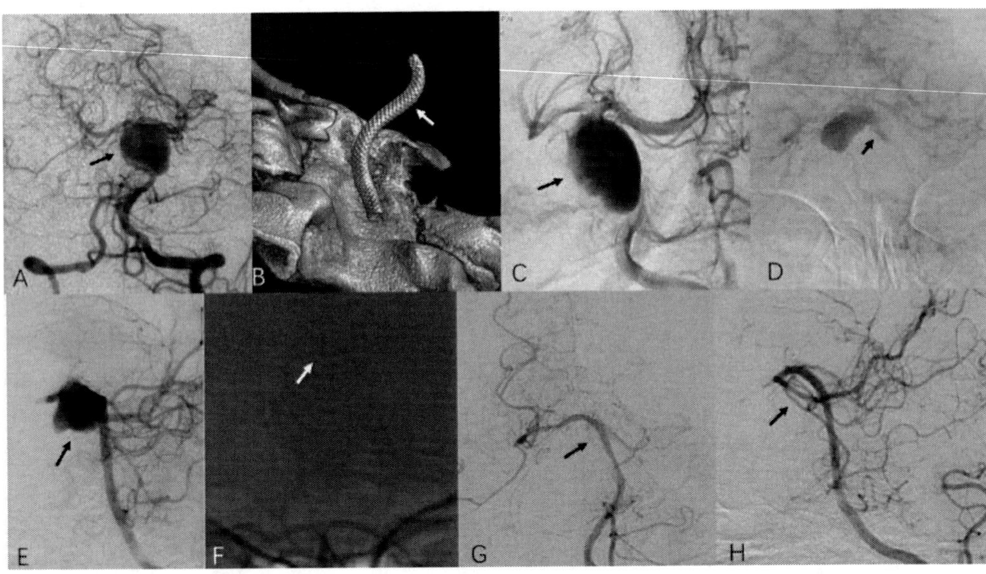

Figure 20. A 20-year-old female patient had headaches. A. Preoperative vertebral artery angiography revealed a giant aneurysm in the upper segment of the basilar artery (arrow). A PED treatment was performed. B. Reconstuction of the Dyna-CT image showed the PED(arrow). C. Immediately after treatment, vertebral artery arteriography revealed contrast retention within the aneurysm. D and E, 2-year follow-up of vertebral artery arteriography showed that most of the aneurysms were occluded due to the PED not completely covering the aneurysm orifice (arrows). F. The non-subtracted image showed placing an additional PED to completely cover the aneurysm orifice (arrow). G and H, vertebral artery angiography showed complete occlusion of the aneurysm at an 8-month follow-up (arrows).

Arterial Dissection

Arterial dissection due to wire, diagnostic catheter or guide catheter–induced intimal damage occurs in 0.6 to 3.6% of coiling cases (Figure 21) [48]. Intimal injury is likely underreported, as many operators do not routinely perform a surveillance angiogram of the access artery after coiling. The vertebral artery is thought to be at greater risk of injury than the internal carotid [49]. Slight vessel dissection is generally asymptomatic, but severe arterial dissection can cause complete occlusion of the major artery placing the patient at increased risk of occlusive or thromboembolic complications [50]. Imaging may directly reveal an injury in the form of a double lumen or intimal flap in arterial dissection, or indirectly in the form of arterial occlusion or stenosis, string sign, aneurysm, or pseudoaneurysm. Initial management of severe arterial dissection consists of stenting and dual antiplatelet therapy with aspirin 100 to 325 mg and clopidogrel 75 mg daily [50, 51]. Dual antiplatelet therapy may be discontinued at 6 months.

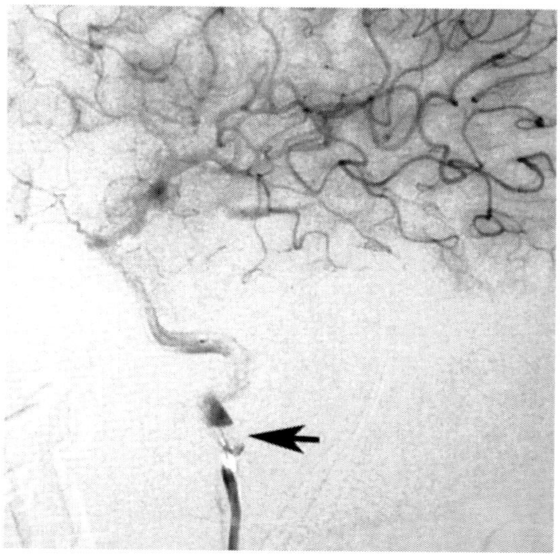

Figure 21. Carotid artery injury during aneurysm coiling. A 56-year-old woman presenting with a posterior communicating artery aneurysm. A digital subtraction angiogram showing an internal carotid artery dissection at the guiding catheter head after aneurysm coiling (arrow).

Vasospasm

Cerebral vasospasm presents most commonly following aneurysmal SAH, but may also complicate embolization procedures. Hyperdynamic therapy, intra-arterial injection of pharmacologic agents, and balloon angioplasty are all potential therapeutic interventions. The major complication rate with endovascular treatment for vasospasm was recently reported at 5% [52]. Although there is balloon angioplasty in literature reports [53], this method is not commonly used. Tips for the avoidance of complications with intracranial angioplasty for vasospasm include limiting treatment to only arteries that are relatively easy to access with a balloon catheter and undersizing the balloon diameter to minimize risk of rupture. Medication is usually effective and intra-arterial injection of nicardipine or verapamil can be used [54].

Deep Vein Thrombosis

Deep vein thrombosis is underestimated in patients undergoing endovascular treatment of cerebral aneurysms. Deep vein thrombosis is a significant source of morbidity and mortality in hospitalized patients. Among 485 patients with SAH, the overall incidence of deep vein thrombosis and pulmonary embolism were 4.3%, and 2.3%, respectively [55]. The following factors were associated with increased deep vein thrombosis and pulmonary embolism risk: increasing age, black race, male sex, teaching hospital, congestive heart failure, coagulopathy, neurological disorders, paralysis, fluid and electrolyte disorders, obesity, and weight loss [56]. Patients that underwent clipping versus coiling had similar deep vein thrombosis and pulmonary embolism rates. Deep vein thrombosis and pulmonary embolism was associated with pulmonary/cardiac complication, infectious complication, ventriculostomy, and vasospasm. Treatment of venous thromboembolism with anticoagulation and/or inferior vena cava filter placement was not associated with immediate complications.

Recanalization

Endovascular coiling of intracranial aneurysms is associated with a recanalization rate of up to 25% [57]. Aneurysm size, presence of intrasaccular thrombus, and primary packing density have been discussed as possible risk factors [58]. The drawback of endovascular treatment is aneurysmal remnants or recurrences, which is safely and durably amenable to flow diversion [58].

Complications of Balloon Test Occlusion

Balloon test occlusion is a commonly used technique to assess the risk of cerebral ischemia prior to arterial sacrifice. When performed without prior test occlusion, sacrifice of the ICA carries a 26% stroke rate and a mortality rate of 12%; by contrast, internal carotid occlusion after test occlusion carried a stroke rate of 16.2% in a recent series [59]. The high stroke rate following a negative balloon occlusion test indicates the need for adjunctive testing prior to vessel sacrifice. neurological complications following balloon test occlusion include thromboembolic stroke in 0.4% of cases, arterial dissection in 1.2%, and aneurysm dissection in 0.2% [60]. Very rarely, overinflation of the balloon can rupture intracranial vessels or result in development of a carotid-cavernous fistula. Balloon inflation in the carotid bulb or basilar artery may also cause a vasovagal response with bradycardia and hypotension, or rarely, cardiac arrest. The vast majority of vasovagal responses respond quickly to balloon deflation, and do not require intra-venous fluid bolus or vasopressor administration.

Radiation Complications

A literature review indicates that skin entrance doses in excess of 2 Gy may occur in 73% of aneurysm embolization, resulting in subacute deterministic changes, including alopecia, skin erythema, or scalp tenderness in up to 40% of these patients [61]. Coil, balloon-assisted coiling, and flow diverter procedures appeared similar with respect to radiation exposure, and fluoroscopy and procedure times. Stent-assisted coiling was associated with a significantly higher radiation exposure and longer procedure and fluoroscopy times compared with other common aneurysm embolization techniques. However, stent-assisted coiling remains the treatment of choice for complex and challenging aneurysms, where extensive neck remodeling is required. But, when coil, balloon-assisted coiling, or flow diverter procedures may offer feasible treatment alternatives, patients and staff could benefit from reduced radiation exposure, and procedure and fluoroscopic times [61].

Other Complications

Other complications are retroperitoneal hemorrhage, and groin hematoma related to femoral artery puncture [62]. Delayed leukoencephalopathy is reported to be an inflammatory or allergic reaction to polymer material that is shed from catheters after aneurysm treatment and oral glucocorticoids seem to be a reasonable first-line treatment strategy [63].

Conclusion

Although endovascular devices and treatment techniques are continuously developing, these minimally invasive procedures still carry treatment-specific risks. Awareness of complications, their predisposing factors, and their prevention and management can further reduce morbidity and mortality.

References

[1] Pierot L, Cognard C, Anxionnat R, Ricolfi F. Ruptured intracranial aneurysms: factors affecting the rate and outcome of endovascular treatment complications in a series of 782 patients (CLARITY study). *Radiology*. 2010;256 (3):916-923.

[2] Vinuela F, Duckwiler G, Mawad M. Guglielmi detachable coil embolization of acute intracranial aneurysm: perioperative anatomical and clinical outcome in 403 patients. *J Neurosurg*. 1997;86 (3):475-482.

[3] Sluzewski M, van Rooij WJ, Rinkel GJ, Wijnalda D. Endovascular treatment of ruptured intracranial aneurysms with detachable coils: long-term clinical and serial angiographic results. *Radiology*. 2003;227 (3):720-724.

[4] Krag CH, Speiser L, Dalby RB. Long-term outcomes of endovascular simple coiling versus neurosurgical clipping of unruptured intracranial aneurysms: A systematic review and meta-analysis. *J Neurol* Sci. 2021 Mar 15;422:117338. doi: 10.1016/j.jns.2021.117338. Epub 2021 Feb 9. Erratum in: *J Neurol Sci*. 2021 May 15;424:117411. PMID: 33596532.

[5] Ye Z, Lv X. The formation mechanism of acute dissection of blood blister-like aneurysm and its implication of endovascular treatment. *Chin Neurosurg J*. 2021 Jun 3;7 (1):32.

[6] Xiong J, Tian J, Li Y, Li N, Lv X. Stent-Assisted Coiling of a Ruptured Supraclinoid Internal Carotid Artery Aneurysm in Tetralogy of Fallot Under Conscious Sedation. *Ann Indian Acad Neurol*. 2021 Jan-Feb;24 (1):116-118.

[7] Xiong J, Wang L, Tian J, Li Y, Gong C, Lv X. Stent-Assisted Coiling of Brain Aneurysms Under Conscious Sedation and Simultaneous Coronary Heart Disease Stenting: A New Concept. *Ann Indian Acad Neurol*. 2020 Jul-Aug;23 (4):572-574.

[8] Lv X, Yu J, Zhang W, Zhao X, Zhang H. Acute hemorrhagic cerebral artery dissection: Characteristics and endovascular treatment. *Neuroradiol J*. 2020 Apr;33 (2):112-117.

[9] Lv X, Ge H, Jin H, He H, Jiang C, Li Y. Endovascular treatment of unruptured posterior circulation intracranial aneurysms. *Ann Indian Acad Neurol*. 2016 Jul-Sep;19 (3):302-6.

[10] Ihn YK, Shin SH, Baik SK, Choi IS. Complications of endovascular treatment for intracranial aneurysms: Management and prevention. *Interv Neuroradiol*. 2018 Jun;24 (3):237-245. doi: 10.1177/1591019918758493. Epub 2018 Feb 21. PMID: 29466903; PMCID: PMC5967192.

[11] Bradac GB, Bergui M, Stura G, et al. Periprocedural morbidity and mortality by endovascular treatment of cerebral aneurysms with GDC: a retrospective 12-year experience of a single center. *Neurosurg* Rev. 2007;30 (2):117-125; discussion 125-116.

[12] Yu SC, Chan MS, Boet R, Wong JK, Lam JM, Poon WS. Intracranial aneurysms treated with Guglielmi detachable coils: midterm clinical and radiological outcome in 97 consecutive Chinese patients in Hong Kong. *AJNR Am J Neuroradiol*. 2004;25 (2):307-313.

[13] White PM, Lewis SC, Nahser H, Sellar RJ, Goddard T, Gholkar A. HydroCoil Endovascular Aneurysm Occlusion and Packing Study (HELPS trial): procedural safety and operator-assessed efficacy results. *AJNR Am J Neuroradiol*. 2008;29 (2):217-223.

[14] Algra AM, Greving JP, de Winkel J, Kurtelius A, Laban K, Verbaan D, van den Berg R, Vandertop W, Lindgren A, Krings T, Ming Woo PY, Chu Wong GK, Roozenbeek B, van Es ACGM, Dammers R, Etminan N, Boogaarts H, van Doormaal T, van der Zwan A, van der Schaaf IC, Rinkel GJE, Vergouwen MDI. Development of the SAFETEA Scores for Predicting Risks of Complications of Preventive

Endovascular or Microneurosurgical Intracranial Aneurysm Occlusion. *Neurology*. 2022 Sep 2:10.1212/WNL.0000000000200978. doi: 10.1212/WNL.0000000000200978. Epub ahead of print. PMID: 36240099.

[15] Soeda A, Sakai N, Sakai H, et al. Thromboembolic events associated with Guglielmi detachable coil embolization of asymptomatic cerebral aneurysms: evaluation of 66 consecutive cases with use of diffusion-weighted MR imaging. *AJNR Am J Neuroradiol* 2003; 24 (1):127–132.

[16] Pelz DM, Lownie SP, Fox AJ. Thromboembolic events associated with the treatment of cerebral aneurysms with Guglielmi detachable coils. *AJNR Am J Neuroradiol* 1998;19 (8):1541–1547.

[17] Derdeyn CP, Cross DT III, Moran CJ, et al. Postprocedure ischemic events after treatment of intracranial aneurysms with Guglielmi detachable coils. *J Neurosurg* 2002;96 (5):837–843.

[18] Kanaan H, Jankowitz B, Aleu A, et al. In-stent thrombosis and stenosis after neck-remodeling device-assisted coil embolization of intracranial aneurysms. *Neurosurgery* 2010;67 (6):1523–1532, discussion 1532–1533.

[19] Krishnakumar H, Mascitelli J, Hassan A, Leary J, Son C. Treatment of cerebral aneurysms with flow diversion or stent assisted coiling in patients on concurrent oral anticoagulation. *Neuroradiol J*. 2022 Nov 21:19714009221114443. doi: 10.1177/19714009221114443. Epub ahead of print. PMID: 36409963.

[20] Bodily KD, Cloft HJ, Lanzino G, Fiorella DJ, White PM, Kallmes DF. Stent-assisted coiling in acutely ruptured intracranial aneurysms: a qualitative, systematic review of the literature. *AJNR Am J Neuroradiol*. 2011 Aug;32 (7):1232-6.

[21] Gaudino C, Navone SE, Da Ros V, Guarnaccia L, Marfia G, Pantano P, Peschillo S, Triulzi FM, Biraschi F. Incidence of intra-procedural complications according to the timing of endovascular treatment in ruptured intracranial aneurysms. *Front Neurol*. 2023 Jan 11;13:1096651.

[22] Ryu CW, Park S, Shin HS, Koh JS. Complications in Stent-Assisted Endovascular Therapy of Ruptured Intracranial Aneurysms and Relevance to Antiplatelet Administration: A Systematic Review. *AJNR Am J Neuroradiol*. 2015 Sep;36 (9):1682-8.

[23] Qureshi AI, Luft AR, Sharma M, Guterman LR, Hopkins LN. Prevention and treatment of thromboembolic and ischemic complications associated with endovascular procedures: part II — clinical aspects and recommendations. *Neurosurgery*. 2000;46 (6):1360-1375; discussion 1375-1366.

[24] Zanaty M, Osorno-Cruz C, Byer S, Roa JA, Limaye K, Ishii D, Nakagawa D, Torner J, Yongjun L, Ortega-Gutiérrez S, Samaniego EA, Allan L, Hasan D. Tirofiban Protocol Protects Against Delayed Cerebral Ischemia: A Case-Series Study. *Neurosurgery*. 2020 Oct 15;87 (5):E552-E556. doi: 10.1093/neuros/nyaa170. PMID: 32415850.

[25] Gentric JC, Brisson J, Batista AL, Ghostine J, Raymond J, Roy D, Weill A. Safety of Abciximab injection during endovascular treatment of ruptured aneurysms. *Interv Neuroradiol*. 2015 Jun;21 (3):332-6. doi: 10.1177/1591019915582001. Epub 2015 May 11. PMID: 25964436; PMCID: PMC4757264.

[26] Brinjikji W, Morales-Valero SF, Murad MH, Cloft HJ, Kallmes DF. Rescue treatment of thromboembolic complications during endovascular treatment of cerebral aneurysms: a meta-analysis. *AJNR Am J Neuroradiol*. 2015 Jan;36 (1):121-5. doi: 10.3174/ajnr.A4066. Epub 2014 Jul 31. PMID: 25082819; PMCID: PMC7965919.

[27] Aggour M, Pierot L, Kadziolka K, Gomis P, Graftieaux JP. Abciximab treatment modalities for thromboembolic events related to aneurysm coiling. *Neurosurgery*. 2010;67 (2 Suppl Operative):503-8.

[28] Shen G, Jia Z, Zhao L, Lu G, Liu S, Shi H. The safety and efficacy of a low dose of tirofiban for early complications during and after stent-assisted coiling of ruptured intracranial aneurysms: A propensity matching study. *Clin Neurol Neurosurg*. 2022 Mar;214:107132. doi: 10.1016/j.clineuro.2022.107132. Epub 2022 Jan 15. PMID: 35151058.

[29] Fourie P, Duncan IC. Microsnare-assisted mechanical removal of intraprocedural distal middle cerebral arterial thromboembolism. *AJNR Am J Neuroradiol* 2003;24 (4):630–632.

[30] Cloft HJ, Kallmes DF. Cerebral aneurysm perforations complicating therapy with Guglielmi detachable coils: a meta-analysis. *AJNR Am J Neuroradiol* 2002;23 (10):1706–1709.

[31] Doerfler A, Wanke I, Egelhof T, et al. Aneurysmal rupture during embolization with Guglielmi detachable coils: causes, management, and outcome. *AJNR Am J Neuroradiol* 2001;22 (10): 1825–1832.
[32] Willinsky R, terBrugge K. Use of a second microcatheter in the management of a perforation during endovascular treatment of a cerebral aneurysm. *AJNR Am J Neuroradiol* 2000;21 (8): 1537–1539.
[33] Fleming JB, Hoh BL, Simon SD, et al. Rebleeding risk after treatment of ruptured intracranial aneurysms. *J Neurosurg* 2011;114 (6):1778–1784.
[34] Byrne JV, Sohn MJ, Molyneux AJ, Chir B. Five-year experience in using coil embolization for ruptured intracranial aneurysms: outcomes and incidence of late rebleeding. *J Neurosurg* 1999; 90 (4):656–663.
[35] Lv X, Chen Z, Liu L, Jiang C, Wang G, Wang J. Rupture of Intradural Giant Aneurysms: The Mode of Treatment, Anatomical, and Mechanical Factors. *Neurol India*. 2019 Sep-Oct;67 (5):1194-1199. doi: 10.4103/0028-3886.271250. PMID: 31744943.
[36] Abdelkhalek H, Abdelhameed EA, Zakarea A, El Malky I. Predictors of flow diverter stent in large and giant unruptured intracranial aneurysms, single-center experience. *Neurol Sci*. 2022 Nov;43 (11):6399-6405. doi: 10.1007/s10072-022-06336-w. Epub 2022 Aug 19. PMID: 35984605; PMCID: PMC9616764.
[37] Lee J, Kim DH, Lee SH, Moon JH, Yang SY, Cho KT, Kim BH. Stent-assisted Coiling vs. Flow Diverter for Treating Blood Blister-like Aneurysms : A Proportion Meta-analysis. *Clin Neuroradiol*. 2022 Dec;32 (4):889-902. doi: 10.1007/s00062-022-01160-3. Epub 2022 Apr 11. PMID: 35403855.
[38] Fiorella D, Albuquerque FC, Deshmukh VR, McDougall CG. Monorail snare technique for the recovery of stretched platinum coils: technical case report. *Neurosurgery* 2005;57 (1, Suppl):E210, discussion E210.
[39] Fessler RD, Ringer AJ, Qureshi AI, Guterman LR, Hopkins LN. Intracranial stent placement to trap an extruded coil during endovascular aneurysm treatment: technical note. *Neurosurgery* 2000;46 (1):248–251, discussion 251–253.
[40] Sugiu K, Martin J-B, Jean B, Rüfenacht DA. Rescue balloon procedure for an emergency situation during coil embolization for cerebral aneurysms. Technical note. *J Neurosurg* 2002;96 (2):373–376.
[41] Nii K, Onizuka M, Kaneko Y, Aikawa H, Tsutsumi M, Kazekawa K. Irretrievable unraveled coil remaining in the vascular lumen between the cerebral aneurysm and puncture site. *J Neuroendovasc Therapy* 2009;3:42–46.
[42] Luo CB, Chang FC, Teng MMH, Guo WY, Chang CY. Stent management of coil herniation in embolization of internal carotid aneurysms. *AJNR Am J Neuroradiol* 2008;29 (10):1951–1955.
[43] Murayama Y, Nien YL, Duckwiler G, et al. Guglielmi detachable coil embolization of cerebral aneurysms: 11 years' experience. *J Neurosurg* 2003;98 (5):959–966.
[44] Lee SH, Suh DC, Park JC, Lee DH. A new retrieval method for an already detached coil mass in the aneurysm sac: 'Thread and catch' technique. *Interv Neuroradiol*. 2018 Apr;24 (2):146-149. doi: 10.1177/1591019917747249. Epub 2017 Dec 14. PMID: 29239684; PMCID: PMC5847014.
[45] Walcott BP, Stapleton CJ, Choudhri O, Patel AB. Flow diversion for the treatment of intracranial aneurysms. *JAMA Neurol* 2016;73 (8):1002-1008.
[46] Bonney PA, Connor M, Fujii T, Singh P, Koch MJ, Stapleton CJ, Mack WJ, Walcott BP. Failure of Flow Diverter Therapy: Predictors and Management Strategies. *Neurosurgery*. 2020 Jan 1;86 (Suppl 1):S64-S73. doi: 10.1093/neuros/nyz305. PMID: 31838530.
[47] Lv X, Yang H, Liu P, Li Y. Flow-diverter devices in treatment of intracranial aneurysms: A Meta-analysis and systematic review. *Neuroradiol J*. 2016;29 (1):66-71.
[48] Cloft HJ, Jensen ME, Kallmes DF, Dion JE. Arterial dissections complicating cerebral angiography and cerebrovascular interventions. *AJNR Am J Neuroradiol* 2000;21 (3):541–545.
[49] Inamasu J, Guiot BH. Iatrogenic vertebral artery injury. *Acta Neurol Scand* 2005;112 (6):349–357.
[50] Engelter ST, Brandt T, Debette S, et al. Cervical Artery Dissection in Ischemic Stroke Patients (CADISP) Study Group. Antiplatelets versus anticoagulation in cervical artery dissection. *Stroke* 2007; 38 (9):2605–2611.
[51] Pham MH, Rahme RJ, Arnaout O, et al. Endovascular stenting of extracranial carotid and vertebral artery dissections: a systematic review of the literature. *Neurosurgery* 2011;68 (4):856–866, discussion 866.

[52] Hoh BL, Ogilvy CS. Endovascular treatment of cerebral vasospasm: transluminal balloon angioplasty, intra-arterial papaverine, and intra-arterial nicardipine. *Neurosurg Clin N Am* 2005; 16 (3):501–516.

[53] American Society of Interventional and Therapeutic Neuroradiology. Mechanical and pharmacologic treatment of vasospasm. *AJNR Am J Neuroradiol* 2001;22 (8, Suppl):S26–S27.

[54] Bauer AM, Rasmussen PA. Treatment of intracranial vasospasm following subarachnoid hemorrhage. *Front Neurol* 2014;5:72.

[55] Pan J, Bonow RH, Temkin N, Robinson EF, Sekhar LN, Levitt MR, Lele AV. Incidence and Risk Model of Venous Thromboembolism in Patients with Aneurysmal Subarachnoid Hemorrhage. *World Neurosurg*. 2023 Jan 16:S1878-8750 (23)00061-X. doi: 10.1016/j.wneu.2023.01.045. Epub ahead of print. PMID: 36657716.

[56] Kshettry VR, Rosenbaum BP, Seicean A, Kelly ML, Schiltz NK, Weil RJ. Incidence and risk factors associated with in-hospital venous thromboembolism after aneurysmal subarachnoid hemorrhage. *J Clin Neurosci*. 2014 Feb;21 (2):282-6. doi: 10.1016/j.jocn.2013.07.003. Epub 2013 Oct 13. PMID: 24128773.

[57] Nguyen TN, Hoh BL, Amin-Hanjani S, Pryor JC, Ogilvy CS. Comparison of ruptured vs unruptured aneurysms in recanalization after coil embolization. *Surg Neurol*. 2007;68 (1):19-23.

[58] Akgul E, Onan HB, Islek I, Tonge M, Durmus Y, Barburoglu M, Azizova A, Erol C, Hakyemez B, Sencer S, Aydin K, Arat A. Flow diverter stents in the treatment of recanalized intracranial aneurysms. *Interv Neuroradiol*. 2021 Aug;27 (4):481-489. doi: 10.1177/1591019921990507. Epub 2021 Jan 28. PMID: 33509011; PMCID: PMC8580529.

[59] McIvor NP, Willinsky RA, TerBrugge KG, Rutka JA, Freeman JL. Validity of test occlusion studies prior to internal carotid artery sacrifice. *Head Neck*. 1994 Jan-Feb;16 (1):11-6. doi: 10.1002/hed.2880160104. PMID: 8125782.

[60] Wang AY, Chen CC, Lai HY, Lee ST. Balloon test occlusion of the internal carotid artery with stump pressure ratio and venous phase delay technique. *J Stroke Cerebrovasc Dis*. 2013 Nov;22 (8):e533-40. doi: 10.1016/j.jstrokecerebrovasdis.2013.05.036. Epub 2013 Jul 11. PMID: 23849747.

[61] Weerakkody RA, Walsh SR, Cousins C, Goldstone KE, Tang TY, Gaunt ME. Radiation exposure during endovascular aneurysm repair. *Br J Surg*. 2008 Jun;95 (6):699-702. doi: 10.1002/bjs.6229. PMID: 18446782.

[62] Lv X, Wang G, Wang J. 2021. *Craniospinal Vascular Diseases and Endovascular Neurosurgery*. Nova Science, NY, USA.

[63] Ridwan S, Kandyba JA, Schug A, Malsagov E, Karageorgos N, Hans FJ. Delayed Leukoencephalopathy and Foreign Body Reaction After Endovascular Treatment in Patients With Intracranial Aneurysms and Aneurysmal Subarachnoid Hemorrhage-A Systematic Review of the Literature. *Front Surg*. 2021 Dec 23;8:732603. doi: 10.3389/fsurg.2021.732603. PMID: 35004833; PMCID: PMC8733731.

Chapter 23

Postprocedural Rupture of Intracranial Unruptured Aneurysms after Deployment of a Flow Diverter

Jinlu Yu*
Department of Neurosurgery, First Hospital of Jilin University, Changchun, China

Abstract

Postprocedural rupture of intracranial unruptured aneurysms after flow diverter (FD) deployment is catastrophic. At present, the cause of this complication is poorly understood. Therefore, we conducted a review. The findings are as follows. The incidence of postprocedural rupture of intracranial unruptured aneurysms after FD deployment is <5%. Although postprocedural aneurysm rupture can occur within days or weeks following FD deployment, it is most likely to occur 1 month after surgery. The causes of postprocedural aneurysm rupture include an increase in intra-aneurysmal pressure caused by a detrimental flow pattern induced by FD deployment, an increase in aneurysmal volume caused by the rapid formation of red thrombi, and progressive destruction of the aneurysm wall by inflammation and autolysis. In patients with postprocedural aneurysm rupture after FD deployment, aneurysm size was an independent risk factor, as large aneurysms had a greater postprocedural rupture rate. To date, there have been no effective means to prevent postprocedural aneurysm rupture after FD deployment, but several management strategies, including steroid administration, adjunctive coiling, overlapping FDs and coiling followed by staged FD deployment, have been attempted. Postprocedural aneurysm rupture after FD deployment may result in fatal hemorrhage and carotid cavernous fistula. If the patient is stable, prompt surgery to reduce intracranial pressure is necessary. Then, the ruptured aneurysm requires isolation from the cerebral circulation by open surgery, covered stent deployment and additional FD deployment. For a carotid cavernous fistula, transvenous embolization can be used. The prognosis of postprocedural aneurysm rupture after FD deployment is poor.

Keywords: intracranial unruptured aneurysm, flow diverter, postprocedural rupture, prognosis

* Corresponding Authpr's Email: jlyu@jlu.edu.cn.

In: Understanding and Managing Cerebral Aneurysms
Editor: Xianli Lv
ISBN: 979-8-89113-608-3

1. Introduction

Flow diverter (FD) deployment is useful for curing large or giant saccular wide-neck, fusiform, dissecting, or recurrent intracranial unruptured aneurysms (Figure 1) [1-3]. An FD provides more than 30% metal coverage; thus, after deployment, progressive thrombosis within the aneurysm and remodeling of the vessel wall can be expected [4-8]. However, FD deployment for unruptured aneurysms has inherent risks, including ischemic and hemorrhagic complications and worsening mass effects [9-13]. Among the hemorrhagic complications, aneurysm rupture after FD deployment is catastrophic, and most patients have no opportunity for further treatment [4, 14-16]. Currently, the cause, prevention and treatment of postprocedural rupture of intracranial unruptured aneurysms after FD deployment are poorly understood. Therefore, we present a literature review of this issue and report our experience.

2. Incidence and Timing

2.1. Incidence

The incidence of postprocedural rupture of unruptured intracranial aneurysms after FD deployment varies among reports but is typically <5% [14, 15, 17-21]. In Brinjikji et al.'s meta-analysis of intracranial aneurysms treated by FDs, 1654 aneurysms among 1451 patients were included in 29 studies, for a rate of 4% [18].

In a multicenter registry study on the embolization of intracranial aneurysms via the Pipeline Embolization Device (PED) (Medtronic, Minneapolis, Minnesota, USA) in China, of 1322 aneurysms in 1171 patients, the incidence rate was 2.1% [19]. According to the European Society of Minimally Invasive Neurological Therapy (ESMINT), a retrospective analysis of delayed aneurysm rupture after FD deployment revealed 1421 aneurysms in 1274 patients, for a rate of 1% [21]. In a multicenter international retrospective study of the PED registry of 906 aneurysms in 793 patients, the incidence rate was 0.6% [14].

The above rates of postprocedural aneurysm rupture were retrieved from the data analyses of aneurysms of various sizes that were treated by FD deployment. Large aneurysms may have a higher risk of rupture after FD deployment. According to the results of the retrospective analysis of the ESMINT cohort, the incidence of delayed aneurysm rupture after FD deployment in the subgroup of aneurysms >10 mm was 2.1%, which was greater than the 1% incidence of delayed rupture in all aneurysms [21]. In addition, in Briganti et al.'s meta-analysis of 18 studies involving a total of 1704 aneurysms in 1483 patients treated with FDs, the incidence of postoperative subarachnoid hemorrhage in patients with large and giant aneurysms was 4%, which was greater than the 1.8% incidence of postoperative subarachnoid hemorrhage in patients with small aneurysms [22].

According to the above clinical trials and studies, the vast majority of enrolled aneurysms were unruptured; therefore, the incidence of postprocedural rupture of intracranial unruptured aneurysms should conform to these data.

2.2. Occurrence Timing

Postprocedural aneurysm rupture can occur in the early or late period following FD deployment [23, 24]. At present, the most widely accepted definition of the early postoperative period is within 1 month after treatment [19]. Most postprocedural aneurysm ruptures occur in the early postoperative period following FD deployment [25]. In Sweid et al.'s study, the rate was 88% in the early postoperative period [20]. In a Chinese study, the rate was 95% [19]. In Rouchaud et al.'s systematic review of 81 aneurysm ruptures after FD deployment, the rate of aneurysm rupture within 1 month postsurgery was 77%, and subsequent rupture rates were as follows: less than 1 day in 10% of cases, 1 to 7 days in 33% of cases, 7 days to 1 month in 35% of cases, and more than 1 month in 23% of cases [9].

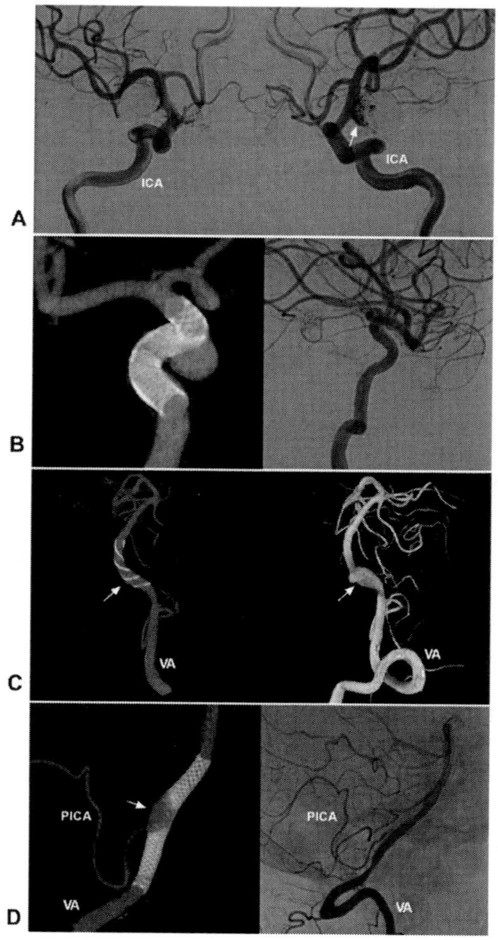

Abbreviations: DSA: digital subtracted angiography, FD: flow diverter, ICA: internal carotid artery, PICA: posterior inferior cerebellar artery, VA: vertebral artery.

Figure 1. Comparison of patient prognosis between patients treated with traditional stents and flow diverters. A: Left panel: DSA image showing that the aneurysm was coiled with the assistance of a traditional stent; Right panel: DSA at the six-month follow-up showing that the aneurysm (arrow) had recurred. B: Left panel: Vaso-reconstructive DSA showing that the FD was deployed to cover the aneurysm; Right: DSA at the ten-month follow-up showing that the aneurysm had healed. C: Left penal: Vaso-reconstructive DSA showing that the LEO stent (Balt Extrusion, Montmorency, France) was deployed to cover the dissection (arrow); Right panel: DSA at the six-month follow-up showing that the dissection (arrow) progressed. D: Left panel: Vaso-reconstructive DSA showing that the FD was deployed to cover the dissection (arrow); Right: DSA at the eight-month follow-up showing that the dissection healed.

3. Causes and Risk Factors

3.1. Rupture Causes

FD deployment can lead to an increase in intra-aneurysmal pressure through the induction of a detrimental flow pattern that presents with an enhanced 'inflow jet" into the aneurysm (Figures 2A-B) [23, 25, 26]. Alterations in intra-aneurysmal shear forces to new points and blood outflow restriction from FD deployment can result in aneurysm rupture [27]. Even with the assistance of adjunctive coiling, the aneurysm can still rupture following FD deployment (Figure 2C). A computational fluid dynamic study showed that unstable flow patterns and greater energy loss after FD deployment may be important risk factors related to aneurysm rupture [28]. Acute aneurysm rupture on the same day as FD deployment is likely due to an increase in intra-aneurysmal pressure (Figure 3).

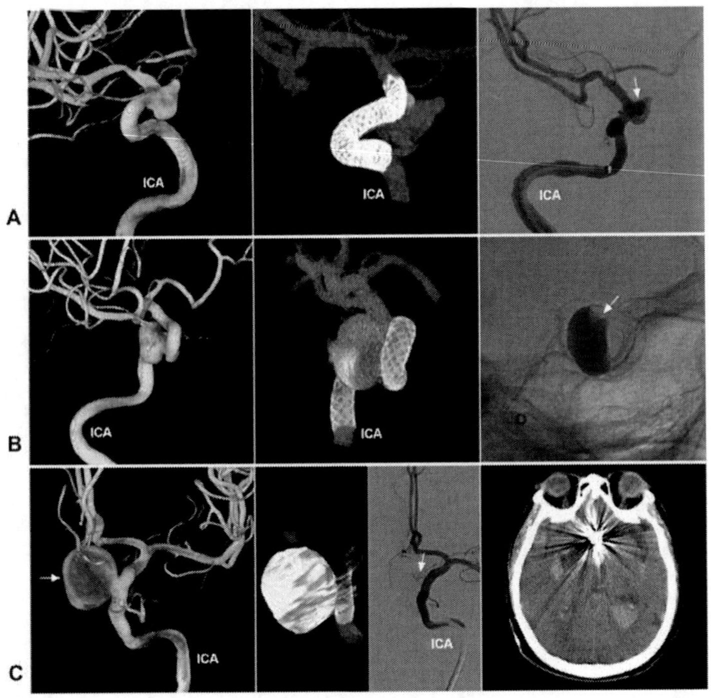

Abbreviations: CT: computed tomography, DSA: digital subtracted angiography, ICA: internal carotid artery, FD: flow diverter.

Figure 2. FD deployment in anterior circulation aneurysms with an enhanced 'inflow jet" or aneurysm filling. A: Left panel: DSA image showing a large aneurysm in the ophthalmic segment of the ICA; Middle panel: Vaso-reconstructive DSA image showing that the FD was deployed to cover the aneurysm neck; Right panel: DSA after FD deployment showing the 'inflow jet" (arrow) into the aneurysm. B: Left panel: DSA image showing a large aneurysm in the clinoid segment of the ICA; Middle panel: Vaso-reconstructive DSA image showing that the FD was deployed to cover the aneurysm neck; Right panel: DSA after PED deployment showing contrast agent retention; the arrow indicates the inflow zone of blood flow. C: Left panel: DSA image showing a large aneurysm (arrow) in the ophthalmic segment of the ICA; Middle left panel: Vaso-reconstructive DSA image showing that the FD was deployed to cover the aneurysm neck and that the aneurysm was coiled; Middle right panel: DSA image showing small aneurysm filling (arrow); Right panel: CT image on the first day after FD deployment showing extensive intracranial hemorrhage, indicating that the aneurysm ruptured.

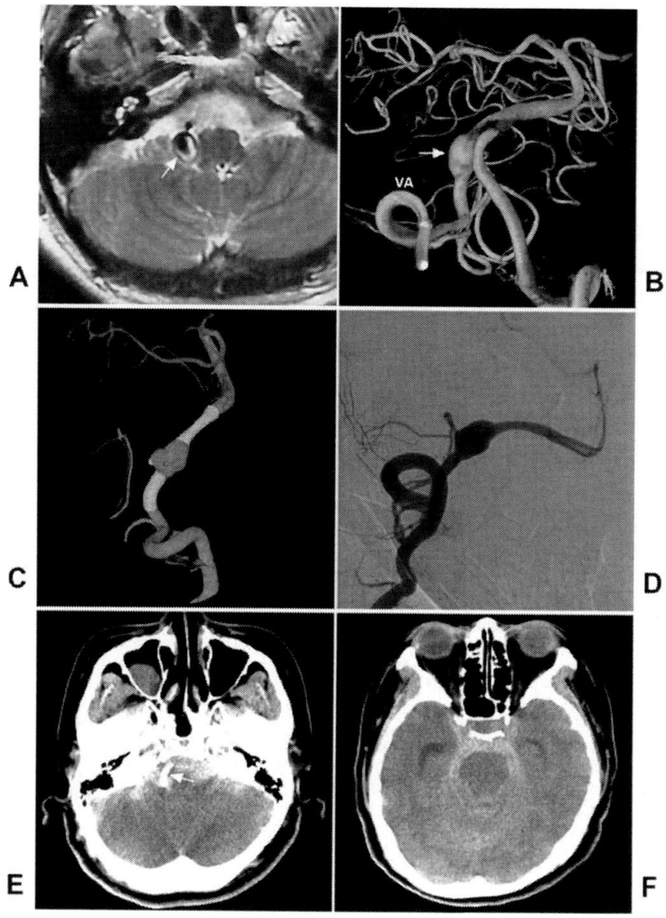

Abbreviations: CT: computed tomography, DSA: digital subtracted angiography, FD: flow diverter, MRI: magnetic resonance imaging, VA: vertebral artery.

Figure 3. Acute VA aneurysm rupture on the same day as FD deployment. A: MR image showing an aneurysm (arrow) beside the brainstem. B: DSA image showing a large irregular dissecting aneurysm (arrow) in the VA. C: Vaso-reconstructive DSA showing that the FD was deployed to cover the aneurysm. D: Immediate DSA after FD deployment showing the aneurysm filling. E-F: Postoperative 6-hour CT image showing subarachnoid hemorrhage. The arrow in E indicates the FD.

After FD deployment, aneurysmal thrombosis occurs [29]. Rapid formation of red thrombi may lead to aneurysm volume expansion, thus producing a mechanical force that tears the aneurysm [23, 30, 31]. Red thrombi are unstable and contain high concentrations of macrophages that provoke a cascade of inflammation and autolysis (Figure 4). Inflammation and autolysis may result in progressive destruction of the aneurysm wall, which may explain postprocedural rupture of intracranial unruptured aneurysms after FD deployment in some cases [31-33]. In Kulcsar et al.'s report of 13 postprocedural aneurysm ruptures, 80% of the aneurysm cavity was occluded by a thrombus, and 2 aneurysms were completely thrombosed [25]. Therefore, an intra-aneurysmal red thrombus may not prevent aneurysm rupture until the red thrombus in the aneurysm is replaced by stable fibrous tissue [31].

However, red thrombus formation, inflammation and autolysis can also occur in large and giant aneurysms embolized by coiling with/without the assistance of low-metal-coverage stents. Why did postprocedural aneurysm rupture occur less frequently? When thrombi form within large and giant aneurysms after coiling, the aneurysm neck is open, and even if covered by a traditional stent, thrombi can migrate toward the neck, thus relieving the pressure within the aneurysm. In contrast, FD deployment may not only restrict thrombus expansion in aneurysms but also increase intra-aneurysmal pressure, and any residual filling of the aneurysm may preserve the potential for postprocedural rupture [31, 34].

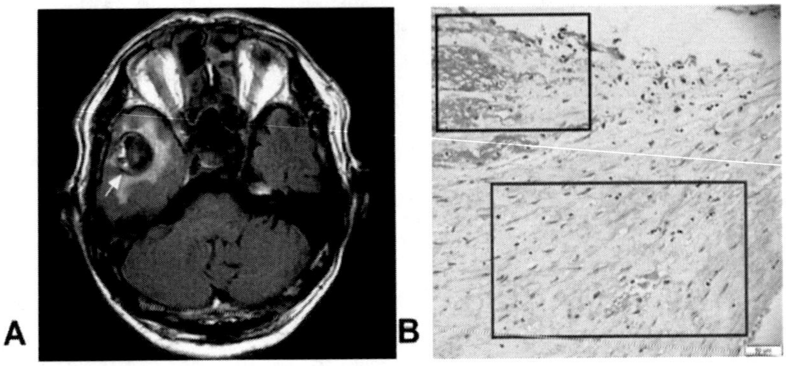

Figure 4. Inflammation in the thrombosed aneurysm wall. A: Magnetic resonance imaging showing a thrombosed aneurysm (arrow) in the temporal lobe with edema. B: Pathological examination (hematoxylin-eosin staining) showing granulation tissue hyperplasia and chronic inflammatory cell infiltration in the thrombus (blue frame) of the aneurysm cavity; in the aneurysm wall (black frame), fibrinoid necrosis and chronic inflammatory cell infiltration can be observed.

3.2. Risk Factors

For postprocedural rupture of intracranial unruptured aneurysms after FD deployment, multiple risk factors should be considered. Aneurysm size is an independent risk factor, and small (<7 mm) and medium (7-<10 mm) aneurysms with regular shapes are safe and rarely rupture after FD deployment [14, 25, 28, 35-37]. After FD deployment, large (10-<25 mm) and giant (>25 mm) aneurysms exhibit more detrimental flow patterns and faster accumulation of thrombi. In addition, the aneurysm wall may become thinner and have more fragile microfissures in large and giant aneurysms (Figure 5) [9, 14, 19, 25, 38].

Therefore, large and giant aneurysms are associated with a greater risk of postprocedural rupture, which has been confirmed by subsequent studies. Kallmes et al. performed a statistical analysis and showed that the rate of aneurysm rupture after FD deployment was greater for giant aneurysms (4.5%) than for large (0.6%) or small aneurysms (0%) ($P < 0.01$) [14]. According to the retrospective analysis of the ESMINT cohort, the size of all delayed ruptured aneurysms was >10 mm [21]. In a Chinese trial, an aneurysm >10 mm in size was found to be an independent predictor of postprocedural aneurysm rupture in the early postoperative period [19].

Antiplatelet therapy is also problematic when the aneurysm is not completely resolved after FD deployment by preventing platelet aggregation and thrombosis (Figure 6) [32]. Other factors, such as FD type and aneurysm location, cannot be considered risk factors [14, 22, 25, 39].

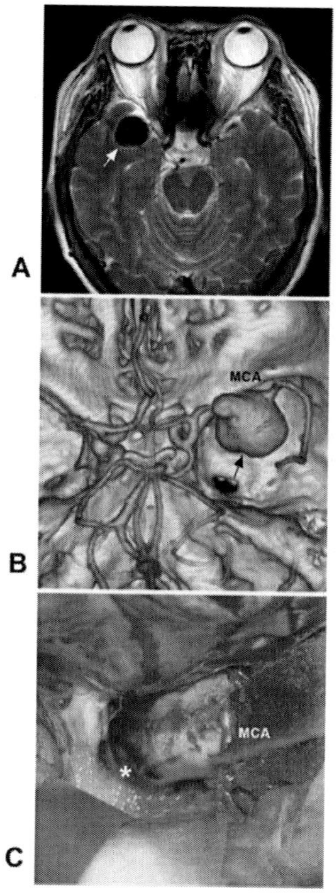

Abbreviations: MCA: middle cerebral artery.

Figure 5. Weakness of the large aneurysm wall. A: Magnetic resonance imaging showing a large aneurysm (arrow) in the Sylvian fissure. B: Computed tomography angiography image showing the aneurysm located at the MCA. C: Intraoperative image showing the weak dissection with an interwall hematoma (asterisk).

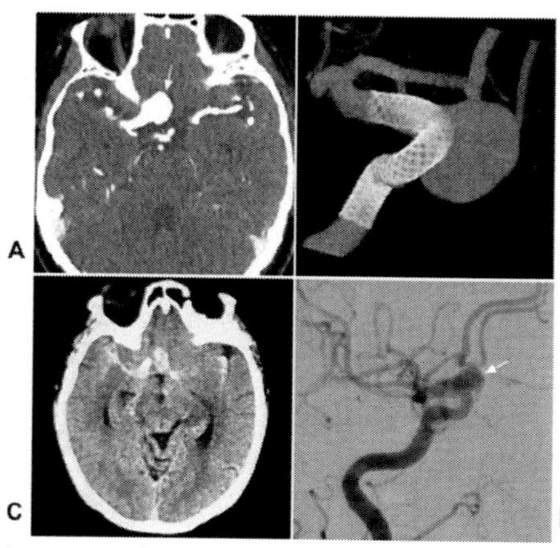

Abbreviations: CT: computed tomography, DSA: digital subtracted angiography, FD: flow diverter.

Figure 6. Delayed aneurysm rupture following FD deployment. A: CT image showing an intracranial unruptured aneurysm (arrow). B: Vaso-reconstructive DSA showing that the FD was deployed to cover the aneurysm in the ophthalmic segment of the internal carotid artery. C: Postoperative one-and-a half-month CT image showing subarachnoid hemorrhage, indicating that the aneurysm ruptured. D: DSA showing that the aneurysm was filled (arrow).

4. Clinical Demonstration

Patients can develop severe headache before postprocedural aneurysm rupture due to aneurysm expansion or microexsanguination [32]. Hampton et al. reported that a patient with a giant aneurysm in the carotid terminus, which ultimately ruptured, experienced worsening headache 5 days after FD deployment [23]. Sentinel headache can persist for a long time. For instance, in Chow et al.'s report, a patient suffered severe intractable headache 8 days after FD deployment, and the headache lasted for 12 days. Twenty days after FD deployment, the patient suddenly collapsed due to aneurysm rupture [31].

After aneurysm rupture following FD deployment, intradural aneurysms can present with subarachnoid hemorrhage, intracerebral hematoma, intraventricular hemorrhage or a combination of these hemorrhages [21]. Cavernous carotid aneurysms can cause the development of a carotid cavernous fistula (CCF) [25].

5. Prevention

Until now, there have been no effective means to prevent aneurysm rupture after FD deployment, but subsequent management can be attempted.

5.1. Steroid Administration

Steroids may help to relieve side effects from the inflammatory response and have been used for symptomatic aneurysms. Roccatagliata et al. reported that in 3 patients with thrombosed aneurysms presenting with acute headache, progressive hemiparesis and acute ophthalmoplegia, symptoms resolved after the administration of corticosteroids as the sole therapy [40]. Osorno-Cruz et al. reported that a patient with bilateral optic tract edema following FD-assisted coiling of a large ophthalmic aneurysm was treated with corticosteroids and repeat FD deployment, and the symptoms improved [41]. Steroid therapy was proposed prior to or at the same time as FD therapy, which might help to stabilize thrombus formation and reduce aneurysm rupture risk. However, the effect of steroids is not predictable [23, 42]. Kulcsar et al. reported 13 cases of aneurysm rupture after FD deployment; although 8 patients received steroids, the aneurysms still ruptured [25]. Therefore, additional studies are needed.

5.2. Adjunctive Coiling

Adjunctive coiling during FD deployment may decrease the risk of aneurysm rupture [25, 43-47]. The reason may be that adjunctive coils can stabilize the thrombus and accelerate aneurysm occlusion [48]. Concerns about aneurysm rupture after FD deployment are so serious that Balt Extrusion issued a medical device alert instructing practitioners not to use the Silk FD (Balt Extrusion, Montmorency, France) without coils [49]. However, adjunctive coiling was not always effective at preventing aneurysm rupture following FD deployment (Figure 2C) [10, 33,

50]. In the review by Rouchaud et al. of ruptured aneurysms after FD deployment, approximately 20% of the aneurysms accepted adjunctive coiling [9].

During coiling, the aneurysm neck should receive increased attention because this region can also rupture. In Ikeda et al.'s report, after aneurysm rupture, an autopsy confirmed that the rupture occurred at the proximal inflow zone near the neck due to direct stress caused by residual blood flow after FD deployment [34]. In addition, the distal outflow zone near the neck was not absolutely safe. According to a study of flow dynamics, high-velocity slipstreams may have an impact on distal but not proximal aneurysm necks after coiling aneurysms, which indicates that coiling aneurysm necks may be necessary [51, 52].

5.3. Overlapping FDs

Overlapping FDs can reduce blood flow to promote aneurysm occlusion and prevent aneurysm regrowth [26, 53, 54]. Therefore, it can be concluded that overlapping FDs may be useful for preventing postprocedural aneurysm rupture in large and giant aneurysms, particularly when jet flow occurs after FD deployment [55]. In Kim et al.'s report, a giant aneurysm initially treated with a single FD and coiling experienced symptom aggravation, which was relieved after an additional FD was deployed, and complete aneurysm occlusion was achieved [56]. To overlap FDs, the longer FD should be as long as possible to cover the aneurysm neck and must be fixed; the additional shorter FD should cover only the aneurysm neck, and the diameter of the second FD should be equal to that of the first [57].

However, the strategy of overlapping FDs is not a panacea. According to our previous review, postprocedural aneurysm rupture can still occur, despite overlapping FDs in some aneurysms [58]. The reason may be that in some aneurysms, although overlapping FDs decrease blood flow into the aneurysm, they conversely increase parent artery resistance, potentially resulting in a greater increase in intra-aneurysmal pressure [34].

5.4. Coiling Followed by Staged FD Deployment

After first-stage coiling, the aneurysm may become small or medium in size. Then, following second-stage FD deployment, minor increases in intra-aneurysmal pressure may reduce the risk of delayed aneurysm rupture (Figure 7). In addition, staged FD deployment is technically easy and safe [59]. However, more evidence is needed for coiling followed by staged FD deployment for the treatment of intracranial unruptured aneurysms.

5.5. Other Methods

Because intra-aneurysmal pressure may increase after FD deployment, controlling postoperative blood pressure may be a practical method. However, further clinical studies are necessary. In addition, a low dose of antiplatelet therapy is important for stabilizing intra-aneurysmal thrombi and aneurysm walls in the early stage; therefore, reducing the dose of antiplatelet agents may be a reasonable way to reduce the risk of aneurysm rupture after FD deployment [34]. The new generation of FDs with modified surfaces may reduce the need for antiplatelet therapy, even if single antiplatelet therapy is sufficient for FD deployment, which may reduce the risk of aneurysm rupture after FD deployment [60].

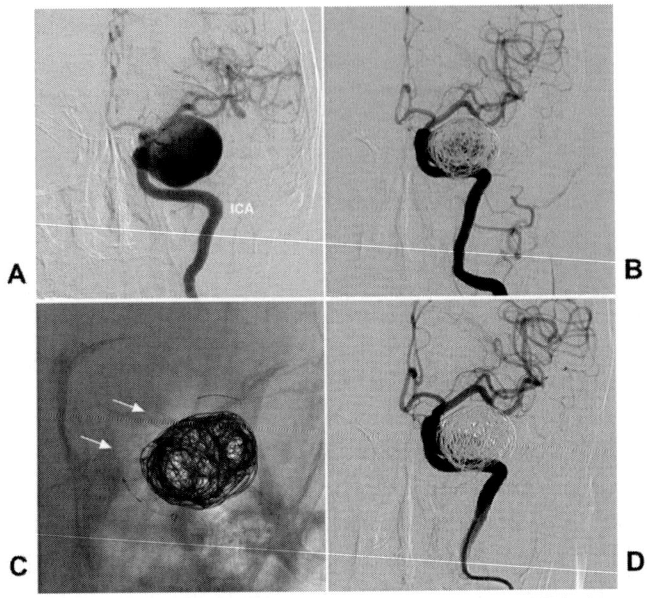

Abbreviations: DSA: digital subtracted angiography, FD: flow diverter, ICA: internal carotid artery.

Figure 7. Coiling followed by staged FD deployment. A: DSA image showing a giant aneurysm in the ophthalmic segment of the ICA. B: DSA showing that the aneurysm was coiled first. C: After three months, FD deployment was performed, and an X-ray image showing the FD (arrows) that covered the aneurysm neck. D: DSA after FD deployment showing less blood flow into the aneurysm.

6. Management and Prognosis

6.1. Management

When aneurysm rupture occurs after FD deployment in a stable patient, prompt treatment is necessary. The increase in intracranial pressure resulting from hemorrhage should be resolved by external ventricular drainage, hematoma drainage, or surgical hematoma evacuation. Then, ruptured aneurysms may require isolation from the cerebral circulation as soon as possible. During open surgery, resolving the aneurysm with clipping is a good choice. However, because aneurysms are often large or giant, open surgery is often difficult, so endovascular treatment can be considered.

If the aneurysm is located in a thick parent artery, such as the intracranial internal carotid artery or vertebral artery, deployment of a covered stent can be attempted. In Chen et al.'s report, a large supraclinoid internal carotid artery aneurysm was treated with FD and adjunctive coiling. After 11 hours, the aneurysm ruptured and was successfully treated with a Willis covered stent (MicroPort, Shanghai, China) [57].

The deployment of a covered stent may be difficult or impossible due to tortuous thin parent arteries or critical side branches [61]. An additional FD deployment can be attempted [62]. However, additional FD deployment cannot definitively prevent subsequent rupture. For

CCF, in addition to covered stents, transvenous embolization with coils, additional FD deployment, and carotid artery occlusion can be performed [24, 63-65].

6.2. Prognosis

Postprocedural rupture of intracranial unruptured aneurysms after FD deployment is often fatal because of the rapid deterioration of the patient [32]. According to our previous review, only 9.5% of patients survived [58]. Patients with infratentorial aneurysm rupture often have poor outcomes (Figure 3). Patients with supratentorial delayed aneurysm rupture who experienced less hemorrhage survived (Figure 2C). Cavernous aneurysm rupture with CCF can result in a good outcome after proper treatment [24, 65].

Conclusion

The incidence of aneurysm rupture following FD deployment is <5%. Most cases of postprocedural rupture occurred 1 month after surgery. The causes include an increase in intra-aneurysmal pressure, an increase in aneurysm volume, and progressive destruction of the aneurysm wall. In patients with aneurysm rupture after FD deployment, aneurysm size was an independent risk factor; the larger the aneurysm was, the greater the risk of postprocedural rupture. Until now, there have been no effective means to prevent postprocedural aneurysm rupture, but steroid administration, adjunctive coiling and overlapping flow diverters can be attempted. After aneurysm rupture, prompt open surgery to reduce the increased intracranial pressure is necessary. Ruptured aneurysms require isolation from the cerebral circulation as soon as possible, including surgical clipping, covered stent deployment, and additional FD deployment. For CCF, transvenous embolization with coils and carotid artery occlusion can be used. The prognosis of aneurysm rupture after FD deployment is poor, and only a few patients survive.

References

[1] Turk, A. S., 3rd, R. H. Martin, D. Fiorella, J. Mocco, A. Siddiqui, and A. Bonafe. 2014. "Flow Diversion Versus Traditional Endovascular Coiling Therapy: Design of the Prospective Large Aneurysm Randomized Trial." *AJNR Am J Neuroradiol* 35, no. 7 (Jul): 1341-5. https://dx.doi.org/10.3174/ajnr.A3968.

[2] Raymond, J., J. C. Gentric, T. E. Darsaut, D. Iancu, M. Chagnon, A. Weill, and D. Roy. 2017. "Flow Diversion in the Treatment of Aneurysms: A Randomized Care Trial and Registry." *J Neurosurg* 127, no. 3 (Sep): 454-462. https://dx.doi.org/10.3171/2016.4.jns152662.

[3] Lv, X., C. Jiang, Z. Wu, W. Jiang, and G. Wang. 2020. "Complex Cerebral Aneurysms: Intra-Luminal Reconstruction Using Pipeline Flow-Diverting Stent and the Obliteration Mechanism." *Neuroradiol J* 33, no. 2 (Apr): 91-97. https://dx.doi.org/10.1177/1971400919894879.

[4] Vollherbst, D. F., H. S. Cekirge, I. Saatci, F. Baltacioglu, B. Onal, O. Koc, R. Rautio, M. Sinisalo, A. Tomasello, P. Vega, M. Martínez-Galdámez, J. Lynch, V. Mendes Pereira, M. Bendszus, and M. A. Möhlenbruch. 2023. "First Clinical Multicenter Experience with the New Pipeline Vantage Flow

Diverter." *J Neurointerv Surg* 15, no. 1 (Jan): 63-69. https://dx.doi.org/10.1136/neurintsurg-2021-018480.

[5] Atallah, E., H. Saad, N. Mouchtouris, K. Bekelis, J. Walker, N. Chalouhi, S. Tjoumakaris, M. Smith, R. H. Rosenwasser, H. Zarzour, N. Herial, J. Feghali, M. R. Gooch, S. Missios, A. Sweid, and P. Jabbour. 2019. "Pipeline for Distal Cerebral Circulation Aneurysms." *Neurosurgery* 85, no. 3 (Sep 1): E477-e484. https://dx.doi.org/10.1093/neuros/nyz038.

[6] Ravindran, K., A. Enriquez-Marulanda, P. T. M. Kan, L. Renieri, N. Limbucci, S. Mangiafico, M. M. Salem, A. Y. Alturki, J. M. Moore, C. S. Ogilvy, and A. J. Thomas. 2018. "Use of Flow Diversion for the Treatment of Distal Circulation Aneurysms: A Multicohort Study." *World Neurosurg* 118 (Oct): e825-e833. https://dx.doi.org/10.1016/j.wneu.2018.07.062.

[7] Dmytriw, A. A., M. Dibas, N. Adeeb, M. M. Salem, A. Salehani, M. Waqas, A. Saad Aldine, V. M. Tutino, C. S. Ogilvy, A. H. Siddiqui, M. R. Harrigan, A. J. Thomas, H. Cuellar, and C. J. Griessenauer. 2022. "The Pipeline Embolization Device: A Decade of Lessons Learned in the Treatment of Posterior Circulation Aneurysms in a Multicenter Cohort." *J Neurosurg* (Mar 11): 1-8. https://dx.doi.org/10.3171/2021.12.jns212201.

[8] Zhang, H., J. Ren, J. Wang, and X. Lv. 2022. "The Off-Label Uses of Pipeline Embolization Device for Complex Cerebral Aneurysms: Mid-Term Follow-up in a Single Center." *Interv Neuroradiol* (Dec 30): 15910199221148800. https://dx.doi.org/10.1177/15910199221148800.

[9] Rouchaud, A., W. Brinjikji, G. Lanzino, H. J. Cloft, R. Kadirvel, and D. F. Kallmes. 2016. "Delayed Hemorrhagic Complications after Flow Diversion for Intracranial Aneurysms: A Literature Overview." *Neuroradiology* 58, no. 2 (Feb): 171-7. https://dx.doi.org/10.1007/s00234-015-1615-4.

[10] Kan, P., A. H. Siddiqui, E. Veznedaroglu, K. M. Liebman, M. J. Binning, T. M. Dumont, C. S. Ogilvy, J. R. Gaughen, Jr., J. Mocco, G. J. Velat, A. J. Ringer, B. G. Welch, M. B. Horowitz, K. V. Snyder, L. N. Hopkins, and E. I. Levy. 2012. "Early Postmarket Results after Treatment of Intracranial Aneurysms with the Pipeline Embolization Device: A U.S. Multicenter Experience." *Neurosurgery* 71, no. 6 (Dec): 1080-7; discussion 1087-8. https://dx.doi.org/10.1227/NEU.0b013e31827060d9.

[11] Liang, F., Y. Zhang, P. Yan, C. Ma, S. Liang, and C. Jiang. 2019. "Outcomes and Complications after the Use of the Pipeline Embolization Device in the Treatment of Intracranial Aneurysms of the Posterior Circulation: A Systematic Review and Meta-Analysis." *World Neurosurg* 127 (Jul): e888-e895. https://dx.doi.org/10.1016/j.wneu.2019.03.291.

[12] Lv, X., H. Ge, H. He, C. Jiang, and Y. Li. 2017. "A Systematic Review of Pipeline Embolization Device for Giant Intracranial Aneurysms." *Neurol India* 65, no. 1 (Jan-Feb): 35-38. https://dx.doi.org/10.4103/0028-3886.198200.

[13] Lv, X., H. Yang, P. Liu, and Y. Li. 2016. "Flow-Diverter Devices in the Treatment of Intracranial Aneurysms: A Meta-Analysis and Systematic Review." *Neuroradiol J* 29, no. 1 (Feb): 66-71. https://dx.doi.org/10.1177/1971400915621321.

[14] Kallmes, D. F., R. Hanel, D. Lopes, E. Boccardi, A. Bonafé, S. Cekirge, D. Fiorella, P. Jabbour, E. Levy, C. McDougall, A. Siddiqui, I. Szikora, H. Woo, F. Albuquerque, H. Bozorgchami, S. R. Dashti, J. E. Delgado Almandoz, M. E. Kelly, R. th Turner, B. K. Woodward, W. Brinjikji, G. Lanzino, and P. Lylyk. 2015. "International Retrospective Study of the Pipeline Embolization Device: A Multicenter Aneurysm Treatment Study." *AJNR Am J Neuroradiol* 36, no. 1 (Jan): 108-15. https://dx.doi.org/10.3174/ajnr.A4111.

[15] Pierot, L., L. Spelle, J. Berge, A. C. Januel, D. Herbreteau, M. Aggour, M. Piotin, A. Biondi, X. Barreau, C. Mounayer, C. Papagiannaki, J. P. Lejeune, J. Y. Gauvrit, and V. Costalat. 2018. "Feasibility, Complications, Morbidity, and Mortality Results at 6 Months for Aneurysm Treatment with the Flow Re-Direction Endoluminal Device: Report of Safe Study." *J Neurointerv Surg* 10, no. 8 (Aug): 765-770. https://dx.doi.org/10.1136/neurintsurg-2017-013559.

[16] Kang, H., B. Luo, J. Liu, H. Zhang, T. Li, D. Song, Y. Zhao, S. Guan, A. Maimaitili, Y. Wang, W. Feng, Y. Wang, J. Wan, G. Mao, H. Shi, K. Wang, and X. Yang. 2022a. "Mortality after Treatment of Intracranial Aneurysms with the Pipeline Embolization Device." *J Neurointerv Surg* 14, no. 1 (Jan). https://dx.doi.org/10.1136/neurintsurg-2020-017002.

[17] Cloft, H. J. 2011. "Flow Diversion for Cerebral Aneurysms: A Cautionary Tale." *AJNR Am J Neuroradiol* 32, no. 1 (Jan): 26. https://dx.doi.org/10.3174/ajnr.A2373.

[18] Brinjikji, W., M. H. Murad, G. Lanzino, H. J. Cloft, and D. F. Kallmes. 2013. "Endovascular Treatment of Intracranial Aneurysms with Flow Diverters: A Meta-Analysis." *Stroke* 44, no. 2 (Feb): 442-7. https://dx.doi.org/10.1161/strokeaha.112.678151.

[19] Kang, H., Y. Zhou, B. Luo, N. Lv, H. Zhang, T. Li, D. Song, Y. Zhao, S. Guan, A. Maimaitili, Y. Wang, W. Feng, Y. Wang, J. Wan, G. Mao, H. Shi, X. Yang, and J. Liu. 2021. "Pipeline Embolization Device for Intracranial Aneurysms in a Large Chinese Cohort: Complication Risk Factor Analysis." *Neurotherapeutics* 18, no. 2 (Apr): 1198-1206. https://dx.doi.org/10.1007/s13311-020-00990-8.

[20] Sweid, A., R. M. Starke, N. Herial, N. Chalouhi, S. Das, M. P. Baldassari, T. D. Alexander, S. Tjoumakaris, M. R. Gooch, D. Hasan, R. H. Rosenwasser, V. Romo, and P. Jabbour. 2020. "Predictors of Complications, Functional Outcome, and Morbidity in a Large Cohort Treated with Flow Diversion." *Neurosurgery* 87, no. 4 (Sep 15): 730-743. https://dx.doi.org/10.1093/neuros/nyz508.

[21] Z., Kulcsar, and Szikora I. 2012. "The Esmint Retrospective Analysis of Delayed Aneurysm Ruptures after Flow Diversion (Radar) Study." *EJMINT* 2012: 1244000088.

[22] Briganti, F., G. Leone, M. Marseglia, G. Mariniello, F. Caranci, A. Brunetti, and F. Maiuri. 2015a. "Endovascular Treatment of Cerebral Aneurysms Using Flow-Diverter Devices: A Systematic Review." *Neuroradiol J* 28, no. 4 (Aug): 365-75. https://dx.doi.org/10.1177/1971400915602803.

[23] Hampton, T., D. Walsh, C. Tolias, and D. Fiorella. 2018. "Mural Destabilization after Aneurysm Treatment with a Flow-Diverting Device: A Report of Two Cases." *J Neurointerv Surg* 10, no. Suppl 1 (Jul): i51-i55. https://dx.doi.org/10.1136/jnis.2010.002873.rep.

[24] Lin, L. M., G. P. Colby, B. Jiang, G. Pero, E. Boccardi, and A. L. Coon. 2015. "Transvenous Approach for the Treatment of Direct Carotid Cavernous Fistula Following Pipeline Embolization of Cavernous Carotid Aneurysm: A Report of Two Cases and Review of the Literature." *J Neurointerv Surg* 7, no. 8 (Aug): e30. https://dx.doi.org/10.1136/neurintsurg-2014-011235.rep.

[25] Kulcsár, Z., E. Houdart, A. Bonafé, G. Parker, J. Millar, A. J. Goddard, S. Renowden, G. Gál, B. Turowski, K. Mitchell, F. Gray, M. Rodriguez, R. van den Berg, A. Gruber, H. Desal, I. Wanke, and D. A. Rüfenacht. 2011. "Intra-Aneurysmal Thrombosis as a Possible Cause of Delayed Aneurysm Rupture after Flow-Diversion Treatment." *AJNR Am J Neuroradiol* 32, no. 1 (Jan): 20-5. https://dx.doi.org/10.3174/ajnr.A2370.

[26] Vakharia, K., M. Waqas, S. A. Munich, J. Lim, A. Gong, F. Chin, K. V. Snyder, A. H. Siddiqui, and E. I. Levy. 2020. "Is Contrast Stasis after Pipeline Embolization Device Deployment Associated with Higher Aneurysm Occlusion Rates?" *World Neurosurg* 133 (Jan): e434-e442. https://dx.doi.org/10.1016/j.wneu.2019.09.032.

[27] Cebral, J. R., F. Mut, M. Raschi, E. Scrivano, R. Ceratto, P. Lylyk, and C. M. Putman. 2011. "Aneurysm Rupture Following Treatment with Flow-Diverting Stents: Computational Hemodynamics Analysis of Treatment." *AJNR Am J Neuroradiol* 32, no. 1 (Jan): 27-33. https://dx.doi.org/10.3174/ajnr.A2398.

[28] Li, W., Z. Tian, W. Zhu, Y. S. Zhang, K. Wang, Y. Zhang, Y. Wang, X. Yang, and J. Liu. 2019. "Hemodynamic Analysis of Postoperative Rupture of Unruptured Intracranial Aneurysms after Placement of Flow-Diverting Stents: A Matched Case-Control Study." *AJNR Am J Neuroradiol* 40, no. 11 (Nov): 1916-1923. https://dx.doi.org/10.3174/ajnr.A6256.

[29] Fox, B., W. E. Humphries, V. T. Doss, D. Hoit, L. Elijovich, and A. S. Arthur. 2015. "Rupture of Giant Vertebrobasilar Aneurysm Following Flow Diversion: Mechanical Stretch as a Potential Mechanism for Early Aneurysm Rupture." *J Neurointerv Surg* 7, no. 11 (Nov): e37. https://dx.doi.org/10.1136/neurintsurg-2014-011325.rep.

[30] Trivelato, F. P., M. T. Salles Rezende, A. C. Ulhôa, L. Henrique de Castro-Afonso, G. S. Nakiri, and D. G. Abud. 2018. "Occlusion Rates of Intracranial Aneurysms Treated with the Pipeline Embolization Device: The Role of Branches Arising from the Sac." *J Neurosurg* (Apr 1): 1-7. https://dx.doi.org/10.3171/2017.10.jns172175.

[31] Chow, M., C. McDougall, C. O'Kelly, R. Ashforth, E. Johnson, and D. Fiorella. 2012. "Delayed Spontaneous Rupture of a Posterior Inferior Cerebellar Artery Aneurysm Following Treatment with Flow Diversion: A Clinicopathologic Study." *AJNR Am J Neuroradiol* 33, no. 4 (Apr): E46-51. https://dx.doi.org/10.3174/ajnr.A2532.

[32] Turowski, B., S. Macht, Z. Kulcsár, D. Hänggi, and W. Stummer. 2011. "Early Fatal Hemorrhage after Endovascular Cerebral Aneurysm Treatment with a Flow Diverter (Silk-Stent): Do We Need to Rethink Our Concepts?" *Neuroradiology* 53, no. 1 (Jan): 37-41. https://dx.doi.org/10.1007/s00234-010-0676-7.

[33] Briganti, F., G. Leone, M. Napoli, W. Lauriola, F. Florio, and F. Maiuri. 2015b. "Early Fatal Hemorrhage after Endovascular Treatment of a Giant Aneurysm with Flow Diverter Device and Coils." *Clin Neuroradiol* 25, no. 2 (Jun): 201-5. https://dx.doi.org/10.1007/s00062-014-0310-x.

[34] Ikeda, H., A. Ishii, T. Kikuchi, M. Ando, H. Chihara, D. Arai, E. Hattori, and S. Miyamoto. 2015. "Delayed Aneurysm Rupture Due to Residual Blood Flow at the Inflow Zone of the Intracranial Paraclinoid Internal Carotid Aneurysm Treated with the Pipeline Embolization Device: Histopathological Investigation." *Interv Neuroradiol* 21, no. 6 (Dec): 674-83. https://dx.doi.org/10.1177/1591019915609121.

[35] Ujiie, H., Y. Tamano, K. Sasaki, and T. Hori. 2001. "Is the Aspect Ratio a Reliable Index for Predicting the Rupture of a Saccular Aneurysm?" *Neurosurgery* 48, no. 3 (Mar): 495-502; discussion 502-3. https://dx.doi.org/10.1097/00006123-200103000-00007.

[36] Ujiie, H., H. Tachibana, O. Hiramatsu, A. L. Hazel, T. Matsumoto, Y. Ogasawara, H. Nakajima, T. Hori, K. Takakura, and F. Kajiya. 1999. "Effects of Size and Shape (Aspect Ratio) on the Hemodynamics of Saccular Aneurysms: A Possible Index for Surgical Treatment of Intracranial Aneurysms." *Neurosurgery* 45, no. 1 (Jul): 119-29; discussion 129-30. https://dx.doi.org/10.1097/00006123-199907000-00028.

[37] Luther, E., D. J. McCarthy, M. C. Brunet, S. Sur, S. H. Chen, D. Sheinberg, D. Hasan, P. Jabbour, D. R. Yavagal, E. C. Peterson, and R. M. Starke. 2020. "Treatment and Diagnosis of Cerebral Aneurysms in the Post-International Subarachnoid Aneurysm Trial (Isat) Era: Trends and Outcomes." *J Neurointerv Surg* 12, no. 7 (Jul): 682-687. https://dx.doi.org/10.1136/neurintsurg-2019-015418.

[38] Lv, X., Z. Chen, L. Liu, C. Jiang, G. Wang, and J. Wang. 2019. "Rupture of Intradural Giant Aneurysms: The Mode of Treatment, Anatomical, and Mechanical Factors." *Neurol India* 67, no. 5 (Sep-Oct): 1194-1199. https://dx.doi.org/10.4103/0028-3886.271250.

[39] Saber, H., R. Y. Kherallah, M. O. Hadied, S. Kazemlou, P. Chamiraju, and S. Narayanan. 2019. "Antiplatelet Therapy and the Risk of Ischemic and Hemorrhagic Complications Associated with Pipeline Embolization of Cerebral Aneurysms: A Systematic Review and Pooled Analysis." *J Neurointerv Surg* 11, no. 4 (Apr): 362-366. https://dx.doi.org/10.1136/neurintsurg-2018-014082.

[40] Roccatagliata, L., P. Guédin, S. Condette-Auliac, S. Gaillard, F. Colas, A. Boulin, A. Wang, S. Guieu, and G. Rodesch. 2010. "Partially Thrombosed Intracranial Aneurysms: Symptoms, Evolution, and Therapeutic Management." *Acta Neurochir (Wien)* 152, no. 12 (Dec): 2133-42. https://dx.doi.org/10.1007/s00701-010-0772-9.

[41] Osorno-Cruz, C., A. Piscopo, A. Raghuram, S. Sanchez, E. Samaniego, and D. Hasan. 2021. "Reversible Bilateral Optic Tract Edema Following Pipeline-Assisted Coiling of a Large Ophthalmic Aneurysm: A Case Report." *Clin Neurol Neurosurg* 211 (Dec): 107029. https://dx.doi.org/10.1016/j.clineuro.2021.107029.

[42] Rehman, A. A., R. C. Turner, S. Wright, S. Boo, and A. T. Rai. 2019. "An Autopsy Report of Basilar Artery Aneurysm Flow Diversion Complicated by Postoperative Day 3 Hemorrhage from Vessel Rupture." *J Neurointerv Surg* 11, no. 5 (May): e2. https://dx.doi.org/10.1136/neurintsurg-2018-014511.rep.

[43] Kang, H., B. Luo, J. Liu, H. Zhang, T. Li, D. Song, Y. Zhao, S. Guan, A. Maimaitili, Y. Wang, W. Feng, Y. Wang, J. Wan, G. Mao, H. Shi, Y. Zhang, and X. Yang. 2022b. "Postoperative Occlusion Degree after Flow-Diverter Placement with Adjunctive Coiling: Analysis of Complications." *J Neurointerv Surg* 14, no. 4 (Apr): 371-375. https://dx.doi.org/10.1136/neurintsurg-2021-017445.

[44] Chen, C. J., M. R. Patibandla, M. S. Park, and M. Y. Kalani. 2019. "Regrowth of a Large Intracranial Aneurysm after on-Label Use of the Pipeline Embolization Device." *J Neurosci Rural Pract* 10, no. 1 (Jan-Mar): 142-144. https://dx.doi.org/10.4103/jnrp.jnrp_273_18.

[45] Liang, S., R. Yuan, and X. Lv. 2020. "A Novel Treatment of a Patient with a Giant Ruptured Middle Cerebral Artery Aneurysm by Acute Coiling Followed by Scheduled Pipeline Flex Placement." *Neuroradiol J* 33, no. 6 (Dec): 517-519. https://dx.doi.org/10.1177/1971400920941192.

[46] Wang, C., B. Luo, T. Li, A. Maimaitili, G. Mao, D. Song, Y. Wang, W. Feng, Y. Wang, H. Shi, J. Wan, J. Liu, S. Guan, Y. Zhao, and H. Zhang. 2022. "Comparison of the Pipeline Embolisation Device Alone or Combined with Coiling for Treatment of Different Sizes of Intracranial Aneurysms." *Stroke Vasc Neurol* 7, no. 4 (Aug): 345-352. https://dx.doi.org/10.1136/svn-2021-001258.

[47] Akiyama, T., H. Imamura, M. Goto, R. Fukumitsu, T. Sunohara, S. Matsumoto, N. Fukui, Y. Omura, T. Fukuda, K. Go, S. Kajiura, M. Shigeyasu, K. Asakura, R. Horii, Y. Naramoto, R. Nishii, Y. Yamamoto, C. Sakai, and N. Sakai. 2022. "Pipeline Flow Diversion with Adjunctive Coil Embolization for Internal Carotid Artery Aneurysms Following an Intradural Component: Results in 46 Consecutive Aneurysms from a Japanese Single-Center Experience." *Neurosurg Rev* 45, no. 3 (Jun): 2221-2230. https://dx.doi.org/10.1007/s10143-021-01719-7.

[48] Nelson, P. K., P. Lylyk, I. Szikora, S. G. Wetzel, I. Wanke, and D. Fiorella. 2011. "The Pipeline Embolization Device for the Intracranial Treatment of Aneurysms Trial." *AJNR Am J Neuroradiol* 32, no. 1 (Jan): 34-40. https://dx.doi.org/10.3174/ajnr.A2421.

[49] Lubicz, B., L. Collignon, G. Raphaeli, J. P. Pruvo, M. Bruneau, O. De Witte, and X. Leclerc. 2010. "Flow-Diverter Stent for the Endovascular Treatment of Intracranial Aneurysms: A Prospective Study in 29 Patients with 34 Aneurysms." *Stroke* 41, no. 10 (Oct): 2247-53. https://dx.doi.org/10.1161/strokeaha.110.589911.

[50] Fischer, S., Z. Vajda, M. Aguilar Perez, E. Schmid, N. Hopf, H. Bäzner, and H. Henkes. 2012. "Pipeline Embolization Device (Ped) for Neurovascular Reconstruction: Initial Experience in the Treatment of 101 Intracranial Aneurysms and Dissections." *Neuroradiology* 54, no. 4 (Apr): 369-82. https://dx.doi.org/10.1007/s00234-011-0948-x.

[51] Kerber, C. W., S. T. Hecht, K. Knox, R. B. Buxton, and H. S. Meltzer. 1996. "Flow Dynamics in a Fatal Aneurysm of the Basilar Artery." *AJNR Am J Neuroradiol* 17, no. 8 (Sep): 1417-21.

[52] Gomez-Paz, S., Y. Akamatsu, J. M. Moore, C. S. Ogilvy, A. J. Thomas, and C. J. Griessenauer. 2020. "Implications of the Collar Sign in Incompletely Occluded Aneurysms after Pipeline Embolization Device Implantation: A Follow-up Study." *AJNR Am J Neuroradiol* 41, no. 3 (Mar): 482-485. https://dx.doi.org/10.3174/ajnr.A6415.

[53] Damiano, R. J., V. M. Tutino, N. Paliwal, D. Ma, J. M. Davies, A. H. Siddiqui, and H. Meng. 2017. "Compacting a Single Flow Diverter Versus Overlapping Flow Diverters for Intracranial Aneurysms: A Computational Study." *AJNR Am J Neuroradiol* 38, no. 3 (Mar): 603-610. https://dx.doi.org/10.3174/ajnr.A5062.

[54] Kerl, H. U., H. Boll, T. Fiebig, G. Figueiredo, A. Förster, I. S. Nölte, A. Nonn, C. Groden, and M. A. Brockmann. 2014. "Implantation of Pipeline Flow-Diverting Stents Reduces Aneurysm Inflow without Relevantly Affecting Static Intra-Aneurysmal Pressure." *Neurosurgery* 74, no. 3 (Mar): 321-34; discussion 334. https://dx.doi.org/10.1227/neu.0000000000000253.

[55] Fan, F., Y. Fu, J. Liu, X. Yang, H. Zhang, T. Li, H. Shi, J. Wan, Y. Zhao, Y. Wang, W. Feng, D. Song, Y. Wang, G. Mao, A. Maimaitili, and S. Guan. 2022. "Multiple Pipeline Embolization Devices for the Treatment of Complex Intracranial Aneurysm: A Multi-Center Study." *Front Aging Neurosci* 14: 905224. https://dx.doi.org/10.3389/fnagi.2022.905224.

[56] Kim, G., J. Kim, S. K. Park, and J. Chung. 2022. "Retreatment of a Recurrent Giant Aneurysm of the Internal Carotid Artery after Treatment with a Flow-Diverting Stent." *J Cerebrovasc Endovasc Neurosurg* (Oct 19). https://dx.doi.org/10.7461/jcen.2022.E2022.06.007.

[57] Chen, X., S. Gui, L. Dong, L. Zhang, H. Ge, P. Liu, Y. Li, and M. Lv. 2022. "Case Report: Covered Stent Placement to Treat Delayed Aneurysmal Rupture after Flow Diverter-Assisted Coil Embolization." *Front Neurol* 13: 964733. https://dx.doi.org/10.3389/fneur.2022.964733.

[58] Hou, K., G. Li, X. Lv, B. Xu, K. Xu, and J. Yu. 2020. "Delayed Rupture of Intracranial Aneurysms after Placement of Intra-Luminal Flow Diverter." *Neuroradiol J* 33, no. 6 (Dec): 451-464. https://dx.doi.org/10.1177/1971400920953299.

[59] Lv, N., H. Ma, Y. Zhou, Z. Li, Y. Zeng, Q. Li, R. Zhao, Y. Fang, P. Yang, Q. Huang, B. Hong, Y. Xu, Z. Lin, and J. Liu. 2022. "Coiling Followed by Staged Flow Diversion for Large and Giant Intracranial Aneurysms." *Front Neurol* 13: 1024447. https://dx.doi.org/10.3389/fneur.2022.1024447.

[60] de Castro-Afonso, L. H., J. P. Machado, G. S. Nakiri, T. G. Abud, L. M. Monsignore, R. K. Freitas, R. S. de Oliveira, B. O. Colli, and D. G. Abud. 2023. "Two Year Follow-up of Distal Unruptured

Intracranial Aneurysms Treated with a Surface Modified Flow Diverter under Prasugrel Monotherapy." *J Neurointerv Surg* (Jul 31). https://dx.doi.org/10.1136/jnis-2023-020397.

[61] Zhu, Y. Q., M. H. Li, C. Fang, H. Q. Tan, W. Wang, P. L. Zhang, Y. S. Cheng, J. B. Wang, and L. T. Ma. 2010. "Application of the Willis Covered Stent in the Treatment of Aneurysm in the Cisternal Segment of the Internal Carotid Artery: A Pilot Comparative Study with Midterm Follow-Up." *J Endovasc Ther* 17, no. 1 (Feb): 55-65. https://dx.doi.org/10.1583/09-2688.1.

[62] Mazur, M. D., P. Taussky, J. D. MacDonald, and M. S. Park. 2016. "Rerupture of a Blister Aneurysm after Treatment with a Single Flow-Diverting Stent." *Neurosurgery* 79, no. 5 (Nov): E634-e638. https://dx.doi.org/10.1227/neu.0000000000001412.

[63] Berge, J., A. Biondi, P. Machi, H. Brunel, L. Pierot, J. Gabrillargues, K. Kadziolka, X. Barreau, V. Dousset, and A. Bonafé. 2012. "Flow-Diverter Silk Stent for the Treatment of Intracranial Aneurysms: 1-Year Follow-up in a Multicenter Study." *AJNR Am J Neuroradiol* 33, no. 6 (Jun): 1150-5. https://dx.doi.org/10.3174/ajnr.A2907.

[64] Oishi, H., K. Teranishi, K. Yatomi, T. Fujii, M. Yamamoto, and H. Arai. 2018. "Flow Diverter Therapy Using a Pipeline Embolization Device for 100 Unruptured Large and Giant Internal Carotid Artery Aneurysms in a Single Center in a Japanese Population." *Neurol Med Chir (Tokyo)* 58, no. 11 (Nov 15): 461-467. https://dx.doi.org/10.2176/nmc.oa.2018-0148.

[65] Nakae, R., M. Nagaishi, I. Takano, Y. Tanaka, A. Hyodo, and K. Suzuki. 2018. "Transvenous Coil Embolization for the Treatment of Carotid Cavernous Fistula after Pipeline Placement: A Case Report." *J Stroke Cerebrovasc Dis* 27, no. 4 (Apr): e65-e69. https://dx.doi.org/10.1016/j.jstrokecerebrovasdis.2017.10.023.

Chapter 24

Current Monitoring in Neurocritical Care for Aneurysmal Subarachnoid Haemorrhage

Padmaja Durga*, MD
Department of Anesthesiology and Intensive Care, Nizam's Institute of Medical Sciences, Hyderabad, India

Abstract

Aggressive intensive care of patients with aSAH using invasive neuromonitoring is associated with improved outcomes. In addition to disturbances in ICP and patients with SAH are frequently have derangement of CPP, cerebral blood flow (CBF), cerebral oxygenation, and cerebral energy metabolism. The incidence of intracranial hypertension in aSAH is around 80%. aSAH patients with longer episodes of ICP above 20–25 mmHg have shown to be associated with an increased risk of clinical deterioration, delayed cerebral ischaemia, unfavorable outcome, and mortality. After ventriculostomy ICP should be maintained above 15 mm Hg to reduce the risk of re-bleeding. CPP closer to 70–90 mmHg is associated with better brain tissue oxygenation, cerebral energy metabolism, and favourable outcome in aSAH but the threshold has not been validated through prospective studies. It is possible to individualize autoregulatory CPP-target using derived parameters from ICP waveform such as pressure reactivity index (PRx), mean flow index (Mx), and oxygen reactivity index (ORx). SAH is associated with varied changes in cerebral blod flow (CBF) from hyperemia to vasospasm to ischaemia. Transcranial Doppler (TCD) ultrasonography is a bedside dynamic monitoring tool to screen for the presence and progression of cerebral vasospasm in patients with SAH. It can be differentiated from cerebral hyperemia through Lindegrad index. In patients with SAH, additional applications of the TCD technique include studies of CBF autoregulation integrity by the carotid artery compression test (transient hyperemic response test) or induced hypertension and indirect evaluation of ICP through the use of the pulsatility index. Adequacy of global cerebral blood flow can be assessed using jugular venous oximetry. Very few studies have evaluated the diagnostic or clinical relevance of jugular venous oximetry in the management of patients with SAH. Concomitant use of brain tissue oxygenation monitoring ($PbtO_2$) may further improve the clinical relevance. $PbtO_2$, measured using commercial devices, can be used as a surrogate measure of CBF. PbtO2 monitoring is a reliable technique for early detection of DCI and brain hypoxia in patients with SAH. Treatment of PbtO2 below 1.33 kPa was effective in reducing secondary ischemic damage. Limitations of PbtO2

* Corresponding Author's Email: Email: padmajanims@yahoo.com.

In: Understanding and Managing Cerebral Aneurysms
Editor: Xianli Lv
ISBN: 979-8-89113-608-3

monitoring are, it provides information only on local tissue changes and its an invasive technique. Near Infrared Spectroscopy (NIRS)is a simple, portable, continuous, real time, non-invasive monitoring of cerebral oximetry. Vasospasm detection, DCI prediction, and prognostication have explicitly been evaluated in the aSAH population using NIRS. Cerebral metabolic dysfunction has been shown to extensively mediate the pathophysiology of brain injury after SAH. Cerebral microdialysis (CMD) is a tool that can measure concentrations of multiple bioenergetics metabolites in brain interstitial fluid. Emerging investigations have suggested that CMD is an effective way to monitor the changes of cerebral metabolic dysfunction after SAH in real-time and can also monitor for the development of vasospasm and delayed neurological deficits. It has been suggested that the use of continuous EEG to assess for non-convulsive seizures in patients who fail to improve. EEG monitoring also helps in detecting cortical spreading depression (CSD) and DCI. Every neuromonitoring technique, in isolation, has limitations. For that reason. The combined use of multiple monitors is termed "multimodality monitoring" (MMM). MMM tools have been developed to enable monitoring of the different steps to achieve cerebral energy metabolism and enables earlier detection of impending brain injury, diagnosis of the specific pathomechanisms and initiation of cause-specific therapies. Precision and personalization in managing Aneurysmal subarachnoid haemorrhage is possible with monitoring targeted therapy.

Keywords: aneurysmal subarachnoid haemorrhage, vasospasm, delayed cerebral injury, intracranial pressure monitoring, cerebral autoregulation, transcranial doppler, near infrared spectroscopy' brain tissue oxygen monitoring, cerebral microdialysis, multimodal monitoring

Abbreviations

aSAH	Aneurysmal subarachnoid hemorrhage
MCA	middle cerebral artery
DCI	delayed cerebral ischemia.
EEG	Electroencephalogram
NIC	neurointensive care
cEEG	Continuous EEG
ICP	Intracranial pressure
NIRS	Near Infrared Spectroscopy
CPP	cerebral perfusion pressure
$CrSO_2$	Cerebral regional oxygen saturation
CBF	cerebral blood flow
$PbtO_2$	Brain tissue oxygen
CMR	cerebral metabolic rate
ED	epileptiform discharges
TCD	Transcranial Doppler
CMD	Cerebral micro dialysis
$AVDO_2$	arterial to jugular vein oxygen concentration difference v
CSD	cortical spreading depolarization
$SjVO_{2)}$	jugular venous oxygen saturation
MMM	Multimodal monitoring

Introduction

Aneurysmal subarachnoid hemorrhage (aSAH) is a severe type of acute brain injury with high mortality and a burden of neurological sequelae. A large part to delayed effects of the hemorrhage, including vasospasm, and delayed cerebral ischemia. (DCI) It also involves several intracranial and systemic perturbations. The perturbations are more evident in poor-grade patients [IV and V on the World Federation of Neurosurgeons (WFNS) scale [1] and are often associated with delayed neurological deficits [2]. Delayed cerebral ischemia deteriorating into cerebral infarction represents the main threat to a favorable outcome [3]. The clinical outcome in the aSAH is a consequence of the primary haemorrhage and several secondary insults in the acute post-haemorrhage period. Some secondary insults are potentially preventable and can be influenced by therapeutic measures. The general goals of management are aimed at early aneurysm occlusion, either clipping or coiling, to prevent re-bleeding and prevention of delayed ischemic neurological deficits through cerebral blood flow augmentation. In the acute phase, the brain is also vulnerable to secondary brain injury resulting from physiological perturbations because of a high incidence of non-neurological complications after SAH. Therefore, optimizing the systemic and cerebral physiology in neurointensive care (NIC) is important. Evolving secondary brain injury can be fairly detected as a neurological deterioration, clinically assessed by repeated neurological examinations and this is more challenging in unconscious patients that require intubation, mechanical ventilation, and sedation. DCI often present an altered level of consciousness, diminishing the reliability of the neurological exam [4, 5]. Patients may also have unrecognized ischemic episodes [6] which are associated with worst long-term deficits and higher mortality [7]. Hence, neuromonitoring is required for patients with aSAH. Aggressive intensive care of patients with aSAH using invasive neuromonitoring is associated with improved outcomes [8]. While the neuromonitoring techniques have been tested in traumatic brain injury and stroke, their application to patients with aSAH is a more recent development. Thus, while the risks and complications are rather well documented, data on accuracy and reliability in patients with aSAH are still inconclusive and none has so far established itself as a reliable modality to circumvent the loss of clinical exam in poor grade aSAH [9, 10].

Intracranial pressure (ICP) and cerebral perfusion pressure (CPP) are monitored in unconscious aSAH patients in neurointensive care, and treatment aims to avoid intracranial hypertension and to ensure sufficient cerebral perfusion. However, even with normal ICP and CPP, disturbances in cerebral blood flow (CBF), cerebral oxygenation, and cerebral energy metabolism are frequent. Several important pathomechanisms beyond intracranial pressure and cerebral perfusion pressure follow aSAH. Understanding physiological, cellular, and molecular pathomechanisms is required for better monitoring and treatment of these processes (Figure 1) There has been a development advanced neuromonitoring tools to assess cerebral blood flow (imaging and invasive probes, TCD), CBF autoregulation (e.g., pressure reactivity index), brain tissue oxygenation ($PbtO_2$ and jugular bulb oximetry), and cerebral energy metabolism (microdialysis) (Table 1) The monitoring not only improved our understanding of disease pathophysiology but also aided in monitoring the treatment's cerebral effects.

Table 1. Monitoring of Physiological variables in ASAH

Physiological variable	Monitoring method	Advantage/Limitations
ICP	EVD	Both monitoring and treatment of ICP by CSF drainage. Limitations: Infections. Clotting of the EVD.
	Intraparenchymal probe	Less invasive than EVD. Limitations: Does not offer ICP treatment with CSF drainage. Zero-drift.
CPP	Any ICP monitor +continuous systemic ABP.	Continuous global estimate of CBF. Limitations: Spatial constraints; does not take into account differences in cerebral autoregulation or vasospasm.
CBF autoregulation	PRx (ICP and ABP)	Measure of the global autoregulatory status. Limitations: Requires ICP-monitor. insensitive to focal disturbances.
	CPPopt (PRx and CPP)	Global CBF surrogate that takes into account autoregulatory status. Limitations: Requires advanced software. Still insufficiently studied in aSAH. Spatial constraints; insensitive to focal disturbances.
	Mx (TCD and CPP)	Easy to use bedside. May detect regional autoregulatory differences. Limitations: User-dependent. Spatial constraints; limited global spatial validity, especially in the posterior circulation
Cerebral blood flow	Radiology (Perfusion-CT, Xe-CT, PET, MRI)	Both global and focal. Limitations: Logistics; Difficult to transport unstable patients to the radiology department. Time constraints; represents only a snapshot.
	TCD	Easy to use bedside. Limitations: Measures velocity, not CBF. User-dependent. Spatial constraints; limited global spatial validity, especially in the posterior circulation. Time constraints; monitoring occurs in a limited time interval.
	Intraparenchymal thermal diffusion probe	Continuous CBF measure. Limitations: Spatial constraints; limited global spatial validity.
Brain tissue oxygenation	Jugular bulb catheter ($SjvO_2$)	Continuous and feasible global measure. Limitations: Spatial constraints; low sensitivity for focal ischemia.
	Intraparenchymal device (BtO_2)	Continuous and feasible focal measure. Limitations: Spatial constraints; limited global spatial validity, especially in the posterior circulation
	NIRS	Non-invasive. Limitations: Spatial constraints; limited global spatial validity, especially in the posterior circulation
Cerebral energy metabolism	CMD	Feasible for continuous evaluation. Limitations: Spatial constraints; limited global spatial validity.
	PET	Possible to investigate focal/global complex aspects of energy metabolism. Limitations:Logistics; Difficult to transport unstable patients to the radiology department. Time constraints; represents only a snapshot.
	EEG	Helpful to diagnose cerebral ischemia and NCSE Complexity; difficult to interpret bedside.

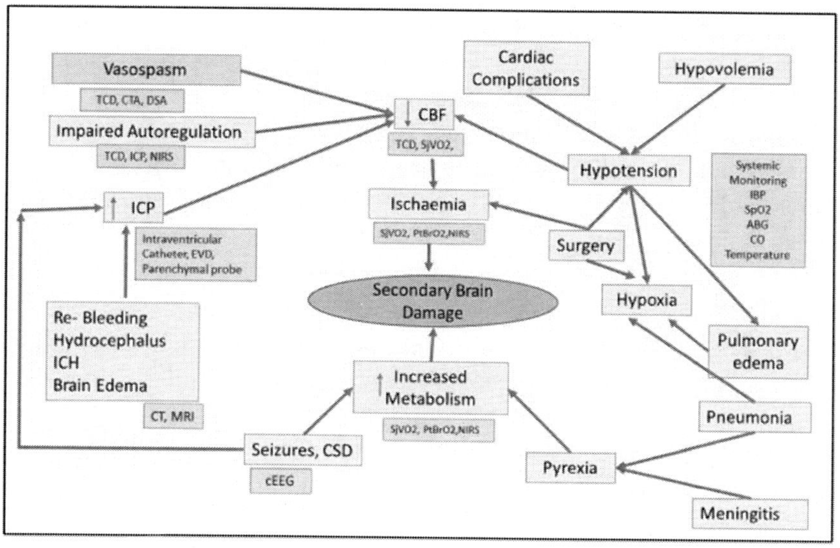

Figure 1. Possible secondary insults after SAH and the available monitoring techniques.

ICP-Monitoring

ICP Changes in aSAH

Intracranial pressure monitoring aims to alert the clinician to rises in ICP and thereby protect cerebral perfusion by maintaining an adequate cerebral perfusion pressure (CPP). There is a rapid increase in ICP following the haemorrhage from the ruptured intracranial aneurysm. Following ictus, there can be acute (<24 h) and delayed (2–14 days post-ictus) secondary ICP elevations due to, e.g., re-bleeding, acute hydrocephalus, intracerebral haemorrhage, subdural hematomas, diffuse global cerebral oedema, and cerebral oedema. High ICP may in turn induce compression of neural structures as well as lead to macro- and microvascular CBF disturbances by lowering CPP [11]. The incidence of intracranial hypertension is high in SAH, and around 80% of the patients exhibited episode of ICP above 20 mmHg for more than 5 min at least once [12, 13]. Due to the lack of clear evidence on ICP-monitoring from aSAH studies, most centres have extrapolated the ICP regime from TBI protocols. There are some critical aSAH-related issues that need to be considered. ICP monitoring is applied in aSAH more liberally in less unconscious patients since ICP may be increased due to CSF disturbances even before ventricular dilatation appears.

ICP Monitoring Techniques

Several ICP monitoring techniques are available [14]. The fluid-filled catheter transducer systems are generally considered the gold standard [15]. Alternatively, various catheter tip ICP monitoring systems are available (e.g., Camino, Codman, and Spiegelberg). Intraventricular placement of catheters is recommended in all patients with SAH presenting with acute hydrocephalus and a depressed level of consciousness. A ventriculostomy through the lamina terminalis applied during aneurysm surgery can also be used for monitoring [16]. ICP measurements and cerebrospinal fluid (CSF) drainage can be performed, and ICP waveform analysis is also possible. The introduction of a ventricular catheter poses risks of bleeding, damage to parenchyma, and an infection rate close to 10%. The Camino and Codman systems are generally safe but may still pose the risk of infection and intra-parenchymal damage [17]. These catheter tip devices allow evaluation of ICP waveforms similar to ventricular catheters, but they cannot drain CSF. These catheters cannot be recalibrated once implanted [18, 19]. This problem might be solved with the Spiegelberg monitor, which uses a small air pouch system and is unique in performing automatic zeroing in situ every hour. The intraventricular version of the system allows CSF drainage. However, because of its inferior frequency properties, many methods of ICP waveform analysis are not possible with the Spiegelberg monitor [20].

ICP-Thresholds in aSAH

The ICP thresholds that warrant treatment are not well investigated in aSAH as in TBI. Some studies show that monitoring thresholds for SAH are in accordance with those established in TBI. There is persuasive evidence that aggressive treatment of increased ICP improves outcomes. aSAH patients with longer monitoring episodes of ICP above 20–25 mmHg have shown to be associated with an increased risk of clinical deterioration, delayed cerebral ischaemia, unfavorable outcome, and mortality [21, 22]. There has been concern about an increased risk of aneurysm re-bleeding if vetriculostomy is performed before aneurysm repair but data are contradicting. After ventriculostomy ICP should be maintained above 15 mm Hg to reduce the risk of re-bleeding [23, 24, 25].

Intracranial Compliance

Intracranial compliance may be reduced earlier than ICP elevation. This makes the patient susceptible to small changes in intracranial volume. In patients with severely compromised intracranial compliance even routine procedures such as turning or suctioning can produce deleterious elevations of ICP. Intracranial compliance can be studied through the relation between ICP and changes in volume of the intracerebral space. One method depends on injection of sterile saline into the ventricular system but it can be associated risk of infection or disruption of intracranial dynamics. An alternative method, relying on inflating and deflating a balloon in the cerebrospinal space, is implemented in the Spiegelberg monitor. Alternatively, altered ICP wave morphology may be a clue to a compromised cerebral compliance (insert ICP wave).

Cerebral Autoregulation and CPP

Arterial Blood Pressure (ABP) and cerebral perfusion pressure (CPP)-monitoring are very important during NICU. The approach to target ABP and CPP in aSAH care is biphasic [26].

Elevated ABP is thought to be an important risk factor for re-bleeding, with highest risk is estimated to occur within the first 24 h post-ictus. Currently, the recommendations for blood pressure management until aneurysm is secured are avoiding systolic blood pressure (SBP) above 160 mmHg (AHA) and https://www.ncbi.nlm.nih.gov/pmc/articles/PMC9932216/ mean arterial blood pressure (MAP) above 110 mmHg (NCC), although more aggressive ABP-lowering management has not shown any definite outcome benefit. After a successful aneurysm occlusion, there is a gradual increase in the risk of cerebral vasospasm, delayed cerebral ischemia (DCI), and brain infarctions during the following 10–14 days. Both AHA and the NCC recommend to maintain euvolemia to prevent cerebral ischemia and to induce arterial hypertension in case of DCI, but without any strict ABP-/CPP-threshold. It has been demonstrated that CPP closer to 70–90 mmHg is associated with better brain tissue oxygenation, cerebral energy metabolism, and favourable outcome in aSAH [27]. There is a need for more prospective studies to validate the thresholds and also determine the best methods achieve the CPP targets, e.g., ABP augmentation by fluids and vasopressors and/or different methods of ICP-lowering.

CPP Targets

During the acute phase, aSAH patients exhibit various degrees of cerebral vasopasm thoughout the vascular tree, which may also vary over time. Fixed CPP-targets cannot be universally applied to these patients as there can be differences in cerebral autoregulation between patients and throughout the temporal course. It is therefore logical that management should be titrated based an individual and temporally dynamic cerebral pressure autoregulatory status. There are several tools which use derived parameters from ICP waveform to assess this function- pressure reactivity index (PRx), mean flow index (Mx), and oxygen reactivity index (ORx) [28]. There are preliminary reports of individualized autoregulatory CPP-target (29)s, but their role in aSAH remains to be determined [27].

CPPopt can be obtained when PRx is plotted against CPP, an autoregulation curve with the optimal plateau phase of stable CBF. CPPopt as a treatment target has shown promising results in TBI studies. However, the evidence to support CPPopt in aSAH is less clear. Some studies have found that CPP below CPPopt is associated with lower CBF and precedes DCI, whereas CPP above CPPopt seems to provoke hyperemia and seizures, but it does not correlate with cerebral energy metabolism or unfavorable outcome [30].

Cerebral Blood Flow

Changes in the CBF Following SAH

There are several changes in the CBF and metabolism following SAH [31]. Under normal conditions cerebral blood flow (CBF) is coupled to cerebral metabolism. The ischaemic damage from the reduced CBF soon after rupture of an aneurysm is offset by reduced cerebral metabolic rate (CMR), particularly in the poor grade patients with SAH. The flow stop occurring in the first short period after aneurysm rupture or direct toxic effects of subarachnoid blood may be responsible for the reduction in the CMR. Thus, in some patients there is relatively high CBF (luxury perfusion) early after SAH. Later the CBF level approaches the metabolic demands of the brain, but in poor-grade patients uncoupling between flow and metabolism may continue for a longer period [31]. In others, CBF is low because of either increased ICP or reduced metabolic rate. Vasospasm may decrease CBF to below metabolic demand depending on the severity and duration.

The normal mean hemispheric CBF is about 50 ml 100 g/1 /min; neurological deficits normally do not occur until CBF decreases below approximately 25 ml 100 g/1 /min. Monitoring of CBF can provide early warning before the occurrence of neurological deficits. Monitoring CBF could assess flow reductions suggestive of cerebral ischaemia, measure the effects of treatment, and evaluate the integrity of autoregulatory mechanisms. In addition to radiographic methods several devices can be used at the patient's bedside to monitor for CBF changes. These radiographic studies, particularly PET, have demonstrated that cellular injury often can occur in the absence of ischemia. Measurement of CBF has long been used in experimental models to define thresholds for ischemia leading to interest in monitoring CBF in patients, in large part because ischemia can underlie secondary cerebral injury. Several techniques are available but none have established the position of a practical bedside monitoring system. Moreover, in SAH regional variation in metabolic rate and CBF is immense, which challenges choice of monitoring.

Using nitrous oxide as a marker, Kety and Schmidt made the first determinations of CBF. Xenon-enhanced CT, 133Xe emission CT, single photon emission computed tomography (SPECT) and positron computed tomography have all been used for measuring CBF in patients with SAH. The CBF measurements can determine the net effect of the initial bleeding and vasospasm on cerebral perfusion. However, these techniques are invasive, and are discontinuous, hence, not capable of detecting all the ischaemic events. They also pose the important safety concern of transporting critically ill patients. Their diagnostic or prognostic values have not been established. Flow can be continually monitored in a single small region of brain using invasive thermal diffusion flowmetry (TDF) or, less commonly, laser Doppler flowmetry (LDF). Laser Doppler flowmetry (LDF) provides reliable measurements of local cortical non-directional CBF [32]. However, the technique is limited by extremely local measurements, arbitrary units of measurements, and artifacts. In patients with SAH the LDF technique has been used concomitant with transcranial Doppler ultrasound (TCD) in the detection of secondary ischaemia and therapeutic management of vasospasm, confirming that high Doppler flow velocities and ischaemia are often not correlated. A thermal diffusion flowmetry technique for continuous and quantitative assessment of regional CBF has been developed, but difficulties in clinical practice with respect to accuracy and reliability have been encountered and again the technique is invasive. Neither technique has gained significant clinical acceptance, as they are invasive nature, have a small field of view, and uncertainly as to where they should be placed, and they are expensive and available only in limited research centres. There are few data regarding ischemic thresholds for these devices and their diagnostic or prognostic values have not been reported in aSAH.

Transcranial Doppler Ultrasound

Transcranial Doppler (TCD) ultrasonography is a bedside dynamic monitoring tool to screen for the presence and progression of cerebral vasospasm in patients with SAH. A low-frequency (2 MHz) pulsed wave probe is used to insonate a major cerebral basal artery through cranial windows: areas of the skull with little attenuation and scattering of the signal because of sparse or no cancellous bone. This allows computer assisted generation of information on peak systolic, end diastolic and mean flow velocities along with a pulsatility index from the recorded waveforms [33]. Although DSA is the gold standard for diagnosing cerebral vasospasm and has a high sensitivity and specificity, the limitations of DSA and CT angiography are that they are invasive methods and require contrast administration with associated risks of transportation of patients. They provide only a snapshot of information about cerebral vasospasm at the time of imaging. TCD measurements help decide whether a clinical worsening results from vasospasm or if other causes should be excluded by, for example, a CT scan. CTA can be performed when TCD readings become elevated and neurological examination is limited [34].

TCD has several applications for aSAH. The transcranial Doppler is the most frequently used bedside monitor for detecting vasospasm of the MCA. After SAH, CBF may deviate considerably from normal [35]. As CBF affects the flow velocities, the assessment of vasospasm from flow velocities alone may be insufficient. Lindegaard and co-workers suggested using a 'Hemispheric Index' between flow velocities in the MCA and internal carotid artery on the same side [36]. It is resistant to changes in CBF and, therefore, predictive of MCA lumen narrowing. An index of more than 3.0 indicates MCA vasospasm and values above 6.0 suggest severe MCA vasospasm [36].

In patients with SAH, additional applications of the TCD technique include studies of CBF autoregulation integrity by the carotid artery compression test (transient hyperemic response test) or induced hypertension and indirect evaluation of ICP through the use of the pulsatility index [37]. Monitoring using transient hyperemic response test has predictive value in vasospasm development [38]. The major advantage is its bedside non-invasive nature allowing serial measurements. Yet there are several limitations. Major drawbacks are the operator dependency along with the lack of an established relationship between flow velocities and delayed neurological deficits [39]. The frequency of angiographically documented vasospasm is higher than in symptomati cases, so also high TCD flow velocities may be well tolerated in some patients [40]. The reported sensitivity and specificity when angiography is used as a reference standard is around 60–100%, [41, 42] positive predictive value (PPV)is (100%) whereas the negative predictive value (NPV) is low (30%) and when symptomatic vasospasm is used as reference standard sensitivity and specificity are 80–100%, PPV is low (39%) but the NPV is high (90%) [43, 44]. A systematic review and meta-analysis that included 17 studies (n = 2870 patients) shows that evidence of vasospasm on TCD was found to be highly predictive of DCI [44, 45]. Combining TCD with other neuromonitoring such as EEG [45] or Brain Tissue Oxygen Tension [46] may increase the prediction of DCI. Because of anatomical variations, the lack of correlation between flow velocities and lumen diameter, and frequent participation in collateral blood flow, TCD is less reliable in detecting vasospasm in the major cerebral arteries other than MCA. Predictive power is improved with the use of transcranial color-coded duplex sonography (TCCS) [47]. Vasospasm in smaller arteries is beyond the detection capacity of TCD. This is rare and does not lead to delayed neurological deficits [48]. Integrity of the CBF autoregulation, the number of arteries involved, and the anatomy of the circle of Willis are some of the factors that determine the clinical condition of the patient. This makes treatment decisions based on TCD findings alone difficult [49]. Consecutive TCD measurements and inclusion of the Lindegaard ratio and the rate of the increase in velocities in interpreting the data improves performance. Steep velocity increases (>25 cm/ s /day) from baseline level are generally accepted as a warning of the development of vasospasm [50]. The use of TCD or TCCS monitoring is recommended to predict and assess the severity of vasospasm after aneurysmal SAH [51] but the evidence for other applications is not strong [9].

Jugular Venous Oximetry

Adequacy of global cerebral blood flow can be assessed using jugular venous oximetry. $CMRO_2 = CBF^* CaO_2\text{-}CvO_2$ where CaO_2 and CvO_2 denote arterial and jugular venous oxygen content, respectively. Assuming an unchanged metabolic rate of oxygen (CMRO2), AVDO2 changes in inverse proportion to CBF. Hence, the arterial to jugular vein oxygen concentration difference (AVDO2) may serve as an indirect measure of relative changes in CBF and this may be replaced by the difference in arterial and jugular venous saturation ($SjVO_2$) [52, 53]. A retrograde catheter can be placed in the internal jugular vein for serial measurements or continuous fibreoptic monitoring of jugular venous oxygen saturation ($SjVO_2$)). A low $SjVO_2$ values indicate hypoperfusion and elevated values relative hyperaemia. The side of monitoring is often debated. Unless the patient has lateralizing pathology the difference in oxygen saturation on the two sides is small. Anatomical data suggest that blood from the cortex might preferably drain into the right jugular vein and blood from the subcortex into the left, right IJV may be preferred. $SjVO_2$ measurements reflect global CBF and cannot detect focal CBF changes. [52, 53) Generally, $SjVO_2$ values of less than 50–60% are considered the threshold for cerebral hypoxaemia. This corresponds to an intraparenchymal brain tissue partial pressure of oxygen ($Pbro_2$) of around 1.3–2 kPa [54]. The $Sjvo_2$ catheter can also used in the assessment of CBF autoregulation and vasoreactivity [53, 54]. Few studies have used Sjvo2 measurements in patients with SAH. A study demonstrated that in nine of 26 patients with SAH at least one episode of $Sjvo_2$ desaturation and abnormal reductions in Sjvo2 was observed in 10% of total serial measurements and ICP is significantly elevated during these episodes [55]. Possible complications from retrograde jugular catheterization are similar to anterograde catheterization including carotid artery puncture, haematoma formation, infection, jugular vein occlusion, and increases in ICP during placement. In head trauma patients, the use of Sjvo2 catheters seems promising but very few studies have evaluated the diagnostic or clinical relevance of jugular venous oximetry in the management of patients with SAH [55, 56]. Concomitant use of brain tissue oxygenation monitoring may further improve the clinical relevance.

Cerebral Oxygenation

Brain Tissue Oxygenation

Brain tissue oxygen (Pbto2) provides a surrogate measure of regional CBF and represents the balance among oxygen supply, diffusion, and consumption. Intraparenchymal oxygen-sensitive or combined oxygen-, carbon dioxide- and pH-sensitive microelectrodes are available for bedside on-line monitoring of brain tissue oxygenation ($Pbro_2$). $PbtO_2$ can be measured commercially using the Licox system or the Neurovent-PTO system, and used as a surrogate measure of CBF [41]. Whereas $Pbro_2$ only provides information on oxygen tension, the combined microelectrodes present indirect information on the metabolic status of the brain.

Excluding the first hour after insertion, $Pbro_2$ monitoring is a reliable technique with good quality of data [57]. $Pbto_2$ has been found to help in the early detection of DCI and brain hypoxia in patients with SAH [58]. A low $Pbro_2$ level is associated with the severity of the haemorrhage, ischaemic events and a poor clinical outcome. A specific hypoxic lower limit, below which the brain is at risk of being damaged, is undetermined. Different authors find different cut-off points. However, a lower $Pbro_2$ level of around 1.3–2 kPa is probably rational, corresponding to Sjvo2 values of around 60% [41]. Treatment of $PbtO_2$ below 1.33 kPa was effective in reducing secondary ischemic damage [59]. $Pbro_2$ monitoring only provides information on local tissue changes, and there are reservations concerning changes in other areas of the brain. $Pbro_2$ monitoring is an invasive technique. Infection is a potential adverse complication but so far no cases have been reported. Prolonged catheter placement might result in oedema in the surrounding tissue and infiltration of the catheter by inflammatory cells making the measurements obtained after several days more difficult to interpret. The diagnostic and prognostic value has not been reported and the influence on patient outcome is undetermined [60].

Near Infrared Spectroscopy

Near Infrared Spectroscopy (NIRS)is a simple, portable, continuous, real-time, non-invasive monitoring of cerebral oximetry. A NIRS device emits light from a light-emitting diode (LED) or a laser in the near-infrared range, usually between 700 and 850 nm, and collects what reaches the photodetectors after absorption and scattering. The absorption is proportional to the concentration of chromophores. The chromophores of interest are oxyhemoglobin (HbO_2) and deoxyhemoglobin (HHb). The percentage of HbO_2 over total haemoglobin thus provides the cerebral regional oxygen saturation (c-rSO_2), which is named variably by different manufacturers and abbreviated (rSO_2, TOI, TCCO, $StcO_2$). The normal baseline probably ranges between 60 and 75%. [61] C-rSO_2 is assumed to reflect the balance between cerebral oxygen consumption (cerebral metabolic rate of oxygen ($CMRO_2$)) and oxygen delivery in the region of interest. NIRS values rely on many assumptions- a fixed arterial: venous ratio [usually 30:70 or 25:75) and a constant scattering which may change following aSAH. Brain oedema creates significant shifts in intracranial photon scattering that may cause unpredictable and profound alterations in the readings. There is little correlation between cerebral ischemia detected by NIRS and cerebral ischemia defined as a $PtiO_2$ of <15 mmHg [62, 63, 64) and low $SjvO_2$ [55]. However, NIRS, $PtiO_2$ and $SjvO_2$ assess different processes that are intimately related but cannot be substituted.

There are several causes for the pathological decline in c-rSO_2, such as arterial hypotension, low cardiac output, systemic hypoxia, hyperventilation, stroke or impending DCI. Conversely, high c-rSO_2 might be secondary to hyperemia, acidosis, hypoglycemia, high levels of sedation or hypothermia. Convulsions might present as low, high or oscillating c-rSO_2. There is a good association between c-rSO_2 and cerebral blood flow (CBF) [65]. NIRS has been shown to detect changes in CBF with ventilation, [66] cardiac output augmentation with either dobutamine or milrinone in DCI patients, resulting in a better c-rSO_2 [67]. Hence, it can be used to personalize targets. NIRS monitoring has been used to evaluate cerebrovascular reactivity- the tissue oxygenation index (TOx) or cerebral oxygenation index (COx), which is calculated as a rolling correlation coefficient between averaged CPP (or MAP) values and the corresponding NIRS signal [68, 69]. It has been validated against the pressure reactivity index (PRx) [70] and TCD-derived reactivity index (Mx) [71].

Vasospasm detection, DCI prediction, and prognostication have explicitly been evaluated in the aSAH population. A decrease of more than 12% in c-rSO_2 from the baseline was associated with a better predictive value than same-side TCD using the traditional threshold value of 200 cm/s to detect severe vasospasm on CT angiography [72] and sensitivity of 86%-94% and specificity of 71%-86% to detect DCI [72, 73]. Impaired cerebrovascular reactivity on the side contralateral to the aneurysm was associated with an OR of DCI of 19 (95% CI: 1.2–320) and a threshold of 0.07 conferred TOx a sensitivity of 58%, and a specificity of 91% to predict DCI [74]. Patients with preserved cerebrovascular reactivity, as defined by a negative or near-zero TOx was associated with good functional outcomes at 90 days (OR, 2.5) [70]. The relationship between c-rSO_2 and outcome in aSAH patients has been examined. Cerebral desaturation (c-rSO_2 <50% for 30 min) was independently associated with DCI and poor functional outcomes (mRS of 4-6 at 3 months (OR 2.72) [75]. It was seen that patients with an unfavourable outcome spent more time with a cerebral desaturation than those with a good outcome (5 h 43 vs. 1 h 47) and patients with episodes of cerebral desaturation lasting more than 2 h were at much higher risk of poor short-term outcomes than those without [76]. Although NIRS seems ideal for timely ischemia detection and to improve management in aSAH, the quality of evidence supporting its use currently remains low [61].

Cerebral Microdialysis

Perturbations in the cerebral metabolic function are common in aneurysmal subarachnoid hemorrhage (aSAH) (Figure 2). Cerebral metabolic dysfunction has been shown to extensively mediate the pathophysiology of brain injury after subarachnoid hemorrhage (SAH). The measurement of alterations of metabolites in the brain can help understand pathophysiological changes occurring after SAH, especially cerebral energy dysfunction [77]. Cerebral microdialysis (CMD) is a tool that can measure concentrations of multiple bioenergetics metabolites in brain interstitial fluid. Microdialysis, a chemical sampling method, which allows endogenous low-molecular weight substances to passively diffuse and equilibrate across a semi-permeable membrane into a dialysate where concentrations can be analyzed, has changed from a 'bench' to a bedside technique. Today bedside equipment, allowing spectro-photometric analysis of some substances of interest, are commercially available. The dialysate is normally collected every hour and thus the measured concentrations are average concentrations in that hour. However, CMD is a regional measuring technique that is influenced by proximity to focal lesions [78]. The microdialysis catheters implanted into the relevant positions in relation to affected tissue, provide prompt information on metabolism and its consequences for cell survival. Ischaemia within the region of the microdialysis catheter is associated with pathological changes in energy-related metabolites (glucose, pyruvate, and lactate), excitotoxines (as glutamate and aspartate) and membrane degrading products, (such as glycerol). Monitoring cerebral metabolism with intracerebral microdialysis (CMD) allows early detection of secondary injury and may guide decisions and affect outcomes in neurocrtitical care of these patients.

Interest has focused on the ability of microdialysis to monitor the development of vasospasm and delayed neurological deficits. Studies have shown that changes in metabolites indicative of ischaemia occurred before the onset of symptoms in 83% of patients with delayed neurological deficits following SAH [79, 80]. Studies concerning which markers are the most sensitive or predictive is still conflicting. Studies have indicated that in patients with SAH the lactate/pyruvate ratio is a more reliable marker than lactate alone and elevated concentrations of glutamate is the earliest marker of vasospasm followed over time by lactate. Increases in lactate/ glucose and lactate/pyruvate followed by increases in glycerol, a high sensitivity (94%), specificity (88%), and PPV (85%) in terms of detecting delayed neurological deterioration can be found [80]. The ischaemic pattern precedes the occurrence of delayed neurological deficits by a mean interval of 11h [77]. Microdialysis was compared with TCD and angiography was found to have the higher specificity and positive likelihood ratio for confirming delayed neurological deficits [81]. Patients with poor-grade SAH or an unfavourable outcome have higher concentrations of markers than less affected patients [82]. There is still a paucity of clinical studies evaluating the actual impact of microdialysis monitoring on patient outcome.

There are important limitations to the microdialysis technique. The most important is the fact that the technique monitors metabolic changes in the vicinity of the catheter only. Unless the catheter is placed in an area where secondary insults are affecting nerve cells, 'normal' concentrations will be measured. In patients with SAH the most informative placement of the catheter seems to be the vascular territory of the artery harbouring the ruptured aneurysm. Informative placement of the catheter is infact difficult because of the fact that vasospasm and infarction after SAH are not limited to the area of aneurysm location, but can be found in other areas of the brain depending on the distribution of the haemorrhage. Alternatively, more than one catheter can be placed [83]. Bleeding and infection are potential adverse complications but so far no cases have been reported. Prolonged catheter placement might result in oedema in the surrounding tissue and infiltration of the dialysis membrane by inflammatory cells making the measurements obtained after several days more difficult to interpret. Microdialysis has several potential area of interest for the future. The measurement of endogenous substances associated with neuronal damage, for example protein S-100, nitric oxide, and free oxygen radicals, and small-molecule mediators of inflammationsuch as IL-6 may provide valuable information for intervention and correlate with DCI and outcome [84, 85, 86]. Intracerebral microdialysis may also provide important bedside information on the effect of interventional therapy and active interventions initiated based on CMD monitoring showed lower DCI incidence [87]. CMD may also provide an opportunity to assess pharmacokinetics of drugs across the blood–brain barrier [88]. Despite the lack of a standard procedure as well as the presence of limitations regarding CMD application and data interpretation for both clinical and experimental studies, Emerging investigations have suggested that CMD is an effective way to monitor the changes of cerebral metabolic dysfunction after SAH in real-time [89]. The combination of CMD and other monitoring tools might be able to further understand the relationship between cerebral metabolic dysfunction and brain injury after SAH, determine the severity of brain injury and predict the pathological progression and outcomes after SAH. More translational preclinical investigations and clinical validation may help to optimize CMD as a powerful tool in critical care and personalized medicine for patients with SAH.

Online Bedside Monitoring of Molecular Injury Patterns-

The newly developed proximity extension assay (PEA) is a very sensitive tool to detect small quantities of protein while using only small volumes of fluid. [90] It is possible to efficaciously detect and study numerous brain protein biomarkers from patients with aSAH [90, 91]. This may enable a deeper understanding of ongoing pathophysiological processes and refine indications and time windows of treatments for neuroprotective pharmacological agents.

EEG Monitoring

Recent technical advances and broader availability have made cEEG feasible for more patients with aSAH. Quantitative EEG software programs allow the expeditious, real-time detection of adverse events such as seizures and DCI possible [92, 93]. Epileptic activity is common following aSAH and this may manifest as focal or generalized, convulsive and non-convulsive seizures. Seizures occasionally occur immediately after ictus or re-bleeding and in case of cerebral ischemia and brain herniation [94, 95]. Convulsive seizures are typically easy to identify, whereas non-convulsive seizures are rather detected with electroencephalography (EEG) in patients in a poor neurological condition without any other clear explanation. The rate of seizures based on clinical criteria has been estimated to occur in between 4 and 26% of the cases, whereas the rate of epileptic activity may be much higher as evaluated with EEG and in particular with the more sensitive method electrocorticography. It has been suggested that the use of continuous EEG to assess for non-convulsive seizures in patients who fail to improve [96]. Ictal-interictal continuum abnormalities, such as sporadic epileptiform discharges, generalized periodic discharges, or seizures, may help predict whether patients are at risk for delayed ischemic events [97, 98]. Alpha/delta ratios are the best predictors of vasospasm and delayed ischemic events and are lower in patients who are at risk for delayed cerebral infarct within the first four days post injury [97]. Alpha/delta ratios in intracortical EEG decrease approximately 42% in patients with vasospasm compared with 17% in those without [99]. Published criteria for predicting DCI based on changes in cEEG spectral features [92] are (1) decreasing relative alpha power variability, (2) decreasing alpha-to-delta power ratio, (3) worsening focal slowing, or (4) late-appearing epileptiform abnormalitie. The burden of epileptiform discharges (ED), measured as number of ED per houri, can be a novel biomarker for predicting those at high risk of DCI [100]. EEGs can also be conducted on comatose patients to determine levels of consciousness, arousability, and awareness. There is potential to quantify patient consciousness using EEG monitoring and neurological examination [101]. Although vasospasm of proximal cerebral arteries has been regarded as the main cause of DCI, vasospasm of distal arteries, microthrombosis, impaired autoregulation, cortical spreading depolarization (CSD), and spreading ischemia are thought to be involved in DCI after aSAH. CSD is characterized by a moving gradient of cortical membrane depolarization with subsequent electrical depression and associated CBF disturbances (inverse neurovascular coupling). This may ultimately result in disturbed cerebral energy metabolism and cell death [102]. EEG monitoring helps in detecting CSD and DCI. There are currently no specific treatments for CSD, but it has generally been suggested beneficial to optimize systemic and cerebral physiology. A recent study showed beneficial effects of cilostazol on DCI and neurological outcome [103]. EEGs can be analyzed along with somatosensory evoked potentials to predict neurological deterioration, which may allow physicians to detect and protect against future neurological damage [104]. Multimodal electrophysiological monitoring including median nerve somatosensory evoked potential (M-SSEP), tibial nerve somatosensory evoked potential (T-SSEP), flash-visual evoked potential (f-VEP), brainstem auditory evoked potential (BAEP) and central conduction time (CCT) have shown to predict outcomes in aSAH [105, 106].

Multimodality Monitoring - Individualizing Neurointensive Care in aSAH

In a classic neurointensive care, ICP and CPP are monitored in unconscious aSAH patients and treatment aims to avoid intracranial hypertension and to ensure sufficient cerebral perfusion. Even in case of normal ICP and CPP, disturbances in CBF, $PbtO_2$, and cerebral energy metabolism are frequent. There are several physiological steps that affect CBF and the cerebral delivery of oxygen (CDO_2) as well as nutrients (glucose and lactate; CDGlc and CDLac). The steps to optimize cerebral energy metabolism divided into the CBF-, oxygenation-, and nutrient-patways together with factors involved in energy metabolism are shown in the figure below (Figure 2).

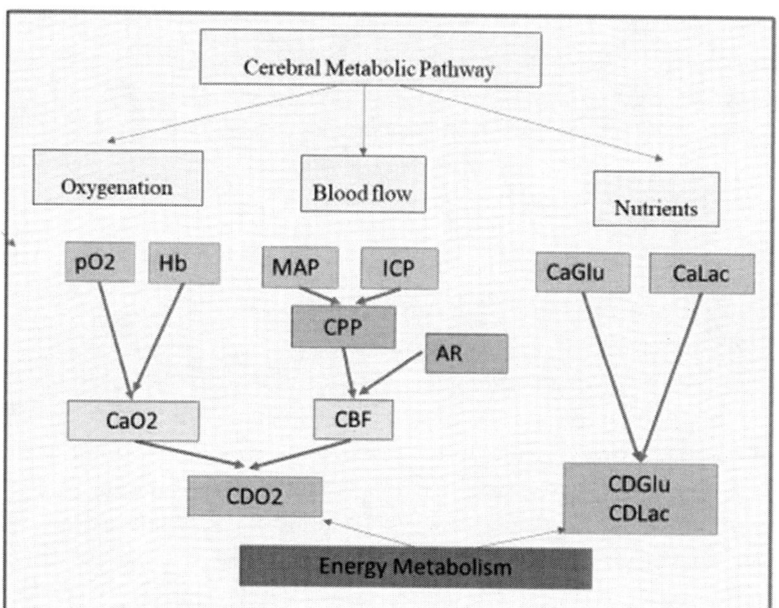

Figure 2. Factors controlling cerebral oxygen metabolism.

Every neuromonitoring technique, in isolation, has limitations. The radiological imaging only gives snapshots of the cerebral status. The global measures such as jugular bulb oxygenation may be too insensitive to detect small, but important, focal cerebral oxygen disturbances. The microdialysis represents only a small brain region and is not suitable to guide a global therapy such as CPP-levels. The combined analysis of the information obtained by the different techniques may provide a more accurate picture of the cerebral situation. For that reason, Multimodal monitoring (MMM) tools have been developed to enable monitoring of the different steps to achieve cerebral energy metabolism. The combined use of multiple monitors is termed "multimodality monitoring" (MMM). Multimodal monitoring includes cerebral pressure autoregulation (pressure reactivity index, mean flow index), CBF (intraparenchymal probes, transcranial Doppler, and radiological imaging), brain tissue oxygenation (jugular bulb, btO2), and cerebral energy metabolism (microdialysis and radiological imaging). A complete MMM setup enables earlier detection of impending brain injury, diagnosis of the specific pathomechanisms and initiation of cause-specific therapies. [105] The various physiological derrangements following aSAH and role of neuromonitoring is given in Table 1. However, the implementation of MMM-based management has been limited to a few research-oriented NIC units. Intracranial pressure (ICP), brain lactate to pyruvate ratio (L/P ratio), and brain parenchymal oxygen tension (pO(2)) were used as surrogates for clinical status in a comatose man after high-grade aSAH resulting in good outcome [105]. Currently, a uniform protocol for management is applied to all aSAH patients [51] despite significant patient heterogeneity. Precision and personalization in managing Aneurysmal subarachnoid haemorrhage is possible with monitoring targeted therapy. MMM protocols could then be of value to further diagnose the cause of energy metabolic disturbance to individualize CBF- and CaO_2-oriented treatments [107, 108].

Multimodal monitoring generates an enormous amount of continuous and imaging data. Clinicians may be confronted with the risk of "information overload" that can lead to medical errors. Hence, the data are not helpful unless annotated so that one can search for "epochs of interest,"such as effects of therapies, and also identify potential artifacts. Ergonomic data displays that present standardized informatics infrastructure including data collection, data visualization, data analysis, and decision support, are essential [109, 110]. The validity of guiding management based on these MMM-tools remains controversial. Altogether, MMM carries great potential, despite existing limitations [108].

Limitations of Neuromonitoring in aSAH

It is important to remember that neurological monitoring is only part of the problem and that systemic physiological monitoring is as important in a patient with SAH as in any patient in the intensive care setting. However, there are several challenges in monitoring these patients. Patients are usually agitated and can accidentally remove the monitoring equipment are well known in the neurointensive care unit. Most of the monitoring techniques discussed will require cooperative or sedated patients. Neuromonitoring may enable a deeper understanding of ongoing pathophysiological processes and refine indications and time windows of treatments for neuroprotective pharmacological agents. But the placement of parenchymal probes for invasive neuromonitoring or non-invasive monitoring does not per se positively affect outcome after aneurysmal SAH. A beneficial effect will only arise if values reflecting a problem in cerebral pathophysiology detected result in structured treatment modification, thus optimizing therapy. The data generated through monitoring is likely enormous and complex, and will most likely be a need to analyze the dynamics of this information with artificial intelligence to understand their complex patterns in future NIC units [111].

Conclusion

The management of aneurysmal subarachnoidal haemorrhage is challenging and often requires an extensive team work. After aSAH, the primary haemorrhage and a number of secondary insults in the acute post-haemorrhagic period determine the outcome. Several neuro-monitoring techniques are available for prompt recognition of preventable and potentially reversible cerebral or systemic complications. These have not only improved our understanding of disease pathophysiology but also aid in monitoring the cerebral effects of treatments. None of the techniques, when considered in isolation, has proved sufficient after SAH. Their validity to guide management in aSAH still remains unclear considering their inherent temporal, spatial, and logistical constraints. There are no guidelines for monitoring or specific monitoring thresholds for aSAH. The 2023 recommendations for the Management of Patients With Aneurysmal Subarachnoid Hemorrhage from the American Heart Association/American Stroke Association recommendations for monitoring of aSAH [112] are given in Table 2.

The success or failure of a monitoring system is contingent upon the successive steps following the measurement of a neuroparameter to the implementation of a response from the neurointensive team. This depends upon human skills and vigilance. Therefore, the successful implementation of any new monitoring system depends on a thorough introduction and continuous training of the professional team. The scientific interest elicited by neuro-monitoring or neuro-imaging techniques should not cloud the issue of their practical relevance. More research is required to address the accuracy and reliability of the neuromoitoring technique, theoretical and practical limitations and risks, impact on decision making and influence on patient outcome.

References

[1] Teasdale GM, Drake CG, Hunt W, Kassell N, Sano K, Pertuiset B, et al. A universal subarachnoid hemorrhage scale: report of a committee of the World Federation of Neurosurgical Societies. *J Neurol Neurosurg Psychiatry*. 1988;51(11):1457.

[2] Crobeddu E, Mittal MK, Dupont S, Wijdicks EF, Lanzino G, Rabinstein AA. Predicting the lack of development of delayed cerebral ischemia after aneurysmal subarachnoid hemorrhage. *Stroke*. 2012;43(3):697-701.

[3] Rosengart AJ, Schultheiss KE, Tolentino J, Macdonald RL. Prognostic factors for outcome in patients with aneurysmal subarachnoid hemorrhage. *Stroke*. 2007;38(8):2315-21.

[4] Vergouwen MD, Vermeulen M, van Gijn J, Rinkel GJ, Wijdicks EF, Muizelaar JP, et al. Definition of delayed cerebral ischemia after aneurysmal subarachnoid hemorrhage as an outcome event in clinical trials and observational studies: proposal of a multidisciplinary research group. *Stroke*. 2010;41(10):2391-5.

[5] Raatikainen E, Vahtera A, Kuitunen A, Junttila E, Huhtala H, Ronkainen A, et al. Prognostic value of the 2010 consensus definition of delayed cerebral ischemia after aneurysmal subarachnoid hemorrhage. *J Neurol Sci*. 2021;420:117261.

[6] Shimoda M, Takeuchi M, Tominaga J, Oda S, Kumasaka A, Tsugane R. Asymptomatic versus symptomatic infarcts from vasospasm in patients with subarachnoid hemorrhage: serial magnetic resonance imaging. *Neurosurgery*. 2001;49(6):1341-8; discussion 8-50.

[7] Schmidt JM, Wartenberg KE, Fernandez A, Claassen J, Rincon F, Ostapkovich ND, et al. Frequency and clinical impact of asymptomatic cerebral infarction due to vasospasm after subarachnoid hemorrhage. *J Neurosurg*. 2008;109(6):1052-9.

[8] Cesarini KG, Hardemark HG, Persson L. Improved survival after aneurysmal subarachnoid hemorrhage: review of case management during a 12-year period. *J Neurosurg*. 1999;90(4):664-72.

[9] Le Roux P, Menon DK, Citerio G, Vespa P, Bader MK, Brophy GM, et al. Consensus summary statement of the International Multidisciplinary Consensus Conference on Multimodality Monitoring in Neurocritical Care: a statement for healthcare professionals from the Neurocritical Care Society and the European Society of Intensive Care Medicine. *Neurocrit Care*. 2014;21 Suppl 2:S1-26.

[10] Le Roux P, Menon DK, Citerio G, Vespa P, Bader MK, Brophy GM, et al. Consensus summary statement of the International Multidisciplinary Consensus Conference on Multimodality Monitoring in Neurocritical Care : a statement for healthcare professionals from the Neurocritical Care Society and the European Society of Intensive Care Medicine. *Intensive Care Med*. 2014;40(9):1189-209.

[11] Connolly ES, Jr., Rabinstein AA, Carhuapoma JR, Derdeyn CP, Dion J, Higashida RT, et al. Guidelines for the management of aneurysmal subarachnoid hemorrhage: a guideline for healthcare professionals from the American Heart Association/american Stroke Association. *Stroke*. 2012;43(6):1711-37.

[12] Florez WA, Garcia-Ballestas E, Deora H, Agrawal A, Martinez-Perez R, Galwankar S, et al. Intracranial hypertension in patients with aneurysmal subarachnoid hemorrhage: a systematic review and meta-analysis. *Neurosurg Rev*. 2021;44(1):203-11.

[13] Magni F, Pozzi M, Rota M, Vargiolu A, Citerio G. High-Resolution Intracranial Pressure Burden and Outcome in Subarachnoid Hemorrhage. *Stroke*. 2015;46(9):2464-9.

[14] Czosnyka M, Hutchinson PJ, Balestreri M, Hiler M, Smielewski P, Pickard JD. Monitoring and interpretation of intracranial pressure after head injury. *Acta Neurochir Suppl*. 2006;96:114-8.

[15] Lundberg N, Troupp H, Lorin H. Continuous recording of the ventricular-fluid pressure in patients with severe acute traumatic brain injury. A preliminary report. *J Neurosurg*. 1965;22(6):581-90.

[16] Kraemer JL, Gobbato PL, Andrade-Souza YM. Third ventriculostomy through the lamina terminalis for intracranial pressure monitoring after aneurysm surgery: technical note. *Arq Neuropsiquiatr*. 2002;60(4):932-4.

[17] Lozier AP, Sciacca RR, Romagnoli MF, Connolly ES, Jr. Ventriculostomy-related infections: a critical review of the literature. *Neurosurgery*. 2008;62 Suppl 2:688-700.

[18] Piper I, Barnes A, Smith D, Dunn L. The Camino intracranial pressure sensor: is it optimal technology? An internal audit with a review of current intracranial pressure monitoring technologies. *Neurosurgery*. 2001;49(5):1158-64; discussion 64-5.

[19] Eide PK. Comparison of simultaneous continuous intracranial pressure (ICP) signals from a Codman and a Camino ICP sensor. *Med Eng Phys*. 2006;28(6):542-9.

[20] Lang JM, Beck J, Zimmermann M, Seifert V, Raabe A. Clinical evaluation of intraparenchymal Spiegelberg pressure sensor. *Neurosurgery*. 2003;52(6):1455-9; discussion 9.

[21] Yang J, Lu J, Li R, Lin F, Chen Y, Han H, et al. Application of Intracranial Pressure-Directed Therapy on Delayed Cerebral Ischemia After Aneurysmal Subarachnoid Hemorrhage. *Front Aging Neurosci*. 2022;14:831994.

[22] Baggiani M, Graziano F, Rebora P, Robba C, Guglielmi A, Galimberti S, et al. Intracranial Pressure Monitoring Practice, Treatment, and Effect on Outcome in Aneurysmal Subarachnoid Hemorrhage. *Neurocrit Care*. 2022.

[23] Voldby B, Enevoldsen EM. Intracranial pressure changes following aneurysm rupture. Part 1: clinical and angiographic correlations. *J Neurosurg*. 1982;56(2):186-96.

[24] Voldby B, Enevoldsen EM. Intracranial pressure changes following aneurysm rupture. Part 2: associated cerebrospinal fluid lactacidosis. *J Neurosurg*. 1982;56(2):197-204.

[25] Voldby B, Enevoldsen EM. Intracranial pressure changes following aneurysm rupture. Part 3: Recurrent hemorrhage. *J Neurosurg*. 1982;56(6):784-9.

[26] Lang EW, Diehl RR, Mehdorn HM. Cerebral autoregulation testing after aneurysmal subarachnoid hemorrhage: the phase relationship between arterial blood pressure and cerebral blood flow velocity. *Crit Care Med*. 2001;29(1):158-63.

[27] Svedung Wettervik T, Hanell A, Howells T, Ronne Engstrom E, Lewen A, Enblad P. ICP, CPP, and PRx in traumatic brain injury and aneurysmal subarachnoid hemorrhage: association of insult intensity and duration with clinical outcome. *J Neurosurg*. 2023;138(2):446-53.

[28] Svedung Wettervik T, Fahlstrom M, Enblad P, Lewen A. Cerebral Pressure Autoregulation in Brain Injury and Disorders-A Review on Monitoring, Management, and Future Directions. *World Neurosurg*. 2022;158:118-31.

[29] Tas J, Beqiri E, van Kaam RC, Czosnyka M, Donnelly J, Haeren RH, et al. Targeting Autoregulation-Guided Cerebral Perfusion Pressure after Traumatic Brain Injury (COGiTATE): A Feasibility Randomized Controlled Clinical Trial. *J Neurotrauma*. 2021;38(20):2790-800.

[30] Svedung Wettervik T, Howells T, Lewen A, Ronne-Engstrom E, Enblad P. Temporal Dynamics of ICP, CPP, PRx, and CPPopt in High-Grade Aneurysmal Subarachnoid Hemorrhage and the Relation to Clinical Outcome. *Neurocrit Care*. 2021;34(2):390-402.

[31] Song JN, Chen H, Zhang M, Zhao YL, Ma XD. Dynamic change in cerebral microcirculation and focal cerebral metabolism in experimental subarachnoid hemorrhage in rabbits. *Metab Brain Dis*. 2013;28(1):33-43.

[32] Rejmstad P, Haj-Hosseini N, Aneman O, Wardell K. Optical monitoring of cerebral microcirculation in neurointensive care. *Med Biol Eng Comput*. 2018;56(7):1201-10.

[33] Manno EM. Transcranial Doppler ultrasonography in the neurocritical care unit. *Crit Care Clin*. 1997;13(1):79-104.

[34] Ivanidze J, Sanelli PC. Vasospasm: Role of Imaging in Detection and Monitoring Treatment. *Neuroimaging Clin N Am*. 2021;31(2):147-55.

[35] Talacchi A. Sequential measurements of cerebral blood flow in the acute phase of subarachnoid hemorrhage. *J Neurosurg Sci*. 1993;37(1):9-18.

[36] Lindegaard KF, Nornes H, Bakke SJ, Sorteberg W, Nakstad P. Cerebral vasospasm diagnosis by means of angiography and blood velocity measurements. *Acta Neurochir (Wien)*. 1989;100(1-2):12-24.

[37] Soehle M, Chatfield DA, Czosnyka M, Kirkpatrick PJ. Predictive value of initial clinical status, intracranial pressure and transcranial Doppler pulsatility after subarachnoid haemorrhage. *Acta Neurochir (Wien)*. 2007;149(6):575-83.

[38] Al-Jehani H, Angle M, Marcoux J, Teitelbaum J. Early abnormal transient hyperemic response test can predict delayed ischemic neurologic deficit in subarachnoid hemorrhage. *Crit Ultrasound J*. 2018;10(1):1.

[39] Lele AV, Wabl R, Wahlster S, Keen J, Walters AM, Fong CT, et al. Associations Between Transcranial Doppler Vasospasm and Clinical Outcomes After Aneurysmal Subarachnoid Hemorrhage: A Retrospective Observational Study. *Cureus*. 2022;14(11):e31789.

[40] Ekelund A, Saveland H, Romner B, Brandt L. Is transcranial Doppler sonography useful in detecting late cerebral ischaemia after aneurysmal subarachnoid haemorrhage? *Br J Neurosurg*. 1996;10(1):19-25.

[41] Fan TH, Rosenthal ES. Physiological Monitoring in Patients with Acute Brain Injury: A Multimodal Approach. *Crit Care Clin*. 2023;39(1):221-33.

[42] Esmael A, Flifel ME, Elmarakby F, Belal T. Predictive value of the transcranial Doppler and mean arterial flow velocity for early detection of cerebral vasospasm in aneurysmal subarachnoid hemorrhage. *Ultrasound*. 2021;29(4):218-28.

[43] Darsaut TE, Keough MB, Chan AM, Farzin B, Findlay JM, Chow MM, et al. Transcranial Doppler Velocities and Angiographic Vasospasm after SAH: A Diagnostic Accuracy Study. *AJNR Am J Neuroradiol*. 2022;43(1):80-6.

[44] Kumar G, Shahripour RB, Harrigan MR. Vasospasm on transcranial Doppler is predictive of delayed cerebral ischemia in aneurysmal subarachnoid hemorrhage: a systematic review and meta-analysis. *J Neurosurg*. 2016;124(5):1257-64.

[45] Chen HY, Elmer J, Zafar SF, Ghanta M, Moura Junior V, Rosenthal ES, et al. Combining Transcranial Doppler and EEG Data to Predict Delayed Cerebral Ischemia After Subarachnoid Hemorrhage. *Neurology*. 2022;98(5):e459-e69.

[46] Craven CL, Sae-Huang M, Hoskote C, Watkins LD, Reddy U, Toma AK. Relationship between Brain Tissue Oxygen Tension and Transcranial Doppler Ultrasonography. *World Neurosurg*. 2021;149:e942-e6.

[47] Turek G, Kochanowicz J, Rutkowski R, Krejza J, Lyson T, Gorbacz K, et al. Accuracy of transcranial colour-coded sonography in the diagnosis of anterior cerebral artery vasospasm. *Neurol Neurochir Pol.* 2012;46(3):233-8.

[48] Newell DW, Grady MS, Eskridge JM, Winn HR. Distribution of angiographic vasospasm after subarachnoid hemorrhage: implications for diagnosis by transcranial Doppler ultrasonography. *Neurosurgery.* 1990;27(4):574-7.

[49] Bartels RH, Verhagen WI, Van der Spek JA, Grotenhuis JA, Brandsma E, Notermans SL. Transcranial Doppler ultrasonography: influence on scheduling of angiography and delayed surgery for ruptured intracranial aneurysms. *J Neurosurg Sci.* 1994;38(1):21-7.

[50] Naval NS, Thomas CE, Urrutia VC. Relative changes in flow velocities in vasospasm after subarachnoid hemorrhage: a transcranial Doppler study. *Neurocrit Care.* 2005;2(2):133-40.

[51] Treggiari MM, Rabinstein AA, Busl KM, Caylor MM, Citerio G, Deem S, et al. Guidelines for the Neurocritical Care Management of Aneurysmal Subarachnoid Hemorrhage. *Neurocrit Care.* 2023 Aug;39(1):1-28.

[52] Dearden NM, Midgley S. Technical considerations in continuous jugular venous oxygen saturation measurement. *Acta Neurochir Suppl (Wien).* 1993;59:91-7.

[53] Mayberg TS, Lam AM. Jugular bulb oximetry for the monitoring of cerebral blood flow and metabolism. *Neurosurg Clin N Am.* 1996;7(4):755-65.

[54] Kiening KL, Unterberg AW, Bardt TF, Schneider GH, Lanksch WR. Monitoring of cerebral oxygenation in patients with severe head injuries: brain tissue PO2 versus jugular vein oxygen saturation. *J Neurosurg.* 1996;85(5):751-7.

[55] Citerio G, Cormio M, Portella G, Vascotto E, Galli D, Gaini SM. Jugular saturation (SjvO2) monitoring in subarachnoid hemorrhage (SAH). *Acta Neurochir Suppl.* 1998;71:316-9.

[56] Heran NS, Hentschel SJ, Toyota BD. Jugular bulb oximetry for prediction of vasospasm following subarachnoid hemorrhage. *Can J Neurol Sci.* 2004;31(1):80-6.

[57] Ekelund A, Kongstad P, Saveland H, Romner B, Reinstrup P, Kristiansson KA, et al. Transcranial cerebral oximetry related to transcranial Doppler after aneurysmal subarachnoid haemorrhage. *Acta Neurochir (Wien).* 1998;140(10):1029-35; discussion 35-6.

[58] Gouvea Bogossian E, Battaglini D, Fratino S, Minini A, Gianni G, Fiore M, et al. The Role of Brain Tissue Oxygenation Monitoring in the Management of Subarachnoid Hemorrhage: A Scoping Review. *Neurocrit Care.* 2023 Aug;39(1):229-240.

[59] Roh D, Park S. Brain Multimodality Monitoring: Updated Perspectives. *Curr Neurol Neurosci Rep.* 2016;16(6):56.

[60] Kieninger M, Meichelbock K, Bele S, Brundl E, Graf B, Schmidt NO, et al. Brain multimodality monitoring in patients suffering from acute aneurysmal subarachnoid hemorrhage: clinical value and complications. *J Integr Neurosci.* 2021;20(3):703-10.

[61] Bensaidane MR, Turgeon AF, Lauzier F, English SW, Leblanc G, Francoeur CL. Neuromonitoring with near-infrared spectroscopy (NIRS) in aneurysmal subarachnoid haemorrhage: a systematic review protocol. *BMJ Open.* 2020;10(11):e043300.

[62] Kerz T, Beyer C, Huthmann A, Kalasauskas D, Amr AN, Boor S, et al. Continuous-wave near-infrared spectroscopy is not related to brain tissue oxygen tension. *J Clin Monit Comput.* 2016;30(5):641-7.

[63] Brawanski A, Faltermeier R, Rothoerl RD, Woertgen C. Comparison of near-infrared spectroscopy and tissue p(O_2) time series in patients after severe head injury and aneurysmal subarachnoid hemorrhage. *J Cereb Blood Flow Metab.* 2002;22(5):605-11.

[64] Forcione M, Ganau M, Prisco L, Chiarelli AM, Bellelli A, Belli A, et al. Mismatch between Tissue Partial Oxygen Pressure and Near-Infrared Spectroscopy Neuromonitoring of Tissue Respiration in Acute Brain Trauma: The Rationale for Implementing a Multimodal Monitoring Strategy. *Int J Mol Sci.* 2021;22(3).

[65] Taussky P, O'Neal B, Daugherty WP, Luke S, Thorpe D, Pooley RA, et al. Validation of frontal near-infrared spectroscopy as non-invasive bedside monitoring for regional cerebral blood flow in brain-injured patients. *Neurosurg Focus.* 2012;32(2):E2.

[66] Westermaier T, Stetter C, Kunze E, Willner N, Holzmeier J, Kilgenstein C, et al. Controlled transient hypercapnia: a novel approach for the treatment of delayed cerebral ischemia after subarachnoid hemorrhage? *J Neurosurg*. 2014;121(5):1056-62.
[67] Mutoh T, Ishikawa T, Suzuki A, Yasui N. Continuous cardiac output and near-infrared spectroscopy monitoring to assist in management of symptomatic cerebral vasospasm after subarachnoid hemorrhage. *Neurocrit Care*. 2010;13(3):331-8.
[68] Steiner LA, Pfister D, Strebel SP, Radolovich D, Smielewski P, Czosnyka M. Near-infrared spectroscopy can monitor dynamic cerebral autoregulation in adults. *Neurocrit Care*. 2009;10(1):122-8.
[69] Moerman A, De Hert S. Recent advances in cerebral oximetry. Assessment of cerebral autoregulation with near-infrared spectroscopy: myth or reality? *F1000Res*. 2017;6:1615.
[70] Silverman A, Kodali S, Strander S, Gilmore EJ, Kimmel A, Wang A, et al. Deviation From Personalized Blood Pressure Targets Is Associated With Worse Outcome After Subarachnoid Hemorrhage. *Stroke*. 2019;50(10):2729-37.
[71] Zweifel C, Castellani G, Czosnyka M, Carrera E, Brady KM, Kirkpatrick PJ, et al. Continuous assessment of cerebral autoregulation with near-infrared spectroscopy in adults after subarachnoid hemorrhage. *Stroke*. 2010;41(9):1963-8.
[72] Park JJ, Kim C, Jeon JP. Monitoring of Delayed Cerebral Ischemia in Patients with Subarachnoid Hemorrhage via Near-Infrared Spectroscopy. *J Clin Med*. 2020;9(5).
[73] Park JJ, Kim Y, Chai CL, Jeon JP. Application of Near-Infrared Spectroscopy for the Detection of Delayed Cerebral Ischemia in Poor-Grade Subarachnoid Hemorrhage. *Neurocrit Care*. 2021;35(3):767-74.
[74] Liu G, Guo Z, Sun X, Chai W, Qi L, Li H, et al. Monitoring of the Effect of Cerebral Autoregulation on Delayed Cerebral Ischemia in Patients with Aneurysmal Subarachnoid Hemorrhage. *World Neurosurg*. 2018;118:e269-e75.
[75] Yousef KM, Balzer JR, Crago EA, Poloyac SM, Sherwood PR. Transcranial regional cerebral oxygen desaturation predicts delayed cerebral ischaemia and poor outcomes after subarachnoid haemorrhage: a correlational study. *Intensive Crit Care Nurs*. 2014;30(6):346-52.
[76] Burzynska M, Uryga A, Kasprowicz M, Czosnyka M, Dragan B, Kubler A. The relationship between the time of cerebral desaturation episodes and outcome in aneurysmal subarachnoid haemorrhage: a preliminary study. *J Clin Monit Comput*. 2020;34(4):705-14.
[77] Nielsen F, Haure P, Madsen J, Steenfeldt Nielsen B, Reides Bjarkam C. Cerebral Microdialysis in Aneurismal Subarachnoid Hemorrhage Patient Reveals a Detrimental Shift in Brain Energy Metabolism, Despite Normal Perfusion Pressure. *Metabolites*. 2020;10(9).
[78] Kofler M, Gaasch M, Rass V, Schiefecker AJ, Ianosi B, Lindner A, et al. The Importance of Probe Location for the Interpretation of Cerebral Microdialysis Data in Subarachnoid Hemorrhage *Patients. Neurocrit Care*. 2020;32(1):135-44.
[79] Helbok R, Kofler M, Schiefecker AJ, Gaasch M, Rass V, Pfausler B, et al. Clinical Use of Cerebral Microdialysis in Patients with Aneurysmal Subarachnoid Hemorrhage-State of the Art. *Front Neurol*. 2017;8:565.
[80] Sarrafzadeh AS, Sakowitz OW, Kiening KL, Benndorf G, Lanksch WR, Unterberg AW. Bedside microdialysis: a tool to monitor cerebral metabolism in subarachnoid hemorrhage patients? *Crit Care Med*. 2002;30(5):1062-70.
[81] Unterberg AW, Sakowitz OW, Sarrafzadeh AS, Benndorf G, Lanksch WR. Role of bedside microdialysis in the diagnosis of cerebral vasospasm following aneurysmal subarachnoid hemorrhage. *J Neurosurg*. 2001;94(5):740-9.
[82] Patet C, Quintard H, Zerlauth JB, Maibach T, Carteron L, Suys T, et al. Bedside cerebral microdialysis monitoring of delayed cerebral hypoperfusion in comatose patients with poor grade aneurysmal subarachnoid haemorrhage. *J Neurol Neurosurg Psychiatry*. 2017;88(4):332-8.
[83] Torne R, Culebras D, Sanchez-Etayo G, Garcia-Garcia S, Munoz G, Llull L, et al. Double hemispheric Microdialysis study in poor-grade SAH patients. *Sci Rep*. 2020;10(1):7466.

[84] Zeiler FA, Thelin EP, Czosnyka M, Hutchinson PJ, Menon DK, Helmy A. Cerebrospinal Fluid and Microdialysis Cytokines in Aneurysmal Subarachnoid Hemorrhage: A Scoping Systematic Review. *Front Neurol*. 2017;8:379.

[85] Helbok R, Ko SB, Schmidt JM, Kurtz P, Fernandez L, Choi HA, et al. Global cerebral edema and brain metabolism after subarachnoid hemorrhage. *Stroke*. 2011;42(6):1534-9.

[86] Sarrafzadeh A, Schlenk F, Gericke C, Vajkoczy P. Relevance of cerebral interleukin-6 after aneurysmal subarachnoid hemorrhage. *Neurocrit Care*. 2010;13(3):339-46.

[87] Winberg J, Holm I, Cederberg D, Rundgren M, Kronvall E, Marklund N. Cerebral Microdialysis-Based Interventions Targeting Delayed Cerebral Ischemia Following Aneurysmal Subarachnoid Hemorrhage. *Neurocrit Care*. 2022;37(1):255-66.

[88] Stovell MG, Helmy A, Thelin EP, Jalloh I, Hutchinson PJ, Carpenter KLH. An overview of clinical cerebral microdialysis in acute brain injury. *Front Neurol*. 2023;14:1085540.

[89] Svedung Wettervik T, Engquist H, Hanell A, Howells T, Rostami E, Ronne-Engstrom E, et al. Cerebral Microdialysis Monitoring of Energy Metabolism: Relation to Cerebral Blood Flow and Oxygen Delivery in Aneurysmal Subarachnoid Hemorrhage. *J Neurosurg Anesthesiol*. 2023 Oct 1;35(4):384-393.

[90] Dyhrfort P, Shen Q, Clausen F, Thulin M, Enblad P, Kamali-Moghaddam M, et al. Monitoring of Protein Biomarkers of Inflammation in Human Traumatic Brain Injury Using Microdialysis and Proximity Extension Assay Technology in Neurointensive Care. *J Neurotrauma*. 2019;36(20):2872-85.

[91] Vlachogiannis P, Hillered L, Enblad P, Ronne-Engstrom E. Temporal patterns of inflammation-related proteins measured in the cerebrospinal fluid of patients with aneurysmal subarachnoid hemorrhage using multiplex Proximity Extension Assay technology. *PLoS One*. 2022;17(3):e0263460.

[92] Rosenthal ES, Biswal S, Zafar SF, O'Connor KL, Bechek S, Shenoy AV, et al. Continuous electroencephalography predicts delayed cerebral ischemia after subarachnoid hemorrhage: A prospective study of diagnostic accuracy. *Ann Neurol*. 2018;83(5):958-69.

[93] Claassen J, Hirsch LJ, Kreiter KT, Du EY, Connolly ES, Emerson RG, et al. Quantitative continuous EEG for detecting delayed cerebral ischemia in patients with poor-grade subarachnoid hemorrhage. *Clin Neurophysiol*. 2004;115 (12):2699-710.

[94] Allen BB, Forgacs PB, Fakhar MA, Wu X, Gerber LM, Boddu S, et al. Association of Seizure Occurrence with Aneurysm Treatment Modality in Aneurysmal Subarachnoid Hemorrhage Patients. *Neurocrit Care*. 2018;29(1):62-8.

[95] Dewan MC, Mocco J. Current practice regarding seizure prophylaxis in aneurysmal subarachnoid hemorrhage across academic centers. *J Neurointerv Surg*. 2015;7(2):146-9.

[96] Banoczi W. ICU-cEEG Monitoring. *Neurodiagn J*. 2020;60(4):231-71.

[97] Foreman B, Albers D, Schmidt JM, Falo CM, Velasquez A, Connolly ES, et al. Intracortical electrophysiological correlates of blood flow after severe SAH: A multimodality monitoring study. *J Cereb Blood Flow Metab*. 2018;38(3):506-17.

[98] Guo Y, Fang S, Wang J, Wang C, Zhao J, Gai Y. Continuous EEG detection of DCI and seizures following aSAH: a systematic review. *Br J Neurosurg*. 2020;34(5):543-8.

[99] Stuart RM, Waziri A, Weintraub D, Schmidt MJ, Fernandez L, Helbok R, et al. Intracortical EEG for the detection of vasospasm in patients with poor-grade subarachnoid hemorrhage. *Neurocrit Care*. 2010;13(3):355-8.

[100] Kim JA, Zheng WL, Elmer J, Jing J, Zafar SF, Ghanta M, et al. High epileptiform discharge burden predicts delayed cerebral ischemia after subarachnoid hemorrhage. *Clin Neurophysiol*. 2022;141:139-46.

[101] Claassen J, Velazquez A, Meyers E, Witsch J, Falo MC, Park S, et al. Bedside quantitative electroencephalography improves assessment of consciousness in comatose subarachnoid hemorrhage patients. *Ann Neurol*. 2016;80(4):541-53.

[102] Sugimoto K, Shirao S, Koizumi H, Inoue T, Oka F, Maruta Y, et al. Continuous Monitoring of Spreading Depolarization and Cerebrovascular Autoregulation after Aneurysmal Subarachnoid Hemorrhage. *J Stroke Cerebrovasc Dis*. 2016;25(10):e171-7.

[103] Sugimoto K, Nomura S, Shirao S, Inoue T, Ishihara H, Kawano R, et al. Cilostazol decreases duration of spreading depolarization and spreading ischemia after aneurysmal subarachnoid hemorrhage. *Ann Neurol*. 2018;84(6):873-85.

[104] Amantini A, Fossi S, Grippo A, Innocenti P, Amadori A, Bucciardini L, et al. Continuous EEG-SEP monitoring in severe brain injury. *Neurophysiol Clin*. 2009;39(2):85-93.

[105] Kolb B, Wolfson D, Da Silva I, Munich SA. Multimodal monitoring to guide neurosurgical intervention in high-grade aneurysmal subarachnoid hemorrhage: illustrative case. *J Neurosurg Case Lessons*. 2022;3(26):CASE22107.

[106] Miro Llado J, Lopez-Ojeda P, Pedro J, Marnov A, Contreras L, Pariente L, et al. Evaluation of multimodal intraoperative neurophysiologic monitoring during supratentorial aneurysm surgery: a comparative study. *Neurosurg Rev*. 2022;45(3):2161-73.

[107] Svedung Wettervik T, Lewen A, Enblad P. Fine tuning of neurointensive care in aneurysmal subarachnoid hemorrhage: From one-size-fits-all towards individualized care. *World Neurosurg X*. 2023;18:100160.

[108] Monteiro E, Ferreira A, Mendes E, Dias CC, Czosnyka M, Paiva JA, et al. Brain Multimodal Monitoring in Severe Acute Brain Injury: Is It Relevant to Patient Outcome and Mortality? *Acta Neurochir Suppl*. 2021;131:83-6.

[109] Zhang J. Human-centered computing in health information systems. Part 1: analysis and design. *J Biomed Inform*. 2005;38(1):1-3.

[110] Zhang J. Human-centered computing in health information systems part 2: evaluation. *J Biomed Inform*. 2005;38(3):173-5.

[111] Vespa PM. Multimodality monitoring and telemonitoring in neurocritical care: from microdialysis to robotic telepresence. *Curr Opin Crit Care*. 2005;11(2):133-8.

[112] Hoh BL, Ko NU, Amin-Hanjani S, Hsiang-Yi Chou S, Cruz-Flores S, Dangayach NS, et al. 2023 Guideline for the Management of Patients With Aneurysmal Subarachnoid Hemorrhage: A Guideline From the American Heart Association/American Stroke Association. *Stroke*. 2023 Jul;54(7):e314-e370.

Index

A

B

C

D

E

F

G

H

I

L

M

N

O

P

R

S

T

U

V

W